The Original Beauty Bible

Unparalleled Information for
Beautiful and Younger Skin
at Any Age

PAULA BEGOUN

BEAUTYPEDIA.COM
YOUR ULTIMATE SOURCE FOR COSMETIC PRODUCT REVIEWS

The Best of the Best
Access Paula's lists of the best products or quickly find the product you're searching for

Free Email Updates
Keep up with what's new on Beautypedia.com by signing up for Paula's FREE Beautypedia Bulletin

Subscribe Today
Subscribers have exclusive access to over 40,000 skin-care and makeup reviews from more than 250 lines plus complete ingredient lists for every skin-care product reviewed

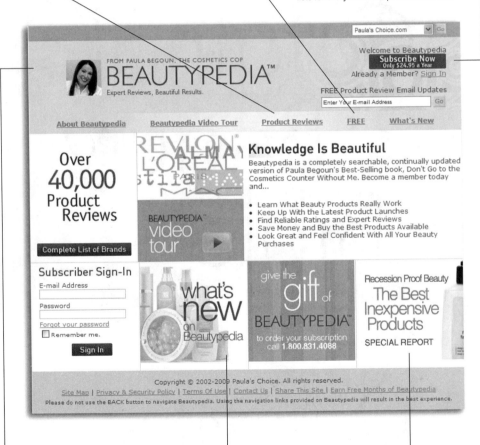

Beautypedia.com
Thousands of precise, researched, and controversial reviews—all online in an easily searchable product database!

Real Time Updates
New full line and individual product reviews added often, so you'll be better informed than ever before!

FREE Special Reports
On a wide range of cosmetic topics, from the best inexpensive products to cosmetics myth-busting

COSMETICSCOP.COM
SUPERIOR SKIN-CARE & EXPERT INFORMATION

Shop
Take a look at Paula's state-of-the-art skin-care line. There are products designed for a broad range of needs and concerns, from acne to wrinkled, sun-damaged skin

FREE email Beauty Bulletins
Sign up for Paula's Beauty Bulletins and stay informed about what's happening in the cosmetics industry. Free product reviews, intriguing special reports, "Dear Paula" Q&As, and more

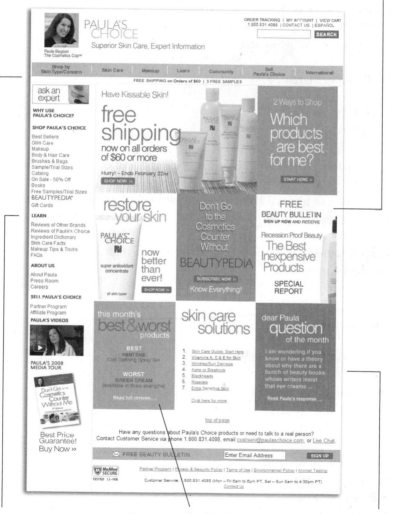

Learn
FInd extensive information on how to determine and manage your skin type, sensible solutions for everything from wrinkles to blemish-fighting, and ingredient updates! Read all about beauty facts and fiction, and pick up expert tips on how to apply makeup to your advantage!

Best & Worst Products
Every month, Paula reviews new products and awards a "best" and "worst" product. Find out if your favorite products meet the Cosmetic Cop's strict criteria!

Dear Paula
Check out the current "Dear Paula" Question of the Month for the latest pressing skin-care questions and beauty concerns. Better yet, submit your beauty questions and concerns to Paula today!

Contributor: Bryan Barron
Editors: Sigrid Asmus, John Hopper, Stephanie Parsons, Seanna Browder
Art Direction, Cover Design, and Typography: Erin Smith Bloom
Printing: RR Donnelley
Research Assistant: Bryan Barron

Copyright © 2009, Paula Begoun
Publisher: Beginning Press
        1030 SW 34th Street, Suite A
        Renton, Washington 98057

1st Edition Printing: March 2009

ISBN: 978-1-877988-33-2
      10 9 8 7 6 5 4 3 2 1

This book is distributed to the United States book trade by:
 Publishers Group West
 1700 Fourth Street
 Berkeley, California 94710
 (510) 528-1444

To the Canadian book trade by:
 Raincoast Books Limited
 9050 Shaughnessy Street
 Vancouver, B.C., V6P 6E5 Canada
 (604) 633-5714

To the Australian book trade by:
 Peribo Pty Limited
 58 Beaumont Road
 Mount Kuring-Gai NSW 2080 Australia
 02 9457 0011

...CRAZY

...APTER TWO—UNDERSTANDING THE HYPE

CHAPTER THREE— FRAUDS & FEARS

CHAPTER EIGHT—SKIN CARE & MOISTURIZERS

CHAPTER NINE—EVERY SKIN TYPE CAN BENEFIT FROM EXFOLIATING

CHAPTER TEN—SKIN-CARE PLANNING:
GOING OVER THE BASICS

CHAPTER ELEVEN—SOLUTIONS FOR WRINKLES

CHAPTER TWELVE—SOLUTIONS FOR
PERIMENOPAUSE & MENOPAUSE

CHAPTER THIRTEEN—SOLUTIONS FOR SKIN LIGHTENING

CHAPTER FOURTEEN—SOLUTIONS FOR DRY SKIN

CHAPTER FIFTEEN—SOLUTIONS FOR ACNE

CHAPTER NINETEEN—SOLUTIONS FOR SEBORRHEA AND ECZEMA

CHAPTER TWENTY—SOLUTIONS FOR CELLULITE

CHAPTER TWENTY ONE—SOLUTIONS FOR WOUNDS, SCARS, OR STRETCH MARKS

CHAPTER TWENTY FIVE—GROWING HAIR

CHAPTER TWENTY SIX—MEDICAL COSMETIC CORRECTIVE PROCEDURES

CHAPTER TWENTY SEVEN—BODY & NAIL CARE

CHAPTER TWENTY EIGHT—PROBLEMS? SOLUTIONS!

CHAPTER TWENTY NINE—MAKING SENSE OF MAKEUP

CHAPTER THIRTY—ANIMAL RIGHTS

NOTE FROM THE PUBLISHER

The intent of this book is to present the author's research, ideas, and perceptions regarding skin care, makeup, cosmetic surgical procedures, and the marketing, selling, and use of cosmetics and skin-care products. The author's sole purpose is to provide consumers with information and advice regarding skin care, the purchase of beauty products, and cosmetic procedures. The recommendations presented are strictly those of the author, reflecting the author's opinions about the subjects and the products described. Some women may find success with a skin-care routine or product that is not mentioned herein. It is everyone's inalienable right to choose and to judge products and procedures on the basis of their own criteria, research, and standards, and to disagree with the author. More important, because everyone's skin can react differently to external stimuli, any product can cause a negative reaction. If you develop sensitivity to a skin-care product or cosmetic, stop using it immediately and consult your physician. If you need medical advice regarding your skin or the various cosmetic procedures available, it is best to consult a dermatologist, board-certified plastic surgeon, or your own medical practitioner.

CHAPTER 1
THE BEAUTY INDUSTRY: UNIVERSALLY CRAZY

WHY A NEW EDITION

As is true with every edition of the books I've written on the cosmetics industry starting in 1984 with *Blue Eyeshadow Should Be Illegal* and then *Don't Go to the Cosmetics Counter Without Me*, and *Don't Go Shopping for Hair Care Products Without Me*, much has changed in the world of makeup and skin. Serious research has increased exponentially on all fronts—from antioxidants, anti-irritants, cell-communicating ingredients, skin-identical ingredients, aquaporins, MMPs, sun protection, and on and on. We know more about why skin wrinkles, how skin heals, what the effects of hormones are on skin function, and how to treat blackheads and acne, not to mention having a better understanding of how sun and oxygen destroy skin.

Cosmetic dermatology and plastic surgery procedures have greatly improved, though the array of options has become more extensive and the risks or benefits more difficult to evaluate. As I compiled the research and began rewriting this book, I was amazed at how far the cosmetics world has advanced as well as dismayed at how much has remained the same. Regrettably, there are still infinite misleading claims, poor formulations, the all-natural farce, the abundance of skin-care myths, and the never-ending fiction that expensive means better.

It was an amazing process to assemble all this information. At first I thought it was going to be a fairly simple update. It turns out that almost 60% of this book was completely rewritten and reorganized. I hope you find it helpful as you try to decipher and decode the complicated world of beauty. I know it can be done, but it isn't easy. What is certain is that the story must start with information supported by peer-reviewed, published studies—and that's what you'll find in this book.

ALL OVER THE WORLD

Over the past several years I have done media interviews and speaking engagements to women's groups around the world. I have done presentations for thousands of women from places as far-flung as Jakarta, Indonesia; Seoul, Korea; Stockholm, Sweden; Mexico City, Mexico; Singapore; Sydney and Melbourne, Australia; Kuala Lumpur, Malaysia, and almost every major city in the United States.

From Toronto to Dallas, and everyplace in between, no matter where I've gone, I've never had to change my topic of discussion. I don't even have to do extra research, because the cosmetics industry is so universally crazy. Everywhere I go, the advertisements are so entirely deceptive and the claims so utterly bogus that women ask me the same questions. They want to know why a product they bought didn't work. Why didn't their wrinkles go away? Why didn't their scar fade? Why didn't their skin discolorations change? Why are they still breaking out or just starting to break out? Why do they still have dry, flaky skin after buying so many products promising to make things better? What is the best skin-care ingredient? Do I know about a recent product launched with some miracle ingredient currently being advertised or in an infomercial? I get the exact same questions all over the world.

What almost always happens during my presentation is I see a look of understanding come over women's faces as they grasp how they have been duped time and time again by the cosmetics industry. There isn't a part of the world where the cosmetics industry works any differently, or where the products are any better (not in India, Japan, or even France), or the claims are any less far-fetched. What women everywhere want is to take the best care of their skin, and what most women fall into is the trap of believing the falsehoods propagated by a vast part of the cosmetics industry.

LET ME INTRODUCE MYSELF...

I am the author and publisher of several best-selling books on the cosmetics industry. My first was *Blue Eyeshadow Should Be Illegal*, published in 1984 (which was revised four times); then came *Don't Go to the Cosmetics Counter Without Me* (currently in its seventh edition); and *Don't Go Shopping for Hair Care Products Without Me* (there have been three editions of that book). Over the years I have been a syndicated columnist with Knight Ridder News Tribune Service, a consultant to other cosmetics companies, and a consultant to dermatologists.

My research and writing have been based strictly on my earnest desire to get beyond the hype and chicanery of the cosmetics industry and to disseminate straightforward information that a consumer can really use to look and feel more beautiful.

My expertise and background, like that of any other consumer reporter who covers a range of topics, is based on extensive research in the subject area. What makes my situation unique is that I also have over 25 years of personal experience from working as a professional makeup artist and aesthetician and from selling makeup and skin-care products at department stores, salons, and my own stores, developing my own line of products, and helping other cosmetics companies develop new products.

I use my reporting background to continually and extensively research the cosmetics industry. I base all my comments on comprehensive interviews with dermatologists, oncologists, cosmetics chemists, and cosmetic ingredient manufacturers, and on information I've gleaned from both medical and science journals as well as cosmetics industry magazines. I am constantly reviewing scientific abstracts and studies. I do not capriciously or abruptly make any conclusions. Everything I report is supported by studies and information from experts in the field, and I document my sources throughout this book. Naturally, there are many who disagree with my assertions, and I do the best I can to present other points of view whenever possible. However, I assure you that more often than not a great number of people in the industry agree with my conclusions, even if they can't state so publicly.

A PERSONAL QUEST

In many ways I'm surprised that reviewing, researching, investigating, and questioning the cosmetics industry is what I still do for a living. When I started out as a makeup artist back in 1978 it was never my intent to end up writing as a consumer advocate about the cosmetics industry, much less to develop my own product line.

At first my mission was personal. I had suffered with acne for many years. By the age of 18 I had been to over a dozen dermatologists. I tried hundreds of skin-care products from both inexpensive and expensive cosmetics lines and still I had acne. How could that be? How could all the stuff I diligently applied to my skin—which salesperson after salesperson and doctor after doctor assured me would work—not work? Sometimes one routine worked a little, but not as well as I had hoped and not for very long. And there were always side effects. Most products made my skin so red and irritated I thought it was going to fall off. Slowly but surely I worked my way through the confusion, and after much research and lots more frustration I began to recognize some fundamental problems with the information provided and the products sold by the cosmetics industry. (I'll never forget the day I learned what was really in the Clinique 3-Step system! Their toner at the time contained acetone, the soap was just soap with yellow coloring, and their yellow moisturizer was waxy thickening ingredients and lanolin.) I also found that many of the same difficulties and frustrations were present in the field of dermatology.

Aside from my skin-care struggles as a teenager, in 1978 I got my first job as a freelance makeup artist in Washington, D.C. Depending on the time of year, when the freelance makeup business was slow I supplemented my income with work at department-store makeup counters. But each new job for a different cosmetics line resulted in me being fired.

My first dismissal came after an argument with the line representative of a department-store cosmetics company where I was working. The representative wanted me to say that a toner could close pores and a moisturizer could heal, when I knew that wasn't true. (If a toner could close pores, everyone who used toners would have flawless, poreless skin, and if moisturizers could heal skin, no one would have a pimple or a wrinkle or a scar.) That job lasted about two months.

Several months later, at another department store and for a different cosmetics company, I was involved in a conflict with several of the cosmetics saleswomen working at the other counters. If a customer wanted a particular type of product and I didn't think the product from the line I was selling was right, or if my line didn't offer one, I would walk her over to another counter that I knew had the right product and sell it to her. That caused a nuclear meltdown. I was told to stay behind my counter and not touch another product from any line other than the one I was assigned! (When I recommended that the woman could walk over to the other counter herself, I got in trouble with the sales representatives from my line.) How ludicrous! A product I wanted to recommend, five feet away from me, was out of reach because it wasn't from the counter I was standing behind. That's not my idea of customer service!

A PERSONAL BEAUTY MIRACLE

My career truly began or at least became possible in November 1976 when the United States Food and Drug Administration required all cosmetics to have complete ingredient listings on their labels in descending order (largest percentage first, smallest percentage last). The FDA also standardized the way ingredients needed to be listed to minimize the confusion that would surely arise if various synonyms or trade names for chemical names were used (Sources: www.fda.gov; and *Contact Dermatitis*, April 2006, pages 94–97). While there are certainly products that fail to follow the regulation by using ingredient names that either hide the real nature of the ingredient or make it sound more natural than it really is, that now happens much less often.

To grasp how significant this regulation was, it took till 1995 for Australia to be the next country to mandate ingredient listings on cosmetics, then Europe in 2000, and finally Canada—are you ready for this—in 2008 (but they have until 2010 to comply). In other words, until fairly recently a product being sold in the U.S. would have ingredient listings while in the rest of the world the exact same product would have no ingredient listing. Clearly there was something the cosmetics industry didn't want consumers to know! But it gave me a mission and a job. I wanted to know and understand what was in the products I was using and eventually I came to share what I had learned in my books and online.

There is a caveat to all this. As wonderful as this worldwide ingredient regulation is, the downside is that it is almost impossible for a consumer to decipher the ingredients on a label. The words are incomprehensible. They are either too technical or multisyllabic, or the plant extracts, which are supposed to be in Latin for botanical accuracy, are in a language no one knows. Though even if you knew the Latin name of the plant that wouldn't necessarily be helpful because each part of the plant has its own properties. Stem, leaf, flower, and roots may be more or less beneficial for skin. Even vitamin C as an ingredient has many derivatives that can show up on a cosmetic ingredient list, such as ascorbic acid, ascorbyl glucoside, L-ascorbic acid, ascorbyl palmitate, sodium ascorbate, potassium ascorbate, calcium ascorbate, tetra-isopalmitoyl ascorbic acid, and tetrahexyldecyl ascorbate, to name a few, each having its own benefits, stability profile, and potency.

Cosmetics companies love to showcase the way the part or form of some plant, mineral, or vitamin their products contain is the best. Vitamin C is one of those ingredients that has often been at the front of this marketing ploy. You may have heard of Ester-C, which contains mainly calcium ascorbate, but also a small amount of other vitamin C metabolites. Supposedly this makes Ester C more bioavailable than other forms of vitamin C. This information only comes from the company selling Ester C and there is no published research showing this to have any merit. On the other hand, there has been research showing Ester C to have no preferred benefit over other forms of vitamin C.

THE BEST INGREDIENTS FOR SKIN?

The question women and reporters worldwide always ask me is: Which ingredient or ingredients are the best for skin? The good news is the same as the bad news, because there isn't just one or even a few—there are hundreds of brilliant ingredients for skin. While that means there are great options to choose from, it also makes the selection process exceedingly difficult. Everyone wants a magic bullet, and the world of cosmetics has nothing even vaguely resembling a single-ingredient miracle. A cosmetics company may showcase an ingredient and make it sound sensational, but the truth is there are lots and lots of sensational ingredients. The next time a salesperson, infomercial, or advertisement wants to convince you of some miracle ingredient, ignore it, they are lying through their teeth.

A cosmetics chemist has access to thousands of ingredients that can go into a formula, and trying to translate them all into a format a consumer can understand is impossible. In the cosmetic ingredient dictionary on my web site at www.cosmetics-cop.com I have included over 3,000 ingredients, yet that is only the tip of a rather big and continually growing ingredient database. I spend endless time analyzing what the research says about the formulations and contents of each product I consider.

STRUGGLING WITH THE COSMETICS INDUSTRY

My final department-store cosmetics-counter job ended when I just couldn't take listening to the distortions and exaggerated claims anymore and decided to go out on my own. I opened my own makeup stores in 1981. I didn't sell blue eyeshadow, wrinkle creams, or toners that claimed to close pores. Along the way, I hooked up with a business partner who was at first thrilled with my ideas and concept, mainly because of the media attention my rather controversial stores attracted.

My stores were generating a lot of attention from the press, and in 1982 I was asked to make regular appearances on a local TV station in Seattle, KIRO-TV. I also started receiving national and international TV and print exposure.

Eventually my ideas and concepts no longer pleased my partner. The department-store counters were crowded with women buying blue eyeshadow, wrinkle creams, and toners, so why shouldn't we sell them too? After all, if you saw women throwing away their money on those sorts of products, at prices ranging from $25 to $250 an ounce for items that cost 75 cents to $4 to produce, you wouldn't want a partner like me either. I sold my shares back to her in 1984 and stayed at KIRO-TV for the next two years. I learned a lot about investigative reporting and writing during my time at KIRO-TV in Seattle.

I left the TV station toward the end of 1985 after finishing my first book, *Blue Eyeshadow Should Be Illegal*. I decided to self-publish after receiving several rejection letters from major publishing companies telling me that, although they liked my manuscript, I wasn't a celebrity or a model, and no one would be interested in my point of view. I disagreed. I believed lots of women (OK, not all of them!) were tired of hearing useless, and at times incorrect, information from models and celebrities who were born beautiful and knew which makeup artists, photographers, and managers to hire, but very little about the cosmetics they promoted.

I was right, and I sold several hundred thousand copies of my first book (after several appearances on *The Oprah Winfrey Show*)! And what happened was wonderful. Women were thanking me for opening their eyes to the reality of what did and didn't work in the world of skin care and makeup—the perfect response. Yet despite all I had written, I still received thousands of letters from women asking me, now that they knew how crazy the cosmetics industry was, what they should buy or what I thought of the product they were using or thinking of using. It was one thing to have an overview of the facts, but quite another to have specific information about a specific product. How could anyone tell if the formulation of a product was effective? How would a person know whether the marketing claims were valid? How could someone find out if a company's assertion about their impressive studies backing up their miracle skin-care product were true? That's when I wrote *Don't Go to the Cosmetics Counter Without Me*, which is now in its seventh edition. I've sold over 2 million copies of this book worldwide and it is now online, in an expanded, continually updated review database, at www.Beautypedia.com.

Meanwhile, the demand to know what works and what doesn't has grown, mainly because the industry has grown. As is true in all the books I write, what I also want to do is to separate cosmetics fact from cosmetics fiction and reality from myth, because the fiction and myths spread by the cosmetics industry are nothing less than startling and frustrating. Compared to the information provided by the cosmetics industry, Mother Goose stories sound like the *Encyclopaedia Britannica*.

Perhaps the most difficult part of my job is keeping a straight face when I hear the crazy things cosmetics salespeople tell consumers. Combating this endless parade of useless and bizarre information can be maddening. But it's my job and, thankfully, it has been far more rewarding than I ever expected.

You need this book because it will help you save money—lots of money!—and help you take the best possible care of your skin. Depending on how you spend money on cosmetics, it can add up to a savings of thousands of dollars. And it may literally save your skin if you happen to be using products that are poorly formulated or just plain bad for skin. The bottom line is simple: Wasting money on products that don't work or don't live up to their claims isn't pretty.

COSMETICS CHEMISTRY—AN ART AND A SCIENCE

Every step of the way I am in awe of how beautifully most cosmetics work. Where would we be without the brilliant work of the cosmetics chemists who make the exquisite products we use? Because of their astonishing skill we have moisturizers that take care of dry skin and aid in making skin healthier and more resilient. There are products that really can fight wrinkles and help improve their appearance in some fairly significant ways. Cosmetics chemists have created mascaras that can build thick, lush lashes without flaking or smearing, and foundations that even out skin tone, making it look flawless. We have sunscreens that protect skin from sunburn as well as from wrinkles and the potential for skin cancer. There is an endless array of sensuous lipsticks that add relatively long-lasting color and definition to the mouth. Not to mention blushes that softly accent cheekbones and eyeshadows that define eyes, and, well, the list is endless.

I want to thank all the cosmetics chemists everywhere who strive to produce better and better products that continue to make the beauty industry so incredibly beautiful. I also want to ask cosmetics chemists to do the best they can, whenever they can, to combat the insane marketing departments they have to work with! After interviewing and talking to hundreds of cosmetics chemists over the years, I know most of you don't believe even a fraction of what the advertisements, salespeople, infomercial hucksters, or editorials in fashion magazines say about the products you create. Your work is rooted in science, not hyperbole. I also know this is a risky business. After all, creating products that no one buys is not going to get anyone a promotion, and the marketing department knows all too well what women love to hear, no matter how ridiculous it may sound. But try anyway, just to bring a bit of fresh air into an otherwise very cloudy business.

CHAPTER 2
UNDERSTANDING THE HYPE

If you don't understand how the cosmetics industry works—the good, the bad, and the ugly—you will be a victim of its advertising manipulations, exaggerations, and deceptions, and that isn't good for your skin or your budget.

I had an interesting discussion with a producer of an infomercial as I was finishing up the last chapter for this book before it went to press. Because of confidentiality I can't tell you which one, but it really doesn't matter because they are all the same and they all mislead or deceive or lie through their teeth in the same way. This producer knew that the script she was going to be videotaping was mostly misleading or untrue. Don't get me wrong: She was very nice and she appreciated my research and critique of the topic, but of course there was nothing she could do about it. And nothing I could do either.

What most women don't realize is how everyone in the cosmetics industry knows that the marketing and advertising for cosmetics is either meaningless, hypocritical, or dishonest. That fashion magazines are hamstrung by their advertisers and can't report "beauty" information objectively. They can't disagree with their advertisers. The reporters, producers, and editors all know it. They all talk about it and then shrug their shoulders and say, well, it's a living. Or they laugh about it. Ultimately, they all know women are being suckered into products that can't possibly perform as the claims on the label assert.

WHY COSMETICS COMPANIES CAN MISLEAD LEGALLY

Reporters all over the world constantly ask me why cosmetics companies mislead and often out and out lie to women, and how they manage to get away with it. The simple answer is that women like to be lied to. We want to believe that the products we buy can get us what we want. We prefer the promise of eternal youth (or some approximation) and clear, flawless skin to reality. No matter how many thousands of products there are, often dozens of them from the same companies, and all guaranteeing some degree of a miracle, it still happens—we just don't seem to have a learning curve. We want the next one we buy to be the answer. Using either scientific mumbo jumbo or concoctions said to come straight from the earth, or a mix of both, they tell us exactly what we want to hear. Most cosmetics companies need to lie just to gain a consumer's attention because the truth is never as enticing as the deception.

While women want to find hope in a jar, regulatory agencies do what they can to protect us. However the official limitations provide no real protection from truly misleading information or lies. One of the most beguiling aspects of the cosmetics industry in the U.S. and Canada is that the Food and Drug Administration (FDA), Health Canada (HC), and most regulatory boards around the world—with the exception of the European Union (EU) member countries—don't require cosmetics companies to prove their claims. "Neither cosmetic products nor cosmetic ingredients are reviewed or approved by FDA before they are sold to the public." (Sources: Center for Food Safety and Applied Nutrition, www.cfsan.fda.gov/~dms/cos-206.html, March 3, 2005; and FDA Authority Over Cosmetics and Health Canada, www.hc-sc.gc.ca/hl-vs/iyh-vsv/prod/cosmet-eng.php). That means cosmetics companies, whether they call their products cosmeceutical or otherwise, get to say just about anything they want about their products without any substantiation or proof whatsoever.

Pharmaceutical and over-the-counter drug regulations are infinitely stricter than those dealing with cosmetics. If a drug company makes a claim about what an antihistamine can do to prevent sneezing, the product must contain particular ingredients in specified amounts to win approval from the FDA. The same is true for aspirin and other analgesics, antacids, decongestants, anti-inflammatories, and all drugs across the board in the world of pharmaceuticals. The same is not true for cosmetics.

The only fundamental FDA restriction on cosmetics companies' claims is the legal prohibition of phrases that directly state or promise a permanent change in the skin or hair. Of course, there are a million ways to make something sound like a permanent change to consumers without sounding permanent to the FDA.

What about federal regulations concerning truth in advertising? That issue generally falls under the jurisdiction of the Federal Trade Commission (FTC) and the Federal Communications Commission (FCC), but it doesn't take much to get around these guys either. For example, I can describe at great length how miraculously my product works as long as I throw in phrases such as "appears to," "seems to," "feels as if," "looks like," "you may experience," and lots more variations on these themes. All of these phrases invalidate any promise about a product's performance. A company is not considered to be lying to the consumer when these kinds of terms are used because the purported results are subjective, not actual. It may "seem" like your cellulite has disappeared, or you may "appear" to look younger, or you can "experience" a clear complexion, but nothing has happened except that you may be convinced something has taken place.

Better Than Botox? That question mark poses a question, not a statement, so the FDA is happy, and meanwhile what the consumer hears is that the product is better than Botox. It doesn't take fancy terminology to keep within regulatory guidelines while still misleading the consumer because reading caveats doesn't get our attention. That's how most cosmetics advertising gets around truth-in-advertising restrictions every time.

Another game in the industry happens when companies step way over the line in their advertising campaigns, either on televison or in fashion magazines, and mislead or lie to consumers. They do this because they know that by the time the FDA or HC can take action the advertisement has run its course and made an impression on consumers. Mission accomplished; the company is on to its next product launch. Also, many cosmetics companies know that the FDC and HC are just so overloaded with work and underfunded that their deceptive ads can easily slip under the radar of these agencies and continue on, safe and sound, without any fear of repercussions.

And beyond the lack of regulation, the language and images are manipulated to create a veneer of scientific authority in advertisements that promise everything from younger skin to smoother thighs. The problem here has to do with the studies the cosmetics companies claim are backed by actual research that proves their assertions to be true. This is the wide-open world of claim substantiation, a whole industry of its own that has given the word deception an entirely new meaning.

THE BUSINESS OF CLAIM SUBSTANTIATION —OUR STUDY SHOWS

Just about every cosmetics company has a study or studies they tout as being proof that their product(s) work. From this perspective there isn't a product—from any line—that doesn't work miracles. But of course you never see their studies of the products that failed (something must have failed, right?). Yet since we aren't getting rid of our wrinkles (somehow plastic surgeons and dermatologists are not going out of business because of new skin-care products), while hundreds of new, seemingly miracle-making products are launched every year, it appears that most of these so-called studies must be little more than shams. It turns out that's exactly what most of them are.

When the EU created their Cosmetics Industry Directive, the entire 27-member nation group was obliged to follow it. One of the new regulations unique to the EU was that cosmetics companies must have on file studies that support their claims (Source: Consolidated Version of Cosmetics Directive 76/768/EEC, http://ec.europa.eu/enterprise/cosmetics/html/consolidated_dir.htm). Almost instantly, the industry of claim substantiation was created. In other words, the EU tried to make a difference but failed miserably; they just created a loophole that cosmetics companies could easily get through.

In the world of skin care today, there is an entire business known as claim substantiation, but its studies definitely do not equate with those done under legitimate scientific research standards. Laboratories, including those at some respected universities and colleges, are expert at setting up a study so that the results support whatever the label or advertisements say that a product can do. One important question about this research that many consumers and physicians aren't aware of—and this includes lots of physicians who are involved in these dubious and often completely bogus studies—is this: "Under what conditions were the studies performed?" In the industry, in place of a plausible answer, what happens goes by many names, such as creative claim substantiation, or substantiation strategies (Source: Society of Cosmetic Chemists, www.scconline.org/website/referrals/consultants.shtml).

These research labs exist solely to provide pseudoscientific material for the cosmetics industry. That way, if the marketing copy claims that a moisturizer provides an 82% increase in moisturization or a 90% increase in the skin's water content, the company may very well be able to point to a study that says this is true. Whether the study is the least bit valid is another question altogether. Quoting these inconclusive, vague studies in a news story or ad can make them sound significant and meaningful, but in truth they are more often than not just more hype and exaggeration generated to sell products. One of these claim-substantiation companies actually advertises its ability to deliver "creative claim generation/substantiation."

For example, in a skin-care study to establish whether or not a product gets rid of wrinkles, the subjects participating often begin by washing their face and then stripping it clear with alcohol. The company then takes the "before" photos and measurements (such as wrinkle depth, skin tone, and water loss, among other parameters). With that starting point, it's hardly surprising that the "before" situation is much worse than the "after" results. What would the results have been if the woman had started by using a gentle cleanser, a good moisturizer, and a sunscreen (for example, effective ones different from those being tested)? Or, what would the effects of any other products have been if compared to those of the product being tested? Perhaps dozens of other products could have performed as well or better.

(Sources for the above: *Cosmetic Claims Substantiation, Cosmetic Science and Technology Series*, vol. 18, ed. Louise Aust, New York: Marcel Dekker, 1998; and the *Cosmetics and Toiletries* article: "The European Group on Efficacy Measurement of Cosmetics and Other Topical Products is considering new cosmetic legislation to regulate claims of efficacy," by G. E. Pierard, Ph.D, Allured Publishing Corp., Boca Raton, FL, 2000.)

During the more than 25 years I've been researching and reviewing the cosmetics industry I have asked every cosmetics company whose product or products we've reviewed to show us their "studies" and in all those 25 years, I have received only five of these studies (and none, and I mean NONE, of those five studies proved the claims the companies were making). There are lots of ways to use pseudo-science to create proof for a claim that, in reality, has very little to do with science and everything to do with marketing

According to an article in *Cosmetics & Toiletries* magazine (December 1999, pages 52–53), "Skin moisturization studies using bioengineering methods are commonplace today. If data generated for a new test product demonstrate a statistically significant difference between the test product and untreated skin in favor of increased hydration, then claims indicating this to the consumer would be substantiated.... For example, [the claim] 'moisturizes your skin for up to 8 hours' would be substantiated by a study where a statistical difference was observed between the test product and untreated skin for up to 8 hours following application of the test product." In essence, in examples like this, what the words "our studies show" are telling you is that, when compared with plain, unmoisturized, washed skin, the moisturizer made skin moist! That isn't exactly shocking. The use of any moisturizer would show the same results.

I've seen this process at work firsthand, and it is disturbing. Whoever is paying the bill hires the research lab. The lab is handed the products and told what to look for and what kind of results are needed—for example, proof of moisturization, exfoliation, smoothness, or some other measurable parameter. Then the lab goes about setting up a study to prove that position. Rarely are these studies done double blind, nor do they use a large group of women, or show long-term results, and rarely (actually never) are the results negative. More to the point, these studies are never published. Unpublished research is nothing more than sheer fantasy and illusion. It's completely unscientific and considered invalid by independent researchers. Yet consumers are led to believe this unverified information is fact when they read about it in editorials in fashion magazines and other media. And the cosmetic companies are quick to point out how many studies they've done, but few are ever published and even fewer are ever substantiated.

This same sleight of hand is used quite effectively in brochures and ads. Many cosmetics counters hand out impressively designed, scientific-looking brochures showing how well a product works on the skin. You might see, for example, a microscopic close-up of a patch of skin paired with an explanation of why it looks bad. Beside it is another close-up of the same patch of skin after the product is applied. See how wonderfully the product worked? The deception here is that you are not given enough "before" information. For example, if the woman had acne, what was she doing before to take care of her skin? Was she using products that clogged pores or aggravated breakouts? Had she never used any effective skin-care products for acne? In that case, any basic skin-care routine for acne could make a difference. And was this person the sole best result of the lot? Were there perhaps others who still had breakouts despite treatment or did their skin get worse? Just because information looks scientific doesn't mean it is.

Next time you see stories about test results showing younger-looking skin, new cell growth, or any other claim that sounds too good to be true, regardless of who is making the claim, stop and think. Ask yourself how many times you have heard this "perfect skin in a bottle" message before. Is this "story" about only a single study, or are there any corroborating studies? Does it sound too good to be true? Where is the entire study? What did it really test? You may also want to ask yourself how many more times you are going to swallow another exaggerated claim about a skin-care product, or spend money believing that you've finally found the "best" product available. (Do you really believe that gorgeous, childlike model in the picture looks like that because of the products being advertised?) Think about how many times you've been sucked in by a cosmetics ad, claim, or fashion magazine story, only to be disappointed again and again, until the next advertising campaign for a new product catches your attention. There are many wonderful things that you can do to take care of your skin! But there are also a ton of things that are an embarrassing waste of money.

A PERFECT EXAMPLE OF HOW "STUDIES" CAN MISLEAD

Boots No7 Restore & Renew Beauty Serum ($21.99 for 1 ounce) is one of my favorite examples of how this game of claim substantiation works and can easily fool the media. Here are the facts:

A television documentary that aired in the United Kingdom in March 2007 featured the results of a blind test that compared the efficacy of this Boots serum to tretinoin. Tretinoin is the active ingredient in Retin-A and Renova and is also available as a generic. The research was carried out by scientists at the University of Manchester, with the conclusion that this Boots serum was just as effective at stimulating collagen production as tretinoin, yet cost considerably less. That sounds great until you learn that Boots paid for the research. That means the University was making money on the study and so everyone had a vested interest in making sure the study made the product look great.

The study was done blind instead of double-blind, which means the researchers knew who was getting what product. This type of study isn't as reliable as double-blind studies because, especially when money is at stake, there is a natural bias toward making sure the product in question comes out in the best possible light. Moreover, comparing tretinoin to a "serum" and saying they do the same thing doesn't tell you if myriad other products would have fared just as well. Maybe using someone else's serum, say from Neutrogena or Olay, could produce the same results. But because Neutrogena or Olay weren't the ones paying for the study no one bothered to see if that would be the case. What is distressing is that sunscreen was left out of the equation, which means women might mistakenly believe that all it takes is the Boots serum and your skin will be fine. And finally, if the Boots product is so spectacular, you have to wonder why does Boots continue to sell dozens of other products with different formulas that claim the exact same benefits?

Similar pseudo-science abounds in the cosmetics industry, and I expose it repeatedly when I review products. Believing the claims a cosmetics company makes based on their studies is a risk you don't want to take because more often than not, the study is nothing more than a marketing ploy and not indicative of anything meaningful.

MYTH BUSTING: 30 MAJOR BEAUTY MYTHS AND THE REAL FACTS

I know 30 myths to bust seems like an awful lot, but believe me, there could have been lots more. I struggled on which ones to include that would be the most helpful. What women are led to believe about skin care and makeup could fill volumes. We are incessantly bombarded with these myths disguised as truths, and like any brainwashing procedure it takes effort and facts to get to what is really possible and what is worth your time and money. So these 30 myths represent a snapshot of the typical erroneous information you get from cosmetics companies that end up hurting your skin and budget because they are a poor way to make decisions about the products you buy.

1. *Myth:* **There are skin-care products that really are better than Botox or better than dermal fillers.**

Fact: **Over the past few years cosmetics companies have positioned their skin-care products by claiming that they can compete with or even outdo medical corrective procedures such as Botox.** The ads in fashion magazines for these types of skin-care products often make claims about how dangerous Botox injections can be. There is nothing scary about Botox (other than the sound of the botulism toxin material used). In fact, the research about Botox's effectiveness and safety is overwhelmingly positive for every disorder they treat with it, and there are many, from cerebral palsy in children to headaches and eye tics. (Sources: *Journal of Neural Transmission*, April 2008, pages 617–623; *Laryngoscope*, May 2008, pages 790–796; *Journal of Headache and Pain*, October 2007, pages 294–300; *Expert Opinion on Pharmacotherapy*, June 2007, pages 1059–1072; and *Pediatrics*, July 2007, pages 49–58.)

On the other hand, there is absolutely no research showing that any skin-care product can even remotely work in any manner like Botox, or like dermal fillers such as Restylane or Artecol, or like laser resurfacing. Regardless of their ingredients or the claims these skin-care products make, it just isn't possible. Even Botox can't work like Botox if you apply it topically rather than injecting it into facial muscles. Nor can dermal fillers plump up wrinkles when applied topically rather than being injected. When performed by professionals, Botox and dermal injections make wrinkles in the treated area disappear almost immediately. Believing that skin-care products can do the same is a complete waste of money. There has never been a single skin-care product that has ever put a plastic surgeon or cosmetic dermatologist out of business! It makes sense, then, even with the increasing number of products claiming to be better than Botox, that there were more Botox injections and dermal filler injections performed in 2007 than ever before—millions and millions of them.

2. *Myth:* **Dermal fillers such as Radiesse and Restylane are completely safe and are the best filler options available.**

Fact: **Absolutely not true!** First, there are more than 30 dermal filler materials being used, and many of them are even more beneficial and definitely longer lasting than Radiesse and Restylane (Sources: *Plastic and Reconstructive Surgery*, November 2007, pages 33S–40S; and *Dermatologic Therapy*, May 2006, pages 141–150; and *Clinical and Plastic Surgery*, April 2005, pages 151–162). Although dermal fillers do work beautifully to fill out depressed areas of the face, such as the nasal labial folds that extend from your nose to your mouth, deep lines between the eyebrows, and marionette lines along the sides of the mouth, they do pose risks. The advertising for these two products, and the repeated mention of them in fashion magazines, have led consumers to believe that these work flawlessly. There are definitely problems (albeit infrequent) associated with these fillers, and with all of the more than 30 fillers currently being used. These problems and adverse events are primarily granulomas and nodules, which are lumps or hard spheres that may occur under the skin. Although these sometimes must be corrected with surgery, for the temporary fillers the adverse events do fade with time while the semi-permanent fillers can stay in place for far longer periods of time. The trade off is duration versus risk, and the decision is yours.

Please don't take this information to mean you shouldn't consider using dermal fillers to successfully treat wrinkles (millions of successful treatments have been performed); it's just that you should be fully informed before you make any decision about any product or procedure you are considering. One more thing: there are absolutely no skin-care products that can work in any way, shape, or form like a dermal filler. (Sources: *Dermatologic Surgery*, June 2008, Supplemental, pages S92–S99, and December 2007, Supplemental, pages S168–S175; *Plastic and Reconstructive Surgery*, November 2007, Supplemental, pages S17–S26; *Dermatology*, April 2006, pages 300–304; *Journal of Cosmetic Laser Therapy*, December 2005, pages 171–176; and *Aesthetic and Plastic Surgery*, January–February 2005, pages 34–48.)

3. *Myth:* **You should choose skin-care products based on your age.**

Fact: **Many products on the market claim to be designed for a specific age group, especially for "mature" women; mature usually refers to women over 50.** Before you buy into any arbitrary age division when choosing skin-care products, ask yourself why the over-50 group is always lumped together. According to this logic, someone who is 40 or 45 shouldn't be using the same products as someone who is 50 (only 5 or 10 years older), yet someone who is 80 should be using the same products as someone who is 50. If you think that doesn't make sense, you're right.

To clear up the confusion, what you need to know is that skin has different needs that are based on skin type, not on age. Not everyone in the same age group has the same skin type. Your skin-care routine depends on how dry, sun-damaged, oily, sensitive, thin, blemished, or normal your skin is, all of which have nothing to do with age. Then there are the issues of rosacea, psoriasis, allergies, and other skin disorders, which again have nothing to do with age. What everyone needs to do is protect the outer barrier of their skin in exactly the same way—avoid unnecessary direct sun exposure (sun protection), don't smoke, don't irritate your skin, and do use state-of-the-art skin-care products loaded with antioxidants and skin-identical ingredients (Sources: *International Journal of Cosmetic Science*, October 2007, pages 409–410; and *Cutaneous and Ocular Toxicology*, April 2007, pages 343–357). Plenty of young women have dry skin, and plenty of older women have oily skin and breakouts (particularly women who are experiencing perimenopausal or menopausal hormone fluctuations).

Some skin disorders, diseases, and functionality problems are associated with older skin, but whether they appear or not depends on the woman and her particular skin. They are not universally true of older skin because even these specific maladies can occur in younger people as well (such as ulcerated skin, wounds that don't heal, itchy skin, and thinning skin). In addition, none of these problems have anything to do with "normal," daily skin-care needs; whatever your age, a healthy skin-care routine for your skin type can do wonders (Sources: *British Journal of Community Nursing*, May 2007, pages 203–204; *Journal of Investigative Dermatology*, December 2005, pages 364–368; and *Journal of Vascular Surgery*, October 1999, pages 734–743).

Turning 50 does not mean a woman should assume that her skin is drying up and that she must therefore begin using "mature" skin-care products. After all, those are almost always just products that are designed for dry skin, and are in no way different from any of the other skin-care products for dry skin on the market. Besides, for many women over 50 (including me), it definitely does not mean that the battle with blemishes is over. Let me just reiterate this: There are no products designed for older women that address any special needs other than dry skin!

4. *Myth:* **Products labeled as "hypoallergenic" are better for sensitive skin.**

Fact: **"Hypoallergenic" is little more than a nonsense word.** In the world of cosmetics, this term is nothing more than an advertising contrivance meant to imply that a product is unlikely or less likely to cause allergic reactions and therefore is better for sensitive or problem skin. To "imply" is never the same as to state a "fact," and in this situation it is patently untrue that products labeled "hypoallergenic" are any better for sensitive skin! There are absolutely no accepted testing methods, ingredient restrictions, regulations, guidelines, rules, or procedures of any kind, anywhere in the world, for determining whether or not a product qualifies as being hypoallergenic. A company can label their product "hypoallergenic" because there is no regulation that says they can't, no matter what proof they may point to—and what proof can they provide given there is no standard to measure against? Given that there are no regulations governing this supposed category that was made up by the cosmetics industry, there are plenty of products labeled "hypoallergenic" that contain problematic ingredients and that could indeed trigger allergic reactions, even for those with no previous history of skin sensitivity. The word "hypoallergenic" gives you no reliable understanding of what you are or aren't putting on your skin (Sources: www.fda.gov; and *Ostomy and Wound Management*, March 2003, pages 20–21).

5. *Myth:* **"Dermatologist tested" on a cosmetics label is a good indication that the product is reliable and can live up to the claims.**

Fact: **You absolutely should not rely on the "dermatologist tested" claim any more than you should rely on the appearance of a doctor's name on a product's label to indicate you are getting a superior formulation**. There are many misleading and deceptive aspects to the term "dermatologist-tested" as it's used on a label, but at the top of the list is that this claim does not tell you what dermatologist did the testing, what he or she tested, how he or she performed the testing, or what the results were. That is, they don't tell you what they found with their supposed testing; they just tell you that they tested it. Without all of the testing information and results, there is no way to determine what it means. More often than not it just means that a cosmetics company paid a doctor to say that it's a good product (and there are lots of doctors on the payroll of lots of cosmetics companies). Or they could actually have performed a test, but only on six people, or used testing methods that guaranteed a positive outcome, which happens more often that you'd think. But that hardly provides results you can rely on. Dermatologist-tested is nothing more than a marketing gimmick because people like to believe that doctors have the consumer's best interest at heart. In the world of cosmetics, however, that is not always the case.

6. *Myth:* **Cosmeceutical companies make better products than cosmetics companies.**

Fact: **The term "cosmeceutical" is, sad to say, a false advertising gimmick created by dermatologists to suggest that their "cosmeceutical" products are somehow better than other products in the cosmetics industry.** What pathetic chicanery and deceit! At the very least what you should expect from the medical world is scientific fact, not these fictitious, sales-oriented machinations. When you hear the word "cosmeceutical," you're supposed to think a product is a blend of cosmetic ingredients and pharmaceutical-grade ingredients and, therefore, it must be better for your skin—right? The fact is, "cosmeceutical" is just a trumped-up word that has no legal or recognized meaning; it definitely has nothing to do with what the product may contain versus the content of any "non-cosmeceutical" cosmetic. A quick comparison of ingredient lists reveals that there is nothing any more unique or pharmaceutical about cosmeceuticals than any other cosmetics in the cosmetics industry. Plus, the FDA does not consider the term "cosmeceutical" to be a valid product class, so the term isn't regulated. So you should view it merely as a marketing term, and nothing more. Anyone can use that term to represent their brand's identity (Source: www.fda.gov).

Organizations like the American Academy of Dermatology have muddied the issue even further by stating "Dermatologists know how to use cosmeceutical ingredients and can advise their patients about the best ways to achieve healthy looking skin" (Source: AAD, www.aad.org). I read dermatology journals every month, and I've been to enough dermatology conferences to know that is absolutely not true. They haven't a clue. But even more to the point, dermatologists don't agree on what makes one product a cosmeceutical and the other not. Depending on who you talk to, products containing retinol (or other retinoids, which are part of the vitamin A molecule), or hydroquinone, or certain botanicals such as green tea, soy, pomegranate, curcumin, or grape, are the gold standard. But *all* these ingredients are available for use by all cosmetics companies—and indeed they show up in all kinds of products and often not in the ones labeled cosmeceutical.

Another description tossed around maintains that a cosmeceutical contains an ingredient that performs some kind of special action on the skin. However, all of those ingredients can be used by any cosmetics company, regardless of their designation or where they're applied.

According to the AAD, "the answer to whether or not cosmeceuticals really work lies in the ingredients and how they interact with the biological mechanisms that occur in aging skin." But again, that's true for any cosmetic. Even doctors can be seduced by their own hype so they can sell skin-care products and market them as something different by using a coined, misleading term.

7. *Myth:* **Age spots are best treated with specialty skin lighteners, whiteners, or products claiming to get rid of brown skin discolorations.**

Fact: **First, the term "age spot" is really a misnomer. Brown, freckle-like skin discolorations are not a result of age; they are the result of years of unprotected sun exposure.** You can demonstrate this for yourself: just compare the skin on the parts of your body that haven't seen the sun (like your backside or the inner part of your arm) with skin on the parts of your body that see the sun on a regular basis. The parts of your body that don't the see sun will have minimal to no skin discolorations. And keep in mind that the bad rays of the sun also come through windows! (Sources: *Journal of Cosmetic Dermatology*, September 2007, pages 195–202; *Dermatology Nursing*, October 2004, pages 401–413; and *Age and Ageing*, March 2006, pages 110–115.)

Second, a number of skin-care products that claim they can make skin whiter or lighter more often than not contain no ingredients that can have any significant, or even minor, impact on melanin production (melanin is the brown pigment in skin). In addition, even when the product does contain an ingredient that can have an effect, it usually contains such a small amount that it won't help at all. Basically, there is no comparison between the effects (or non-effects) of using one of these products and using a sunscreen plus a product containing hydroquinone.

Because unprotected sun exposure is the primary trigger for most brown, freckle-like skin discolorations, the primary way to reduce, prevent, and possibly even eliminate skin discolorations is diligent, daily application of a well-formulated sunscreen. Be sure not to forget the back of your hands and your chest (and be sure to reapply every time you wash your hands, because sunscreen does wash off).

No other aspect of controlling or reducing brown skin discolorations is as important as being careful about not getting a tan, and never exposing your skin to the sun without using a sunscreen rated SPF 15 or more—and more is usually better. And make sure that the sunscreen includes the UVA-protecting ingredients of titanium dioxide, zinc oxide, avobenzone (which can also be on the label as butyl methoxydibenzoylmethane), Tinosorb, or Mexoryl SX (which can also be on the label as ecamsule), because they prevent the UVA damage that triggers brown spots (Source: *Journal of the American Academy of Dermatology*, December 2006, pages 1048–1065).

Though I rarely express my own personal, anecdotal experience (I always rely on scientific studies rather than guess why a positive or negative result is taking place), in this case I will share what I do. I have found that using a sunscreen with only titanium dioxide and zinc oxide as the active ingredients has the most impressive results. The difference in my face, arms, and hands has been significant ever since I made that change several years ago. There is some research that supports this personal experience, but I wish there were more science to back it up. I suspect the reason why the results may be superior is the coverage zinc oxide or titanium dioxide provides (more like a blanket over skin), "blocking" the sun rather than chemically converting the rays as synthetic sunscreen agents do. Keeping the sun from penetrating into skin is the best protection possible for skin (Sources: *The Lancet*, August 2007, pages 528–537; *Skin Pharmacology and Physiology*, June 2005, pages 253–262; www.aad.org/public/publications/pamphlets/common_melasma.html; and www.emedicine.com/DERM/topic260.htm).

Beyond the use of sunscreen, hydroquinone has the highest efficacy for lightening skin, with a long history of safe use behind it, more so than any other skin-lightening ingredient. There are other alternatives that show promise for lightening skin, but they have been the subject of far less research and their effectiveness often pales in comparison to that of hydroquinone. It is interesting to note that when applied to the skin some of these alternative ingredients actually break down into small amounts of hydroquinone, which explains why they have an effect. These alternative ingredients include *Mitracarpus scaber* extract, *Uva ursi* (bearberry) extract, *Morus bombycis* (mulberry), *Morus alba* (white mulberry), and *Broussonetia papyrifera* (paper mulberry), all of which contain arbutin, which can inhibit melanin production. Technically, these extracts contain hydroquinone-beta-D-glucoside. Pure forms of arbutin, such as alpha-arbutin, beta-arbutin, and deoxy-arbutin, are considered more potent for skin lightening, but again the research is at best limited. Other ingredients that have some amount of research on their potential skin-lightening abilities are licorice extract (specifically glabridin), azelaic acid, and stabilized vitamin C (L-ascorbic acid, ascorbic acid, and magnesium ascorbyl phosphate), aloesin, gentisic acid, flavonoids, hesperidin, niacinamide, and polyphenols. However, no one knows how much is needed in a cosmetic lotion or cream to have an effect, and most of the research has been done in vitro, not on human skin.

To sum it up, there is a very specific game plan you can follow to get the most impressive results; it starts with avoiding sun exposure, daily use of a well-formulated sunscreen (365 days per year), and using a skin-care product that contains hydroquinone. In addition, an exfoliant (such as AHAs and BHA) can be helpful; certain laser, intense-pulsed light, and radio wave treatments from a dermatologist or plastic surgeon can also be extremely helpful. But, and this is an important but: If you don't also use a sunscreen daily you will be wasting your time and money! (Sources: *Journal of Cutaneous Medicine and Surgery*, May–June 2008, pages 107–113; *Journal of Investigative Dermatology Symposium Proceedings*, April 2008, pages 20–24; *Bioscience, Biotechnology, and Biochemistry*, December 2005, pages 2368–2373; *Experimental Dermatology*, August 2005, pages 601–608; *Journal of Bioscience and Bioengineering*, March 2005, pages 272–276; *International Journal of Dermatology*, August 2004, pages 604–607; *Journal of Drugs in Dermatology*, July–August 2004, pages 377–381; *Dermatologic Surgery*, March 2004, pages 385–388; and *Facial and Plastic Surgery*, February 2004, pages 3–9.)

8. *Myth:* Women outgrow acne; you're not supposed to break out once you reach your 20s and beyond!

Fact: **If only that were true, my skin-care struggles in life would have been very different.** In fact, women in their 20s, 30s, 40s, and even 50s can have acne just like teenagers, and the treatment principles remain the same. Not everyone who has acne as a teenager will grow out of it, and even if you had clear skin as a teenager, there's no guarantee that you won't get acne later in life, perhaps during menopause. You can blame this often-maddening inconsistency on hormones! What is true is that men can outgrow acne, because after puberty men's hormone levels level out, while women's hormone levels fluctuate throughout their lifetime, which is why many women experience breakouts around their menstrual cycle (Sources: *International Journal of Dermatology*, November 2007, pages 1188–1191; *American Journal of Clinical Dermatology*, May 2006, pages 281–290; and *International Journal of Cosmetic Science*, June 2004, pages 129–138). There are actually lots of myths about acne; see the following for a few corollaries to Myth #8.

9. *Myth:* Acne is caused by eating the wrong foods.

Fact: **This is both true and false.** The traditional foods thought to cause acne, such as chocolate and greasy foods, have no effect on acne, and there is no research indicating otherwise. However, there is the potential that individual dietary allergic reactions can trigger acne, such as eating foods that contain iodine, like shellfish, although there is an ongoing controversy about that. A bit more conclusive is new research showing that milk, especially skim milk, can increase the risk of acne. The same may be true for a diet high in carbohydrates; a high glycemic load can increase breakouts, while a low glycemic load can reduce their occurrence. (Glycemic load is a ranking system for the amount of carbohydrates in a food portion; too many carbs in your diet could trigger breakouts.) Experimenting for a few months to see which of these food groups either hurt or help your skin is worth the effort (Sources: *Molecular Nutrition and Food Research*, June 2008, pages 718–726; *Dermatologic Therapy*, March–April 2008, pages 86–95; *Journal of the American Academy of Dermatology*, May 2008, pages 787–793; and *Dermatology Online Journal*, May 30, 2006).

10. *Myth:* **If you clean your face better you can clear up your acne.**

Fact: **Over-cleaning your face can actually make matters worse.** Acne is caused primarily by hormonal fluctuations that affect the oil gland, creating an environment where acne-causing bacteria (*Propionibacterium acnes*) can flourish. Don't confuse scrubbing or "deep cleaning" with helping acne, because it absolutely doesn't. Over-cleansing your face triggers inflammation that can actually make acne worse. What really helps breakouts is using a gentle cleanser so you don't damage your skin's outer barrier or create inflammation, both of which hinder your skin's ability to heal and fight bacteria, along with using gentle exfoliation. An effective exfoliating product that contains salicylic acid or glycolic acid can make all the difference in reducing acne when used with a topical disinfectant containing benzoyl peroxide. None of these products should contain any irritating ingredients whatsoever, and particularly not alcohol, menthol, peppermint, or eucalyptus. (Sources: *Journal of the European Academy of Dermatology Venereology*, May 2008, pages 629–631; *Expert Opinion in Pharmacotherapy*, April 2008, pages 955–971; *International Journal of Dermatology*, March 2008, pages 301–302; *Journal of Cosmetic Dermatology*, March 2007, pages 59–65; *Cutis*, July 2006, Supplemental, pages 34–40; and *Skin Pharmacology and Physiology*, June 2006, pages 296–302.)

11. *Myth:* **Makeup causes acne.**

Fact: **Probably not.** There is no research indicating that makeup or skin-care products cause acne, and there is no consensus on which ingredients are problematic. In the late 1970s there was some research performed on rabbit skin using 100% concentrations of ingredients to determine whether or not they caused acne. Subsequently, it was determined that this study had nothing to do with the way women wear makeup or use skin-care products, and it was never repeated or considered useful in any way. Still, women do experience breakouts after using some skin-care or makeup products (or a random combination of both—I know I do). Such breakouts can be the result of an irritant or an inflammatory response, a random skin reaction, or a result of problematic ingredients unique to a person's skin type. That means you have to experiment to see what might be causing your breakouts. There is no information from medical research or the cosmetics industry to help or point you in the right direction. And just so you know, "noncomedogenic" is a meaningless word the cosmetics industry uses to indicate that a product is less likely to cause breakouts; the problem is no standards or regulations have been set up to describe this category.

12. *Myth:* **Stress causes acne.**

Fact: **Generally, it is believed that stress can trigger acne, but no one is exactly sure how that works, and there is conflicting research.** While it never hurts to reduce angst and worry in your life, stress as a causative factor for acne is hard to pinpoint. Plus, the way to treat acne doesn't change because of the stressors in your life. (Sources: *Archives of Dermatologic Research*, July 2008, pages 311–316; *European Journal of Dermatology*, July–August 2008, pages 412–415; *American Journal of Clinical Dermatology*, May 2006, pages 281–290; and *International Journal of Cosmetic Science*, June 2004, pages 129–138.)

13. *Myth:* **Toothpaste works to prevent or quickly heal a pimple.**

Fact: **Absolutely not true!!!** This would be funny if so many people didn't believe it. None of the ingredients in toothpaste can have a positive effect on acne or change a blemish once you have it, and actually it can make matters worse. The bacteria in your mouth are not related to the bacteria (*P. acnes*) in your pores that cause acne. And although the fluoride or sodium monofluorophosphate in your toothpaste can help fight bacteria in your mouth, on your skin they can actually cause pimples and redness in the areas they come in contact with. This is known as perioral dermatitis (Sources: *Journal of the American Dental Association*, September 2003, page 1165; *Journal of the American Academy of Dermatology*, June 1990, pages 1029–1032; and *Archives of Dermatology*, June 1975, page 793). The other ingredients in toothpaste might have minimal abrasive properties, but they provide nothing that a gentle rubbing with a washcloth can't do far better. Another issue for skin is that the flavorings added to toothpaste present additional problems that you should avoid on your skin (Source: *Contact Dermatitis*, October 2000, pages 216–222).

14. *Myth:* **Applying collagen and elastin to skin will add to the collagen and elastin content of skin, which will eliminate wrinkles.**

Fact: **Collagen and elastin in skin-care products can serve as good water-binding agents, but they cannot fuse with your skin's natural supply of these supportive elements.** In most cases, the collagen molecule is too large to penetrate into the skin. But even when it is made small enough to be absorbed it cannot bind with the collagen existing in skin, and there isn't a shred of research indicating otherwise. What do exist are myriad studies showing that collagen is a very good moisturizing ingredient, which is great for skin, but it is neither unique nor the only formulary option. It is important to point out that even if you were to take the collagen that is used in medically administered dermal injections and rub it on your skin, it wouldn't be absorbed, and it wouldn't change wrinkles by bolstering the existing collagen. There is even less research showing that elastin has any benefit when applied topically (Source: *International Journal of Cosmetic Science*, April 2005, pages 101–106).

Keep in mind that even if collagen or elastin could be absorbed, and even if they could combine with your existing collagen or elastin, without guidelines you would just keep adding collagen and elastin to your skin, and eventually it would stick out in places you wouldn't want it to, stick out in lumps if too much was absorbed in one place, and plump up your fingers because that's what you use to apply the product that contains these ingredients. When a physician uses collagen injections to plump up lips and lines on the face, he or she can inject only so much collagen into your face before you end up with overblown lips and a distorted facial expression.

Protecting your skin from sun damage, daily exfoliation with a well-formulated AHA or BHA product, and treating your skin to a range of ingredients (antioxidants, cell-communicating ingredients, and skin-identical ingredients) that it needs to look and feel its best will protect its natural collagen supply and allow it to build new collagen—something healthy, protected skin loves to do and does quite well.

15. *Myth:* **Eye creams are specially formulated for use around the delicate eye area.**

Fact: **There is no evidence, research, or documentation validating the claim that the eye area needs ingredients different from those you use on your face, neck area, or décolletage.** Even if there were ingredients that were special for the eye area, that isn't evident in the labels for eye-care products; their formulations seem to be chosen at random, with no consistency in the industry. All cosmetics companies put whatever ingredients they want to into their eye products. Typically, they give you half as much but charge you twice as much as the same product being sold for your face. The ingredient labels on these "specialty" products more than prove the point. Eye creams are a whim of the cosmetics industry designed to evoke the sale of two products when only one is needed.

One more point: Occasionally a physician, aesthetician, or someone selling skin-care products will defend their eye creams by telling me that the eye area doesn't need ingredients that cause irritation. Well, I agree wholeheartedly with that statement, but the same is absolutely true for the face, or anywhere else on your body. You shouldn't be applying formulations with needlessly irritating ingredients—period! That means that all your eye area needs is a well-formulated product, and that can certainly be the same product you use on your face.

16. *Myth:* **There is (or will be) a product out there that really can eliminate wrinkles.**

Fact: **Regrettably, there is no magic potion or combination of products in any price range that can make wrinkles truly disappear, or prevent them, except daily use of a well-formulated sunscreen (and never getting a tan).** The wrinkles you see and agonize over (not to be confused with fine lines caused by dryness, which are easily remedied with a good moisturizer) are the result of cumulative sun damage and the inevitable breakdown of your skin's natural support structure. Skin-care ingredients, no matter who is selling them or what claims they make for them, cannot replace what plastic surgeons and cosmetic dermatologists do. There are literally thousands of anti-wrinkle products being sold and we buy more of them than almost any other beauty product. Yet as I stated before, despite this onslaught of products, plastic surgeons and dermatologists are not going out of business.

An interesting study in *Skin Research and Technology* (May 2007, pages 189–194) compared the effects of an inexpensive moisturizing face cream with an expensive one in a luxurious jar. Eighty Swedish women ages 35–64 years were randomly divided into three groups: Group A treated their facial skin for six weeks with the expensive cream in its luxury jar, Group B used an inexpensive moisturizer presented in the same luxury jar, and Group C used the expensive cream contained in a neutral jar. The evaluations were made by the subjects, by a clinical trained observer, and by measuring the skin surface relief using optical profilometry (a method that measures the contours and roughness of surface skin). All the results showed no differences between the three groups related to the effects on wrinkles and smoothness, and there was no assessment of their skin feeling younger or more beautiful. Facial appearance was the same and profilometry showed reduced surface microrelief with all the products.

Don't take this to mean that there aren't skin-care products that can significantly help improve skin, because there are, including sunscreen, exfoliants (AHAs or BHA), moisturizers loaded with antioxidants and cell-communicating ingredients, retinoids (components of Vitamin A), and numerous others. It's just that anti-wrinkle skin-care products can't perform according to the exaggerated claims on the label. After all, if they worked as promised then cosmetics companies wouldn't be launching new anti-wrinkle products every few months.

17. *Myth:* **Expensive cosmetics are better than inexpensive cosmetics.**

Fact: **The absolute truth is that there are good and bad products in all price categories.** The amount of money you spend on skin-care products has nothing to do with the quality or uniqueness of the formula. An expensive soap by Erno Laszlo is no better for your skin than an inexpensive bar soap such as Dove (though I suggest that both are potentially too irritating and drying for all skin types). On the other hand, an irritant-free toner by Neutrogena can be just as good as, or maybe even better than, an irritant-free toner by Orlane or La Prairie (depending on the formulation), and any irritant-free toner is infinitely better than a toner that contains alcohol, peppermint, menthol, essential oils, eucalyptus, lemon, or other irritants, no matter how natural-sounding the ingredients are and regardless of the price or claim. I've seen lots of expensive products that are little more than water and wax, and inexpensive products that are beautifully formulated. And in all price ranges I've seen products come in jar packaging, which is like throwing your money away, since jar packaging can't keep important, air-sensitive ingredients such as antioxidants stable. Spending less doesn't hurt your skin, and spending more doesn't help it. It's all about the formulation, not the price.

18. *Myth:* **European products, especially from countries like France, Switzerland, and Italy, are formulated better than products from other countries. European women just know how to take care of their skin.**

Fact: **Having spent a good deal of time in Europe doing presentations to women about skin care and reviewing European cosmetic brands I can say without hesitation that is utterly not true.** The facts are on the ingredient label and European products have all the same problems that cosmetic products have all over the world, including jar packaging, which doesn't keep air-sensitive ingredients such as plant extracts, vitamins, and many cell-communicating ingredients stable after opening; the use of irritating ingredients or overly drying ingredients; antiquated formulations; and overpriced concoctions that are little more than just wax and water. None of that creates superlative skin care by any definition.

The other notion, that European women take better care of their skin, is a strange ongoing myth. Although European women are not as overweight as American women (actually no country in the world has a bigger obesity problem than the U.S., but that's another discussion), they do not take better care of their skin. They smoke, they tan, they use poorly formulated products, and they believe the same false claims women all over the world get sucked into believing.

19. *Myth:* **Natural ingredients are better for skin than synthetic ingredients.**

Fact: **Whatever preconceived notion someone might have about natural ingredients being better for the skin, or whatever media-induced fiction someone might believe, this is not true.** There is no factual basis or scientific legitimacy for the belief that natural is better. Not only is the definition of "natural" hazy, but the term is loosely regulated, so any cosmetics company can use it to mean whatever they want it to mean. Just because an ingredient grows out of the ground or is found in nature doesn't make it automatically good for skin, and the reverse is also true: Just because it is synthetic doesn't make it bad.

"Consumers should not necessarily assume that an 'organic' or 'natural' ingredient or product would possess greater inherent safety than another chemically identical version of the same ingredient," Dr. Linda M. Katz, director of the Food and Drug Administration's Office of Cosmetics and Colors stated. "In fact, 'natural' ingredients may be harder to preserve against microbial contamination and growth than synthetic raw materials" (*New York Times*, November 1, 2007).

"But people should not interpret even the USDA Organic seal or any organic seal of approval on cosmetics as proof of health benefits or of efficacy," said Joan Shaffer, USDA spokeswoman (Source: www.ams.usda.gov/nop/FactSheets/Backgrounder.html). The National Organic Program is a marketing program, not a safety program. Steak may be graded prime, but that has no bearing on whether it is safe or nutritious to eat.

20. *Myth:* **Packaging doesn't matter when it comes to skin-care products; I just love products that come in beautiful containers, especially jars.**

Fact: **Packaging plays a significant role in the stability and effectiveness of the products you use.** Because many state-of-the-art ingredients, from cell-communicating ingredients, antioxidants, and plant extracts to skin-identical ingredients, are unstable in the presense of air, jar packaging, once opened, permits air to enter freely, which causes these important ingredients, the very ingredients that make a product most beneficial for skin, to break down and deteriorate. Jars also mean you are sticking your fingers into the product, which can transfer bacteria and further cause the great ingredients to break down. Think about how long an unprotected head of lettuce lasts in your refrigerator. Or after opening a can or jar of food, how long does it take before becoming a moldy mess? Airtight packaging, or any packaging that reduces the product's exposure to air, is essential when you are buying the best products for your skin. You should also avoid clear packaging that lets light into the product. Light of any kind is a problem because it causes sensitive ingredients to break down. If that isn't enough to make you reconsider jar packaging, it's worth noting that *The Guidelines on Stability of Cosmetic Products*, March 2004, by the CTFA and COLIPA (respectively, the American and European cosmetic governing associations most cosmetic companies in Europe and the US belong to) states "Packaging can directly affect finished product stability because of interactions which can occur between the product, the package, and the external environment. Such interactions may include... Barrier properties of the container [and] its effectiveness in protecting the contents from the adverse effects of atmospheric oxygen...."

(Sources: *Free Radical Biology and Medicine*, September 2007, pages 818–829; *Ageing Research Reviews*, December 2007, pages 271–288; *Dermatologic Therapy*, September–October 2007, pages 314–321; *International Journal of Pharmaceutics*, June 12, 2005, pages 197–203; *Pharmaceutical Development and Technology*, January 2002, pages 1–32; *International Society for Horticultural Science*, www.actahort.org/members/showpdf?booknrarnr=778_5; and Beautypackaging.com, www.beautypackaging.com/articles/2007/03/airless-packaging.php.)

21. *Myth:* **Blackheads are caused by dirt and can be scrubbed away.**

Fact: **Blackheads may make skin look dirty, but they are unrelated to dirt.** Blackheads are formed when hormones cause too much sebum (oil) production, dead skin cells get in the way, the pore is impaired or misshapen, and the path for the oil to exit through the pore is blocked, creating a clog. As this clog nears the surface of the skin, the mixture of oil and cellular debris oxidizes and turns, you guessed it, black. You cannot scrub away blackheads, at least not completely. Using a topical scrub removes the top portion of the blackhead, but does nothing to address the underlying cause, so they're back again before too long. Instead of a scrub, try using a well-formulated BHA (salicylic acid) product. Salicylic acid exfoliates inside the pore lining, dissolving the oil and dead skin cells that lead to constant blackheads.

22. *Myth:* **Oily skin can be controlled externally (from the outside in) with the right skin-care products.**

Fact: **Possibly, but right now this is mere conjecture, involving an extremely complicated and difficult to understand process.** Oil production is triggered primarily by androgens and estrogen (male and female hormones, respectively), and altering hormone production topically is not something available in the realm of cosmetics.

However, the sebaceous gland itself also produces active androgens that can increase sebum excretion. What can happen is that stress-sensing skin signals (think skin inflammation and irritation) can lead to the production and release of androgens and cause more oil production, which can clog pores (Sources: *Experimental Dermatology*, June 2008, pages 542–551; and *Clinical Dermatology*, September–October 2004, pages 360–366). These factors make topical irritation and inflammation bad for skin, but that still doesn't affect the production of hormones inside the body, the primary source for triggering the pore to make too much oil.

What you can do is use a retinoid (vitamin A or tretinoin) to improve the shape of the pore so that the oil can flow more evenly, preventing clogging. There is some research that niacinamide in skin-care products can help, but no one is quite sure why. You also can avoid making matters worse by not using products that contain oils or thick emollient ingredients. You can absorb surface oil by using clay masks as part of your skin-care routine (though the effect is completely temporary), but you need to avoid masks that contain irritating ingredients. How often you should use a mask depends on your skin type; some people use one every day, others once a week. Masks of this kind may be used after cleansing, left on for 10–15 minutes, and then rinsed with tepid water.

23. *Myth:* **Dry skin is caused by a lack of water, either by not having enough in skin or simply not drinking enough water.**

Fact: **Ironically, dry skin is not as simple as just a lack of moisture.** The studies that have compared the water content of dry skin to that of normal or oily skin show that there doesn't appear to be a statistically significant difference. Healthy skin requires a water content of about 15%, and adding too much moisture, like soaking in a bathtub, is bad for skin because it disrupts the skin's outer barrier (the intercellular matrix) by breaking down the substances that keep skin cells functioning normally and in good shape.

What is thought to be taking place when dry skin occurs is that the intercellular matrix (the substances between skin cells that keep them intact, smooth, and healthy) has become depleted or damaged, bringing about a rough, uneven, and flaky texture that allows water to be lost. But adding water won't keep that moisture in skin unless the outer barrier is maintained or repaired, and again too much water just causes problems.

To prevent dry skin, the primary goal is to avoid and reduce anything that damages the outer barrier, including sun damage, products that contain irritating ingredients, alcohol, drying cleansers, and smoking. All of the research about dry skin is related to the ingredients and treatments that reinforce the substances in skin that keep it functioning normally.

(Sources: *British Journal of Dermatology*, July 2008, pages 23–34; *Journal of the European Academy of Dermatology and Venereology*, September 2007, pages S1–S4; *Journal of Cosmetic Dermatology*, June 2007, pages 75–82; *Dermatologic Therapy*, March 2004, Supplement 1, pages 43–48; and *International Journal of Cosmetic Science*, April 2003, pages 63–95, and October 2000, pages 371–383.)

As for drinking lots of water each day (a beauty tip that refuses to fade away), if all it took to get rid of dry skin was to drink more water, then no one would have dry skin and moisturizers would stop being sold. Keeping your liquid intake up is fine, but if you take in more water than your body needs, all you will be doing is running to the bathroom all day and night. The causes of and treatments for dry skin are far more complicated than water consumption. If anything, though rare, drinking too much water can be dangerous, causing a potentially deadly condition called hyponatremia.

24. *Myth:* **Dry skin causes wrinkles.**

Fact: **Dry skin and wrinkles are not related.** The inseparable association of dry skin with wrinkles continues to endure in the mind of the consumer. Nonetheless, the simple truth is that dry skin and wrinkles are not related in the least. I know that statement may be hard to accept because we're so conditioned by advertising and product claims to think otherwise, but believing the myth can hurt your skin by inducing you to concentrate on treating your dry skin or loading up on moisturizers hoping it will get rid of wrinkles. It just doesn't work that way.

Abundant research has made it perfectly clear that wrinkles and dry skin are not related in terms of cause and effect. Extensive studies and analyses have shown that dry skin is frequently a by-product or result of other assaults on skin that are the real cause of wrinkles. In other words, dry skin is primarily a symptom of other factors that cause wrinkles.

If dry skin doesn't cause wrinkles, what does? Wrinkles are permanent lines etched into skin from sun damage and internal causes (genetic changes, muscle movement, estrogen loss, and fat depletion). Nowhere, at least outside of ads and product claims, is dry skin ever mentioned as a cause of wrinkles. (Sources: *Fertility Sterility*, August 2005, pages 289–290; *Current Molecular Medicine*, March 2005, pages 171–177; *Cutis*, February 2005, Supplemental, pages 5–8; *Rejuvenation Research*, Fall 2004, pages 175–185; *Journal of Dermatology*, August 2004, pages 603–609; and *Contact Dermatitis*, September 2002, pages 139–146.)

Sun damage is by far the most notable cause of wrinkling, which is easily proven by something referred to as the backside test of aging. In other words, compare the areas of your skin that rarely, if ever, see the sun with the parts of your body exposed to the sun on a daily basis. Those areas with minimal sun exposure (such as your backside) are rarely, if ever dry, and they also have minimal to no signs of wrinkles or aging skin. They will also have far more of the firmness, elasticity, and color of "younger" skin because they have not been subjected to years of cumulative exposure to sunlight.

25. *Myth:* **Everyone needs a day cream and a night cream: Skin requires special care at night.**

Fact: **The ONLY difference between a daytime and nighttime moisturizer is that the daytime version should contain a well-formulated sunscreen.** What you often hear cosmetics salespeople say is that the skin needs different ingredients at night than during the day. Yet there isn't a shred of research or a list anywhere of what those ingredients or formulas should be. Skin is repairing itself and producing skin cells every nanosecond of the day—and night. Helping skin do that in as healthy a manner as possible doesn't change based on the time of day. Skin needs a generous amount of antioxidants, cell-communicating ingredients, and skin-identical ingredients all day and all night. Think about it like your diet: Green tea, grapes, flax, and all the other aspects of healthy eating are good for you day or night.

For daytime wear, unless your foundation contains an effective sunscreen, it is essential that your moisturizer feature a well-formulated, broad-spectrum sunscreen rated SPF 15 or higher. Well-formulated means that it contains UVA-protecting ingredients, specifically titanium dioxide, zinc oxide, avobenzone (also called butyl methoxydibenzoylmethane or Parsol 1789), Tinosorb, or Mexoryl SX (also called ecamsule). Regardless of the time of day, your skin needs all the current state-of-the-art ingredients it can get.

26. *Myth:* **Your skin adapts to the skin-care products you are using and you need to change to new products every now and then.**

Fact: **Skin doesn't adapt to skin-care products any more than your body adapts to a healthy diet.** If spinach and grapes are healthy for you they are always healthy, and they continue to be healthy, even if you eat them every day. The same is true for your skin; as long as you are applying what is healthy for skin it remains healthy. This is especially true for sunscreen and products that contain antioxidants, cell-communicating ingredients, and skin-identical ingredients (I explain those groups of products later in this book).

27. *Myth:* **I should just use what I like on my skin, that's the most important thing.**

Fact: **That would be a huge mistake because lots of women often like what isn't good for them.** For example, you may like getting a tan, but that can cause skin cancer and most certainly will cause wrinkles and skin discolorations. You may like smoking cigarettes, but that will cause skin cells to die and will cause the growth of unhealthy, malformed skin cells. You may like that daytime moisturizer you are using, but if it doesn't contain sunscreen it leaves your skin wide open to sun damage. Or you may prefer a moisturizer packaged in a jar, yet because almost all of the important state-of-the-art ingredients, especially antioxidants, plant extracts, vitamins, and cell-communicating ingredients, deteriorate in the presence of air, the jar packaging will not keep these ingredients stable, so you would be short-changing your skin soon after the product is opened. What it takes to help your skin be at its best and to function normally and really fight wrinkles or acne or any other skin problem is far more complex than just using what you "like." This doesn't mean that you shouldn't like what you use, but do take the time to select products that are truly healthy and beneficial for skin. That is, take the time to read the ingredient list and consult reliable reviews of the products you're considering, because you can't determine the benefits intuitively.

Think of it like your diet. If you were given the choice between eating what you like, say chocolate cake versus spinach and broccoli, you would eat a lot more chocolate cake than any green vegetable. But we eat the green veggies not so much because we like them but because we have learned they are better for us. It's impossible to accurately judge effectiveness and value based just on how you feel about the product.

28. *Myth:*You should buy all your skin-care products from one cosmetics brand because the products are designed to work together.

Fact: **That may be good for the company's sales, but it doesn't help your skin and in many cases will only end up causing problems.** Almost every skin-care line in the world has good and bad products or products that are inappropriate for special skin-care concerns. Lots of companies may have products containing problematic ingredients, some because they use irritating ingredients or ingredients that can't remotely live up to their claims, others because of what they *don't* contain such as effective sun protection or products in stable packaging. Much like shopping for food, you have to pick and choose what works and an entire line may not be suited to meet that need.

29. *Myth:* If it tingles or feels cooling on my skin it must be doing something.

Fact: **Any noticeable sensation, even for a brief period of time, is almost always damaging to your skin.** That familiar tingling, cooling sensation is actually just your skin responding to irritation, resulting in inflammation. Products that produce that sensation can actually damage your skin's healing process; make scarring worse; cause collagen and elastin to break down; cause dry, flaky skin; and increase the growth of bacteria that cause pimples.

Inflammation is the real culprit responsible for wrinkles and skin aging. Whether the inflammation in skin is brought about by the sun, smoking, pollution, or irritating ingredients used on the skin, the resulting reaction generates unpleasant and undesirable side effects ranging from dry, itchy skin to acne; reduced ability for the skin to heal; and collagen destruction. When the skin is being irritated from most any source you end up hurting your skin, not helping it.

A tingling or cooling sensation is a signal that your skin is being irritated and inflamed. It is being caused by problematic skin-care ingredients that can include overly abrasive cleansers, alcohol, fragrant plant extracts, peppermint, menthol, eucalyptus, and on and on, and their continued use will greatly reduce your chances of having the kind of skin you want. (Sources: *Skin Pharmacology and Physiology*, June 2008, pages 124–135; *Biochemistry and Pharmacology*, June 2007, pages 1786–1795; *Contact Dermatitis*, June 2006, pages 303–312; and *British Journal of Dermatology*, July 2005, pages 124–131.)

There are times when cooling ingredients are helpful. Ingredients such as menthol, peppermint, camphor, and mint are counter-irritants (Sources: *Archives of Dermatologic Research*, May 1996, pages 245–248; Code of Federal Regulations Title 21–Food and Drugs, revised April 1, 2001, 21CFR310.545, www.fda.gov; and www.naturaldatabase. com). Counter-irritants are used to induce local inflammation in an effort to reduce inflammation in deeper or adjacent tissues. In other words, they substitute one kind of inflammation for another, which is never good for skin, but can provide relief when itching is a temporary nuisance not abated by gentle scratching. Irritation or inflammation, no matter what causes it or how it happens, impairs the skin's immune and healing response (Source: *Skin Pharmacology and Applied Skin Physiology*, November–December 2000, pages 358–371). And although your skin may not show it or doesn't react in an irritated fashion, if you apply irritants to your skin the damage is still taking place and is ongoing, so it adds up over time (Source: *Skin Research and Technology*, November 2001, pages 227–237).

30. *Myth:* **The product I'm using contains ingredients that are known to irritate skin, like alcohol, lavender, bergamot, and peppermint, but I don't feel anything, so those ingredients aren't a problem for me.**

Fact: **Even though you don't feel a substance reacting on your skin, that doesn't mean it isn't doing damage.** For example, we don't feel the UVA rays of the sun. We can be sitting in the shade or inside next to a window and the sun's UVA rays are penetrating through, reaching our skin and causing serious, cumulative damage. Whether or not your skin reacts in the short term doesn't mean damage isn't happening beneath the surface, which is why it is so important to always treat your skin gently. Irritating, drying, and sensitizing ingredients cause problems underneath the skin that will take a toll in the long run, whether your skin shows it or not.

I know I said 30 myths in the title for this chapter but I couldn't resist! Let me add one more:

31. *Myth:* **My grandmother or mother had (has) beautiful skin so I just use what they've always used.**

Fact: **While your lineage may include naturally perfect skin, using skin-care products formulated even more than ten years ago would be a mistake.** It would be similar to saying, my grandmother was a great writer or researcher so I'm going to use the same typewriter or computer they used. No one is going to use a computer for more than five years anymore than they would use a typewriter and still be as productive as they would be using a current state-of-the-art computer. The same is true for skin-care products. What we know nowadays about formulations, ingredients, how skin functions at its best, sun damage, exfoliation, healing, and on and on is rarely addressed in products developed before the millennium.

The brilliant advances in cosmetic chemistry, dermatology, and ingredient technology now allow for the creation of all types of products that have elegant textures, silky applications, superb finishes, and truly effective ingredients that can make a difference in every aspect of your skin-care needs. There are many excellent things to emulate about your grandmother or mother, but the skin-care products they used in the past shouldn't be one of them.

ADVERTISING VICTIMS

Pervasive and endless advertising, along with the bias of fashion magazine cosmetics stories, fuels most cosmetics purchases to one degree or another. Advertising must work or the cosmetics industry wouldn't spend billions of dollars on television, print (particularly fashion magazines), and radio advertising to get you to buy their products. If you don't understand how advertising manipulates your purchases, you will always be a victim of its wiles and contrivances.

Lots of consumers make decisions about what they are going to buy based strictly on advertising. Is it any wonder that the advertising industry in the United States is a multi-billion-dollar business? Procter & Gamble alone spends $1.3 billion annually to advertise its products to the American public. L'Oreal and Estee Lauder each spend about the same. Companies spend these vast sums on advertising because they want (and get) more sales. Cosmetics companies sign celebrities to multimillion-dollar endorsement contracts because they know certain faces can sell millions of dollars worth of products.

We may think we recognize the influence advertising can have on us, and even feel we are above this kind of blatant artifice. But whether we like to admit it or not, we are greatly influenced by the power of advertising.

Celebrity endorsements are a powerful advertising tool in the cosmetics industry. Celebrities are visible everywhere in infomercials, fashion magazines, and TV ads because we as consumers equate being beautiful, or the ability to act, or any celebrity status with knowledge and integrity. An endorsement by someone with a well-known face carries weight. Enticing as it is to believe that listening to celebrities can help you have better skin and a better look, that's not the way it is. Do we really believe that the celebrities in the ads for Revlon or Estee Lauder are there because they love the company's products? Or is it more realistic to see the truth: that these models sign million-dollar contracts to smile brightly, showing their tacit, paid-for approval? A celebrity whose name is attached to a specific line has signed some type of lucrative contract; she's not endorsing the products because she loves them.

Fashion magazines often comment about products celebrities use separate from a signed endorsement. But actresses and models don't all use the same products (or the same makeup artist, plastic surgeon, or dermatologist). They use lots and lots of different products in all price ranges from a vast array of lines, and, like all women, they can be fickle. What they use today may not be what they use tomorrow. Celebrities look for "perfect" products just like the next person and are just as subject to being misled and wasting money as anyone else. Besides, what someone else is using doesn't necessarily have anything to do with your own skin-care or makeup needs.

Perhaps the most insidious and consistent form of cosmetics advertising ploy is show-casing an impossibly perfect, incongruously young woman (or several of them), groomed and photographed at the perfect moment by the best in the fashion world, and seeming to show how well a product works. As if their perfection is a result of any product or product line! In essence, this is fear advertising. Fear that everyone else has the answer, that everyone else is more beautiful and has more perfect skin than you do because they're using products that you aren't. This is a compelling, though completely false, message. The women hired for these ads weren't chosen because they used the product and became beautiful, they were selected from head shot photos provided by modeling agencies.

Fashion and women's magazines in general are another major source of cosmetics information. Yet the information from these pages is all one-sided. Cosmetics companys' advertising dollars are the bread and butter of these magazines and the editors aren't going to provide objective critical information about a main source of income. I can't tell you the number of reporters who tell me they can't print what I tell them even though I provide documented, published research proving what I'm explaining. They always say the same thing: Fashion magazines can't upset their advertisers, and their editors won't let the content through. There is little to no negative information about any cosmetic product or industry trend. Many women's magazines love to feature their "best" cosmetic buys, but if you look closely you'll notice they never include the worst cosmetic buys. If they know what's best why not tell us what they didn't like? Of course that is never going to happen, and this puts you at the mercy of misleading, prejudiced information.

What you need to keep in mind about almost all products, whether from the cosmetics industry or any other industry, is that they all have their pros and cons. The truth is that it is the task of the company paying for the ad, or the salesperson selling you the product, to portray the product in absolutely glowing, positive terms. You might still buy the product, but if you're reading this book at least you will have some facts to base your decision on, not just pretty pictures and catchy words.

As far as cosmetics are concerned, the only objective information is found on the ingredient list. Of course, that's the only part of the package that never gets featured in the magazines or on television, yet it is the only place where the law requires the manufacturer to tell you the truth.

BRAND-NAME LOYALTY

Ask yourself: Why should you be loyal to a cosmetics company if the cosmetics company isn't even loyal to itself? For example:

- **Estee Lauder owns** Aramis, Aveda, Clinique, Bobbi Brown, Prescriptives, M.A.C., Origins, Jo Malone, La Mer, Tommy Hilfiger fragrances, Bumble and Bumble, American Beauty, Flirt, Good Skin, Grassroots, Michael Kors Beauty, Darphin, Ojon, and Donna Karan Cosmetics.

- **L'Oreal owns** Maybelline New York, Garnier, Lancome, Helena Rubinstein, Bio-Medic, Vichy, Biotherm, Shu Uemura, Kiehl's, Soft Sheen-Carson, Redken, Matrix, Kerastase, Giorgio Armani, Inneov, Sanoflore, CCB Paris, Dermablend, The Body Shop, Skinceuticals, Ralph Lauren, and La Roche-Posay.

- **Procter & Gamble owns** Cover Girl, Max Factor, Olay, DDF, Aussie, Camay, Clairol, Gillette, Head & Shoulders, Ivory, Fredric Fekkai, Noxzema, Pantene, SK-II, and Zest.

- **Johnson & Johnson owns** Neutrogena, Aveeno, Clean & Clear, RoC, Rogaine, Lubriderm, Purpose, and Ambi.

Brand-name loyalty just does not make any sense. Clinique makes great mascaras, some great foundations, and some great moisturizers, but several of their toners contain alcohol, which is too irritating and drying for all skin types. Clinique also has several moisturizers packaged in jars that won't keep the important ingredients stable. Lancome has some excellent blushes and mascaras but their foundations with sunscreen typically don't contain UVA-protecting ingredients, while their moisturizers are overly fragranced and most all of them lack state-of-the-art ingredients many other lines include. Neutrogena offers some wonderful makeup products and sunscreens but most of their cleansers are extremely drying and irritating, and some of their sunscreens don't contain UVA-protecting ingredients. Revlon has some great foundations, good mascaras, and terrific lip pencils, but they have failed repeatedly at eyeshadows and their attempts at mineral makeup. Staying with one line, in any price range, is usually a disservice to your skin and budget.

Even our own experience tells us that all the products within one product line aren't great. Haven't we all purchased expensive (and inexpensive) products that didn't work or that we didn't like? Yet the success of the major product lines in establishing brand-name loyalty is astonishing. It is particularly apparent in the way a woman responds to questions about what brand of makeup she is currently using. A customer usually whispers or acts embarrassed when she admits to using a drugstore brand, but if she's using an expensive brand you can hear her across the room. The reality is that the cost of a cosmetic has nothing to do with whether it will work for you. We have all used both inexpensive and expensive makeup that worked beautifully for skin, as well as inexpensive and expensive makeup that looked awful and was bad for skin.

COSMECEUTICALS: DOCTORS GET IN ON THE ACT

It is sobering to know that doctors are the second leading channel for distribution of skin-care products. More than 10,000 physicians sell skin-care products through their offices. Just when I thought it couldn't get any worse, now that doctors are in the mainstream of cosmetic sales their objectivity has gone in the same direction as the rest of the cosmetics industry. That is extremely distressing because while most women would never assume a physician would mislead them, I see it all the time. Products sold at a physician's office are not automatically better and are often more overpriced than the rest of the industry. You often get the same sales pressure from a physician that you do at the cosmetics counter or from infomercials. Notably, several doctors are famous because of their presence on infomercials or in advertisements. However, do not mistake salesmanship with medical information; they are not the same.

For example, take the invention of "cosmeceuticals," a term physicians created to describe the products they sell. Cosmeceuticals are loosely defined as products that combine the benefits of a cosmetic and a pharmaceutical. The term is used to give the impression that these products have more effective or more active ingredients than just ordinary cosmetics.

As more and more doctors get into selling or endorsing skin-care products, you will hear more and more about cosmeceuticals. Dr. Tina Alster is the spokesperson for Lancome; Dr. Karyn Grossman is the spokesperson for Prescriptives; Dr. Patricia Wexler's namesake products, Patricia Wexler M.D. Dermatology, launched as the next best way to seeing Wexler herself, at least if you shop at Bath & Body Works; Skin Effects by Dr. Jeffrey Dover is at CVS; Dr. Sheldon Pinnell's SkinCeuticals line has been purchased by L'Oreal; and, of course, there's Dr. N.V. Perricone, Dr. Murad, and Dr. Howard Sobel, with his DDF line that's now owned by Procter & Gamble.

Despite all this display of medical pedigree, the term cosmeceutical is not in any way regulated or controlled, and anyone can slap that label on their products to promote them as being more "medical."

Do cosmeceuticals really differ from any other cosmetics? The answer is no, because no matter how a product is labeled and marketed many skin-care treatments contain ingredients that affect the function of skin. Effectiveness isn't reserved just for cosmeceuticals, it is completely within the realm of any well-formulated product.

Regardless of the name—cosmeceutical or otherwise—a skin-care product is only as good as what it contains and the ability of those ingredients to help your skin function better; or, in the vernacular, to act younger. In fact, moisturizers, just like any other skin-care product claiming to have an effect on wrinkles or sagging skin, should absolutely contain an elegant mix of antioxidants, cell-communicating ingredients, and intercellular substances, because they help skin keep a normal level of hydration, build collagen, reduce skin discolorations, and prevent cellular damage.

(Sources: Packaged Facts, U.S. Cosmeceuticals to 2008, www.the-infoshop.com; *SKINmed*, July–August, pages 214–220; *Dermatologic Surgery*, July 2005, pages 873–880; *Photochemistry and Photobiology*, January–February 2005, pages 38–45; *Archives of Dermatological Research*, April 2005, pages 473–481; *Business Week Online*, "An Ugly Truth About Cosmetics," November 30, 2004; *Biological & Pharmaceutical Bulletin*, April 2004, pages 510–514; *Bioorganic and Medicinal Chemistry*, December 2003, pages 5345–5352; and *American Journal of Clinical Dermatology*, March–April 2000, pages 81–88, and September–October 2000, pages 261–268.)

WHY WE BELIEVE

Almost no one has perfect skin, but perfect skin is what we are all after.

I'm often asked why we believe all of this foolishness, given the copious amounts of information to the contrary and the endless redundancy. (How many anti-wrinkle products can an industry launch until we realize they just can't live up to their claims, especially since they keep on creating new ones?) Here we are, thousands upon thousands of products later, and we still wonder which one really works. Even the cosmetics companies themselves don't believe their own half-truths and party lines, or they wouldn't keep creating new products with the same old claims if the ones they launched earlier really worked.

Our willingness to believe the ads and celebrities and the infomercials and the cosmetics salespeople, not to mention the aestheticians and the dermatologists, all selling some new miracle product has little to do with being foolish or unintelligent. It is much more complicated than that, both from emotional and sociological perspectives. There are extremely compelling reasons why we get taken in by empty, meaningless ads and claims time after time.

For women (and to some degree men) our skin tells the world where we stand in terms of beauty and age, and in nearly every culture around the world being young and attractive is a strong part of a person's identity and societal status. Skin displays the ravages of time, via sun damage, gravity, and genetically determined signs of aging, well before any of us want to see it. For women in cultures around the world, flawless and wrinkle-free skin on the face is considered an obligatory component of beauty. Thus begins our quest to achieve what women the world over want, to look and feel beautiful.

Reason No. 1. For the most part, skin-care products and, more specifically, wrinkle creams feel good and take very good care of skin. We all need to clean our faces, and many of us have to fight dry, oily, or combination skin. Most sunscreens really do work, many acne products can have benefit, and there are products with elegant, brilliant formulations. One way or another, without skin-care products we would be left with more problems than we started with. So the reason we buy the stuff in the first place is because a lot of these products take great care of our skin. They don't perform the miracles they suggest; they aren't worth the big bucks they frequently cost, but in general they do help. The fact that lots of skin-care products perform well can lead one to believe that another brand or price range may perform even better and this is where the seduction begins.

Reason No. 2. Even though many skin-care products do their job, many also fail miserably. Women frequently buy the wrong products for their skin type, and more often than we'd like to think the formulations are so irritating and poorly conceived they cause complications, making matters worse, or, at the very least, they simply do not eliminate the skin problems they were bought for. That's why so many women are constantly searching for the right products and making constantly changing choices. They believe the right products for their skin type are out there somewhere if only they could find them! Skin problems are a recurrent headache. It is the rare individual who doesn't have to be concerned about acne, wrinkles, dry skin, oily skin, irritation, or a combination of these. Almost no one has perfect skin, but perfect skin is what we are all after.

Reason No. 3. Beauty myths die a long, hard death. Once we believe something about our skin (dry skin causes wrinkles, everyone needs a moisturizer, face creams can't be used on other parts of the face or neck, natural ingredients are better for skin than synthetically derived ones, and on and on), it is very hard to change our minds. I bust many myths throughout this book, but they are endless, and the industry relentlessly and continually hammers them into our heads so that letting go of them is almost impossible. It takes information, and some of that information is boring, technical, and hard to grasp. But once you've mastered some of the basics, none of the bogus facts you hear or see will catch you off guard again.

Reason No. 4. Everything the ads, brochures, and cosmetics salespeople tell us sounds very convincing. Given the amount of money cosmetics companies spend on packaging, promotions, and advertising, it should! Just remember that all that glitters is not gold. The glitter and shine at the cosmetics counters sure looks like gold, but it rarely (if ever) is. Do not be convinced again and again that because something "sounds" good, it is, or that expensive means better—because it isn't.

Reason No. 5. It is very difficult to believe cosmetics companies would deceive us, especially when what they are selling is so beguiling and beautifully packaged. This desire to trust in a company's higher purpose is part of what we all want to presume. It is tiresome to be cautious about everything. And the spokesmodels for these companies look so convincing and sweet; surely they wouldn't lie to us—yet that is exactly what they are doing to one degree or another. The empirical evidence as well as the vast amount of published research should convince us to be more circumspect. After all, consider a cosmetics company that is selling 30 anti-wrinkle products. Clearly they can't believe their own hype, since if even one of those products lived up to the claims why would they need the 29 other versions they sell? Sure, some companies offer the same type of product for different skin types or personal preferences, and that's fine. It just doesn't explain or justify dozens of other products making the same anti-wrinkle claims.

Reason No. 6. We want to believe that what they tell us is true. It is reassuring to assume that the $10 or $50 or $150 you just spent is somehow going to take care of your skin-care or makeup problems. Surely all those scientists and dermatologists must have invented something that works by now!

We also want to believe that there are wrinkle creams that get rid of wrinkles and astringents that close pores and lipsticks that last all day, but be skeptical. If wrinkle creams can work, why do any of us have wrinkles? If astringents or toners can close pores, why do any of us have open pores? If lipstick really can last all day, why must we constantly reapply it? It is OK to accept reality, because being realistic will not make you any less beautiful or prevent you from taking good care of your skin.

Reason No. 7. Most cosmetics companies aren't out and out lying to us but they aren't telling the truth either. Even the most extreme ads hedge their promises and claims with vague language that doesn't really say anything specific. When you see an ad for a wrinkle cream that reduces fine lines, restores suppleness, and rejuvenates the skin, you must remember that any moisturizer can make that claim and not be lying. The company may really have a study showing that their skin-care product performed well, even though the study is paid for by the company selling the product, or was poorly controlled or designed, didn't compare the product against a placebo or a competing brand, tested the products on ten or fewer women, and is little more than a publicity stunt.

Reason No. 8. Cosmetics salespeople are trained and paid to sell you their products and many do this very well. By far the best tactic in cosmetics sales is to reinforce a woman's insecurity. This emotional battleground is the salesperson's best weapon and one that the consumer is least equipped to avoid or resist. See if these routines sound familiar:

(A) The salesperson reminds the consumer that she could look as good as some well-known celebrity or model. The salesperson offers a lipstick and says, "This product is used by [insert name of a well-known celebrity or model]." What Oprah or Jennifer Aniston uses is something we pay attention to, as is evidenced in fashion magazine after fashion magazine.

(B) The salesperson helps the consumer notice all the problems her skin is having (after all, she's the expert—she's supposed to notice these problems). She may ask, "Aren't you concerned about how dry your skin is, particularly around your eyes?" or "You aren't using a special serum [shocked reaction]? Everyone needs a special serum to protect their skin from the environment, stress, hormones, or makeup."

(C) The salesperson suggests that if a woman continues to make the same skin-care mistakes over and over, she will pay for it down the road: "You can't start too soon using this product because it can only get worse if you wait, and then it may be too late to do anything about it." Time is of the essence, so act now is the pitch we've all run into if we've spent any time at a cosmetics counter or listening to a cosmetics sales spiel on television.

It is essential to know that cosmetics salespeople are not necessarily trained in skin care or makeup; they are trained to sell products. To assume these people have a scientific or even a basic knowledge about skin is a serious mistake. A 1992 study by the city of New York's Department of Consumer Affairs assessed the statements and claims made by cosmetics salespeople and stated that "more than one in three [cosmetics salespeople] stretched the truth beyond recognition, making claims the company attorneys would never allow." Another one-third gave ambiguous or cryptic responses to skin-care questions, and the rest just recommended products.

I know I come down hard on cosmetics salespeople. It isn't that I haven't met some wonderful cosmetics salespeople, because I have. Many times these remarkable women and men have given me insight into the cosmetics industry that otherwise would have been impossible for me to obtain. I would also like to acknowledge from experience that, for the most part, particularly at department stores, selling cosmetics is not an easy or lucrative way to earn a living.

Unfortunately, I have also had some difficult encounters with cosmetics salespeople. I have listened to and overheard hundreds of crazy conversations about skin care and makeup application that are nothing more than sales pressure and absurdly incorrect information. It is generally hard to distinguish sales technique from valid information, but it is safe to assume that when you are buying skin-care or makeup products from a cosmetics salesperson, or even an aesthetician, you are far more likely to encounter salesmanship than factual information.

Reason No. 9. It's hard to question advice you receive from a cosmetics representative of any kind. For one thing, it isn't customary for women to refute or challenge what they hear, either directly or indirectly. Asserting your doubts and scrutinizing what you are told when dealing with cosmetics salespeople (or any salesperson) is difficult, but once you do, you will start noticing that the information being doled out is baseless and mostly unbelievable. As you start questioning what you hear, the salesperson inevitably gets caught in the pretense and fumbles about, trying to find a plausible explanation. For example, next time a cosmetics salesperson or aesthetician tells you the product they want you to buy gets rid of wrinkles ask them what all the other "anti-wrinkle" products they sell are for. Once you've finished reading this book, you will know more than most of the women and men selling makeup and skin-care products.

Reason No. 10. **Fashion magazines make everything sold by the cosmetics industry look and sound amazing.** Articles in fashion magazines almost without exception glorify cosmetics, with only occasional, buried hints of objectivity. Cosmetics companies have a stranglehold on the way fashion magazines present information on skin care and makeup. What makes this so pathetic is that reading fashion magazines is the primary way women get advice, news, and reports on their beauty needs. Gloria Steinem, in an article in *Ms.* magazine, once explained why she would no longer accept advertisements for cosmetics. She said her advertisers demanded that their ads be placed near compatible and positive editorial stories, that they must not be near material that challenged the nature of the product, and that stories in the entire magazine must not contain anything the advertiser found objectionable or displeasing. That concisely explains why you never see a negative article about the cosmetics or fashion industry in the pages of fashion magazines.

THE 10 BEAUTY COMMANDMENTS EVERYONE SHOULD KNOW

There are many ways to take beautiful care of your skin, but the first step is to acquire a clear understanding of how the so-called "beauty" industry works so you don't repeatedly get waylaid by bad or ineffective products and misleading, absurd claims. Let's start at the beginning with some basic guidelines that can help you get through most of this information. Get to know these commandments before you go shopping at another cosmetics counter, see another infomercial, have a friend introduce you to a new multilevel cosmetics line, talk to your dermatologist, have a facial, or read another fashion magazine. Once you've taken these basics to heart, you will have a better perspective on what you are really buying at the cosmetics counters, what these products can and can't do, whether what you are using is worth the money, and, most important, whether any of this can hurt your skin.

One confession: This is just a partial list. There are many more "thou shalts" and "thou shalt nots," and I go through each and every one of these throughout this book, presenting the information you need to make an educated decision about your skin care, body care, and makeup.

1.   THOU SHALT NOT believe expensive cosmetics are better than inexpensive cosmetics.
2.   THOU SHALT NOT believe there is any such thing as a natural cosmetic (or that natural means better).
3.   THOU SHALT NOT believe in miracle ingredients that can cure skin-care woes.
4.   THOU SHALT NOT covet thy neighbor's perfect skin (or believe her perfect skin came from a particular product or cosmetics line; skin is more complicated than that).
5.   THOU SHALT NOT believe everything a cosmetics salesperson tells you.

6. THOU SHALT NOT believe in the existence of anti-wrinkle, firming, toning, lifting, or filling-in creams, lotions, or masks that can permanently erase wrinkles.

7. THOU SHALT NOT be seduced by every new promotion, new product, or new product line that the cosmetics industry creates.

8. THOU SHALT NOT get a tan; sun is your enemy, not your friend; it is the primary reason that skin wrinkles and develops skin cancer (and it isn't just about getting a sunburn—turning the skin brown is equally as damaging when done on a regular basis).

9. THOU SHALT NOT buy a cellulite cream, nor shalt thou assume it's possible to dissolve fat from the outside in, because you absolutely cannot. If these products worked, who would have cellulite?

10. THOU SHALT NOT see pictures of pubescent, anorexic models (who spend two hours getting their hair and makeup done and another two hours posing while the photographer and a corps of assistants determine the most flattering lighting, after which the resulting picture goes through a battery of digitally enhanced touch-ups and adjustments) and believe you will get the same (or even similar) results from using the products being advertised. That is, unless you happen to be pubescent, anorexic, and a model and can somehow stay in the right lighting all the time.

CHAPTER 3
FRAUDS & FEARS

BE AFRAID, BE VERY AFRAID

Over the years I've spent a good deal of my time battling the endless bombardment of inaccurate and absurd information disseminated by cosmetics companies and cosmetics salespeople from every corner of the industry. Over the past several years the Internet has given rise to another form of cosmetics insanity, coming from grass-roots organizations trying to keep the cosmetics industry from killing us.

These Web sites and possibly well-intentioned people take a piece of information, a piece of a study, or a scientific point of view and make it sound like fact. They also tend to only use information that "proves" their point (that is, most cosmetics are killing us) by selectively using only the data that show they are right while ignoring any evidence to the contrary. I wish the world was that black and white, because decision-making would be so much easier, but that isn't the case. Issues are more complex than the answers that are often presented, and getting to the facts can take a masters degree in way too many disciplines.

What almost always complicates matters is that there is a grain of a truth that gets blown out of proportion. Trying to balance out seemingly contradictory information is a challenge. It's one of the reasons I get criticized for being long-winded and writing too much. My goal is to get all the facts out on the table and that takes a lot of words.

Although I am extremely critical of the cosmetics industry I also prefer a rational, balanced point of view. I prefer fact to supposition, I prefer critical analysis to a knee-jerk reaction, and I absolutely prefer reality to fiction. There is no question the cosmetics industry has its faults, but trying to kill us is not one of them.

It doesn't take much to make a consumer afraid of just about anything; a little bit of science can sound so dire. For example, dihydrogen monoxide (DHMO) is a colorless and odorless chemical compound, also referred to by some as dihydrogen oxide, hydrogen hydroxide, hydronium hydroxide, or simply hydric acid. Its basis is the highly reactive hydroxyl radical, a substance that has been shown to mutate DNA, denature proteins, disrupt cell membranes, and chemically alter critical neurotransmitters. The atomic components of DHMO are found in a number of caustic, explosive, and poisonous compounds such as sulfuric acid, nitroglycerine, and ethyl alcohol. Dihydrogen oxide? That's simply H_2O—plain, everyday water.

We need to use safe ingredients that work on our skin to make it look and feel better. The cosmetics industry overwhelmingly complies with "safe" ingredients. Finding effective products (regardless of their origin) and getting past the fear-mongering generated by so many earnest as well as unscrupulous companies and Web sites can go a long way to helping you do that.

MINERAL OIL AND PETROLATUM

The notion that mineral oil and petrolatum (Vaseline) are bad for skin has been around for some time, with Aveda being the most visible company to mount a crusade deriding these ingredients. But now there are dozens of others. According to many companies that produce "natural" cosmetics, mineral oil and petrolatum are terrible ingredients because they come from crude oil (petroleum) and are used in industry as metal-cutting fluids (among other uses) and, therefore, can harm the skin by forming an oil film and suffocating it.

This foolish, recurring misinformation about mineral oil and petrolatum is maddening. After all, crude oil is as natural as any other earth-derived substance. Moreover, lots of ingredients are derived from awful-sounding sources but are nevertheless benign and totally safe. Salt is a perfect example. Common table salt is sodium chloride, composed of sodium and chloride, but salt doesn't have the caustic properties of chloride (a form of chlorine) or the unstable explosiveness of sodium. In fact, it is a completely different compound with the harmful properties of neither of its components.

Cosmetic/pharmaceutical-grade mineral oil and petrolatum are considered the safest and most nonirritating ingredients in the world of skin care. Yes, they can keep air off the skin to some extent, but that's what a good antioxidant is supposed to do; and they don't suffocate skin, at least not any more than any plant oil. In fact research shows plant oils and mineral oil have pretty much the same function on skin.

Moreover, petrolatum and mineral oil are known for being efficacious in wound healing, and are also considered to be among the most effective moisturizing ingredients available. The confusion around mineral oil is also caused by some cosmetics companies and people who use the information about non-purified mineral oil as a scare tactic. The mineral oil used in skin-care products is certified as either USP (United States Pharmacopeia) or BP (British Pharmacopeia). This is the type that's used in skin-care products, and it's completely safe, soothing, non-irritating, and perfectly healthy for skin.

(Sources: *Journal of Dermatologic Science*, May 2008, pages 135–142; *International Journal of Cosmetic Science*, October 2007, pages 385–390; *European Journal of Ophthalmology*, March–April 2007, pages 151–159; *International Wound Journal*, September 2006, pages 181–187; *Ostomy Wound Management*, December 2005, pages 30–42; *Dermatitis*, September 2004, pages 109–116; *Cosmetics & Toiletries*, January 2001, page 79; *Cosmetic Dermatology*, September 2000, pages 44–46; and *Cosmetics & Toiletries*, February 1998, pages 33–40.)

PARABENS AND PRESERVATIVES

You may not think of them as an essential part of your skin care and cosmetics, but without question skin-care and cosmetics products need preservatives. This is especially true for products that contain plant extracts—just think about how long a bunch of broccoli lasts in your refrigerator before it becomes a mushy, discolored mess.

Whether it is a cleanser, lotion, toner, blush, foundation, or mascara, without preservatives these everyday items would become overloaded with bacteria, mold, and fungus, making them harmful to skin, eyes, and mucous membranes. However, as necessary as preservatives are to the safety of cosmetics, they've had their share of woes over the years. For example, back in the early '90s, it was discovered that when formaldehyde-releasing preservatives (such as 2-bromo-2-nitropane 1-3 diol, or DMDM hydantoin) are combined with amines (such as triethanolamine), something called nitrosamine forms, and nitrosamine (in its various forms) is, in fact, carcinogenic. This problem was viewed as inconsequential for cosmetics because the amount of preservatives used in cosmetics is minute. No test has shown it to cause problems for people applying makeup or using skin-care products. Studies relating to carcinogenic properties of nitrosamine were done by feeding it orally to laboratory rats. Still, it is not a pleasant thought to associate a "carcinogen" with your cosmetics in any way, shape, or form. As a result, and despite their effectiveness, formaldehyde-based preservatives are not as popular as they once were.

Another group of preservatives, called parabens, is now in a predicament similar to that of formaldehyde-releasing preservatives, and this has become a common subject for questions from my readers. These parabens may come in the form of butylparaben, ethylparaben, isobutylparaben, methylparaben, or propylparaben, and they have been linked distantly (meaning in limited studies and with only a handful of subjects or animal studies) to breast cancer due to their weak estrogenic activity and their presence in breast-cancer tumors, as well as to low sperm-count rates in men. But even from a distance that has some people worried, especially considering that, by some estimates, more than 90% of all cosmetics products contain one or more parabens. In fact, parabens are the most widely used group of cosmetic preservatives in the world because of their efficacy, low risk of irritation, and stability.

What started the concern about parabens was a study published in the *Journal of Steroid Biochemistry and Molecular Biology*, January 2002, pages 49–60, that evaluated the estrogenic activity of parabens in human breast-cancer cells. The very technical findings of the study, which involved both oral administration and injection into rat skin, did show evidence of a weak estrogenic effect on cells in a way that could be problematic for binding to receptor sites that may cause proliferation of MCF-7 breast-cancer cells.

A single study identified parabens in human breast-tumor samples supplied by 20 patients. This study was concerned primarily with the use of deodorants that contained parabens rather than with cosmetics in general, but it has been extrapolated to the cosmetics industry as a whole, prompting many consumers to check the ingredient lists of the products they're using. But more to the point, the presence of parabens in human breast tumors doesn't mean they caused the tumors.

Pervasive fear was generated by these well-circulated facts. What didn't make the e-mail spam rounds is that all the researchers who are studying this issue, as well as health organizations around the world, agree that the information to date is hardly conclusive and at best vague, and that potentially parabens require more study (Sources: *Journal of Applied Toxicology*, January–February 2004, pages 1–4, September–October 2003, pages 285–288, and March–April 2003, pages 89–59; and *Journal of the National Cancer Institute*, August 2003, pages 1106–1118).

With regard to deodorants in general, it turns out parabens are rarely used as the preservative. A scientific review paper published in the *Bulletin du Cancer*, September 2008, pages 871–880, concluded that "After analysis of the available literature on the subject [of deodorants causing cancer], no scientific evidence to support the hypothesis was identified and no validated hypothesis appears likely to open the way to interesting avenues of research."

On the other side of the coin, there is research showing that parabens are absorbed through intact skin and are not broken down (Source: *Journal of Applied Toxicology*, July 2008, pages 561–578), but once again the association as to its effect is just not known.

It is also important to realize that parabens are used in food products as well (Source: *Food Chemistry and Toxicology*, October 2002, pages 1335–1373), which could very well be the source, not cosmetics. What is surprising to some is that parabens actually have a "natural" origin. Parabens are formed from an acid (p-hydroxy-benzoic acid) found in raspberries and blackberries (Source: *Cosmetics & Toiletries*, January 2005, page 22). So much for the widely held belief that natural ingredients are the only answer for skin-care products!

As yet, no one has any idea (or has evaluated) whether it is the consumption of parabens or their application to the skin that is responsible for their presence in human tissue. And no one knows what the presence of parabens in human tissue means.

In terms of the low male sperm count in relation to parabens, research published in *Birth Defects Research, Part B, Developmental and Reproductive Toxicology*, April 2008, pages 123–133, concluded that parabens had no effect on sperm count in an in vivo experiment (meaning it was done on real guys).

Does this mean you should stop buying products that contain parabens? I mean who wants this stuff being absorbed through their skin whether there is conclusive research or not? That's a good question, but the answer isn't simple and the studies are hardly conclusive on any front. Clearly it is a serious issue, and the FDA is conducting its own research to determine what this means for human health (Source: The Endocrine Disruptor Knowledge Base (EDKB), http://edkb.fda.gov/index.html). But a definitive answer is far from close.

As a point of reference, and just to keep the concern over parabens in perspective, it is important to realize that parabens are hardly the only substances that have estrogenic effects on the body. The issue is that any source of estrogen, including the estrogen our bodies produce or the types associated with plant extracts, may bind to receptor sites on cells, either strongly or weakly. This can either stimulate the receptor to imitate the effect of our own estrogen in a positive way, or it can generate an abnormal estrogen response. It is possible that a weak plant estrogen can help the body, but it is also possible for a strong plant estrogen to make matters worse. For example, there is research showing that coffee is a problem for fibrocystic breast disease, possibly because coffee exerts estrogenic effects on breast cells. (Sources: *Journal of the American Medical Women's Association*, Spring 2002, pages 85–90; *Annals of the New York Academy of Science*, March 2002, pages 11–22; and *American Journal of Epidemiology*, October 1996, pages 642–644.)

To quote some studies directly: "Although parabens can act similarly to estrogen, they have been shown to have much less estrogenic activity than the body's naturally occurring estrogen. For example, a 1998 study (Routledge et al., in *Toxicology and Applied Pharmacol-*

ogy) found that the most potent paraben tested in the study, butylparaben, showed from 10,000- to 100,000-fold less activity than naturally occurring estradiol (a form of estrogen) [found in our water systems]. Further, parabens are used at very low levels in cosmetics. In a review of the estrogenic activity of parabens (Golden et al., in *Critical Reviews in Toxicology*, 2005), the author concluded that based on maximum daily exposure estimates, "it was implausible that parabens could increase the risk associated with exposure to estrogenic chemicals" (Source: www.fda.gov).

Ironically, the endocrine-disrupting potencies of ingredients like parabens or phthalates (also discussed in this chapter) "are several orders of magnitude lower than that of the natural estrogens" (Source: *Environment International*, July 2007, pages 654–669). Human endocrine-disrupting sources have their origin in plants, such as marijuana (Source: *Toxicology*, January 2005, pages 471–488), or in medicines such as acetaminophen (Tylenol) (Source: *Water Research*, November 2008, pages 4578–4588).

A study conducted at the Department of Obstetrics and Gynecology at Baylor College of Medicine in Houston, Texas, investigated the estrogenic effects of licorice root, black cohosh, dong quai, and ginseng "on cell proliferation of MCF-7 cells, a human breast cancer cell line...." The results showed that "Dong quai and ginseng both significantly induced the growth of MCF-7 cells by 16- and 27-fold, respectively, over that of untreated control cells, while black cohosh and licorice root did not" (Source: *Menopause*, March–April, 2002, pages 145–150). Another study concluded that "Commercially available products containing soy, red clover, and herbal combinations induced an increase in the MCF-7 [breast cancer] proliferation rates, indicating an estrogen-antagonistic activity...." (Source: *Menopause*, May–June 2004, pages 281–289). Despite this evidence, when was that last time you read a media report or received a forwaded e-mail about the breat cancer risk from soy or ginseng?

One more point about the risk of breast cancer related to underarm deodorant. In October 2002, a study conducted at the Seattle-based Fred Hutchinson Cancer Research Center, published in the *Journal of the National Cancer Institute*, looked at the issue of underarm deodorant use and breast cancer. The study compared the use of underarm deodorant in 810 women who had been diagnosed with breast cancer, and 793 women who were not affected by the disease. When the two groups were compared, researchers found no evidence of an increased risk of breast cancer linked to using antiperspirant or deodorant, or using antiperspirant or deodorant after shaving with a traditional razor blade. In short, the researchers believed their study proved there was no link between underarm deodorants and breast cancer risk.

NANOTECHNOLOGY

Getting to the truth about the use of nanoparticles in cosmetics, like many issues in the cosmetics industry—with its confusing screen of distorted information—isn't easy. But getting it right is important, particularly because the sunscreen ingredients titanium dioxide and zinc oxide, so essential to the health of skin, are involved. Nanotechnology is about changing any material from its original size and making it much, much smaller. This technology is used in a wide variety of industries, from medicine to agriculture to cosmetics. In the case of cosmetic products and over-the-counter drugs such as sunscreens, making particles nano-sized has two chief advantages: it can make the product more aesthetically pleasing (this is often the case with mineral sunscreens—making the particles of the active mineral smaller allows them to be applied without leaving a noticeable white cast), and it can enhance penetration of certain ingredients, such as vitamins and other antioxidants.

You may have seen concerns expressed in the media, online, and by certain lobbying groups about the use of nanoparticles in cosmetic products, both in general and in particular, when it comes to using nanoparticles of titanium dioxide and zinc oxide as the active ingredients in sunscreens. What's been reported about these benign sunscreen ingredients often sounds scary, with some reports going so far as to state that nanoparticles of these sunscreen actives reach the bloodstream and are potentially dangerous. Some articles about sunscreen nanoparticles have even stated these can interact with sunlight and cause cellular damage to skin. As alarming as this sounds, these assertions are not supported by any published information and they are without support from the medical world or the FDA.

Reviews of scientific data by major regulatory agencies have concluded that nanoparticles of titanium dioxide and zinc oxide remain on the surface of the skin and in the outer dead layer (stratum corneum) of skin. They are not absorbed into the bloodstream and do not affect living skin cells. Studies coming to these conclusions have tested these nanoparticles on healthy, intact human skin and on various types of human and animal skin samples.

Based on these conclusions and those of other studies I have reviewed from toxicologists, the question of nanoparticle risk from the mineral sunscreen actives is not a human health issue. There is no proof that these sunscreen actives absorb into skin. And in fact, regardless of any potential risk, you would never want that to happen since sunscreen actives need to remain in the surface layers of skin in order to protect it from UV damage.

Further, in terms of the potential risk that titanium dioxide could generate free radicals in the presence of sunlight, it has been shown that adding antioxidants to the mix (whether they're in your sunscreen or already naturally present in skin) eliminates this risk, and other research has established that both zinc oxide and titanium oxide are stable substances that don't elicit free-radical damage at all.

(Sources for this information: www.tga.gov.au/npmeds/sunscreen-zotd.htm#pdf; *Experimental Dermatology*, August 2008, pages 659–667; *Environmental Science and Toxicology*, July 2007, pages 5, 149-153; *Critical Reviews in Toxicology*, March 2007, pages 251–277; *Skin Pharmacology and Physiology*, January 2007, pages 148–154; and *Skin Pharmacology and Applied Skin Physiology*, September–October 1999, pages 247–256.)

Interestingly, a study from Taiwan demonstrated that applying nanoparticles of titanium dioxide to pinprick sites actually had an antibacterial effect in the presence of sunlight. The nanoparticles actually kept the pinprick wound sites from becoming infected (Source: *Artificial Organs*, February 2008, pages 167–174)! That would not be the expected outcome if nanoparticles of titanium dioxide were inherently harmful to skin cells.

OXYGEN FOR THE SKIN

The cosmetics industry is overflowing with people who have no clue what they are doing, and the issue of oxygen in skin-care products demonstrates that perfectly. After selling us products to ward off oxygen's effects on the skin (the word antioxidant means anti-oxygen), the beauty industry then turns around and sells us products that claim to provide oxygen to the skin. Doesn't the beauty industry have anything better to do? (No, it doesn't, especially if there is an interested consumer willing to make a purchase.)

Many cosmetic products contain antioxidants, ingredients that keep oxygen off the face, such as vitamin C, superoxide dismutase, selenium, curcumin, plant extracts, and vitamin E, among dozens and dozens of others. At the same time, the cosmetics industry also sells products that contain hydrogen peroxide (H_2O_2) or some other oxygen-releasing ingredient that supposedly delivers an oxygen molecule when it comes into contact with skin. It makes sense to wonder if the extra oxygen would just trigger free-radical damage and cause more problems for the skin. But if you were also using products that contained antioxidants, wouldn't they "scavenge" up that free-radical oxygen? The answer is that if the product could deliver extra oxygen to the skin it would indeed generate free-radical damage and, based on data from almost every imaginable published study on the subject, that's bad for skin.

So why the concern about supplying more oxygen to the skin? Oxygen depletion is one of the things that happens to older skin, regardless of whether it's been affected by sun damage or any other health issue. Why or how that happens is a complete unknown, though it is thought to have something to do with blood flow and a reduction in lung capacity as we age. Nevertheless, delivering extra oxygen to the skin doesn't reverse it. After all, there is plenty of oxygen in our environment. The earth's atmosphere is 21% oxygen; the oceans, lakes, and rivers are about 88% oxygen. Oxygen is a constituent of most rocks and minerals, and makes up 46.7% (by weight) of the solid crust of the earth. Oxygen makes up 60% of the human body, and is in every cell and organ. It is a constituent of all living tissues; almost all plants and animals, including humans, require oxygen to maintain life. However, oxygen is utilized by the body almost exclusively through respiration. Oxygen on the surface may affect the very top layer of skin, but so what? How much extra oxygen does skin need? Again, no one knows. Can it be absorbed? No. Plus, none of this addresses the issue about oxygen generating more free-radical damage, which is one of the processes that makes the veins and capillaries of the body stop working efficiently.

That brings us to this question: How did the caprice of oxygen booths get started? Oxygen booths (hyperbaric chambers) are used medically to repair skin ulcers and wounds that have difficulty healing. According to the American Diabetes Association's *Diabetes Forecast* (June 1993, page 57), "When you have a stubborn [wound] that won't heal, the white blood cells that fight the infection in the [wound] use 20 times more oxygen when they're killing bacteria. Also, the more oxygen your body has to work with, the more efficiently it lays down wound-repairing connective tissue. Yet just when you need more oxygen, you may have less. If you have neuropathy (diabetic nerve damage), that may cause changes in blood flow, resulting in islands of low oxygen levels in your foot. Less oxygen means slower healing, and a [wound] that doesn't heal could eventually lead to an amputation. So it seems that you should try to get extra oxygen in your blood when you have a foot ulcer, to bring the oxygen levels in the tissues around the ulcer up to normal, or even higher. But sitting in your living room and breathing in 100% oxygen won't do the trick. Under normal circumstances, only so much oxygen will dissolve in your blood." Pressure is needed to allow the oxygen to be used by the body; and sitting in a hyperbaric booth serves that purpose. The article continues, "But it is the inhaled oxygen, which is then absorbed by your blood after you breathe it, that speeds wound healing, not the oxygen drifting past the wound. You may have seen advertisements for devices that encase a person's leg and deliver oxygen to the skin. This is not hyperbaric oxygen therapy, and it's not effective—your skin doesn't absorb oxygen that way. These devices may even reduce the amount of oxygen that gets to your leg."

Moreover, leg ulcers and wounds are a temporary condition, but skin aging is ongoing. The notion that oxygen treatments affect aging, wrinkles, or any other skin malady is a joke. Nary a study exists anywhere to support those ideas, though there is a ton of research showing that the oxidative process generated by oxygen is partly responsible for wrinkles and skin aging in general.

PROPYLENE GLYCOL

Propylene glycol (along with other glycols and glycerol) is a humectant or humidifying and delivery ingredient used in cosmetics, meaning it helps other ingredients absorb better into the skin. Despite research to the contrary, you can find Web sites and spam e-mails stating that propylene glycol is really industrial antifreeze and the major ingredient in brake and hydraulic fluids. These sites also state that tests show it to be a strong skin irritant. They further point out that the Material Safety Data Sheet (MSDS) on propylene glycol warns users to avoid skin contact because systemically (in the body) it can cause liver abnormalities and kidney damage.

As ominous as that sounds, it is so far from the reality of cosmetic formulations that almost none of it holds any water or poses real concern. It is important to realize that the MSDS sheets are talking about 100% concentrations of a substance. Even water and salt have frightening comments regarding their safety according to their MSDS reports. It is true that propylene glycol in 100% concentration is used as antifreeze, but—and this is a very big *but*—in cosmetics it is used in only the smallest amounts to keep products from melting in high heat or freezing when it is cold. It also helps active ingredients penetrate the skin. In the minute amounts used in cosmetics, propylene glycol is not a concern in the least. Women are not suffering from liver problems (as some Web sites have asserted) because of propylene glycol in cosmetics.

And finally, according to the U.S. Department of Health and Human Services, within the Public Health Services Agency for Toxic Substances and Disease Registry, "studies have not shown these chemicals [propylene or the other glycols as used in cosmetics] to be carcinogens" (Source: www.atsdr.cdc.gov).

Polyethylene glycol (PEG) is another ingredient "natural" Web sites have attempted to make notorious. They gain a great deal of attention by attributing horror stories to PEG. For example, several Web sites state the following: "Because of their effectiveness, PEGs are often used in caustic spray-on oven cleaners, yet are also found in many personal care products. Not only are they potentially carcinogenic, but they contribute to stripping the skin's Natural Moisture Factor, leaving the immune system vulnerable." There is no research substantiating any of this. Quite the contrary: PEGs have no known skin toxicity. The only negative research results for this ingredient group indicate that large quantities given orally to rats can cause tumors. How that got related to skin-care products is a mystery to me.

PHTHALATES

Dibutyl phthalate (DBP) was at one time a very common ingredient in many nail polishes. It is used as a plasticizer and is a key component in some fragrances because of its unique properties. But phthalates have become one of the demon ingredients in cosmetics since the Centers for Disease Control and Prevention (CDC, www.cdc.gov) published the *National Report on Human Exposure to Environmental Chemicals—Results for Mono-butyl phthalate [which is] (metabolized from Dibutyl phthalate)*. Basically, the CDC found measurable levels of phthalate in the urine of the participants in a study looking at the issue of phthalates. However, the CDC stated that "Finding a measurable amount of one or more phthalate metabolites in urine does not mean that the level of one or more phthalates causes an adverse health effect. Whether phthalates at the levels of metabolites reported here are a cause for health concern is not yet known; more research is needed" (Sources: CDC, www.cdc.gov/nceh/dls/report/results/Mono-butylPhthalate.htm; and *Environmental Health Perspectives*, December 2000, volume 108, issue 12).

Adult health is one thing, but since then growing research has shown a far more serious concern when children have a detectable amount of phthalates in their system. A study published in the medical journal *Pediatrics* (February 2008, pages 260–268) was shocking to many women when it found a link between baby skin-care products and phthalates being absorbed by the infant; the report concluded: "Phthalate exposure is widespread and variable in infants. Infant exposure[s] to lotion, powder, and shampoo were significantly associated with increased urinary concentrations of monoethyl phthalate, monomethyl phthalate, and monoisobutyl phthalate, and associations increased with the number of products used. This association was strongest in young infants, who may be more vulnerable to developmental and reproductive toxicity of phthalates given their immature metabolic system capability and increased dosage per unit body surface area."

In 1985, the Cosmetic Ingredient Review (CIR) board (www.cir-safety.org/) deemed dibutyl phthalate safe for use in cosmetic products. In 2001, the CIR reviewed new data on the use of three phthalate esters (also known as phthalates) in cosmetics, and on November 19, 2002, the CIR board announced its decision to not reopen the safety assessment of the dibutyl phthalate group of ingredients. Their summary on this issue states that "New data on acute and short-term toxicity were consistent with previously available data." They went on to say that "The developmental effects of phthalates seen in rodents raise questions about the potential for human health risk. However, these effects seen in rodents are at much higher exposure levels than humans are likely to encounter and they are subject to the species difference in the metabolism of phthalate diesters." They also concluded that human exposure to dibutyl and diethyl phthalate was below the reference dose levels set by the U.S. Environmental Protection Agency.

Other research concluded similarly, saying "that levels of concern are minimal to negligible in most situations…" (Source: *Reproductive Toxicology*, August–September 2004, pages 761–764). And a study reported in *Regulatory Toxicology and Pharmacology*, December 2008, pages 232–242, concluded that "The results of the cumulative risk assessments for both a US and a German population show that the hazard index is below one. Thus it is unlikely that humans are suffering adverse developmental effects from current environmental exposure to these phthalate esters."

Despite the fact that the CTFA and CIR maintain that phthalates are safe, the Food and Drug Administration (FDA), Health Canada, and other governmental health agencies around the world remain suspicious. Though the FDA and Health Canada have not restricted the use of phthalates, both agencies have made strong comments regarding their risk and safety. An FDA report titled *Aggregate Exposures to Phthalates in Humans* stated that "Manufacturers consistently argue that there is no evidence that anyone has been harmed by phthalates. As we note, however, and as confirmed by the NTP [National Toxicology Program] panel and FDA, no study has ever examined the impact of phthalates [on human reproduction] … Lack of evidence can hardly be used as evidence of safety when no one has ever [studied the issue on humans]."

The report went on to observe, "The increasing incidence of hypospadias, undescended testes, testicular cancer, and declining sperm counts in the US and many other parts of the world suggests that a closer look at many reproductive tract toxicants and endocrine disrupters is urgently needed in people. With respect to phthalates, however, evidence from relevant animal studies and from limited studies of non-reproductive tract impacts in hospitalized patients is sufficient to require phasing out the use of many of the phthalates." The Health Canada panel reached a similar conclusion, stating "the status quo is not an acceptable option" (Source: *Aggregate Exposures to Phthalates in Humans*, July 2002, www. fda.gov/ohrms/dockets/dailys/02/Dec02/120502/02d-0325-c000018-02-vol1.pdf).

This explains why many cosmetics companies are actively seeking or have already begun using alternatives to phthalates. It could be argued that, at the levels presently used, phthalates pose no health risk. Although there is no concrete human evidence to suggest phthalates are harmful, the lack of studies in this area continues to leave the issue open to debate and perhaps does indicate that a "better safe than sorry" approach is wise.

SODIUM LAURYL SULFATE

Are sodium lauryl sulfate (SLS) and sodium laureth sulfate (SLES) serious problems in cosmetics? I have received more e-mails and letters than I care to count about this concern.

I believe that this entire mania was generated by several Neways members' web sites, and has been carried over as if it were fact into other so-called "all natural" cosmetics lines.

It seems that most of this issue is based on the incorrect reporting about a study at the Medical College of Georgia. As a reminder, here is what is being quoted: "A study from the Medical College of Georgia indicates that SLS is a systemic, and can penetrate and be retained in the eye, brain, heart, liver, etc., with potentially harmful long-term effects. It could retard healing and cause cataracts in adults, and can keep children's eyes from developing properly." This is supposedly quoted from a report given to a Research to Prevent Blindness conference. While the report on animal models extrapolates concerns about the use of SLS, it draws no hard conclusions, stating the amount of SLS used was 10% greater than that used in shampoos and that the research was done on animals, not people. The doctor who conducted the study and delivered the final report is Dr. Keith Green, Regents Professor of Ophthalmology at the Medical College of Georgia, who received his doctorate of science from St. Andrews University in Scotland. I had an opportunity to talk with Dr. Green, who stated that he was completely embarrassed by all this. He told me in a telephone interview back in 1997 that his "work was completely misquoted. There is no part of my study that indicated any [eye] development or cataract problems from SLS or SLES and the body does not retain those ingredients at all. We did not even look at the issue of children, so that conclusion is completely false because it never existed. The Neways people took my research completely out of context and probably never read the study at all." He continued in a perturbed voice, saying, "The statement like 'SLS is a systemic' has no meaning. No ingredient can be a systemic unless you drink the stuff and that's not what we did with it. Another incredible comment was that my study was 'clinical,' meaning I tested the substance on people, [but] these were strictly animal tests. Furthermore, the eyes showed no irritation with the 10-dilution substance used! If anything, the animal studies indicated no risk of irritation whatsoever!" That lack of outcome is in fact why, as of 1987, Green no longer pursued this research. When I asked if anyone has done any follow-up studies looking at SLS and SLES in this regard, Dr. Green said, "No one has done this because the findings were so insignificant."

Yet the resulting mass e-mails continued for some time, carrying on the SLS and SLES myth with a slightly different bent. According to Health Canada, in a press release dated February 12, 1999 (www.hc-sc.gc.ca/), "A letter has been circulating [on] the Internet which claims that there is a link between cancer and sodium laureth (or lauryl) sulfate (SLS), an ingredient used in [cosmetics]. Health Canada has looked into the matter and has found no scientific evidence to suggest that SLS causes cancer. It has a history of safe use in Canada. Upon further investigation, it was discovered that this e-mail warning is a hoax. The letter is signed by a person at the University of Pennsylvania Health System and includes a phone number. Health Canada contacted the University of Pennsylvania Health System and found that it is not the author of the sodium laureth sulfate warning and does not endorse any link between SLS and cancer. Health Canada considers SLS safe for use in cosmetics. Therefore, you can continue to use cosmetics containing SLS without worry."

Further, according to the American Cancer Society's Web site, "Contrary to popular rumors on the Internet, Sodium Lauryl Sulfate (SLS) and Sodium Laureth Sulfate (SLES) do not cause cancer. E-mails have been flying through cyberspace claiming SLS [and SLES] causes cancer ... and is proven to cause cancer. ... [Yet] A search of recognized medical journals yielded no published articles relating this substance to cancer in humans."

That's not to say that sodium lauryl sulfate isn't a potent skin irritant, because it is. That's why it's considered a standard comparison substance for measuring skin irritancy of other ingredients. Thus in scientific studies, when they want to establish whether or not an ingredient is problematic for skin, they compare its effect to the results of SLS. In amounts of 2% to 5% it can cause allergic or sensitizing reactions in lots of people (Sources: *European Journal of Dermatology*, September–October 2001, pages 416–419; *American Journal of Contact Dermatitis*, March 2001, pages 28–32). But irritancy is not the same as the other dire, erroneous warnings floating around the Web about this ingredient!

STEM CELLS IN SKIN-CARE PRODUCTS?

You may have seen advertisements for skin-care products claiming that they use stem cell research or can somehow stimulate stem cells to fight wrinkles. What is absurd about this claim is that while stem cell research for any human benefit is only in its infancy, in the area of wrinkles or skin care it is nonexistent. These ads are a classic example of how a cosmetics company can take serious science and manipulate it to sell products. Scientific literature makes it clear that stem cells are indeed the basis for every organ, tissue, and cell produced in the human body, and it is possible that stem cells may be able to repair or replace damaged tissue, thereby reversing diseases and injuries such as cancer, diabetes, cardiovascular disease, and blood diseases, to name a few (Source: *Experimental Gerontology*, November 2008, pages 986–987). But notice the wording: "may be." We just don't know, and neither does any cosmetics company.

Research on adult stem cells, as well as on embryonic stem cells (though the latter is far more controversial) holds great potential. In fact, adult blood-forming stem cells from bone marrow have been used in bone-marrow transplants for over 30 years. Certain kinds of adult stem cells seem to have the ability to differentiate into a number of different cell types, given the right conditions. If this differentiation of adult stem cells can be controlled in the laboratory, these cells may become the basis for therapies for many serious common diseases. Scientists are experimenting with different research strategies to generate tissues that will not be rejected, an unfortunate problem with some surgical procedures and transplants.

Many complicated questions remain to be answered about stem cells. The following are just a few posed by the National Institutes of Health (www.nih.gov). "How many kinds of adult stem cells exist, and in which tissues do they exist? What are the sources of adult stem cells in the body? Are they 'leftover' embryonic stem cells, or do they arise in some other way? Why do they remain in an undifferentiated state when all the cells around them have differentiated? Do adult stem cells normally exhibit plasticity, or do they only transdifferentiate when scientists manipulate them experimentally? What are the signals that regulate the proliferation and differentiation of stem cells that demonstrate plasticity? Is it possible to manipulate adult stem cells to enhance their proliferation so that sufficient tissue for transplants can be produced? Does a single type of stem cell exist—possibly in the bone marrow or circulating in the blood—that can generate the cells of any organ or tissue? What are the factors that stimulate stem cells to relocate to sites of injury or damage?" As you can see, there are far more questions than answers, and the answers certainly aren't found in any skin-care product any where in the world.

BOTANICALS OR ALL NATURAL?

Is it worthwhile to look for natural ingredients in skin-care products? Leaving aside the fact that the process of removing a plant from the ground, cleaning off the dirt and insects, getting the key parts of the plant extracted, and then stabilizing and preserving it in a cosmetic renders it fairly unnatural, the answer is yes and no. There are bountiful numbers of wonderful plants and plant extracts that have beneficial effects on skin—and there are plenty of plant extracts that present problems for skin, too. Even so, let's say a natural or botanical ingredient is effective as a disinfectant; if so, that doesn't make it better than a synthetically derived disinfectant, it just makes it an alternative. One shortcoming of natural ingredients in skin-care products that the cosmetics industry hasn't addressed is that each natural ingredient has a large range of limitations. These include what happens as a result of the purification process it goes through to get into a product, which part of the plant is effective, bad crops, possible contamination with pesticides, and maintaining consistent concentrations. In many ways synthetic ingredients are often more reliable for the skin; chief among them is that developers have control over the outcome and functionality.

It is also important to reiterate that just because an ingredient is found growing in nature doesn't mean it's good for the skin. Lots of plants are poisonous if ingested and lots of plants can irritate the skin. While plants sound great—pure and natural and all that—and while sesame oil and licorice extract sound far better than capric/caprylic triglyceride (a fatty acid) and glycyrrhetinic acid (a derivative of licorice), they aren't better *or* worse. Each individual ingredient, of which there are thousands, has its pros and cons, and it would be a delusion to assume otherwise.

DRINKING COLLAGEN TO FIGHT WRINKLES?

Most likely many of you have seen ads or spoken to women who are drinking or selling beverages laced with collagen. The sales pitch for these drinks is that drinking collagen will rebuild and enhance the collagen in your skin and that Japanese women have been doing it for years (so of course it must be valid, right? And of course women who don't drink collagen must look wrinkled?). I can see why this would be easy to accept. For more than two decades women have believed that collagen added to skin-care products will add to the collagen in your skin, so why wouldn't the same be true from the inside out? After all, if you drink dairy products rich in calcium you do get better bone growth. If you drink colas and other soda drinks you lose calcium and have an increased risk of osteoporosis (Source: *Osteoporosis International*, December 2005, pages 1803–1808).

Does drinking collagen offer similar possibilities for skin? Most of this attention is a result of a collagen drink called Toki. It is marketed in a pyramid-style business plan so your neighbor or co-worker may be the one tempting you with frivolous, scientific-sounding claims to get you to purchase the drink or the company's associated supplements (there is always something else you need), or try to get you to sell the stuff yourself.

Aside from claims that are too good to be true, Toki asserts that they have impressive, independent studies demonstrating the success of their drink. At best, their research is dubious. Despite the company's contention about having unbiased research, it isn't the truth. The studies they have were paid for by the company distributing their products, namely Lane Labs, based in Allendale, New Jersey. If you end up believing even a portion of their misleading sales pitch you will find yourself out $175 for a 30-day supply. Surely that kind of expenditure requires more than the claims Toki has cooked up.

It is also questionable whether or not Toki actually contains collagen at all. The ingredients on the label are rice germ extract, soybean extract, hijiki seaweed extract, lemon juice, citric acid, artificial lemon flavoring, magnesium stearate, silica, and soybeans. None of those substances have anything to do with collagen. Plant-based sources of collagen are questionable at best, as humans and animals are the only known source of ingestible collagen.

Are Toki or other collagen drinks any better than collagen supplements (which also happen to cost a lot less) at providing potential benefit? You'll be happy to know spending more money will not enhance the outcome. Either way, you won't see your wrinkles diminish or disappear with Toki, so keeping the $175 monthly cost (that's $2,100 a year!) in your pocket may be far more helpful to you in the long run.

In this case, getting past the hype and marketing shenanigans takes information, because anything involving the human body is complicated. Just in case you don't want to make your way through this section, the short answer is, Don't waste your money. Collagen drinks are not miracles for your skin. The distance between the hype and the truth is just too big for any budget to handle.

The same complexity holds true for collagen as a beauty supplement, too, because there is some research showing the intake of collagen can have benefit for skin and bones. But there is no science showing it gets rid of wrinkles, at least not unbiased research.

What is collagen? Collagen is made of protein and functions primarily as a support structure in the body, comprising 30% of its mass. There are many forms of collagen in the human body but only four types account for over 90% of the total. They are: Collagen I, found in skin, tendons, capillaries and veins, bone, and organs. Collagen II is the primary component of cartilage, while Collagen III is the main component of reticular fibers, and Collagen IV is the mainstay of the cell membrane.

When collagen is broken down it can produce gelatin, which can be used in foods (think Jell-O), or in cosmetics (think products that claim to get rid of wrinkles or in nail-care products claiming to grow nails). Pure collagen can be used in skin-care products as a way to keep skin hydrated. But eating Jell-O no more adds collagen to your skin than applying gelatin ever helped anyone grow a nano-inch of nail length. And no one has ever shed a wrinkle from putting collagen on their skin.

So does ingesting pure collagen translate to creating building blocks, the way eating calcium works on the body, or is it more akin to believing that if you feed a cow chocolate it will produce chocolate milk? The answer is that consuming collagen may have a good effect, as eating calcium-rich foods or supplements will, but NOT in terms of helping wrinkles. Thinking otherwise would be like assuming a broken leg will be repaired by eating calcium.

When you eat or drink collagen (from meat or in supplements) it is digested and broken down into the individual amino acids it is made up of, just as it would be with any animal protein you eat. But regardless of the source the collagen would not be distributed directly to the collagen in your skin. It's just not possible, any more than the chocolate in the cow analogy. Still, eating foods containing collagen does seem to be able to help the entire body's formation of collagen, and that's good news (Sources: *Archives of Dermatological Research*, October 2008, pages 479–483; *Knee Surgery, Sports Traumatology, and Arthroscopy*, August 2006, pages 750–755; *Journal of Nutritional Science*, March 2006, pages 211–215; and *American Journal of Physiology Endocrinology and Metabolism*, June 2005, pages 864–869).

One other point that makes matters even more complicated: Some of these collagen drinks say they contain a form of or are able to stimulate the body's production of collagen peptide (a fragment of collagen broken down by enzymes). Collagen peptides have been shown to improve general bone density, have anti-arthritic properties, and even anti-bone-tumor properties (Sources: *Clinical Immunology*, January 2007, pages 75–84; *Matrix Biology*, November 2006, pages S69–S70; and *Journal of Bone and Mineral Metabolism*, November 2004, 547–553). But this is a complex topic and there is no direct research indicating dosage, or information comparing modalities. There is also research showing that some forms of collagen can stimulate arthritis and that only specific forms can offer help (Source: *Molecular Immunology*, November, www.pubmed.gov). Medicating in this arena needs to be done with your physician's advice.

Despite the confusion and the complex manner in which various forms of collagen work in the body (for better and, in some cases, for worse), what you need to know is that drinking collagen is not going to alter your wrinkles, firm your skin, or delay a trip to the cosmetic surgeon for any of the numerous corrective procedures that really do make an anti-wrinkle difference. I'll drink to that!

CHAPTER 4
ORGANIC COSMETICS DO "NATURAL" ONE BETTER

ORGANIC COSMETICS

If you were thinking all-natural was the answer to your skin care woes, "organic" has now taken over and has become the new cosmetics buzzword. Consumers are inundated with organic claims on all manner of products, and with frequent media stories surrounding the potential health risks and unknowns of anything remotely synthetic, it's no wonder that curiosity about organic products is at an all-time high and that product sales are skyrocketing. Celebrities and cosmetics companies are launching skin-care products labeled organic faster then you can say "But is this really good for my skin?"!

Organically speaking, what does the term "organic" mean in the world of cosmetics, and principally for skin care? Shockingly, it doesn't really mean anything because there is no comprehensive definition, and so different organizations and businesses have sprung up, each trying to become the authoritative source giving the stamp of approval—for a fee of course. Then there's the battle the organic lines have with other lines, each saying theirs is the real deal and everyone else is fibbing. Is it any wonder that many consumers looking for genuine organic products are completely bewildered? As it is, you can basically call your product organic and there is really no one to stop you, no matter what it contains. That's expected to change as organic harmonization details are hammered out, but as this book goes to print, the term is still used loosely.

Mostly those using the term "organic" or "all natural" are perpetuating the myth that synthetic ingredients are automatically bad and natural ingredients are automatically good. Today it seems that only organic ingredients are good and even natural ingredients are now bad unless they are obtained organically. Making people afraid of something, whether it's a single ingredient or an entire category of ingredients, is part of the way natural and organic products are marketed.

The truth is more complicated. Consumers are waylaid by the labels, trusting (albeit blindly) that the one they've chosen is the right brand. In reality, what ends up happening more often than not is just an exchange of one marketing scheme, as with traditional cosmetics companies, for a new one where products are labeled to say they include organic plants.

As you venture out to shop for a great skin-care routine, thinking that healthy-sounding product labels mean the products will take the utmost care of your skin, let me help you with some background. Arming yourself with the facts surrounding organic products will give you the best balance for your budget and your skin.

ORGANIC FOOD'S RELATION TO COSMETICS

Since October 2002, according to the U.S. Department of Agriculture (USDA), national regulations have been on the books that specify exact standards for determining what precisely is meant when food (not cosmetics) is labeled "organic," whether it is grown in the United States or imported from other countries. As is stated on the USDA Web site, "Organic food is produced by farmers who emphasize the use of renewable resources and the conservation of soil and water to enhance environmental quality for future generations. Organic meat, poultry, eggs, and dairy products come from animals that are given no antibiotics or growth hormones. Organic food is produced without using most conventional pesticides, fertilizers made with synthetic ingredients or sewage sludge, bioengineering, or ionizing radiation. Before a product can be labeled 'organic,' a government-approved certifier inspects the farm where the food is grown to make sure the farmer is following all the rules necessary to meet USDA organic standards. Companies that handle or process organic food before it gets to your local supermarket or restaurant must be certified, too."

What does any of this have to do with cosmetics? Many consumers are already attracted to any cosmetic that claims to be natural, no matter how bogus the claim. To make their products stand out from the rest, cosmetics companies are starting to use the term "organic" on their product labels. But as *Consumer Reports* (August 2003, page 61) stated, "With no hearings or public discussion, the USDA extended its rules on organic labeling to cosmetics. There are now shampoos and body lotions labeled 70% organic based on the fact that their main ingredient is … water in which something organic, such as an organic lavender leaf, has been soaked."

Tim Kapsner, Senior Research Scientist at Aveda, made a salient point by stating that "In absence of a true industry standard, companies applied the USDA organic food standard for beauty and personal care products ingredients and products. But the USDA's food standards were never designed for this industry, and its strict guidelines limit certain types of 'green chemistry' and pose significant challenges for those seeking to create certified organic products."

Note: For more detailed information on the USDA organic standards, visit their Web site at www.ams.usda.gov/nop or call the National Organic Program at (202) 720-3252.

GREEN CHEMISTRY DEFINED

As mentioned above in the quote from the Aveda chemist, green chemistry is typically described as "the design of chemical products and processes that reduce or eliminate the use or generation of hazardous substances. Green chemistry applies across the life cycle, including the design, manufacture, and use of a chemical product" (Source: www.epa.gov/gcc/). It is also known as sustainable chemistry, and the goals of those utilizing this method to manufacture products include reducing waste, saving energy, and eliminating negative environmental impact. It's a movement that has all the right goals in mind, including working with all types of raw material suppliers to ensure that the ingredients they develop are as "green" as possible. This includes hazardous chemicals (think bleach, ammonia, disinfectants, preservatives). Green chemistry does not discourage these necessary yet hazardous chemicals, but rather looks for ways to make them less dangerous.

Keep in mind that the majority of hazardous chemicals pose minimal risk to us or the environment when they are used as directed and disposed of properly. Green chemistry doesn't rely solely on natural ingredients, but this type of product formulation is far more realistic and ends up being more helpful for skin, relying on the best of both worlds—nature and science. Green chemistry advocates strive to use as many natural and sustainable ingredient sources as possible, but as any cosmetics chemist will tell you it is impossible to make a 100% natural product that can successfully fight acne, skin discolorations, sun damage, sun protection, or other skin problems. For example, at the very least, synthetic preservatives are needed to control the growth of bacteria and potentially harmful microbes even in products composed of natural ingredients. Natural preservatives just don't have the efficacy, formulary compatibility, or cost-effectiveness required to make safe, reliably preserved products (Source: David C. Steinberg, *Preservatives for Cosmetics*, Second Edition, Allured Publishing, 2006).

Work on furthering the concepts and practice of green chemistry has been part of the Environmental Protection Agency's agenda since the early 1990s. You can expect to see more examples of and claims for green chemistry as it becomes more mainstream—and much of this progress is dictated by consumer demand for safer products.

THE ORGANIC MARKET: FULL STEAM (DISTILLATION) AHEAD!

The forecast for continued strong sales of products labeled as organic is nothing less than robust. As a category, organic (and natural) products are worth $7.3 billion. From 2005 to 2007 there was a 53% increase in launches of organic products, including many new brands that appeared in well-known retail outlets such as Wal-Mart, Walgreens, and Target. Companies large and small are jumping on the organic bandwagon, whose wheels and fuel (meaning contents) are presumably composed of organic materials.

As you might expect, at least those of you who have been reading my reviews and investigations over the years, the problem is that almost without exception the formulas are not as organic as they're made out to be and the overuse of irritating, skin-damaging ingredients is the rule rather than the exception. When you add the routine inclusion of numerous synthetic ingredients in many products erroneously labeled as "organic" to that, it's clear consumers are setting themselves up to fall for false claims and an unhelpful, potentially damaging skin-care routine.

What about the numerous products on the market indicating they use Fair Trade ingredients? The concept of Fair Trade is another that has an ethical and emotional pull for consumers seeking natural products with sustainable ingredients. It is their assurance that some of the ingredients in the products they're considering were obtained from farmers or indigenous people who were treated and compensated fairly for the natural ingredients they supply. In order for a product to advertise it contains Fair Trade ingredients, those ingredients must be certified by the Fairtrade Labeling Organisation International, an umbrealla group made up of 23 member organizations who've set worldwide Fair Trade standards. The cosmetics industry is taking this claim seriously, and why shouldn't they? Sales of Fair Trade ingredients have increased seventy-fold in the last 10 years (Source: www. cosmeticsdesign.com).

CHECK THE LABELS FOR THE TRUTH

It takes only a quick look at the ingredients list on a cosmetic to notice that there are a lot of words that are completely unrelated to anything resembling a plant, much less a plant that can be labeled "organic." Plenty of synthetic ingredients are found in products from cosmetics lines that boast about their all "natural" and now "organic" content, even those that have followed the proper channels to be certified organic. Despite this discrepancy, the hope and desire for "healthier-sounding" products will be an emotional pull for lots of consumers, particularly women shopping for themselves and their families. Add to that the perception of organic products as more environmentally friendly and they become even more difficult to resist.

Things become even more confusing when you consider that most "natural" cosmetics lines are sold at supermarkets that showcase organic produce and food products. When specialty grocery stores sell products that have strictly regulated organic labeling, many customers will never notice that the products in the other half of the store, where the cosmetics are sold, are backed by no such regulation, despite the similar labeling.

ORGANIC IN NAME ONLY?

It may surprise you to learn that, as of late 2008, there are still no FDA-approved standards that must be met before labeling cosmetic products as organic. The same is true in Canada, except in the province of Quebec. Another element that's complicating this issue is the fact that even though lots of cosmetics actually do contain organic ingredients, it's rarely the case that the entire formula is organic. Why? There are various reasons, but mostly it's because a number of synthetic ingredients, such as preservatives, are essential components of many cosmetic formulas (there are no natural preservatives that can keep all microbes such as fungus, mold, and bacterium at bay). They're there for a reason: The organic ingredients are not stable and will deteriorate without them. Plus, in contrast to organic food, a certain amount of synthetic ingredients are required in cosmetics to help keep the ingredients mixed together and stable, and to apply smoothly on the skin and look appealing. What good is an organic or all-natural skin-care product if it's unappealing to use on a daily basis?

It also helps to remember that you can't put avocados (or any other food item) on your face to "feed" your skin. Natural or organic does not mean better skin care. Blueberry or grape juice doesn't make for great skin care, won't fight acne, won't deal with skin discolorations, and won't protect from the sun. Plus what it takes to get a plant out of the ground and processed to remove the insects and dirt, and then get it into your product, stabilized and ready for packaging, and eventually ready for you to use, isn't the most natural process in the world.

To make a long story short, these factors help explain why, until acceptable standards are in place, any cosmetic can sport an organic label without having to prove the claim—and many cosmetics companies are doing just that. Remember, most creams, lotions, gels, serums, toners, shampoos, conditioners, and cleansers are about 60% to 90% water, and by the current lax regulations that makes almost any product organic.

Ultimately what's more important than getting labeling standards in place is the fact that lots of plant extracts and essential oils have irritating properties that won't help skin in the least (think lemon, lavender, peppermint, menthol, lime, camphor, cinnamon and more). So what difference does it make if they're organically grown or not? Environmental impact and sustainable farming notwithstanding, peppermint is a problem for skin, whether it's grown with or without pesticides. It may resonate with you emotionally and morally that your skin-care product purchase helps organic farmers during challenging times (it does for me), but if what's inside the finished product isn't going to help your skin, then it's important to know that there are other ways for you to help the environment without lowering your skin-care standards. In summation, there are other ways to support the "Green" movement that don't involve buying poorly formulated or irritating cosmetic products.

ORGANIC OUTRAGE: THE INDUSTRY BATTLES ITSELF

Because the cosmetics industry at large knows the organic movement isn't a passing fad, there is a consortium of natural product–based companies attempting to standardize the definition and labeling of United States–sold cosmetics as organic. They are doing this not only out of frustration at seeing so many products mislabeled as "organic," but also no doubt because of what has occurred with regard to organic cosmetics in Europe in recent years.

According to the Web site www.cosmeticsdesign-europe.com, the Organic Farmers and Growers, a leading UK certification body, developed a cosmetics and body-care standard for companies that wanted to lure consumers with an organic label. Products that meet this group's standards (which are rigorous, but still respectful of current European cosmetics regulations, including the issue of animal testing) are allowed to sport the group's logo on their products, indicating to consumers that they meet organic standards. According to a July 2007 report in *Organic Monitor*, "With the absence of any major regulations and private standards for natural & organic cosmetics in the USA and Canada, North American companies are increasingly making products according to European standards." For more information on this group, visit www.organicfarmers.org.uk.

In late 2008, after six years of deliberation, leading European certification groups proposed a harmonized set of organic standards to the cosmetics industry. Known as the Cosmetics and Natural Standard (COSMOS), the groups behind this harmonization already account for over 1,000 certified cosmetic companies selling over 11,000 certified products in over 38 countries. Previously certified products will only need to go through the certification process again if they desire the COSMOS seal. Otherwise, the existing standard for which these products were originally certified will remain valid. Products that haven't been certified by COSMOS are expected to begin the process in spring 2009. For more information on this topic, visit www.cosmos-standard.org.

In order for a European-sold and–manufactured product to qualify as natural, it must contain no more than 5% synthetic content. Companies selling such products won't be required to disclose the percentage of natural ingredients that are organic. European-sold and –manufactured products wishing to gain organic approval must contain at least 95% organic content. Further, if an organic source is available for any natural ingredient in the product, it must be used rather than the non-organic source. All organic ingredients must also be processed via "green" manufacturing to ensure a minimum of synthetic chemical involvement.

Although those standards are a positive step for harmonization, keep in mind that this addresses only the issue of plant origin and ingredient processing, not good skin care. Again, we aren't talking about diet. You can't put broccoli or lettuce on your face and have it be lunch for your skin.

On the flip side, another group of U.S.-based cosmetics companies (including Estee Lauder brands, Jason Natural, and L'Oreal), not widely known for being champions of organic products, created the Organic and Sustainable Industry Standards (OASIS), whose guidelines are said to best those of organic certification groups such as Ecocert and the organic seal program run by the United States Department of Agriculture. Under OASIS guidelines, a cosmetic product the manufacturer wants to be labeled organic must contain at least 85% organic content. Plans are in place to tighten this requirement to 95% by 2012, bringing the goal of an almost entirely organic cosmetic product closer to the homes of consumers everywhere. OASIS also has certification systems in place for 100% organic products and allows the statement of "Made with Organic" if a product has no less than 70% organic content.

Sounds good, right? Well, another organic-minded group doesn't think so. The Organic Consumers Association (OCA) is taking the group to task for allowing synthetic ingredients to be present in products labeled organic, as well as not having a monitoring system in place to alert people to the presence of chemical by-products when certain ingredients, such as surfactants, undergo a process known as ethoxylation.

The OCA based its organic standards on those of the National Organic Program, which is chiefly concerned with organic food. Members of OASIS have pointed out that the standards of the National Organic Program do not apply to cosmetics because the ingredients and manufacturing necessary to make cosmetic products (organic or not) are outside the simplistic scope of what it takes to grow and certify food as organic. And that is an understatement—a pomegranate doesn't have to sit in your bathroom for a few months before you are done using it!

Nevertheless, the Organic Consumers Association didn't want to back down. They sent cease and desist letters to OASIS companies selling products labeled as organic but containing nonorganic cleansing agents or synthetic antioxidants. OASIS is arguing that their standard permits use of such nonorganic ingredients in cosmetic products because there are currently no suitable organic alternatives. OCA is arguing that in addition to allowing synthetic ingredients in products labeled organic, OASIS consists of "conventional industry members" who have the goal of diluting organic standards to their advantage.

For OCA to assert that their own "standards" don't serve them over and above the consumer is sheer aggrandizement. It's the pot calling the kettle black and nothing more. Traditional cosmetics companies are not doing a disservice to consumers. OASIS is trying to define organic cosmetic standards for the entire industry, something that is currently lacking. What difference does it make if L'Oreal or Burt's Bees spearhead development and integration of organic standards?

As usual, this all comes down to the smaller natural-product companies not wanting larger corporations to use their financial clout and resources to make changes before they can do so (or without their approval), or to act first to get the advantage of their marketing manipulation.

I realize some small business owners' egos may be bruised if OASIS succeeds with their standardization efforts but it is important to keep in mind that large companies with extensive research and development facilities and staff can work more effectively on finding organic solutions to the need for synthetic ingredients (if they are needed). Smaller companies behind the OCA, such as Dr. Bronner's, can only dream of achieving such a feat. One thing is certain: Paying closer attention to organic standards, regardless of affiliation, will pave the way for more accountability and regulation for a term that has been undefined and misused for far too long.

What needs to be at the forefront of organic standards is thinking about what the consumer needs, not marketing claims. It always comes down to creating formulations that are the best for skin. If it serves skin without risk, any ingredient, synthetic or organic, ought to be included in your product. To stick with the claim that only natural ingredients are good will cheat skin of some incredibly important benefits (Sources: *The Rose Sheet*, March 10, 2008, page 3; March 24, 2008, page 3; and March 31, 2008, pages 3–4).

It is worth mentioning that there are smaller cosmetics companies (such as Juice Beauty) that are also members of OASIS; the group is not just for large, internationally distributed cosmetics companies.

OTHER ORGANIC & PRO NATURAL GROUPS

In addition to the United States pro-organic groups mentioned above, there are a few other groups in Europe and the United States that deserve mention.

Ecocert is an independent, accredited organic certification group based in France. They've been on the scene since 1991. Although the group is based in Europe, they work with over 75 countries and inspect the majority of organic food companies in France and a good portion of such facilities elsewhere, too. Ecocert has branches in several major countries, including Spain, Germany, Japan, and Canada. For more information about Ecocert, visit www.ecocert.com.

Cosmebio is a professional association linked to companies selling organic cosmetics. This group is associated with Ecocert and uses their "Bio" label on certified products meeting their standards for organic content and processing. Products that have the "Bio" label contain a minimum of 95% natural ingredients or ingredients of natural origin. They also must have a minimum of 10% organic ingredients. For more information about Cosmebio, visit www.cosmebio.org (Note: this Web site is in French but can be translated).

BDIH is a natural products certification group based in Germany. They are part of the Federation of German Industries and Trading Firms for pharmaceuticals, health-care products, dietary supplements, and cosmetic products. They developed standards in co-operation with cosmetic ingredient manufacturers specializing in natural ingredients, and their guidelines can be found at this Web address: www.kontrollierte-naturkosmetik.de/en/the_guidelines.htm. A product that conforms to this group's standards can be legitimately labeled with their "Certified Natural Cosmetics" seal.

The Natural Products Association (NPA) was founded in 1936 and is the United States' largest non-profit company overseeing the natural products industry. They represent all manner of natural products, from health and beauty aids to foods. In late 2008, NPA announced that they had certified two cosmetics lines with their Natural Standards Program. Those two lines are Aubrey Organics and Burt's Bees (the Burt's Bees certification wasn't too surprising given that Burt's Bees Chief Marketing and Strategic Officer is also the chairman of the Natural Standard Program committee). In order to gain the NPA's seal on products, companies must prove at least 95% of their ingredients are derived from natural sources, which is on par with but not as rigid as EcoCert and emerging European standards.

Please keep in mind that certification has nothing, and I mean absolutely nothing, to do with skin-care benefit. This is all about the source of ingredients, not the all-important research concerning the benefits and the results consumers are looking for in their skin-care products. A stamp of approval on a piece of steak from the USDA does not tell you how a diet of steak may impact your arteries, heart, or brain. Exactly the same principle holds true for skin care, no matter whose name or certification is on the product.

SHOPPING FOR ORGANIC COSMETICS

My preference is that you would never go shopping for any skin-care product without the research and analysis from me and my team about its long-term benefit for your skin. After all, discussing and debating whether a product is organic sidesteps other essential issues, like the need for sun protection, and the skin's need for antioxidants, skin-identical ingredients, and cell-communicating ingredients, even if many of the most stable and most "bio-available" of these are synthetically derived from natural sources. And that's not to mention providing help for exfoliation, fighting acne, rosacea, skin discoloration, and yes, even wrinkles. The entire discussion about organic ignores the need for great skin-care products. Meanwhile the research shows pretty clearly that when the world of synthetic cosmetic ingredients is combined with natural ones that work and don't irritate the skin, you are in the right place to take the best possible care of your skin.

You also need to be aware that there is no substantiated, published research anywhere proving that organic ingredients are superior to nonorganic or synthetic ingredients. Choosing organic is not essential, but it is a preference many consumers have.

If organic is the only way you are willing to go, and until formal standards are available in the United States and the rest of the world, the best approach is to buy products certified by the USDA or Ecocert or one of its related groups. These aren't perfect systems, but when a product bears one of these organization's seals it gives you an honestly transparent way to decipher just how natural and organic the product you're considering is.

As burgeoning groups work to solidify organic standards that can be followed globally, shopping by seal and also by the company's reputation for integrity is the best consumers can do. Of course, unless your attitude is organic-or-nothing, there is every reason to completely ignore any claims of that nature (pun intended) and instead focus on finding the products with ingredients that copious research has shown are truly beneficial for your skin. If some of those products happen to contain organically certified ingredients, great. But if not, consumers don't need to lose sleep over missing out on this segment of the worldwide movement to go Green.

CHAPTER 5
SKIN TYPE?

WHAT IS SKIN TYPE?

Simply put, skin type is the description and interpretation of how and why your skin looks, feels, and behaves as it does.

The four most common and relatively helpful skin-type categories used by the cosmetics industry are:

1. **Normal (no apparent signs of oily or dry areas)**
2. **Oily (shine appears all over skin, no dry areas at all)**
3. **Dry (flaking can appear, no oily areas at all, skin feels tight and may look dull)**
4. **Combination (oily, typically in the central part of the face, and dry or normal areas elsewhere)**

Often blemish-prone skin is included under the oily or combination skin types, though it is sometimes listed as a skin type all by itself. Occasionally, sensitive skin may be listed as an individual skin type. However, I feel strongly that all skin types should be considered sensitive, and I'll explain why in just a moment.

As nice and neat as those four (or six) categories may be, and they are an excellent starting point, the truth is that understanding your skin type is more often than not far more complicated, which is why lots of women find identifying the skin type an elusive, changing puzzle that never settles down in one specific direction. Yet understanding your skin type is incredibly important, and just not in the way the cosmetics industry approaches it or the way we've been indoctrinated to think about it. First, skin type is never static. The variations of what is taking place on your skin can not only change season to season but month to month and even week to week. Adding to the complexity is the strong possibility of skin disorders such as rosacea (which affects more than 40% of the Caucasian population), eczema, skin discolorations, precancerous conditions, blackheads, sun damage, and whiteheads. Four or six categories of skin type just can't cover it.

When it comes to determining your skin type you need to forget what you've been taught by cosmetics salespeople, aestheticians, fashion magazines, and even some dermatologists. The typical categories of normal, oily, dry, and combination are good basics, but they don't address every nuance, and they can change and fluctuate with everything from the weather to your stress levels.

Why is recognizing all the nuances of your skin type so important? **Because different skin types require different product formulations.** Even though many skin types often need the same active ingredients such as sunscreen agents, antioxidants, cell-communicating ingredients, and so on, the base they are in (lotion, cream, gel, serum, or liquid) should match the needs of your skin type. Skin type is the single most important factor influencing the decisions we make about the kinds of skin-care routines and products we buy. But we need to be careful about the way we categorize our skin or the very products we thought would help could actually make matters worse.

WHAT INFLUENCES SKIN TYPE?

Almost everything can influence skin type, which is why it can be so tricky to attribute a single skin type to what you see on your face. Both external and internal elements can and do impact the way your skin looks and feels. To effectively evaluate your skin and determine the correct skin-care routine, here are some of the factors that need to be considered:

Internal Influences:
- Hormonal changes (pregnancy, menopause, menstrual cycle, and more all cause skin conditions to fluctuate from oily to breakouts, skin discolorations, and dryness)
- Skin disorders (rosacea, psoriasis, dermatitis, with each one posing its specific concerns)
- Genetic predisposition of skin type (oily versus dry, prone to breakouts, sensitive skin)
- Smoking (cause of necrotic skin that cannot be corrected by skin-care products)
- Medications you may be taking (some birth-control pills can increase oily skin and breakouts while other types can actually improve the appearance of acne)
- Diet (there is research showing a diet high in antioxidants and omega-3 and omega-6 fatty acids can improve the appearance of skin)

External Influences:
- Climate/weather (cold, warm, moist, dry)
- Your skin-care routine (over-moisturizing or over-exfoliating, using irritating or drying products, using the wrong products for your skin type can create skin problems that weren't there before)
- Unprotected or prolonged sun exposure (the major cause of wrinkles and skin discolorations)
- Secondhand smoke (see above)
- Pollution (creates additional free-radical activity that damages collagen and the skin's genetic stability)

These complex and often overlapping circumstances all contribute to what takes place on and in your skin, which in turn determines your skin type.

WILL MY SKIN TYPE CHANGE?

Absolutely! Another problem with skin typing is the assumption that your skin (and skin type) will be the same forever, or at least until you age. That, too, is rarely the case. If your skin-care routine focuses on skin type alone, it can become obsolete the moment the season changes, your work life becomes stressful, or your body experiences hormonal or diet fluctuations or other physical changes, and whatever else life may bring.

To complicate things even more, in any given period you may have multiple skin types! It is not unusual for women to have a little bit of each skin type simultaneously or at different times of the month or week. An overview of how your skin behaves and changes is necessary to assess what your skin needs so you can then respond by applying the appropriate products to those problems areas.

WILL I EVER HAVE "NORMAL" SKIN?

It depends on how you define normal. As far as the cosmetics industry is concerned, every woman can and should have normal skin. Yet acquiring normal skin is like trying to scale a peak with a slippery, precarious slope. At some point you are going to take a wrong step. And if you have normal skin, at some point it isn't going to be normal any more. Like the rest of our bodies, skin is in a constant state of change. Even women with seemingly perfect complexions go through phases of having oily, dry, or blemish-prone skin—and then there are all the issues related to sun damage or merely growing older. In reality, no one is likely to have normal skin for very long, no matter what she does. Chasing after normal skin can set you on an endless skin-care buying spree, running around in circles trying everything and finding nothing that works for very long or that makes matters worse.

In any case, identifying skin type is highly subjective. Many women have really wonderful skin but refuse to accept it. The smallest blemish or wrinkle or the slightest amount of dry skin distresses them. Or some women see a line or two around their eyes and immediately buy the most expensive anti-wrinkle creams they can find in the hope of warding off their worst imagined nightmare. This is one of those times where being realistic is the most important part of your skin-care routine.

COMBINATION SKIN IS THE MOST CONFUSING SKIN TYPE

Identifying your skin type is made a lot more difficult by the all-encompassing combination skin type. Almost everyone at some time or another, if not all the time, has combination skin. Physiologically, the nose, chin, center of the forehead, and the center of the cheek all have more oil glands than other parts of the face. It is not surprising that those areas tend to be oilier and break out more frequently than other areas. Problems occur when you buy extra products for combination skin, because many ingredients that are appropriate for the T-zone (the area along the center of the forehead and down the nose where most of the oil glands on the face are located) won't help the cheek, eye, or jaw areas. You may need separate products to deal with the different skin types on your face because you should treat different skin types, even on the same face, differently.

UNSEEN SKIN TYPES BELOW THE SURFACE

Another limitation of skin type is that it cannot address skin-care needs that may not be apparent on the skin's surface. For example, sun damage is not evident when you are younger, but sun protection is imperative for all skin types. Oily and dry skin present at the same time, along with some redness, may be an early sign of rosacea, not just a sign of combination skin, and rosacea is a condition that cannot be treated with cosmetics and is not easily diagnosed. What you see on the surface of the skin does not always indicate the type of skin-care products you should buy.

SKIN-CARE PRODUCTS CAN INFLUENCE SKIN TYPE AND NOT IN A GOOD WAY!

One other important point: The skin-care products you use can influence your skin type. Judging skin type simply by looking at your face and feeling your skin won't necessarily identify the underlying situation. For example, if you use an emollient cleanser and follow it with a drying, alcohol-laden toner, and then an emollient moisturizer with a serum underneath, that could very well be causing you to have noticeably combination skin. Using a moisturizer that is too emollient for your skin could be causing breakouts. Using skin-care products that contain irritating ingredients could cause dryness, irritation, and redness. You may think you have a particular skin type, but you may be looking at your skin's reaction to the products you are using.

EVERYONE HAS SENSITIVE SKIN

More than 60% of women worldwide feel they have sensitive skin (Sources: *Skin Research and Technology*, November 2006, pages 217–222; and *British Journal of Dermatology*, August 2001, pages 258–263), and though many physicians feel that this is at best an exaggeration, the truth is these women do have sensitive skin and I would suspect the number is much higher.

Regardless of your primary skin type, ethnic background, or age, minor or major irritating skin conditions can be present, even those you can't feel. The skin can burn, chafe, or crack, and you may have patchy areas of dry, flaky skin related to weather conditions, hormonal changes, the skin-care products you use, or sun exposure. Skin can also break out in small bumps that look like a diaper rash. Skin can itch, swell, blotch, redden, and develop allergic reactions to cosmetics, animals, dust, or pollen.

If that isn't enough to make you itch just a little, then think about the number of cosmetics most women use daily. The average woman uses at least 12 different skin-care, makeup, and hair-care products a day, with each one, on average, containing about 20 different ingredients. That means her skin is exposed to about 240 different cosmetic ingredients on any given day. The fact that any of us have skin left is a testimony to the skin's resiliency, the safety of the majority of cosmetic ingredients, and the talent of cosmetics chemists. Whether we like it or not, most of us will react to something along the way, perhaps even daily.

Your skin is the protective armor that keeps the elements and other invaders from entering the body. We protect most of our anatomy with clothing, but our faces are left painfully exposed to everything. It's no wonder the skin on our faces acts up now and then. Sensitive skin is probably the most "normal" type of skin around.

Everyone has the potential to have or develop sensitive skin given what it goes through, so women of every skin type should heed the precautions for sensitive skin. What are the precautions? There is really only one and it goes for all skin types: Treat your skin as gently as you possibly can. Whether you think of your face as oily, dry, or mature, you still need to be gentle with your skin and avoid things that cause irritation.

MATURE SKIN FOLLY: SKIN TYPE HAS NOTHING TO DO WITH YOUR AGE

Older skin is different from younger skin; that is indisputable. Yet it is a mistake to buy skin-care products based on a nebulous age category. Treating older or younger skin with products supposedly aimed at dealing with specific age ranges does not make sense because not everyone with "older" or "younger" skin has the same needs, yet it's a trap many women (especially older women) fall into. An older person may have acne, blackheads, eczema, rosacea, sensitive skin, or oily skin, while a younger person may have dry, freckled, or obviously sun-damaged skin. Products designed for older, "mature" skin are almost always too emollient and occlusive, and those designed for younger skin are almost always too drying. The key issue with skin type needs to be the actual condition of your skin, not your age.

In fact, regardless of age, all skin types, young and old, need sun protection, lots of antioxidants, ingredients that mimic skin structure, and cell-communicating ingredients. These types of ingredients are of the utmost importance for skin care, and age doesn't change or alter that in any way. While wrinkles may tend to separate younger from older skin, your skin can still be oily at 60 and you can still struggle with breakouts. Not everyone in their 40s, 50s, 60s, or 70s has the same skin-care needs. In a way it's simple: You need to pay attention to what is taking place on your skin, and that varies from person to person.

DOES SKIN COLOR OR ETHNICITY AFFECT SKIN CARE?

Regardless of skin color or ethnic background, all skin is subject to a range of problems. Almost always these skin problems have nothing to do with skin color or ethnic background. Whether it is dry or oily skin, blemishes, scarring, wrinkles, skin discolorations, skin disorders, skin sensitivity, or even risk of sun damage, all men and women of all colors and ethnic backgrounds share similar struggles and require the same products to improve the situation. So, while there are some distinctions between varying ethnic groups when it comes to skin problems and skin-care options, overall these differences are minor in comparison to the number of similarities.

Think of this in relationship to diet. Despite differences in ethnic backgrounds what constitutes a healthy diet is the same for everyone. As humans, all of us need a diet high in antioxidants, omega-3 and omega-6 fatty acids, whole grains, lean protein, and on and on.

The same is true for your skin: What is healthy or helpful for skin is the same regardless of skin color or ethnicity. (Sources: *The American Journal of Clinical Nutrition*, October 2007, pages 1225–1231; *Pharmacological Research*, March 2007, pages 199–206; and *Journal of Nutrition, Health and Aging*, September–October 2006, pages 377–385.)

According to an article in the *Journal of the American Academy of Dermatology* (February 2002, pages 41–62), "People with skin of color constitute a wide range of racial and ethnic groups—including Africans, African Americans, African Caribbeans, Chinese and Japanese, Native American Navajo [and other] Indians, and certain groups of fair-skinned persons (e.g., Indians, Pakistanis, Arabs), and Hispanics.... There is not a wealth of data on racial and ethnic differences in skin and hair structure, physiology, and function. What studies do exist involve small patient populations and that often have methodological flaws. Consequently, few definitive conclusions can be made. The literature does support a racial differential in epidermal melanin [pigment] content and melanosome dispersion in people of color compared with fair-skinned persons. Other studies have demonstrated differences in hair structure and fibroblast size and structure between black and fair-skinned persons. These differences could at least in part account for the lower incidence of skin cancer in certain people of color compared with fair-skinned persons; a lower incidence and different presentation of photo aging; pigmentation disorders in people with skin of color; and a higher incidence of certain types of alopecia [loss of hair] in Africans and African Americans compared with those of other ancestry."

One arena where differences do exist was explained in *Contact Dermatitis* (December 2001, pages 346–349). They noted that "There is a widespread, but largely unsubstantiated, view that certain skin types may be more susceptible to the effect of skin irritants than others. One expression of this would be that certain ethnic groups may also be more likely to experience skin irritation.... In this study, we have investigated 2 carefully matched panels of Caucasian and Japanese women volunteers to determine their topical irritant reaction, both acute and cumulative, to a range of materials. The results indicated that the acute irritant response tended to be greater in the Japanese panel and this reached statistical significance with the stronger irritants. Cumulative irritation was investigated only with the weaker irritants and, although again the trend was to a higher response in Japanese compared to Caucasian panelists, this rarely reached significance." But in the long run, irritation is a problem for all skin types so all women need to treat their skin gently and not use products with sensitizing ingredients.

Throughout this book I will point out the special needs, concerns, and treatment options that affect men and women of color when they differ from those of Caucasian skin types. But beyond that, nearly everything in this book, and especially the chapter on inflammation and irritation, is true for everyone.

DETERMINING YOUR SKIN TYPE

Ideally, you should be using products that don't create or reinforce undesirable skin types. Among the offending products are bar soaps and bar cleansers (both can artificially make skin dry and irritated), occlusive moisturizers (these can clog pores and make breakouts worse), and skin-care products that contain irritating ingredients (causing redness, inflammation, and flaking), including astringents and toners loaded with alcohol and other potentially irritating ingredients. All of these can wreak havoc on the skin. It would be best, then, if the cleanser, toner, and moisturizer you were using matched your skin-care needs—meaning they would be as gentle and brilliantly formulated as possible. Even if that isn't the case, from this point forward you will be better able to understand your skin type and know how to treat your skin appropriately with what is actually helpful for your skin.

Do not judge your skin type after you wash your face. Because the initial sensation you experience after washing your face can be your reaction to the water or the cleanser, you need to wait at least four hours after you've washed your face to accurately judge what is taking place on your skin. (Although with the right cleanser you can mitigate any discomfort after washing your face.) Try to do this assessment on a day when you are not wearing makeup so your foundation and powder won't affect your evaluation.

Next, look in the mirror. Are there areas on your face that are noticeably shiny? Are those areas all over or just over the nose, cheeks, forehead, and chin? If you're not sure, take a Kleenex and dab at your face. Wait another hour and dab again. If the Kleenex has oil smears on it, then you are presently dealing with some amount of oily skin (or possibly a moisturizer that is too emollient for you, but as you read the information about your skin type I can help you work through all this).

Do any areas of your face appear dry or matte? If the answer to this question is yes, then you are dealing with dry skin. For more information, see the chapter Solutions for Dry Skin.

1. **Are some areas of your face both dry and oily?** Then you are dealing with combination skin (though this condition can often be a result of using skin-care products that are both too emollient for your skin type and too drying, but we will work through all this). For more information, see the chapter Solutions for Combination Skin.

2. **Whether your skin is dry or oily, do you notice areas of redness over the nose and cheek area that are accompanied by red bumps that look like blemishes but aren't really pimples?** Are there noticeable surfaced capillaries over these sections as well as areas of extreme sensitivity? Do you flush easily? If you've answer yes to these questions you may possibly have rosacea. Rosacea is a medical condition requiring the attention of a dermatologist. For more information about rosacea, see the chapter Solutions for Rosacea.

3. **Do some areas of your skin tend to break out with small to medium size blemishes, particularly around the time of your menstrual cycle?** If you've answered yes to this, you have mild to moderate acne. For more information, see the chapter Solutions for Blemishes.

4. **Do some areas of your skin have more significant, consistent breakouts that are sometimes deep and painful and/or that lead to scarring?** If you've answered yes to this you have more severe acne. For more information, see the chapter Solutions for Blemishes.

5. **Do areas of your skin, particularly around your nose, chin, cheeks, or forehead, have noticeable blackheads?** If you've answered yes to this you can have a mix of skin problems but dealing with blackheads takes some special steps. For more information, see the chapter Getting Rid of Blackheads.

6. **Eventually all of us will see the impact of unprotected sun exposure on our skin.** If you see wrinkles and skin discolorations appearing, the primary cause will be sun damage that started from the first moments our skin was exposed to the sun when we were babies. Someone at the age of 20 or 30 may have serious sun damage, but the results of that damage won't show up until later in their 30s, 40s, and 50s. Some amount of sun damage is universal for almost everyone, and it continues from the moment your skin sees daylight. Even diligent, daily use of a well-formulated sunscreen only filters up to 97% of the sun's rays (but most of us weren't even thinking about sunscreen when we were younger). Generally, we can all assume we have some amount of sun damage, so everyone's skin has this condition. That means everyone needs skin-care products with ingredients that fight or prevent sun damage. For more information, see the chapters on Solutions for Wrinkles, and Sun Essentials

7. **Do you notice skin discolorations on your face such as areas of new freckling or, for women of color, areas of gray or dark pigment?** More often than not, these discolorations are a condition called melasma (also known as chloasma or pregnancy masking). Typically, these skin discolorations are either caused by sun damage or hormonal fluctuations. For more information about these conditions, see the chapter on Skin Discolorations.

8. **As I explained previously, because everyone has sensitive skin to one degree or another, you must only use products that are gentle, nondrying, and nonirritating.** So add sensitive skin to your skin type. For more information about what can trigger irritation, see the chapter on Irritation and Inflammation.

9. **Do you have patches of raised, red, dry, white scaly, crusted skin around your hairline, nose, eyes, or cheeks?** This may be a skin disorder called psoriasis or some other dermatitis, which requires medical diagnosis and treatment, potentially with prescription products.

If you have consistently puffy, swollen eyes, you may have allergies to dust or mold, or hay fever, though even food allergies can trigger swelling around the eye. You may want to discuss with your doctor the option of taking an antihistamine (there are great over-the-counter options) to see if that helps the condition. Regrettably, despite the claims, there are no skin-care products that can alter puffy eyes. All you can do is stop using products or engaging in activities that might be causing the problem, such as smoking, drinking too much alcohol, or using skin-care products around the eye (or anywhere on the face) that contain irritating ingredients.

As you modify and adjust your skin-care routine with products that are appropriate for your skin type, you will notice only positive changes that get you closer to the skin you want. Remember that skin type isn't static: Even with appropriate, well-formulated skin-care products, your skin type can change depending on the season, your hormones, your stress level, and just the fact that skin does go through changes. You should reevaluate your skin as you notice differences, so keep this list close by so you can fully understand what you are dealing with and not blindly apply products that have no chance of helping.

CHAPTER 6
SKIN'S ENEMY: IRRITATION AND INFLAMMATION

IT HURTS EVERYONE

I started my career as a cosmetics consumer advocate by warning women about the damage being done to their skin by using irritating skin-care ingredients that trigger chronic inflammation when used day in and day out. Over the years my fears about irritation and the resulting inflammation it causes have been reconfirmed over and over by numerous scientific studies. Indeed, chronic irritation and the inflammation that results are a bigger problem for the skin than even I had suspected. Irritation immediately causes inflammation whether you can see it or not, and just as quickly can cause an abrupt breakout response. Or it can cause redness, flaky skin (which can clog pores), or rashes, and it can even cause capillaries to surface on the face.

Chronic and even acute irritation and inflammation can destroy the skin's integrity by breaking down the skin's protective barrier, and that, over time, damages the skin's collagen and elastin components. Inside the skin, inflammation impairs the skin's immune and healing responses. Additionally, breaking down the skin's protective barrier can allow the introduction of bacteria, thus raising the risk of more breakouts. Any way you look at it, irritating the skin in any manner is almost always not a good idea, and especially not when it happens every day with sun exposure or the skin-care products we use.

(Sources: *Inflammation Research*, December 2008, pages 558–563; *Skin Pharmacology and Physiology*, June 2008, pages 124–135 and November–December 2000, pages 358–371; *Journal of Investigative Dermatology*, April 2008, pages 15–19; *Journal of Cosmetic Dermatology*, March 2008, pages 78–82; *Mechanisms of Ageing and Development*, January 2007, pages 92–105; and *British Journal of Dermatology*, December 2005, pages S13–S22.)

INFLAMM-AGING

I wish I had invented that term but I came across it in a research journal I was reading (Source: *Rejuvenation Research*, Fall 2006, pages 402–407). Much of the research on "aging" and wrinkling has to do with inflammation and what it does to skin. As a result of this research it is becoming clear that anything generating inflammation is bad for skin. Irritation generates inflammation and that puts it into the category of things to avoid. (Sources: *Skin Research and Technology*, November 2001, pages 227–237; and *Contact Dermatitis*, November 1998, pages 231–239.)

What causes skin irritation from a skin-care perspective? Many elements are responsible for hurting skin, including hot water, cold water, sun exposure, pollution, irritating skin-care ingredients, soaps, and drying cleansers, plus just scrubbing the skin. You may think that none of those things bothers your skin. However, it is startling to learn that even if your skin doesn't feel or appear irritated after exposure to those things, it is still being irritated and the skin breakdown is nonetheless taking place. That means if you are out in the sun, sitting in a sauna, or using a skin-care product that contains potentially irritating or sensitizing ingredients, the irritation damage is still taking place even though the skin doesn't show it. (Sources: *Journal of Biochemical and Molecular Toxicology*, April 2003, pages 92–94; *Skin Research and Technology*, January 2003, pages 50–58; and *Dermatotoxicology*, edited by Hongbo Zhai and Howard I. Maibach, Seventh Edition, CRC Press, Boca Raton, FL 2007.)

We can get a clearer idea of how this underlying, hidden damage from irritating skin-care routines or products takes place by likening it to what happens to skin in response to unprotected sun exposure. Being exposed to the sun day after day from early childhood results in cumulative damage that takes place beneath the skin's surface and doesn't show itself on the face until after many years of exposure. Diet offers another good comparison. Overeating or eating foods that aren't healthy can cause serious health problems; you don't feel or even notice that the food is hurting you until sometime in the future, yet the damage is still taking place day in and day out.

Avoiding the obvious substances and elements that irritate skin is crucial for healthy skin. This includes not smoking, avoiding unprotected sun exposure at all costs, and not using irritating or harsh skin-care products. Not paying attention to the irritation potential of certain ingredients in skin-care products can be damaging to the health of your skin. What skin-care ingredients irritate skin? That list is presented in the next section. Keep in mind that throughout this book when I indicate something is a possible skin irritant, it means it can be irritating to everyone's skin, even if your skin doesn't appear to have a reaction. Some ingredients always create irritation beneath the skin's surface and cause damage, and that is not good for anyone's skin.

Note: Some irritating ingredients can also have positive results for skin, such as AHAs, BHA, Retin-A, Renova, sunscreen ingredients, some antioxidants, and some preservatives that keep products stabilized. All of those can be considered essential for many skin types and product formulations, yet they do pose a risk of irritation. In this case, it's simply a tradeoff in which the positive benefits outweigh the potential negatives. On the other hand, some ingredients are not only irritating but also have no positive impact on skin, meaning they don't help it in any way and are best avoided. Those are the ones I consistently warn about and advise you to avoid.

HOW TO BE GENTLE

Being gentle to your face is one of the most important parts of any skin-care routine. Along with diligent sun protection (which is really about reducing the inflammation in skin caused by the sun), using gentle, nonirritating skin-care products is part of how you can achieve the best daily and long-term skin-care results possible—so you can have the skin you've always wanted. (Sources: *American Journal of Clinical Dermatology*, May 2004, pages 327–337; *Dermatologic Therapy*, January 2004, pages 16–25; *Cosmetics & Toiletries*, November 2003, page 63; *Global Cosmetics*, February 2000, pages 46–49; and *Contact Dermatitis*, February 1995, pages 83–87.)

We do many things to our skin and buy an assortment of skin-care products that can cause serious irritation. Yet it is far easier than you may think to eliminate these skin-"care" culprits. With that in mind, here is a list of typical skin-care and makeup ingredients and specific cosmetic products and tools to avoid or use cautiously. The skin can react negatively to all of the following products, procedures, and ingredients.

Irritating Skin-Care Steps and Products to Avoid
- Overly abrasive scrubs (including many at-home microdermabrasion scrubs)
- Astringents containing irritating ingredients
- Toners containing irritating ingredients
- Scrub mitts
- Cold or hot water
- Steaming or icing the skin
- Facial masks containing irritating ingredients
- Loofahs
- Bar soaps and bar cleansers (Sources: *International Journal of Dermatology*, August 2002, pages 494–499; *Skin Research and Technology*, May 2001, pages 98–104; and *Dermatology*, March 1997, pages 258–262).

The Most Common Irritating Ingredients to Avoid:
(These are of greater concern when they appear at the beginning of an ingredient list.)
- Alcohol or sd-alcohol followed by a number (Exceptions: Ingredients like cetyl alcohol or stearyl alcohol are standard, benign, waxlike cosmetic thickening agents and are completely nonirritating and safe to use.)
- Camphor
- Citrus juices and oils
- Eucalyptus
- Excessive fragrance
- Menthol
- Menthyl lactate
- Menthoxypropanediol
- Mint
- Peppermint
- Sodium lauryl sulfate
- Arnica
- Bergamot
- Cinnamon
- Clove

- Eugenol
- Grapefruit
- Lavender
- Linalool
- Wintergreen
- Witch hazel
- Ylang-ylang

These ingredients are extremely common; you would be surprised how often they show up in skin-care products for all skin types. Ingredients like camphor, menthol, mint, and alcohol are sometimes recommended because they are considered anti-itch ingredients. The theory works like this: When your skin itches, the nerve endings are sending messages begging you to scratch. If you place these irritating ingredients over the area that itches, the nerve hears the irritation message louder than it hears the itch message and interprets this as a reason to stop itching. That reasoning is fine if minor, sporadic, occasional itching is your problem. If it is not and those ingredients are present in skin-care products meant for everyday use, they introduce a constantly irritating assault to the skin, and cause dryness, rashes, increased oil production, redness, and breakouts. None of those side effects are attractive.

Skin doesn't have to hurt, tingle, or be stimulated even a little to be clean. (If the skin tingles, it is being irritated, not cleaned.) The major rule for all skin types is, if a product or procedure irritates the skin, don't use it again.

Exceptions to the rule: When you initially begin to use an AHA or BHA product or Retin-A, Renova, azelaic acid, or Differin, stinging or tingling can occur. You may need to cut back if it is more than a little tingling, or stop altogether if these symptoms persist for more than a few weeks or worsen with repeated use.

ANTI-IRRITANTS AND ANTI-INFLAMMATORIES

Avoiding irritating ingredients is important for the health of your skin, but it is also helpful to use skin-care products containing ingredients that mitigate or counter the effects of irritation on skin. Anti-irritants and anti-inflammatories are a group of ingredients known for reducing or relieving skin irritation and inflammation. Because irritation and inflammation are well known to be problematic for skin, anti-irritants as well as anti-inflammatories have become popular and necessary terms and components in the cosmetics world and in most medical fields, particularly in dermatology. Many ingredients perform the function of anti-irritants or anti-inflammatories, and better ones are being discovered all the time. Interestingly enough, most antioxidants function as anti-irritants because one of the skin's responses to free-radical damage is irritation and inflammation. These ingredients go a long way toward helping the skin deal with its daily struggle against sun exposure, pollution, skin-care routines (topical disinfectants, sunscreens, and exfoliants can be irritating to skin), and seasonal environmental extremes (Sources: *Exogenous Dermatology*, June 2004, pages 154–160; and *Toxicology Letters*, December 2003, pages 65–73).

HEAT IS A PROBLEM

Because irritation is a problem for skin, anything that irritates the skin should be avoided as much as possible. Heat is one of those things that should be avoided. As good as hot water, direct steam, or dry saunas feel on the skin, they end up causing more problems for the health of the skin. For years, I have recommended washing the face with tepid water. This is because hot water burns the skin and cold water shocks it, and both leave it irritated and dry. These two temperature extremes can also injure skin cells, dehydrate the skin, and cause capillaries to surface. Extreme temperatures in any form cause problems for the skin, but heat is the more attractive alternative (most people avoid a cold shower or bath).

Dry heat is clearly dehydrating. Whether the dry heat comes from a dry sauna or an arid desert climate, it pulls water right out of the skin cell. That's bad for any skin type, but especially for someone with dry skin.

Wet heat is a bit more deceptive. We all know how great the skin feels initially when we exit a hot shower, Jacuzzi, or sauna. It feels plump and saturated with water because the skin absolutely loves drinking up all the water it can. After even a short soak in a tub, your skin can swell and become engorged with water. When you leave a bathtub and your fingers are all thick and wrinkly, it isn't because they are dry, but because they are distorted and swollen with water-saturated skin cells. Because the surface layer of skin likes water so much, hot water can enter the skin, stay there, and cause a burn-like reaction. As a general rule, if water feels hot to the touch, it's too hot for the skin, especially the face. Be very skeptical about facial treatments that involve the use of heat or washing your face with hot (or cold) water; down the line, they could cause more trouble for your skin than you want.

DON'T SMOKE

In this day and age it seems almost silly to remind people that smoking is killing them, killing their teeth, skin, lips, heart, lungs, and causing myriad other associated health complications. Don't we all know this? I have never seen any research anywhere to the contrary. Yet people worldwide continue to smoke. It is shocking and distressing to see this behavior. Addiction or not, stopping smoking is indisputably a primary step in fighting aging and wrinkling.

Smoking is, at the very least, equal to, if not worse than the sun in the direct damage it causes to the skin's surface. In actuality, it is probably even more insidious than sun exposure when it comes to damaging healthy skin. Not only does smoking cause serious free-radical damage and block the body's ability to utilize oxygen, it also creates necrotic (dead) skin tissue that cannot be repaired. Even more unattractive is the breakdown of the elastic fibers of the skin (elastosis), which gives rise to yellow, irregularly thickened skin. At least sun provides some benefit such as vitamin D production and warmth! Smoking provides no benefit of any kind whatsoever.

Moreover, smoking causes a progressive cascade of damage inside the body (restricted blood flow, reduced capacity of the blood to take in oxygen, impairment to the body's immune system) that eventually shows up on the surface of skin, making it look haggard and dull. It also creates serious deep wrinkling around the lips and lip area.

While smoking can make skin look prematurely wrinkled and aged, it's unattractive for many other reasons as well, including the permeating smell of smoke on clothing, breath that smells like smoke, and yellow stains on hands, nails, and teeth. Smoking isn't pretty and it can be deadly. Quitting smoking is one of the most healthful, beautiful things you can do for your skin and body.

(Sources: *Journal of Dermatologic Science*, December 2007, pages 169–175; *Experimental Gerontology*, March 2007, pages 160–165; *Journal of Dermatological Science*, March 2007, pages 169–175; *Skin Pharmacology and Applied Skin Physiology*, January–February 2002, pages 63–68; *Journal of the American Academy of Dermatology*, July 1999, "Cigarette Smoking-Associated Elastotic Changes in the Skin," and May 1996, "Cutaneous Manifestations and Consequences of Smoking"; and *International Journal of Cosmetic Science*, April 1999, pages 83–98.)

FRAGRANCE IN SKIN-CARE PRODUCTS

Essential oils are only essential for your nose, not your skin. They are one of the two groups of ingredients almost universally added to cosmetics (the other being preservatives) that are often the culprits when our skin becomes irritated or sensitized by a cosmetic product. An article in the January 24, 2000, issue of *The Rose Sheet* discussed an advisory report issued by the Scientific Committee on Cosmetic Products and Non-Food Products, a European Commission agency. The report stated that "Information regarding fragrance chemicals used in cosmetic products that have the potential to cause allergic reactions should be provided to consumers." According to the article, "It is seen that a significant increase in fragrance allergy has occurred and that fragrance allergy is the most common cause of contact allergy...."

Concurring with this conclusion is an editorial by Pamela Scheinmann, MD, entitled "The Foul Side of Fragrance-Free Products" (Source: *Journal of the American Academy of Dermatology*, December 1999, page 1020). She states that "Products designated as fragrance-free should contain no fragrance chemicals, not even those that have dual functions." She continues by saying that "hypoallergenic, dermatologist tested, sensitive skin, or dermatologist recommended are no more than meaningless marketing slogans." A large body of evidence comes to the same conclusion and expresses this same concern.

Lots of women assume that the risk to skin from fragrance in skin-care products applies only to synthetic fragrance "chemicals" and not to fragrant plant extracts and oils. When it comes to the health of your skin this would not be a wise assumption. Regardless of the source, most fragrances, natural or synthetic, can cause problems for skin one way or the other. For example, lavender smells wonderful and it may have some anti-microbial properties, but other than that there is no research showing it has any benefit for skin (Sources: *Phytotherapy Research*, June 2002, pages 301–308; and *Healthnotes Review of Complementary and Integrative Medicine*, www.healthwell.com/healthnotes/Herb/). But more importantly, it can be a skin irritant (Source: *Contact Dermatitis*, August 1999, page 111) and a photosensitizer (Source: *Family Practice Notebook*, www.fpnotebook.com/DER188.htm). Research also indicates that components of lavender, specifically linalool, can be cytotoxic, meaning that topical application causes skin-cell death (Source: *Cell Proliferation*, June 2004, pages 221–229).

Essential oils are a group of volatile fluids derived primarily from plants and used in cosmetics primarily as fragrant additives. These components most often include a mix of alcohols, ketones, phenols, linalool, borneol, terpenes, camphor, pinene, acids, ethers, aldehydes, and sulfur, all of which have extremely irritating and sensitizing effects on skin. Even a seemingly benign ingredient like lavender can cause cell death. It's not that some of these ingredients can't have benefit. But why choose them when there are so many other plant extracts that don't have the capacity to irritate skin and provide superior results without any downside?

Why does the cosmetics industry at large continue to add fragrance (synthetic and natural) to products even when there is a lot of information showing it to be a problem for skin? The cosmetics industry knows that, emotionally and psychologically, most women prefer cosmetics that smell nice, even if the consumer says they want to avoid fragrance. When a cosmetics company produces products without fragrance, you will instead get the scent of the ingredients, which are not in the least as appealing as an added sweet, floral, or citrusy fragrance. This is why, in order to kill two marketing birds with one cosmetic stone, companies often list the fragrance components as essential oils or plant extracts rather than listing fragrance or perfume on the label. As lovely as essential oils sound, they are still nothing more than fragrance. So while you don't see the word "fragrance" on the list, and you may approvingly think wintergreen, lemon, cardamom, ylang-ylang, bergamot, rose, geranium, and many, many other fragrant plant oils sound pleasant and healthy, your skin won't be happy about it.

(Sources: *Chemical Research in Toxicology*, January 2008, pages 53–69; *British Journal of Dermatology*, August 2007, pages 295–300; *Contact Dermatitis*, July 2007, pages 1–10; *Journal of Infection and Chemotherapy*, December 2006, pages 349–354; *American Journal of Clinical Dermatology*, April 2003, pages 789–798; *Contact Dermatitis*, October 2001, pages 221–225; *American Journal of Contact Dermatitis*, June 1999, pages 310–315; and September 1998, pages 170–175.)

As for preservatives, they are impossible to avoid in water-based cosmetics because without them our skin-care products would become contaminated with mold, fungus, and bacteria and pose a serious problem for our skin in just a short period of time. However, you can and should stay away from cosmetics, particularly skin-care products, that contain fragrance. It smells nice, but fragrance serves no purpose for skin. Even fragrant ingredients that may also offer a positive benefit are easily replaced with ingredients that can perform the same function without the irritation aspect of the fragrant component. It sounds simple enough to avoid products with fragrance, perfume, or parfum by just reading the ingredient list and then not buying those products. But ingredient lists aren't always that easy to decipher.

The next time you admire the fragrant quality of a skin-care product you're about to apply to any part of your body or face, think twice. Similarly, aromatherapy shouldn't be a skin-care treatment, however therapeutic it is for the sense of smell and emotions. Fragrance might be nice for your spirits, but it is a health risk for skin. And it doesn't matter if the source of the fragrance is essential oils or plant extracts; as far as the health of your skin is concerned, they are all the same.

ALLERGIC REACTIONS

Allergic reactions are not the same thing as what happens when your skin is irritated. Almost anything can illicit an allergic reaction. On the skin, an allergic reaction to a substance can look nearly identical to an irritant reaction, but when it comes to what is going on beneath the surface of your skin it is a completely different reaction. How can you tell the difference when your skin is reacting because it is being irritated versus an allergic reaction? Generally, an allergic response includes persistent redness, itching, and some amount of swelling, causing skin to look more distended. For more information please see the chapter on Solutions for Allergy Prone Skin.

DIET, BEAUTY SUPPLEMENTS, AND WRINKLES

Up until a few years ago I would have said we know diet is important to the skin's health. After all when you don't eat, you die, and that looks particularly bad! But the research pinpointing what kind of diet works the best just wasn't there. That has changed, with research showing what aspects of your diet can fight wrinkles and possibly reduce your risk of skin cancer from the inside out. It all boils down to the theory of reducing inflammation because chronic inflammation prematurely ages the skin. In essence consuming an anti-inflammatory diet is one of the more beautiful things you can do for yourself.

Eating an anti-inflammatory diet has many health benefits, too many to list, but for the sake of this book it's all about the positives for skin. Think multicolor when you choose what to eat: the reds of peppers, apples, cranberries, pomegranates, and strawberries; greens from broccoli, kiwi, kale, green tea, and chilis; blues from blueberries; brown from cocoa and coffee (without sugar), and black from blackberries and black tea; coral from salmon; purple from grapes and purple-colored cabbage; and on and on. Include monounsaturated fats such as olive oil, nuts, and avocados; and sources of omega-3 fatty acids, which are present in cold-water fish such as wild Alaskan salmon, sardines, and anchovies, as well as walnuts and flaxseed. In addition, add a bit of flare to your meals with ginger, turmeric, curry, tamarind, cumin, and cardamon, all of which have potent anti-inflammatory properties.

In terms of taking antioxidant supplements for your general health or cancer prevention, the research is truly mixed. Some studies suggest that taking supplements is not helpful, especially a specific one for a specific problem. Others vehemently disagree, especially those in the vitamin supplement business—and then there are those who say the research isn't there to base an opinion on one way or the other. If anything, there is research suggesting that taking supplements may be problematic but no one is sure what that research means.

What does seem clear is that supplements alone do not make up in any way for an unhealthy diet. The claims for "Beauty supplements" that say they can enhance collagen production and fight wrinkles do not hold water; the research isn't there unless it's been paid for by the company selling the supplement. What you absolutely must know is that a pill of any kind doesn't alter the need for a complete, healthy diet. Always check with your doctor before adding any type of supplement to your diet.

(Sources: *Journal of Investigative Dermatology Symposium Proceedings*, 2008, pages 15–19; *Lipids in Health and Disease*, October 2008, page 36; *Nutrition and Cancer*, February 2008, pages 155–163; *The Journal of Nutrition*, September 2007, pages 2098–2105; *American Journal of Clinical Nutrition*, January 2007, pages 314S–317S; *Annals of Internal Medicine*, September 2006, pages 372–385; *Skinmed*, November–December 2004, pages 310–316; and *International Journal of Cosmetic Science*, December 2002, pages 331–339.)

Along with an anti-inflammatory diet, the best advice is to avoid environmental and emotional "irritations" and stress, and to use skin-care products that don't irritate skin. That can go a long way to prevent many of the pro-inflammatory elements you have to deal with so they don't accumulate and cause more damage.

CHAPTER 7
SUN SENSE AND SENSIBILITY

GETTING NAKED

Protecting skin from the sun has become an intense controversy for two major reasons. Reason number one is our basic need for vitamin D, which is produced by the skin's exposure to sun, meaning that it may be problematic to limit exposure. Reason number two concerns sunscreens and the types of active ingredients that are used to create an SPF (Sun Protecting Factor) rating for these products, some of which might have unwanted systemic consequences. I know, just when you thought you had the sun protection concept down solid a curve ball comes straight across home plate!

However, when it comes to skin, what is absolutely not in question and has not changed is one major yet basic fact: sun damage is by far the most significant cause of wrinkling, skin aging, and skin cancers. Aside from abundant research proving these damaging effects to be true, you can do your own research by taking a test. It's called the backside test of aging. In other words, just compare the areas of your body that rarely, if ever, see the sun with the parts of your body exposed to the sun on a daily basis. You will see that those areas that get minimal sun exposure (such as your backside, inside of your arm, breasts, middle back, and thighs) only very rarely appear dry, flaky, thin, show brown discolorations, have wrinkles, or any of the other signs of "aging." Meanwhile, skin chronically exposed to the sun without protection looks "older" than skin that hasn't been exposed to the sun or has been protected in some manner.

Of course this personal test only works if you are over the age of 30 because that is about the time the accumulated sun damage you've been getting from unprotected and prolonged sun exposure begins to show up. If you are under the age of 30, check out the skin of someone you know over the age of 40; the differences are always astounding. Those areas of the body that get the least amount of sun exposure have far more firmness, elasticity, even color, and the appearance of "younger" skin because they have not been subjected to years of cumulative exposure to sunlight. You can't fight wrinkles and not be exceedingly cautious and even downright neurotic about protecting your skin from the sun.

UNDERSTANDING UV

Before you can understand how to deal with the sun, it is helpful to know what exactly you are dealing with. Sun feels great, especially when you're outdoors and it's shining. But even on a cloudy day, when you can't see the sun, the sun's rays are ever present and ever attacking the skin. Basically, the sun's infrared rays (IR) do the important work of keeping us warm, and the visible rays provide daylight. At the same time, the sun's ultraviolet radiation (UVR) is also important, because its effects are serious for skin and eyes.

In essence, the UVR irradiation present in sunlight is an environmental human carcinogen on par with smoking and pollution. Unprotected exposure to the sun, or to sun lamps that duplicate the sun's effect on skin, is nothing less than toxic. Research on this topic is abundant and clear, particularly when it comes to the appearance of wrinkles, skin discolorations, dryness, flaky skin, immune system impairment, and skin cancer.

UVR is divided into three different bands: UVA, UVB, and UVC. Virtually all UVC radiation is filtered out by the atmosphere so that none actually reaches the earth's surface (although ozone depletion has some researchers worried about this one, too). In direct contrast to UVC, UVA rays reach the earth in significant amounts. UVB reaches the earth, too, though some of this radiation is filtered by the ozone. It is a testament to UVB's destructive effect on skin that even small amounts not blocked by the ozone layer can cause significant damage.

UVB radiation, the rays of the sun that cause sunburn, has a considerable capacity to cause instant skin damage. UVB damages the skin's genetic structure, causing mutations and abnormal growth patterns.

UVA are the silent rays of the sun. You don't feel them, but they are omnipresent and cause the skin's tanning response. As attractive as a tan looks, the free-radical damage that takes place at the same time and is generated by the UVA rays is insidious and relentless.

Even though UVB rays are much stronger than UVA radiation, UVA radiation is the larger danger for skin. That's because the earth is bombarded with about 100 times as much UVA as UVB radiation. So while UVA may be weaker compared to UVB, the amount present in the atmosphere still creates a potent impact on the skin.

What this adds up to is a huge headache for your skin. Looking younger without protecting yourself from the sun is simply impossible. UVA and UVB combined can cause skin cancer, cataracts, and other eye damage, and suppresses the body's (and skin's) immune system, stopping it from working properly. Unprotected or prolonged sun exposure, even with protection, causes the outer layer of skin to become thick, wrinkled, and discolored, while the lower layers of skin are slowly destroyed, causing thinning and more severe wrinkling. Capillaries near the suface of skin can become thinner, break, and become visible, especially on the cheeks, nose, and chin.

Pollution's effect on the ozone layer of the atmosphere, located many miles above the earth's surface, is serious business for many reasons, but this discussion is about what that means for skin. When intact, the ozone layer filters out much of the sun's UVB radiation, though it has relatively little effect on UVA. It is the sunburning UVB rays that increase when the ozone layer is eroded, which means more serious burns for those who dare to go outside without protection.

By the way, UVB rays can't get through glass, so there's no risk of sunburn when you sit in a car or next to a window, but that's the good news. The bad news is that UVA rays can get through windows. Normal glass doesn't protect skin from UVA damage, so sitting in a car or next to a window that lets daylight through offers no UVA protection whatsoever. (Sunglasses are very important, but I discuss that later in this chapter.)

(Sources: *Future Oncology*, December 2008, pages 841–856; *Journal of Pathology*, January 2007, 241–251; *Journal of Investigative Dermatology*, January 2002, pages 117–125;

Clinical Experimental Dermatology, October 2001, pages 573–577; *Journal of the American Academy of Dermatology*, July 2001, pages 610–618; *Experimental Gerontology*, May 2000, pages 307–316.)

SUNTANNING IS NOT PRETTY

There is no such thing as a safe tan from the sun or sun lamps. ALL tanning other than from a self-tanner is a problem. Actually, any and all unprotected sun exposure is damaging to skin. Most of us think sun damage occurs from baking in the sun and getting a deep, dark tan. That is only part of the picture. Sun damage begins the moment you walk out of the house, anytime during the day, whether it is sunny or cloudy (at least 40% to 50% of the sun's rays penetrate cloud cover). It may take 20 minutes for some of us to get burned, an hour or two for some of us to start tanning, but the damage associated with wrinkling and skin cancer begins the moment your skin is exposed to daylight. It is the repeated sun exposure, just several minutes a day, 365 days a year, *even when sitting near a sunny window* (UVA radiation comes through windows), that adds up to a great deal of damage, both aesthetically and physically.

Turning any shade that is darker than your own natural skin color from the sun, whether you have very light or very dark skin or use a sunscreen, is the skin's defensive response to sun damage. It may look nice, but it isn't nice for the skin. Melanocytes are skin cells that contain the brown-colored protein called melanin. These brown skin cells determine a person's natural skin tone. Surprisingly, the difference between the lightest skin color and the darkest is only a very small amount of melanin. With exposure to sun, the melanocytes produce more melanin, and tanned skin is the result. But here's another shock: Despite the fact that tanning is a protective response, it isn't all that helpful. By some estimates, a tan provides an SPF of only about 2. Sorry, there just isn't any way a tan of any kind can be considered healthy. As one dermatologist described it, a tan is the same as a callus on your foot. Yes, it protects the foot, but who wants that kind of protection and why would you continue doing what caused the callus in the first place?

The yellow and red melanin found in light-skinned people provides the least amount of sun protection while the brown melanin found in darker skin tones provides the most sun protection, which is why darker skin tones are less susceptable to skin cancers. But because melanin isn't a very reliable sunscreen overall, both dark- and light-skinned people need protection from UV rays because any tanning or burning causes skin damage to one degree or another. Those with darker skin color will still suffer negative effects from sun exposure. Ashen skin color, mottled skin, wrinkles, and even skin cancer can happen to those with dark skin. Skin cancer is less likely, but the risk of skin damage and wrinkling is certain.

(Sources: *Pigment Cell and Melanoma Research*, October 2008, pages 509–516; *Dermatologic Surgery*, April 2008, pages 460–474; *Photochemistry and Photobiology*, March–April 2008, pages 528–536; *Free Radical Biology and Medicine*, March 2008, pages 990–1000; *Skin Research and Technology*, November 2007, pages 360–368; *Pigment Cell Research*, August 2006, pages 303–314; and *Biological and Pharmaceutical Bulletin*, December 2005, pages 2302–2307.)

SUNSCREEN: ANTI-AGING FRIEND OR FOE?

Just when it seems the message about sunscreen's importance as part of a person's daily routine has been widely accepted, along comes more scary information that has consumers wondering whether their sunscreens are as bad for skin as the sun itself. An article questioning sunscreens appeared in an issue of the fashion magazine *Allure*. To *Allure*'s credit, the article was balanced. Its summation was that you shouldn't skip sunscreen: it does far more good than harm, and the harm doesn't equate to the fear lots of people feel when they don't know the whole story. Funny, that's a lot like many things in life isn't it? Our fears and reactions come from a one-sided piece of information.

The article in *Allure* centered on a study published in the October 2006 issue of *Free Radical Biology & Medicine*. The study found that while sunscreens can protect skin from the free-radical damage sunlight causes, in a short amount of time it causes free-radical damage on its own. Of course, the big question is: are we trading free-radical protection for free-radical damage, thus canceling out the importance of applying sunscreen?

Lots of doctors and researchers took issue with the results of the study for several reasons: it wasn't done double-blind, it wasn't conducted on people, the results haven't been duplicated by other studies, and the study didn't use commercial sunscreen products, just individual active sunscreen ingredients. That last point is important because as any cosmetics chemist will tell you, how a sunscreen is formulated has a significant impact on how the active ingredients function on skin (from spreading and adhering properly to their stability). Testing individual sunscreen ingredients and extrapolating the results to apply to regular sunscreen formulas is like tasting individual ingredients used to make a cake instead of the finished product and then being surprised that the flour doesn't taste sweet.

On the flipside, other studies have shown the protective effect of certain sunscreen actives against free-radical formation—and a growing body of research is demonstrating that adding antioxidants to sunscreens offsets the negative effect sunscreen can have on skin, especially if it is not reapplied at regular intervals during long periods of sun exposure.

Well-known dermatologist Dr. Leslie Baumann was quoted in the *Allure* article as agreeing with the questionable study. She stated, "We've actually been talking about this for a couple of years." Dr. Sheldon Pinnell of Skinceuticals fame also weighed in, stating "It's known that some sunscreens behave in this manner. They get inside the skin and absorb energy, and that energy becomes free radicals...." Lots of dermatologists would disagree with Pinnell's assertion, and even Pinnell believes that any free-radical damage sunscreen may cause (including by virtue of how the active ingredients work) is counteracted by antioxidants, whether in your sunscreen or in other skin-care products you apply. So as it turns out, there really isn't cause for concern.

The only thing that is crystal-clear about the *Free Radical Biology & Medicine* study is that more research is needed to determine whether sunscreen actives as formulated in consumer sunscreens cause measurable free-radical damage on intact human skin. Until conclusive information is available, it is not a wise decision to stop using sunscreen due to fear of free-radical damage. Even if some sunscreen actives do cause free-radical damage, we know it can be offset by antioxidants. We also know that going without sunscreen exposes skin to a long list of problems, the least of those being free-radical damage!

I'll close this topic with a quote in the *Allure* article from Amy Lewis, assistant Clinical Professor of Dermatology at Yale School of Medicine: "Right now we have one small, inconclusive study versus huge amounts of data that show that lack of sun protection causes DNA damage, melanoma, basal-cell and squamous-cell skin cancer, and horrible deformed moles and wrinkles, and there is great evidence for prolonged use of sunscreen to protect against all of those things. If these chemicals cause something, the sun exposure you're trading it for is going to cause *more* free radicals." I couldn't have said it better myself!

VITAMIN D AND SUN

One of the controversies surrounding sun exposure that has cropped up over the past few years is the issue of vitamin D deficiency. Sunlight is the primary source of vitamin D, and vitamin D deficiencies can be a serious health problem. As luck would have it, sunlight is the most abundant, natural source that helps our bodies.

DOES SUNSCREEN INHIBIT VITAMIN D PRODUCTION?

Some people worry that if they use sunscreen it will cancel out their body's ability to absorb vitamin D from the sun. Here, the controversy is between those who feel that exposing our skin to the sun without sunscreen is dangerous, versus those who believe that sunscreen will cancel out the body's ability to manufacture vitamin D from sun exposure. This concern over sunscreen has been expressed in the pages of several reputable resources. (Sources: *Photochemistry and Photobiology*, March–April 2007, pages 459–463; *American Journal of Clinical Nutrition*, December 2004, pages S1678–1688S; and *Archives of Dermatology*, December 1988, pages 1802–1804.)

There are mixed opinions on this one (I know, it's always complicated). Regarding this issue, a June 1999 article in *Cosmetic Dermatology* (page 43) discussed a presentation given by Mark Naylor, MD, assistant professor in the Department of Dermatology at the University of Oklahoma, which described some research on use of sunscreen: "Prospective sunscreen trials examining whether sunscreen contributes to vitamin D deficiency found that regular sunscreen users were not vitamin D deficient." Other research has echoed that assertion. (Source: *Journal of Photochemistry and Photobiology*, December 2007, pages 139–147.)

There is also the issue that no sunscreen, regardless of its active ingredients or how often or liberally it is applied, can provide 100% protection from UV radiation. The tiny amount of UVB light that sunscreens do not shield us from is enough to begin the synthesis of vitamin D, although—depending on your skin color, environment (how much daily sunshine is there), and climate—supplemental vitamin D will likely still be necessary.

There is no question that we need vitamin D, either from the sun or supplementation, because research has found a large percentage of the population is deficient in vitamin D, especially as we age. If skin wrinkles, premature aging of the skin, and skin cancers are an issue for you, then the answer is clear: you need to do both—diligently protect your skin from the sun and take a vitamin D supplement.

(Additional sources for the above: *The Journal of the American Osteopathic Association*, August 2003, pages 3–4; *American Journal of Clinical Dermatology*, March 2002, pages 185–191; *Dermatology*, January 2001, pages 27–30; *British Medical Journal*, October 1999, page 1066; and *Archives of Dermatology*, April 1005, pages 415–421).

Note: Before beginning any new vitamin supplement program, make sure to consult your physician.

SUNTANNING MACHINES

Capitalizing on the controversy around vitamin D and the sun are tanning-bed salons and a lobbying group supporting the billion-dollar tanning-bed industry. Now they feel they have a legitimate reason to encourage you to spend money absorbing UV radiation from their machines, or at least that's the claim they proudly promote. Yet according to the FDA, the FCC (Federal Communications Commission), the American Academy of Dermatology, the Skin Cancer Foundation, and many other medical and regulatory sources worldwide, suntanning machines are nothing more than skin cancer machines, and should be made illegal. The research for this is startling.

Suntanning machines radiate the most damaging effects of the sun only inches away from your body, and, worse, they are available day after day, month after month, in areas of the country where you would not normally see the sun on a daily basis. In addition, they allow exposure of body parts that are usually covered. They pose the same serious risk of skin cancer that unprotected exposure to the sun allows, only more so—by intensifying the actual amount of UVA and/or UVB radiation the skin receives. (Sources: *Dermatological Surgery*, April 2008, 460–474; *International Journal of Dermatology*, December 2007, pages 1253–1257; *Journal of the American Academy of Dermatology*, December 2005, pages 1038–1044; and *Journal of the American Academy of Dermatology*, May 2001, pages 775–780.)

Many studies have found that people who used tanning beds have significantly higher rates of melanoma than those who don't (Sources: *British Journal of Dermatology*, July 2007, pages 215–216, and *Cancer Epidemiology, Biomarkers, and Prevention*, March 2005, pages 562–566). But there is also research that tanning beds do not pose an increased risk of melanoma (Source: *Cancer Causes and Control*, September 2008, pages 659–669). Whether or not there is an increased risk of melanoma, there is a 100% increase in other problems that are dire for the health and appearance of your skin.

As the battle ensues over whether or not tanning beds help reduce vitamin D deficiency or increase the risk of melanoma, it leaves the consumer confused and frustrated with what they should do. It is important to realize that most experts worldwide believe tanning beds should be made illegal. In essence, the key point in the conflicting information is the issue of melanoma. Tanning beds may be a source of vitamin D, but so are vitamin D supplements and those are far cheaper and don't pose a risk of skin cancer. What often gets left out of the debate is the overwhelming information and research about other types of substantial damage to skin that take place when men and women use tanning machines. Whether it's in terms of wrinkles, DNA mutations, thinning skin, immune suppression, or other types of skin cancers (squamous and basal cell), the evidence of damage is undeniable. (Sources: *British Journal of Dermatology*, June 2008, pages 128–133; *Photochemistry and Photobiology Science*, May 2006, pages 160–164; *Journal of the American Osteopathic Association*, August 2003, pages 371–375; *Journal of the National Cancer Institute*, February 2002, page 155; and the World Health Organization publication *Tanning Sunbeds, Risk and Guidance*; 2003.)

Indoor tanning salons have grown significantly in popularity during recent years and the number of people using them has grown as well. It is a multi-billion dollar industry. Despite the potential dangers of these devices, federal regulations have struggled to place minimal restrictions on the labeling of indoor tanning lamps. Indoor tanning salons work vigorously to dispel notions of any link to skin cancer, often falsely promoting various health benefits of indoor tanning. The first lawsuit for injuries resulting from indoor tanning was recently filed against an indoor tanning salon, and other such litigation is poised to follow. Much like the court cases that have found liability in the context of cigarettes, cases like this, which identify similarities between the indoor tanning and cigarette industries, can be one way to make a statement regulatory boards can't (or won't) do (Source: *Michigan Law Review*, November 2008, pages 365–390).

CAN SUNSCREEN AFFECT SKIN NEGATIVELY?

If you thought the dispute about vitamin D was complicated, the controversy about ingredients in sunscreens just takes it beyond the pale. Let me state clearly from the beginning that I am as frustrated by the conflicting research as anyone. We know sun damages skin but what are we to do if sunscreen ingredients pose the same problem or worse? The sunscreens under scrutiny include almost all of the synthetic sunscreen ingredients used in SPF products, such as octylmethoxy cinnamate, 4-methylbenzylidene camphor, phenylbenzimidazole, sulphonic acid, and 2-phenylbenzimidazole, padimate-O, homosalate, oxybenzone, avobenzone, butyl methoxydibenzylmethane, benzophone-3, and Mexoryl.

Many of these ingredients are in question because they have the ability to enter the bloodstream and disrupt the endocrine system, which regulates the releases of hormones into the body, or cause cell mutation in vitro. Synthetic sunscreen ingredients can often mimic estrogen, and so the question is how does that affect systems in the body?

Ironically, the endocrine-disrupting potencies of sunscreen ingredients "are several orders of magnitude lower than that of the natural estrogens" (Source: *Environment International*, July 2007, pages 654–669). Other human endocrine-disrupting sources have a plant origin, such as marijuana (Source: *Toxicology*, January 2005, pages 471–488), or are found in medicines such as acetaminophen (Tylenol) (Source: *Water Research*, November 2008, pages 4578–4588).

Another potential detriment for synthetic sunscreen ingredients is that, upon absorption, these can generate free-radical damage. Synthetic sunscreen ingredients interact with the very light they are meant to direct away from skin cells. Several published studies show oxidative damage in vitro from various sunscreen ingredients. But on the other hand, sunscreen also reacts with the UV radiation and traps it, mitigating harmful effects. Some scientists argue that it is just by this trapping of radicals that synthetic sunscreen ingredients offer their protection.

What's a person to do? Good question, though regrettably there isn't an easy answer.

In truth, all synthetic sunscreen agents, even nano-particled titanium dioxide and zinc oxide, have some intimidating negative research about their potential effects on skin. These aren't junk science articles either—they are all from very notable publications involving both in vivo and in vitro experiments, and include reports in such well-respected journals as *The Lancet, Journal of Investigative Dermatology*, and *Mutation Research*. Rather than elaborate on each specific paper (which would take pages and pages), let me sum up the major issues.

Some in vitro studies have indicated that there is a possibility that certain sunscreen ingredients can be absorbed into skin, and there are a handful of in vivo studies as well. However, there are still many researchers who believe that most sunscreen ingredients stay on the surface of skin (where skin cells are dead) and do not penetrate into the lower layers of skin where the real damage occurs. If that's the case, it means the negative effects seen for surface skin in test tube studies may be irrelevant. Even when absorption has been shown, the related risk has not been demonstrated.

All these issues are significant and deserve more research, but none of the findings indicate that anyone should give up using sunscreen or that the presence of these substances is causing problems. Besides, it is important to realize that no one sunscreen ingredient stands out as more of a potential risk than any other. Finally, it is imperative to recognize what a massive amount of research does show: That not wearing sunscreen, as well as prolonged sun exposure, are both related to lots of serious skin problems.

(Sources: *Aquatic Toxicology*, November 2008, pages 182–187; *American Journal of Clinical Nutrition*, August 2008, pages 570S–577S; *Environmental Health Perspectives*, July 2008, pages 893–897; *Journal of the American Academy of Dermatology*, May 2008, pages S155–S159; *Journal of the European Academy of Dermatology and Venereology*, April 2008, pages 456–461; *International Journal of Andrology*, April 2008, pages 144–151; *Toxicology*, July 2007, pages 140–148; *Advanced Drug Delivery Reviews*, July 2007, pages 522–530; *Critical Reviews in Toxicology*, March 2007, pages 251–277; 2007 *CIR Compendium, Cosmetic Ingredient Review*, 2007, pages 37–38; www.cosmeticinfo.org; *Current Drug Delivery*, October 2006, pages 405–415; *Toxicology In Vitri*, April 2006, 301–307; *Toxicological Sciences*, April 2006, pages 349–361; *Skin Pharmacology and Physiology*, July–August 2005, pages 170–174; *Toxicology*, December 2004, pages 123–130; *Journal of Controlled Release*, June 2002, pages 225–233; November 2002, pages S131–S155; http://ec.europa.eu/health/ph_risk/committees/sccp/docshtml/sccp_out145_en.htm; and *Encyclopedia of Pharmaceutical Technology*, Second Edition, Volume 1, page 519.)

TITANIUM DIOXIDE AND ZINC OXIDE

Titanium dioxide and zinc oxide are often referred to as "nonchemical" sunscreen ingredients, but this is misleading at best. All ingredients used in skin-care products are chemicals and have a direct impact on skin. What these two substances do have in common is that they are inert minerals used as sunscreen ingredients. They also have minimal to no risk of causing an allergic reaction, and are considered by most researchers to be benign and safe for skin; they also protect skin from a good portion of the UVA spectrum. Both their minimal risk of irritation and their ability to protect skin from most of the sun's rays makes them a great choice to consider.

One drawback these two ingredients share is that when they are present in concentrations large enough to impart an SPF 15 without out any other sunscreen ingredient, they tend to leave a white look on the skin. Ingredient manufacturers are working to make better, microfined versions of titanium dioxide and zinc oxide to help reduce or eliminate this problem. There are also versions of titanium dioxide and zinc oxide that are broken down via nanotechnology, and these leave a far less noticeable white appearance on skin. While that option would be great, there are those who consider any ingredient reduced in size by nanotechnology seriously problematic for skin. (See the "Nanotechnology" section in this book for more information on this subject.) Though controversial, there is no evidence that nanoparticled titanium dioxide or zinc oxide is a health risk for skin. In many ways these two sunscreen agents are about as good as it gets in terms of protection and gentleness on the skin.

(Sources: *Skin Pharmacology and Physiology*, June 2008, pages 136–149; *Pharmazie*, January 2008, pages 58–60; *British Journal of Dermatology*, November 2001, pages 789–794, and *Lasers in Surgery and Medicine*, September 2001, pages 252–259.)

SUN STRATEGY

Whether or not you decide to protect your skin from the sun with sunscreen is a personal decision. Given the controversies surrounding sunscreen ingredients (including nano-sized titanium dioxide and zinc oxide) and vitamin D deficiencies, it is not automatically a slam-dunk decision. Nonetheless, what is 100% certain is that not using sunscreen on a daily, regimented basis, and combining that with prolonged exposure to the sun, getting a tan or sunburn, and using tanning machines (with or without sun protection) damages the skin, causes premature wrinkles, some forms of skin cancer, skin discolorations, loss of elasticity, and suppression of the immune system. Using sunscreen, wearing sun-protective clothing, and avoiding prolonged, direct sun exposure is the only way to reduce that inevitable fate for your skin. For me, that is enough to make a compelling argument for wearing sunscreen and being sun smart. No one but you can protect your skin from the sun. (Source: *Journal of the American Academy of Dermatology*, May 2008, pages S149–S154.)

So the decision is yours. I am still going to encourage sun protection and sun avoidance along with vitamin D supplementation because these are by far the best anti-wrinkle, anti-aging miracle we have in the world of skin care. Everything else is an afterthought, and potentially helpful, yet no other options will nullify or alter the ravages of the sun. The following information in this chapter is to help you make decisions about what to use, when to use it, and how to use it.

> *Skin damage from the sun begins within the first minute*
> *your skin is exposed to sunlight.*

WHAT ABOUT SPF?

A sunscreen's SPF rating is incredibly important, but it is not the only guide when you are buying sunscreens. All the SPF number lets you know is how long you can stay in the sun without burning while wearing that product. For example, let's say you're like me and you can stay in the sun for about 15 minutes before your skin starts to turn pink. Applying a sunscreen rated SPF 15 will allow you to stay in the sun 15 times longer (three and three-quarters hours: 15 times 15 minutes) without getting pink. In other words, the SPF number, 15 in this case, multiplied by the amount of time you can normally stay in the sun without getting pink, is how long you can stay in the sun after you've applied the sunscreen. If you normally can stay in the sun 25 minutes without getting pink, applying an SPF 15 sunscreen would let you stay in the sun six and one-quarter hours (15 times 25 equals 375 minutes) without burning.

UVA VERSUS UVB

It's vital to know that the SPF rating refers only to protection from UVB radiation. The European Union has adopted a UVA rating system, but it is controversial and has not yet been adopted in other parts of the globe. The FDA is working on one but there is no telling when that will be done, and England and Japan have a separate system all to themselves. What this adds up to is that no one quite agrees on how to measure UVA protection. As this book goes to press, there is no way to judge the UVA protection in a skin-care product with sunscreen unless you check the ingredient listing. However, only a handful of ingredients can protect skin from the UVA spectrum. So that SPF 15, SPF 30, or SPF 70 sunscreen must absolutely contain the UVA-protecting ingredients of either titanium dioxide, zinc oxide, avobenzone (also called butyl methoxydibenzyl methane), Tinosorb, or ecamsule (Mexoryl), or you will not be getting the best protection. And your skin deserves the best!

APPLYING SUNSCREEN: HOW MUCH, WHEN, AND WHERE

Now that so many products contain sunscreen (foundation, concealers, moisturizers, and even face powders), the next question is, What about application? That's a great question! The major issue for the use of any well-formulated sunscreen (SPF 15 or greater with UVA-protecting ingredients) is liberal application. Why? Because protection is determined not only by the SPF number and the UVA ingredients the product contains, but also by how thick and evenly it is applied, and when, where, and how often the sunscreen is reapplied. But studies show there is a mismatch between the expectations versus the reality of actual use. (Sources: *Lancet*, August 11, 2007, pages 528–537; and *Journal of Photochemistry and Photobiology*, November 2001, pages 105–108.)

Research indicates sunscreen users are only applying 50% of the recommended amount, so they are only receiving 50% of the SPF protection. And that means expensive sunscreen may be dangerous to your skin's health. After all, how likely are you to liberally apply an expensive sunscreen? Not applying sunscreen liberally can negate any benefit you may assume you are getting from the SPF number on the label.

You may have seen recommendations that you should apply sunscreen 20 minutes before you go outside and then again 20 minutes later or whenever you get to where you are going. This is all about the issue of application. Because research has made it clear we aren't wearing enough of the stuff, dermatologists have recommended these use options to get us to comply, and really put on enough to take great care of our skin.

Keep in mind that everyday liberal application, applied 20 minutes before you step outside (not once you get to the car, or get to the beach, or do anything—but before you leave the house) is the key element in getting the best protection possible. But within your skin-care routine, exactly when does sunscreen get applied? If you are applying several skin-care products, ranging from toners to acne medications to moisturizers, the rule is that the last item you apply during the day is your sunscreen. If you apply sunscreen and then apply, say, your moisturizer or an acne product, you could inadvertently be diluting or breaking down the effectiveness of the sunscreen you've just applied.

Any skin-care product, or even just water (and almost all moisturizers are more than 50% water), applied over a sunscreen reduces its effectiveness to one degree or another. This is why you have to reapply sunscreen after swimming or perspiring. If you use moisturizers, which are always lipid soluble, over your sunscreen these will break down the sunscreen via dilution or removal, and that is a serious problem. What about applying foundation (one that doesn't contain sunscreen) over the sunscreen you've just applied? That depends on several more factors, such as how much you apply, how thick or oily it is, or what kind of sunscreen you are using. To eliminate any dilution and to add more protection, you can choose to wear a foundation during the day that contains sunscreen. Voila, no more worries.

If you are using more than one product containing sunscreen, such as an SPF 15 moisturizer and an SPF 8 foundation, it is important to understand that does not add up to an SPF of 23. You would get some increased SPF protective value, but there is no way to know what amount of increased protection that would be. If you want to get the protection of SPF 30, then that is the SPF number you should look for. If you are mixing SPF products, both must contain UVA-protecting ingredients.

What if your foundation is the product you've chosen for sun protection? Then the trick is to be sure you've applied it evenly and liberally. If you apply it too thinly or blend most of it off instead of using it full-depth, you would not get the amount of protection listed on the label.

I am concerned about the pressed powders with sunscreen. Although I don't doubt the validity of these product's SPF ratings, I worry that most women do not apply pressed-powder foundations liberally enough to get the amount of protection stated on the label.

If you lightly dust the powder over the skin there is no way you will get the SPF protection the label indicates. You must be sure you apply the pressed powder in a manner that completely and evenly covers the face. I believe that pressed powders are an iffy way to get sun protection for the face, but they *are* a great way to touch up your makeup during the day and reapply more sunscreen at the same time.

A few more important facts:

- Even on a cloudy day the sun's rays are ever-present and ever attacking the skin.
- Sitting in the shade or wearing a hat protects you only from a small portion of the sun's rays. Plus, other surrounding surfaces such as water, snow, cement, and grass reflect the rays up from the ground to your skin, giving you a double whammy of damage.
- Altitude is a sun enhancer; for every 1,000-foot increase in altitude, the sun's potency increases by 4%.

Time of day does matter. All UV radiation is strongest between 10 A.M. and 2 P.M. Clouds filter some, but not most, of the UVR, which is why you are still likely to get burned on an overcast day, and the UVA rays are still strongly present, too.

WATER RESISTANT NOT WATERPROOF

In 2002, the FDA issued regulations regarding sunscreen that require companies to eliminate the use of the word "waterproof" as a valid claim. In truth, no sunscreen can be waterproof because it must be reapplied if you have been sweating or immersed in water for a period of time. The only approved terms for use on sunscreens, reflecting studies that prove they have limited ability to stay in place when people are in water or sweating, are "water-resistant" or "very water-resistant." A product that is water-resistant means the label's SPF value has been measured after application and 40 minutes of water immersion; it must keep the same SPF value to use the term water-resistant. A very water-resistant product means the SPF value on the label must remain intact after 80 minutes of water immersion.

If you are swimming or sweating, you absolutely should use a sunscreen that's labeled water resistant or very water-resistant. Water-resistant sunscreens are formulated quite differently from regular sunscreens so pay attention to the label: if it doesn't say water resistant, don't use it for exercise or swimming. (Source: *Photodermatology, Photoimmunology, and Photomedicine*, December 2008, pages 296–300.)

For normal wear, I do not recommend daily application of water-resistant sunscreens. The acrylate-type ingredients that help keep sunscreens on when swimming or sweating also make them somewhat tacky or sticky under makeup. For regular application, when you aren't exercising outside or taking a dip, a regular sunscreen with SPF 15 and good UVA protection is the best choice.

SUNBURN

Most of us know about what it feels like to get a sunburn. Spending even a short time in the sun can be all it takes to get a serious, painful burn. Sunburn is an actual radiation burn of your skin. The ultraviolet light from the sun damages the DNA of your skin cells, causing apoptosis, which then triggers release of pro-inflammatory chemicals in your skin called cytokines, leading in turn to redness, swelling, and pain. Even if you get out of the sun once your skin starts turning pink, the sunburn continues to develop for 12 to 24 hours after the initial damage takes place.

It goes without saying that it would be best if we all knew enough to take care of our skin and never get a sunburn, or tan for that matter, but that isn't realistic. So knowing how to take care of sunburn is essential, both to keep from making the problem worse and to help skin heal.

All burns need to be cooled to dissipate the heat simmering in the lower layers of skin and to reduce the resulting inflammation.

If your burn is serious or extremely painful, do not hesitate to find the nearest hospital emergency room. Heat trauma from sunburn can be a serious threat to your health.

Do not cover the burn with thick salves or ointments (butter is the worst). That will trap the heat and cause more damage.

Get the skin in contact with cool compresses immediately, but do not put ice directly on the skin—that's too cold and can cause a different kind of burn. Then keep applying cool compresses on and off for several hours.

You can put pure aloe vera gel in your refrigerator and then apply that to skin. Aloe is helpful but not for the exaggerated reasons the cosmetics industry tells you. Aloe vera is nonocclusive and has some anti-inflammatory benefits that are very helpful for sunburned skin, and is far, far better than applying occlusive or overly fragrant moisturizers, which can impede healing—though Aloe vera is not a miracle plant, but it has its positive traits.

Do not soak the skin with water. Do not immerse yourself in a tub of water or shower for a long period of time. Too much water in the skin inhibits the skin's healing response. (Source: *Journal of Investigative Dermatology*, May 2003, pages 750–758.)

It may also be an option to take ibuprofen as an anti-inflammatory.

SUN RISK FROM USING AHAS, BHA, OR TRETINOIN?

The major signs of sun-damaged skin are that the outer layer of skin becomes thickened, wrinkled, and brown in patches. To some extent that does serve as protection, but it isn't very good protection (it barely rates an SPF 2 or 4), nor is it very attractive! Both AHAs and BHA can help remove some of that thickened, wrinkled exterior—AHAs and BHA because they exfoliate the built-up damaged surface layer of skin, and tretinoin or products containing it because they change abnormal cell production back to some level of normalcy. That change to the exterior of the skin does leave it more vulnerable to the effects of sun exposure. Yet it is far better to improve the appearance of damaged skin by removing that layer than it is to leave it in place for inadequate and unattractive sun protection. After all, it isn't the AHAs or the tretinoin that cause the skin to be more sensitive to sunlight. All they do is remove the old, sun-damaged skin, allowing healthier "younger" skin to be on the surface. Sunscreen is always important, always, but it becomes even more essential to protect the fresh skin cells you are revealing if you are using AHAs or tretinoin on a regular basis.

WHY YOU MAY STILL GET TAN WHEN USING SUNSCREEN

There are many reasons why you may still be getting some tan despite diligent use of sunscreen. One likely cause is the fact that even the best of sunscreens still let some sun rays through. A high SPF number is not about better or deeper protection, but only longer protection—an SPF 30 means you can stay in the sun 30 times longer than it would normally take you to get a slight burn. For most skin types that would provide over 18 hours of sun exposure without getting sunburned. That's impressive, but it is also only a measure of the length of time the protection lasts.

High SPF numbers give the false impression they can provide enhanced protection when that is not the case. A well-formulated sunscreen with an SPF 30 still only protects your skin from about 97% to 98% of the sun's rays. That means 2% to 3% of the sun's rays are still getting through, and that can trigger melanin production, the skin's tanning response. This is especially true for those with darker skin tones or for those who have a lot of previous sun damage, because for them hypermelanin production is more likely to take place.

Here is a chart to give you an idea of the numbers:

SPF 2	50% UV protection
SPF 4	70% UV protection
SPF 8	88% UV protection
SPF 15	94% UV protection
SPF 30	97% UV protection
SPF 50	98% UV protection
SPF 70	98% UV protection

Further, most people misunderstand or have poor information about how to get the best sun protection. Please review the "Applying Sunscreen" and "Sun Strategy" sections in this chapter. It is essential to apply sunscreen liberally and to be sure that the active ingredients on the label include one of the UVA-protecting ingredients: avobenzone, butyl methoxy-dibenzylmethane, Tinosorb, ecamsule (Mexoryl), titanium dioxide, or zinc oxide.

HOW HIGH SHOULD YOU GO?

If SPF 70 doesn't give you significantly better protection (as seen from the chart above), why do many dermatologists recommend using higher SPF numbers then necessary? After all, we know that an SPF 70 can give about 700 minutes of protection (assuming you aren't swimming or sweating) and that even in Alaska during the summer solstice you are not going to get that much exposure to the sun. The answer has to do with application. Because most consumers don't apply sunscreen liberally, they aren't getting optimal protection, or even half of what the label indicates. A higher SPF number means there have to be more sun-protecting ingredients in the product so that even if you don't apply it liberally you would be depositing more sunscreen ingredients on the skin. It is a logical approach with a caveat: More sunscreen ingredients can prove to be more irritating, especially for the face.

SPF-RATED CLOTHING

After you've dressed in the morning and because you take great care of your skin, you apply a well-formulated sunscreen to the areas of your body that will be exposed to the sun. You are confident that the parts of your body covered by clothing are protected from the sun and therefore don't need sunscreen. Think again. Just because some of your body is under wraps doesn't mean it is protected from sun damage. While clothing can be an excellent form of sun protection, if the fabric is sheer, lightweight, or has any transparency (meaning it lets daylight through) it also lets the sun's damaging rays through. "The most important determinant is tightness of the weave. Fabric type is less important. Thickness is also less important than regular weave. Protection drops significantly when the fabric becomes wet. Color plays a minor role with dark colors protecting [slightly] better than light colors. A crude test of clothing is to hold it up to visible light and observing penetration. The FDA defines clothing with an SPF rating as a medical device. One approved line of clothing with a SPF 30 or greater rating is Solumbra" (1-800-882-7860) (Source: *eMedicine Journal*, July 31, 2001, volume 2, number 7; and www.fda.gov).

Sun damage is not to be taken lightly, and lightweight clothing can be a problem. When in doubt, apply sunscreen all over and then get dressed.

HOW LONG DO SUNSCREENS LAST?

How long does sunscreen last in the container? Should you throw it away after a year or two if you haven't used all of it? Sunscreens don't last forever, on your skin or in the bottle. The FDA considers sunscreens to be over-the-counter (OTC) drugs, meaning they are subject to much more stringent guidelines and regulations than cosmetics. According to the FDA's OTC regulations, sunscreens should be stamped with an expiration date if they have less than three years of acceptable stability testing. If they do have three years' worth of acceptable stability testing they do not need to be stamped with an expiration date. That confusing bit of legislation makes the expiration date almost impossible for the consumer to understand. In the long run, you will do best to look for a sunscreen product that is stamped with an expiration date so you know how long it has been on the shelf, although those without expiration dates are not a problem in terms of meeting FDA guidelines.

SUN PROTECTION FOR DIFFERENT SKIN TYPES

Many cosmetics lines sell an endless array of cleansers, toners, anti-wrinkle treatments, eye creams, throat creams, face creams, and facial masks yet never mention the indispensable need for regular, consistent use of a sunscreen. Almost every line does have "sun-care" products, but they are often promoted separately from the "daily care" routines. I've personally spoken to hundreds and hundreds of cosmetics salespeople about their products and repeatedly found a gross lack of information about sun protection. I'm always told how important moisturizers, eye creams, serums, toners, cleansers, and eye-makeup removers are, but almost never do I hear about the value of daily sunscreen use.

There are indeed many ways to get good sun protection, regardless of your other skin-care needs. This is so important that I consider it unconscionable to discuss any skin-care routines, skin-care problems, or skin-care concerns without also including a discussion of sun protection. If you've been intrigued by a new miracle skin-care line, but a sunscreen is not mentioned, that company clearly does not take skin care seriously or ethically. You should not be wasting your money and hurting your skin by considering a company that would ignore such a vital component of healthy skin care.

Now that you understand the importance of using sunscreen on a daily basis, finding the right product is not easy. Perhaps the trickiest part of sunscreen use is finding one that doesn't cause problems, particularly if you have normal to oily skin, acne-prone skin, or sensitive skin. Active sunscreen agents including avobenzone, benzophenones, octyl methoxycinnamate, oxybenzone, padimate O, and many others can cause irritation on the skin, creating patches of dryness, itching, rashlike breakouts, redness, and swelling. Because these particular sunscreen agents can be potentially irritating, many dermatologists feel that titanium dioxide and zinc oxide are the best sunscreen ingredients, since they are practically benign on the skin and are excellent screens for both UVA and UVB radiation. I wish the subject could end here and I could unequivocally recommend titanium dioxide and zinc oxide as the only sunscreen ingredients to look for, but that isn't the case. As safe and effective as titanium dioxide and zinc oxide are they can be occlusive, meaning they can block and clog pores.

The issue for any ingredient that can cause breakouts is threefold: how occlusive it is (meaning blocking oil flow out of the pores), how irritating it is on the skin (perhaps causing rashlike breakouts), and how much the ingredient duplicates what the pore already produces, adding more fuel to the fire. Titanium dioxide and zinc oxide pose the first problem for skin. Are you guaranteed to break out if you use a sunscreen with titanium dioxide? Absolutely not, but it is a possibility. Everyone's skin reacts differently to any and all cosmetic ingredients. One other issue with a sunscreen that uses only titanium dioxide and/or zinc oxide as the active ingredient is a cosmetic one, as these products tend to leave a white appearance and can feel somewhat heavy on the skin. That can be a problem for all skin types. In response to that shortcoming, many sunscreen products combine titanium dioxide with other sunscreen agents, which reduce the amount of potentially irritating ingredients while also decreasing some of titanium dioxide's occlusive tendency.

SUNSCREENS FOR OILY SKIN

The search for a sunscreen that is appropriate for oily skin can be a frustrating, lifelong pursuit. Even those I've created for my line can pose problems for some people. There are difficulties of several kinds. First, the types of ingredients that can be used to suspend sunscreen agents are not exactly the best for oily skin. Regardless of the claim on the label, there are risks that the base formulation can clog pores or feel slippery or greasy on the skin. There's also the problem that the sunscreen ingredients themselves can cause an irritated breakout reaction, a response to the synthetically derived sunscreen agents. (Regrettably, that is the nature of almost all active ingredients used in cosmetics—"active" meaning they actually do something on the skin. Whether they are AHAs, Renova, benzoyl peroxide, hydroquinone, or sunscreen ingredients, if they work, they can be irritating.) In the case of titanium dioxide and zinc oxide, even though they are relatively innocuous and have minimal to no risk of irritation on skin, they can still clog pores, being the thick and occulsive ingredients that they are. Finally, given the wide variety in formulations, there is no way to quantify which ingredients are more problematic than others for causing problems. What's my advice? The only true answer is to experiment. I wish there was a slam-dunk solution I could offer, but there are no product lines that can legitimately make the claim that their sunscreen won't cause breakouts (and those of you with this problem already know that).

For oily skin, or any skin type for that matter, wearing a foundation with a high SPF is an excellent idea, particularly for women with oily skin who don't want to wear layers of skin-care products. This is also an option for women who are just tired of wearing layers and layers of skin-care products and makeup. Luckily, there are now many well-formulated foundations and tinted moisturizers with good SPF numbers containing avobenzone, titanium dioxide, or zinc oxide (with the latter two being far more common than foundations with avobenzone). The one negative about using a foundation with sunscreen is that you need to apply it generously; thin, sheer applications don't work. Plus, as the foundation shifts during the day it is essential to touch it up with a pressed powder containing an SPF 15 that includes the UVA-protecting ingredients of avobenzone, titanium dioxide, or zinc oxide.

If you wear a foundation with a good SPF you might forget to use a sunscreen on your hands, neck, throat, chest, or any other area of your body that is exposed to the sun on a daily basis. If so, those brown "age spots" and crepy skin texture are related to sun damage. Like wrinkling on the face, wrinkling on the rest of the body can't be mitigated without daily use of sunscreen, and that means reapplying your sunscreen every time you wash your hands and taking care to put sunscreen on any exposed parts of your body, day in and day out.

FOR THE LITTLE ONES

When choosing a sunscreen for your child it is always best to follow the advice of your pediatrician. It is very easy to be enticed to buy sunscreen products with pictures of cute babies on the label. However, despite these marketing tactics, products aimed at children and babies are not formulated any differently than products for adults. All sunscreen formulations with an SPF are alike, and do not differ in any way because of the age of the intended user. The only difference I've ever noted in baby products is the use of fragrance and bogus claims that the formula is "mild as water." Oddly, more fragrance is usually included in the baby products, but that only makes them more problematic because fragrances are irritating for all skin types. As for being "mild as water," let me assure you that your child won't feel that way if he or she gets sunscreen active ingredients in the eyes.

What is of greater concern is the fact that many sunscreens claiming to be for children do not contain the UVA-protecting ingredients of avobenzone (butyl methoxydibenzoylmethane), Tinosorb, Mexoryl (ecamsule), titanium dioxide, or zinc oxide. If one of these ingredients is not present in the active ingredient list on the label, do not buy it. And if you already own one, now that you know better, do not use it again and throw it out immediately. Yes, UVA protection is that essential.

If you are looking for a less irritating sunscreen for your child, choose one that contains only pure titanium dioxide or zinc oxide as the active ingredient; these are definitely the best options for a baby's sensitive skin.

THE ART OF SELF-TANNING

Self-tanners are the only way to get a tan that is safe for the skin. All self-tanners are virtually equal in that they use the same ingredient, dihydroxyacetone (DHA), to chemically turn the skin brown. Some products contain a greater concentration of DHA than others, and the higher the concentration the faster the skin will turn color and the darker it will be. The key to a good result is the application, which is always tricky. It takes experimentation to figure out how much to use, how dark to go, what areas to go over lightly (like knees and elbows), what areas to avoid (like palms of hands and armpits), and where to start and stop the application (do you stop at your ankles or continue down to your toes?). All of these are questions you need to answer for yourself, depending on your own personal preferences and blending techniques.

Note: If you choose to buy a self-tanner, whether it contains a sunscreen or not, please be aware that self-tanned brown skin does not offer any protection from the sun. All of the rules for wearing sunscreens still apply when you are using these products.

During the summer months, fashion magazines are replete with advertisements and stories about the best self-tanners and the optimal application for obtaining the best results. Varying products proclaim they are streak-free, won't turn orange, dry in five minutes, tan in under an hour, or have special color indicators. Those claims are often unreliable or misleading. Essentially, any self-tanner can be streak-free if *you* apply it evenly. A product that has "color indicators" simply refers to one with a temporary color that helps you see where you've applied it. That is helpful but still not foolproof, because the tint can dissipate quickly in some areas, leaving you wondering where you've applied it. (However, products that aren't transparent are definitely a great place to start, helping improve your odds of putting it on right.)

As far as the color of the tan you get, there are basically no color differences between products. That's because, as stated earlier, almost all self-tanners contain the same ingredient, dihydroxyacetone, which turns skin brown. DHA is a simple sugar involved in plant and animal carbohydrate metabolism, so you can even think of it as being all natural. How fast your skin turns color also has to do with how much DHA the product contains. The true color differences correlate with how much DHA the product contains and how your own skin reacts to this ingredient. DHA browns the skin through its interaction with the amino acid arginine, which is found in surface skin cells (Source: *Chemical Engineering News*, June 2000). Drying time is irrelevant, because the tanning effect actually depends on the chemical changes taking place in your skin cells. That's why, if you aren't patient and your skin rubs against your clothes (whether the self-tanner is completely dry or not), it will cause smudging or an uneven appearance.

Products that claim to turn your skin tan in less than an hour may actually be a problem, because if you make a mistake in application (and that is almost inevitable at first) it will also be almost instantaneously noticeable. A self-tanner that takes a few applications to achieve the color you want may be a better option as you learn how your skin reacts and hone your technique.

Regardless of the claims made about any self-tanner, it turns out that which product you choose isn't anywhere near as important as your technique and diligence. The following list will help you get the absolute best results with minimum problems. Just let me warn you, trying to do this fast will make your skin look more strange than tan.

1. It takes time, so apply self-tanner in the evening, allowing yourself at least a half hour, although an hour would be best. (For those who think the time it takes to apply self-tanner is inconvenient, remember how many hours it used to take in the sun to get the same amount of color? And with self-tanners there's no risk of wrinkles or skin cancer.)

2. Self-tanners grab on to dead surface skin cells, and you may have more of these in some areas than others. To help achieve a uniform appearance, take a shower or bath and exfoliate your skin, either with a washcloth or some baking soda, or both. Don't overscrub, but do pay extra attention to your knees, ankles, feet, elbows, and neck.

3. After showering and completely drying off, apply a minimal thin layer of moisturizer over the areas where you will be applying self-tanner. This will help the self-tanner glide on more easily and not stick over dry patches. A little extra moisturizer over ankles, knees, and elbows can prevent those areas from looking patchy. I have seen some recommendations that suggest mixing self-tanner with your moisturizer, but don't do it because that will encourage streaking (unless you can precisely mix the two together), and it will take longer for the self-tanner to absorb and dry. Besides, there are several body moisturizers that contain a tiny amount of the self-tanning ingredient dihydroxyacetone, and these can be great for experimenting with a really subtle yet buildable tan.

   Body Sense: *Perspiration can make self-tanners streak, so take a cool shower or bath to keep yourself from sweating. Your skin must be completely dry to get the best results. Do not apply self-tanner in a steamy, hot bathroom.*

4. It is best to apply the self-tanner while naked, but wearing an old bathing suit (one you don't plan to wear outside) can help you determine where you want your tan to be. Either way, have a game plan of where you want to stop and start the color. (Do you want tan armpits, the entire arm tan? What about the heels of your feet, your ears, or the palms of your hands?) Remember that self-tanners will stain clothing and bed linens until they are completely absorbed into the skin and take effect in the skin cells.

Body Sense: *Applying self-tanner on your back requires a friend with a helping hand, although you can use a long-handled paintbrush. I vote for the friend (or significant other) as the paintbrush poses some issues of dripping and uneven application.*

5. Apply self-tanner to one section of your body at a time. Be more concerned about even application than rubbing it all the way in. Avoid areas of your body where you do not want to have color.

6. To prevent tan palms, you can try using surgical or plastic gloves to apply the self-tanner. This can work well, but can also make application trickier. Another option is to wash your hands after you've applied the self-tanner to a section of your body, or just to wash them every few minutes. If you wait too long you will have strange-looking palms. It helps to have a nail brush handy to be sure you get the self-tanner off of your cuticles and the area between your fingers.

7. Different parts of your body "pick up" self-tanner more easily than others. For example, some people find that their legs turn brown more easily than their arms or torso, while others find that their faces and necks change color fastest. Experience will help you determine which is true for you. Be careful around your nose, eyes, ears, hairline, and lips. A cotton swab can help blend a thin, even amount smoothly over those areas. To keep your hair from turning color, apply a layer of conditioner or Vaseline over the hairline.

8. Wait at least 15 minutes before getting dressed. Do not exercise or swim for at least three hours.

9. If you make a mistake and end up with streaky or dark areas of skin, consider using my 2% Beta Hydroxy Acid Liquid over these spots. Then, in the morning, manually exfoliate those areas with a wet washcloth, and Voila! Bye-bye streaks!

10. Problem Areas. As an option for your hands (which can be particularly tricky to get looking natural) apply self-tanner as you would a moisturizer, but then quickly wipe your palms off on a slightly soapy washcloth. Then take a Q-tip dipped in cleanser, eye-makeup remover (one that is not greasy so it doesn't spread or smear), or nail-polish remover and carefully use it to wipe around the nails and cuticle area and between your fingers. Another option is to use a makeup sponge to apply self-tanner to the back of your hands, tops of your feet, temples, and hairline. By holding the sponge deftly between two fingers, you only need to worry about preventing this small area from becoming the wrong color.

Body Sense: *Skin-care products such as AHAs, BHA, topical scrubs, Retin-A, and topical disinfectants can affect the self-tanner's action on your skin or even eliminate the color by exfoliating the surface skin cells (self-tanners only interact with the surface of skin). It is best not to apply these products the evening you apply a self-tanner. However, if you must do so, wait at least two to three hours before you do.*

11. Reapply self-tanner as you feel the need. Generally it will start wearing away in about three to four days as the surface layers of skin shed. If you shave your legs daily, the

self-tanner will fade much faster and may look uneven. If that's the case, reapply self-tanner to legs after shaving.

All of these are valid application techniques, but none of them come with a guarantee, which is why it takes experimenting and going slow to get the best results.

TANNING PILLS?

Tanning pills come in two forms: those that contain tyrosine and those that contain a concentrated dose of beta-carotene. Let's start with tyrosine. The FDA has debunked tyrosine as a tanning accelerator. The marketing pitch is that tyrosine is needed by your body to produce melanin, which is a true statement. Ergo, the logic (albeit flawed) follows: taking pills with tyrosine will increase melanin production. It just isn't true—only exposure to UVA or UVB sun rays can activate tyrosine and other elements in skin to initiate (or trigger) melanin production, the pigment we see as a tan.

The FDA reports in their *Office of Cosmetics and Colors Fact Sheet* (June 27, 2000), "Lotions and pills marketed as 'tanning accelerators' generally contain tyrosine (an amino acid), often in combination with other substances. Tanning accelerators are marketed with the claim that they enhance tanning by stimulating and increasing melanin formation. FDA has concluded that these 'tanning accelerators' are actually unapproved drugs, and the agency has issued warning letters to several manufacturers of these products. There are no scientific data showing that they work; in fact, at least one study has found them ineffective." Companies that sell these types of tyrosine pills or lotions play on the fact that tyrosine is an amino acid that is a precursor for the production of melanin. Yet no research supports the oral consumption of tyrosine as having any effect on the color of skin. In another report, the FDA stated "In fact, an animal study reported a few years ago demonstrated that ingestion or topical application of tyrosine has no effect on [melanin production]. The [FDA] has … issued warning letters to several major manufacturers of these products (Source: www.fda.gov/ora/inspect_ref/igs/cosmet.html).

Another self-tanning pill, called Elusun, shows up on many Internet sites. Elusun's claims are at best misleading and, at worst, potentially dangerous. Elusun says that it can prevent the skin from aging during sun exposure, a claim that's not only completely false information, but also a truly harmful statement. Without sunscreen that contains UVA-protecting ingredients, all sun exposure is damaging, and no oral vitamin or supplement can change that.

Does Elusun color the skin? Yes, by giving the body high doses of beta-carotene (an FDA-approved vitamin supplement and food-coloring agent). Beta-carotene is the stuff that makes carrots orange and, if you consume enough of it, it can alter the skin's color. However, according to the FDA, megadoses of beta-carotene "enter the blood stream and are partially deposited in skin tissue, giving the skin a tan-like color … [but they are not] approved for [tanning] use, and products containing them are considered adulterated. Some reports of adverse reactions associated with 'tanning pills' have mentioned stomach cramps, hepatitis, nausea, diarrhea, and deposition of the color in the retina of the eye." Megadoses of beta-carotene can be harmful (Source: www.fda.gov/ora/inspect_ref/igs/cosmet.html).

Aside from pills that contain beta-carotene, there are others that contain another food-coloring substance called canthaxanthin. This ingredient works much like beta-carotene, but according to the FDA, "At least one company submitted an application for the approval of canthaxanthin-containing pills as a tanning agent, but withdrew the application when side effects, such as the [formation] of crystals in the eye, were discovered."

The FDA also states on its Web site that "In recent years, 'suntan accelerators' have appeared on the market. They claim to enhance tanning by stimulating and increasing melanin formation…. One type of suntan accelerator is based on bergapten (5-methoxypsoralen) which is found in bergamot oil and is a well-known phototoxic substance (responsible for Berloque dermatitis). Bergapten increases the skin's sensitivity to ultraviolet light, intensifies erythema [redness] formation, and stimulates melanocytes to produce melanin. It has also been reported to be photo-carcinogenic in animals" (Source: www.fda.gov/ora/inspect_ref/igs/cosmet.html).

SKIN CANCER AND SUN DAMAGE

According to the Centers for Disease Control and Prevention (CDC) and the American Academy of Dermatology, one million new cases of skin cancer are diagnosed each year. That gives skin cancer the unfavorable distinction of being the most common form of cancer in the United States. As reported by Dr. Darrell S. Rigel of the New York University School of Medicine, the chance for an American to develop melanoma in their lifetime is 1 in 84. Those aren't the kinds of odds you want to gamble on, at least not when it comes to losing portions of your skin or your life.

Most skin cancers fall into three categories: basal cell carcinomas, squamous cell carcinomas, and melanomas. Basal cell carcinomas and squamous cell carcinomas are caused by repeated, unprotected sun exposure (Sources: *Cancer Epidemiological Biomarkers and Prevention*, September 2008, pages 2388–2392; *Dermatology*, February 2008, pages 124–136; *American Journal of Clinical Dermatology*, May–June 2000, pages 167–179).

However, there is some controversy as to whether melanomas are caused by unprotected sun exposure. Despite the disagreement, what is not in question is that other types of skin cancers are caused by unprotected or prolonged sun exposure. (Sources: *Archives of Dermatology*, December 2000, pages 1447–1449; and *Journal of the American Medical Association*, June 2000, pages 2955–2960.)

As a general theory, scientists believe that exposure to UVA and some UVB radiation triggers mutations in replicating skin cells, causing their genetic coding to go haywire. The cells forget how to maintain the normal cell turnover process because of the radiation damage. Fortunately, nonmelanoma skin cancers are relatively easy to treat if detected in time, and are rarely fatal. Melanomas are a much more dangerous and life-threatening form of cancer.

An article in the *Journal of Epidemiology* (December 1999, Supplement, pages 7–13) summed up the issue quite nicely: "Skin cancer is the most commonly occurring cancer in humans…. Descriptive studies show that incidence rates of the main types of skin cancer, basal cell carcinoma, squamous cell carcinoma and melanoma are [highest] in populations in which ambient sun exposure is high and skin transmission of solar radiation is high, suggesting strong associations with sun exposure. Analytic epidemiological studies confirm that exposure to the UV component of sunlight is the major environmental determinant of skin cancers and associated skin conditions and evidence of a causal association between cumulative sun exposure and SCC, solar keratoses and photodamage is relatively straight-forward…. Complementary to [population and research] data is the molecular evidence of ultraviolet (UV) mechanisms of carcinogenesis [cancer] such as UV-specific mutations in the DNA of tumor suppressor genes in skin tumors. With increased UV irradiation resulting from thinning of the ozone layer, skin cancer incidence rates have been predicted to increase in the future—unless, as is hoped, human behavior to reduce sun exposure can offset these predicted rises."

Other than sun protection, you should be aware of some early, telltale signs of skin cancer. Early detection of skin cancer can save your skin and your life. If you perceive a change in your skin that you are not sure about, talk to your doctor; even a minor difference in a mole or a freckle, or a blemish that doesn't look "normal," can be an indication of skin cancer.

The five most typical characteristics of skin cancer are:

1. An open sore of any size that bleeds, oozes, or crusts and remains open for three or more weeks. A persistent, nonhealing sore is one of the most common signs of early skin cancer.

2. A reddish patch or irritated area that doesn't go away and doesn't respond to cortisone creams or moisturizers. Sometimes these patches crust over or flake off, but they never go away completely.

3. A smooth growth with a distinct rolled border and an indented center. It can look like a small blemish or wound, but tends to grow and doesn't heal.

4. A shiny bump or nodule with a slick, smooth surface that can be pink, red, white, black, brown, or purple in color. It can look like a mole, but the texture and shine are what make it different.

5. A white patch of skin that has a smooth, scarlike texture. The area of white skin can have a taut, clear appearance that stands out from the appearance of the surrounding skin.

The American Academy of Dermatology has a list of the "A, B, C, Ds" of identifying skin cancer, as follows:

A. Asymmetry: One half of the lesion or suspect area is unlike the other half.

B. Border: There is an irregular, scalloped, or poorly circumscribed border around a suspected skin lesion or mole.

C. Color: Color varies from one area to another, with shades of tan, brown, black, white, red, or blue.

D. Diameter: The area is generally larger than 6 mm (diameter of a pencil eraser).

ACTINIC KERATOSIS

If you have had any amount of unprotected sun exposure and you are between the ages of 30 and 80 you might have noticed uneven, rough-feeling, slightly raised, occasionally crusty, and generally light brown or light pink patches on your chest, hands, arms, or neck. These discolorations are called actinic keratosis or solar keratosis, and are distinct from other types of brown discolorations that show up on skin. According to the Skin Cancer Foundation, "One in six people will develop an actinic keratosis in the course of a lifetime." The more typical brown spots that appear on skin due to sun exposure are called melasmas. Melasmas look more like brown freckling and are not raised, rough, or crusted, and are considered benign. Actinic keratosis, though not cancerous, are problematic because they are considered indicative of a precancerous skin condition and require evaluation by a dermatologist. If you are in doubt whether a brown patch on your skin is a melasma or an actinic keratosis, it is best to ask your doctor. (Source: *Journal of Oral Maxillofactory Surgery*, June 2008, pages 1162–1176.)

Prevention is the best method of averting the occurrence of these types of brown patches, and that means daily and liberal use of effective sunscreens. Unfortunately, because most of us were not aware of appropriate sun protection for much of our lives, many of us have a pretty good chance of seeing one of these patches crop up somewhere on our bodies.

There are a number of ways to deal with removing actinic keratosis. The primary techniques are curettage, cryosurgery, and photodynamic therapy, plus topical chemotherapy options (Sources: *Dermatology Therapy*, September–October 2008, pages 412–415; and *American Journal of Clinical Dermatology*, May–June 2000, pages 167–179).

Deciding what to do depends primarily on the status of the lesion and how much the appearance bothers you. This requires a discussion with your dermatologist to evaluate your various options.

A typical method of removal is to scrape or cut the lesion off with procedures called curettage, electrodesiccation, or even simple scraping with a surgical razor. Curettage refers to cutting out the lesion with a curette, a spoon-shaped implement that has a sharp edge. Electrodesiccation uses an electric current to remove the skin tissue while it simultaneously controls bleeding. In both instances a biopsy is done to check on the status of the lesion. Both of these methods can cause scarring, and recurrence of the lesions is a problem.

Cryosurgery uses extreme cold, in the form of liquid nitrogen, to get rid of the unwanted tissue. This method doesn't cause bleeding or scarring but it can leave behind a white mark that often doesn't regain normal skin color. There is also a strong likelihood of recurrence.

When there are numerous actinic keratosis lesions present, two topical medications are sometimes used. The first, 5-fluorouracil (brand name Efudex), a chemotherapy agent for some cancers, is applied to the spots twice a day for three to five weeks. The side effects of this treatment can be significant, though temporary. Inflammation, burning, stinging, crusting, and some discomfort or pain are typical, but healing takes place one to two weeks after treatment is discontinued. It is considered a highly effective treatment.

Another chemotherapy agent used topically, masoprocol cream, 10% (brand name Actinex), is similar to 5-fluorouracil in terms of application and results, although there is a far higher risk of contact dermatitis with masoprocol than with 5-fluorouracil.

Immune response modulators are capable of selectively destroying abnormal skin cells. In a small study group "six men with actinic keratosis were treated with imiquimod 5% cream (trade name Aldara) three times a week for 6-8 weeks. In the event of a local skin reaction treatment was modified to two times per week. Results: All the AK [actinic keratosis] lesions were successfully cleared.... Histologically [under the skin], no apparent signs of persisting AK could be detected, and no recurrences were reported during follow up" (Source: *British Journal of Dermatology*, May 2001, pages 1050–1053). Aldara is a potential option to discuss with your physician.

Chemical peeling uses trichloroacetic acid (TCA), which is applied under light sedation. Much like any other cosmetic chemical peel, this causes the top layers of the skin to slough off, to be replaced within a few weeks by growth of new skin. A TCA peel is used when deeper penetration is needed to remove the lesion. The downsides to this method are the need for sedation, which makes it rather inconvenient, and the prolonged healing time; the upside is that the eventual results are considered quite good.

The newest treatment recently approved by the FDA is called photodynamic therapy. This is an interesting procedure that involves the topical application by a physician of a prescription-only cream containing aminolevulinic acid (brand name Levulan Kerastick). About 14 to 18 hours after the cream has been applied, the area is exposed to a particular light source, called BLU-U or Blue Light, for approximately 15 to 20 minutes. This is considered a very successful treatment with little risk to skin. However, after the aminolevulinic acid has been applied, the skin becomes abnormally sensitive to daylight or bright indoor lighting until the treatment is completed. It is critical to wear sunlight-protective clothing and to avoid any exposure to the sun because sunscreens will not protect you. It is also important to avoid sitting close to any light source. Side effects during treatment usually include burning, a crawling feeling on skin, itching, numbness, and stinging sensations, darkening or lightening of treated skin, crusting, scabs, and red itchy bumps. However, once treatment is discontinued the reaction and brown spots are gone and tend not to return.

AFTER-SUN CARE

I worry about the concept of "after-sun care." It sounds as if you can undo all the sun damage you incurred during the day. I admit it's a great marketing concept, but it is risky business for someone to buy into the notion that skin can be repaired following unprotected sun exposure. If you leave your skin defenseless and exposed to the sun's rays, and then slather some lotion, toner, or serum on afterward, hoping you can miraculously or even in a minor way heal, eliminate, correct, or cancel the devastating injury to your skin (and all sun exposure over time is devastating), you would be hoping in vain. Slathering on moisturizer does not help skin heal. Take a look at Chapter 8, which focuses on understanding moisturizers to see how you can best help skin in any situation.

BUYING SUNGLASSES

Wearing sunglasses on a regular basis is critical for the health of your eyes. The lens of the eye turns out to be a pretty good absorber of UVA rays, but, unlike the skin, the lens cannot slough off damaged cells. That means there is no way for the lens to ever repair itself. Protecting the eyes isn't just a cosmetic or a costume; it is about keeping your sight undiminished for as long as possible. Your eyes need protection from ultraviolet radiation, and whether you buy inexpensive or expensive sunglasses, it is a waste of money if they don't supply it.

Eyes exposed to sunlight are at risk for cataracts, sunburn (the eyeball itself can get sunburned), irritation, skin cancer of the eyelid, and dry eyes. Fortunately, most sunglasses do protect us well from the sun, but there is no easy way to know which ones do and which ones don't. Some sunglasses come with labels indicating they offer UV radiation protection, but there are no regulations or standards in this field. It doesn't hurt to buy sunglasses with a UV protection label, but there are some things you need to check out to make sure you purchase a pair that does more than just look good.

I strongly recommend buying sunglasses that hug the face and have wide rims and side-pieces. This way, you shield the eyes from any sunlight coming in from above, below, or around the sides, as well as protect more of the delicate skin around the eyes from sun damage.

The American Academy of Ophthalmology (www.aao.org/) offers a few extremely helpful guidelines for finding the best protection:

1. Select sunglasses that block ultraviolet rays. Don't be deceived by color or cost. The ability to block UV light is not dependent on the darkness of the lens or the price tag. You should always buy sunglasses with this feature. Shop for sunglasses that block 99% or 100% of all UV light. Some manufacturers' labels say "UV absorption up to 400nm." This is the same thing as 100% UV absorption.

2. Ideally, your sunglasses should wrap all the way around to your temples, so the sun's rays can't enter from the side.

3. Even if you wear contacts with UV protection, remember your sunglasses.

4. Be sure that the lens tint is uniform, not darker in one area than another.

5. Another test to be sure the glasses are well made is to hold them out from you at arm's length. Look through them from this distance at a straight line such as the edge of a bookcase or wall. Then slowly move the glasses across the straight line. If the straight edge distorts, sways, curves, or moves, the lenses have imperfections and you should not buy them.

6. Tinted sunglasses have an impact on what kind of sun exposure you get, aside from their impact on the face. Red- and yellow-tinted lenses can cut haze, but may not adequately protect from sun exposure, though if they had a UV coating they would work to protect against sun damage. Check them in daylight or consult an ophthalmologist. Gray, green, and brown tints are known for providing good viewing as well as good sun protection. Black and blue tints can be too dark, impairing good vision.

CHAPTER 8
SKIN CARE & MOISTURIZERS

WHAT IS A MOISTURIZER? (THE ANSWER WILL SURPRISE YOU)

A moisturizer should moisturize, right? But then what does an anti-wrinkle or anti-aging product do? What about a treatment or serum? Moisturizer is an overused term that has lost meaning over the years. With all the anti-aging, anti-wrinkling, lifting, firming, nourishing, organic, works-like-Botox, eye cream, intensive treatment, throat cream, and neck cream products touting their miracle formulations, it's hard to know where moisturizers fit into the picture. In actuality, to be of any value for skin, and regardless of the name or claim, "moisturizers," whether they are in cream, lotion, serum, or even liquid form, or labeled as some miracle anti-something or other formulation, must be filled with ingredients that maintain skin's structure by reducing free-radical damage (environmental assaults on the skin from sun, pollution, and air), reinforce the skin's barrier function, and help all forms of skin cells (immune cells, collagen, elastin) function more normally. When moisturizers contain the well-researched, effective groups of ingredients that can do these things they can maintain the skin's natural moisture balance, and they are as close to "anti-aging" and repairing as any skin-care product you can get. Those categories of ingredients that can help skin do this are antioxidants, cell-communicating ingredients, skin-identical ingredients, and anti-irritants.

The days of plain, water-and-wax moisturizers are over, although many lines still sell such formulations to unwary customers. Using these antiquated formulations is like using computers made in the 1980s. That would be cheating your skin by not giving it the best that's out there to help it (dare I say it) look younger.

WHAT EVERY SKIN TYPE NEEDS

Remember these terms – Antioxidants, Cell-Communicating Ingredients, and Skin-Identical Ingredients

Regardless of the name on the label, and whether it's a moisturizer, anti-wrinkle or anti-aging product, serum, treatment, or whatever clever term that appears on the label, what all these products should contain are antioxidants, cell-communicating ingredients, and skin-identical ingredients. All skin types need these ingredients to be as healthy as possible. And I mean ALL SKIN TYPES! As long as the product you are using contains a selection of these types of ingredients you are going to be taking the best possible care of your skin when it comes to using a "moisturizer." What about your skin type? The only thing that differentiates a "moisturizer" or anti-wrinkle product or anti-aging treatment, serum, or other option for your skin type is the texture of the product. Gels and liquids are best for oily and combination skin, serums and light lotions are best for normal to slightly dry skin, and more emollient lotions and creams are best for dry to very dry skin. Texture is all about skin type—but the brilliant ingredients for healthy skin remain the same for everyone, regardless of product texture or personal preference.

FREE-RADICAL DAMAGE

Antioxidants are all about reducing something called free-radical damage, a term you may already be familiar with. Free-radical damage occurs on a molecular, unseen, unfelt, atomic level but it is nevertheless one of the most destructive internal processes affecting the body, which causes both the body and the skin to "age." It is also responsible for many serious health problems that range from cancer to cardiovascular disease, atherosclerosis, hypertension, restricted blood flow, diabetes, and neurodegenerative diseases such as Alzheimer's and Parkinson's disease, as well as rheumatoid arthritis. For the skin, sun exposure is the major cause of free-radical damage. (Sources: *Free Radical Biology and Medicine*, March 2008, pages 990–1000; *Ageing Research Reviews*, December 2007, pages 271–288; *International Journal of Biochemistry and Cell Biology*, January 2007, pages 44–84; and *International Journal of Cosmetic Science*, February 2005, pages 17–34.)

What are free radicals and why are they running amok? Molecules are made of atoms, and a single atom is made up of protons, neutrons, and electrons. Electrons need to be in pairs in order to function properly. However, when oxygen molecules are involved in a chemical reaction, they can lose one of their electrons. This oxygen molecule that now only has one electron is called a free radical. With only one electron the oxygen molecule must quickly find another electron, and it does this by taking the electron from another molecule. When that molecule in turn loses one of its electrons, it too must seek out another, in a continuing, spiraling reaction. Molecules attempting to repair themselves in this way trigger a cascading event called "free-radical damage."

What causes a molecule to let go of one of its electrons, generating free-radical damage? The answer is any compound or element that contains or generates an unstable oxygen molecule, such as carbon monoxide, hydrogen peroxide, sunlight, smoking, and pollution.

Free-radical damage causes mutation and damage to the DNA in your cells, and damaged DNA means your skin, now unable to generate healthy or new collagen, creates malformed skin cells; it also greatly impedes skin's ability to heal. Free-radical damage is not a pretty process for skin or any part of your body.

You may be asking: With all that free-radical damage taking place (and you can never stop it completely), and all this oxygen, car exhaust, sunlight, and city air around us, how is it that we don't fall apart right now? The answer to that is antioxidants and the way they function.

ANTIOXIDANTS

Antioxidants are an essential part of any state-of-the-art moisturizer. An immense body of research continues to show that antioxidants are a potential panacea for skin's ills, and ignoring their benefit while shopping for moisturizers (or any products with names like anti-aging or anti-wrinkle or treatment) means you'll be shortchanging your skin. What makes antioxidants so intriguing is that they seem to have the ability to reduce or prevent some amount of the oxidative damage that destroys and depletes the skin's function and structure while also preventing some of the degenerative effects in skin caused by sun exposure.

The number of antioxidants that can show up in a skin-care product is almost limitless. Yet despite endless cosmetics companies launching new miracle ingredients on a constant, unrelenting basis there is no single best one, and many work well together. These vital elements for skin can range from alpha lipoic acid, beta-glucan, coenzyme Q10, grape seed extract, green tea, soybean sterols, superoxide dismutase, vitamin C (ascorbyl palmitate and magnesium ascorbyl palmitate), and vitamin E (alpha tocopherol, tocotrienols) to pomegranate, cucurmin, turmeric, and on and on and on.

Although antioxidants have great ability to intercept and mitigate free-radical damage, it is ironic that they share a particular weakness: they deteriorate when repeatedly exposed to air (oxygen) and sunlight. Ironic, yes but it's actually testament to how antioxidants work in the presence of oxygen and light. Because of this issue, an antioxidant-laden moisturizer packaged in a jar or clear (instead of opaque) container will likely lose its antioxidant benefit within weeks (or days, depending on the formula) after it is opened. This means you should seek out moisturizers with antioxidants that are packaged in opaque tubes or bottles, and check to be sure that the opening the product is dispensed from is small in order to minimize exposing the product to air.

Antioxidants, with their molecular weapons against free-radical damage, are considered so vital to our understanding of the origins of wrinkles, cancer, aging, illness, and disease that they have become a profound area of research. Free-radical damage is what antioxidants are supposed to take care of, either by stopping new damage, or by reversing earlier damage caused by free radicals. And antioxidants can potentially repair damage by allowing healthy cells to proliferate.

When skin isn't damaged by the sun's rays (which generate free-radical damage), it contains a natural supply of antioxidants. With unprotected exposure to the sun these vital elements are depleted and don't regenerate. Supplying your skin with these substances in a product you leave on your face provides your skin with what it needs to function normally and "act younger."

(Sources: *Clinics in Dermatology*, November–December 2008, pages 614–626; *Skin Therapy Letter*, September 2008, pages 5–9; *Journal of Drugs in Dermatology*, July 2008, pages S7–S12; *Dermatologic Therapy*, September–October 2007, pages 322–329; *Dermatologic Surgery*, "The Antioxidant Network of the Stratum Corneum," July 2005, pages 814–817; *Journal of Pharmaceutical and Biomedical Analysis*, February 2005, pages 287–295; and *Cosmetic Dermatology*, December 2001, pages 37–40.)

SKIN-IDENTICAL INGREDIENTS

We are trained by the cosmetics industry to worry about getting more moisture to our skin, yet dry skin is not about putting moisture in the skin but rather helping our skin to keep the water it has. You can give skin all the moisture in the world but it won't be absorbed where you need it. Think about what happens when you soak in a bathtub. That's a lot of moisture your skin is getting, but the skin doesn't become less dry just because you've taken a long bath; if anything, soaking in a tub disrupts the barrier of your skin, making skin drier.

You may have heard of the term humectants, meaning ingredients in skin-care products that attract water to skin. While those can be helpful, what good is attracting water to the skin if the structure isn't there to keep the water from leaving?

The term "skin-identical ingredients" refers to the substances between skin cells (technically referred to as the intercellular matrix) that keep skin cells connected and help maintain skin's fundamental external structure. Think of your skin as consisting of bricks, with the mortar being the material that holds these bricks together. Skin cells are the bricks, and the mortar (cement) between them is made up of skin-identical ingredients. An intact, stable, healthy, and strong mortar structure is what allows skin to look smooth, soft, moist, supple, and young.

Unfortunately, the mortar, especially in the external barrier of our skin, is easily compromised by sun damage (that's the major culprit), irritation, overcleansing, overscrubbing, dry climate, air conditioning, indoor heaters, skin disorders, and on and on. When the skin's mortar (the intercellular matrix) breaks down, water loss, flakiness, and inflexible, stiff, uncomfortable-feeling skin is the result.

It is of vital importance for all skin types to maintain or restore the skin's mortar (intercellular matrix) to help skin fight off environmental stresses and most certainly look younger. These substances that keep skin intact are what I refer to as skin-identical ingredients. Antioxidants are one group of skin-identical ingredients, but skin-identical ingredients also encompass an additional assortment of substances, such as ceramides, lecithin, glycerin, polysaccharides, hyaluronic acid, sodium hyaluronate, sodium PCA, amino acids, cholesterol, glycerol, phospholipids, glycosphingolipids, glycosaminoglycans, glycerides, fatty acids, and many, many more. All of these give skin what it needs to keep skin cells together. Just adding water alone can do nothing if the intercellular matrix is damaged. When a moisturizer contains a combination of these, it can help reinforce the skin's natural ability to function normally, improve skin's texture, fight environmental stress (sun, pollution, and more), and along with antioxidants and cell-communicating ingredients, eliminate dry skin with regular use.

CELL-COMMUNICATING INGREDIENTS

Cell-communicating ingredients are getting a lot of attention for their role in helping skin function more normally. Medical journals refer to these as "cell signaling" substances—but I think "cell communicating" is more descriptive of what they do in relation to skin care.

Where antioxidants work by intervening in a chain-reaction process called free-radical damage, "grabbing" the loose-cannon molecule that causes free-radical damage to reduce its impact on skin, cell-communicating ingredients, theoretically, have the ability to tell a skin

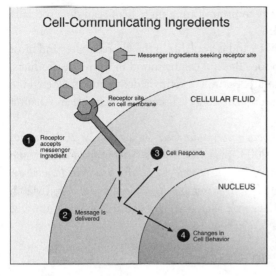

Cell-Communicating Ingredients

Messenger ingredients seeking receptor site

Receptor site on cell membrane

CELLULAR FLUID

1. Receptor accepts messenger ingredient

3. Cell Responds

NUCLEUS

2. Message is delivered

4. Changes in Cell Behavior

cell to look, act, and behave better, more like a normal healthy skin cell would, or to stop other substances from telling the cell to behave badly or abnormally. This is exciting news because antioxidants lack the ability to "tell" a damaged skin cell to behave more normally.

Years of unprotected or poorly protected sun exposure causes abnormal skin cells to be produced. Instead of normal, round, even, and completely intact skin cells being regenerated, when damaged cells form and reproduce they are uneven, flat, and lack structural integrity. As a result of these deformities, they behave poorly. This is where cell-communicating ingredients (examples are niacinamide and adenosine triphosphate) have the potential to help.

Every cell has a vast series of receptor sites for different substances. These receptor sites are the cell's communication hookup. When the right ingredient for a specific site shows up, it has the ability to attach itself to the cell and transmit information. In the case of skin, this means telling the cell to start doing the things a healthy skin cell should be doing. If the cell accepts the message, it then shares the same healthy message with other nearby cells and so on and so on.

As long as there is a receptor site and the appropriate, healthy signaling substance, a lot of good, healthy communication takes place. But a cell's communication network is more complex than any worldwide telephone system ever imagined. The array of receptor sites and the substances that can make connections to them make up a huge, complex, and varied group with incredible limitations and convoluted pathways that we are still finding out about. As far as skin care is concerned, it's an area of research that is in its infancy. No doubt you will be hearing more and more about cell-communicating or cell-signaling ingredients being used in skin-care products, despite the lack of solid research. The good news is that, theoretically, this new horizon in skin care is incredibly exciting.

RETINOL

When it comes to cell-communicating ingredients for skin, the two we know the most about are vitamin A and niacinamide, with vitamin A (retinol is the name for the entire vitamin A molecule) having by far the most research. We know that there is a receptor site on a skin cell for a form of vitamin A called all-trans retinoic acid—also known as tretinoin. When vitamin A is absorbed into the skin it is broken down by enzymes there and becomes retinoic acid. In this form, it can send information to the skin cell telling it to behave more normally and to make healthier skin cells and, to some extent, the skin cell listens and responds accordingly. That is what a all cell-communicating ingredients can do, especially vitamin A when it becomes retinoic acid.

Tretinoin is considered a drug by the FDA and is available in the United States and most other Western countries only by prescription. Retinol can be found in skin-care products, most typically in the form of retinyl palmitate. Retinol or retinylaldehye are considered the more active forms but they can also be more irritating. I discuss niacinamide in Chapter Fifteen, *Solutions for Acne*.

(Sources: *International Journal of Biochemistry and Cell Biology*, July 2004, pages 1141–1146; *Nature Medicine*, February 2003, pages 225–229; *Microscopy Research and Technique*, January 2003, pages 107–114; *Skin Pharmacology and Applied Skin Physiology*, September–October 2002, pages 316–320; *Journal of Investigative Dermatology*, March 2002, pages 402–408; *Experimental Cell Research*, March 2002, pages 130–137; and www. signaling-gateway.org.)

PEPTIDES

Peptides are a group of cell-communicating ingredients that are showing up in lots of skin-care products these days. They are tiny portions of proteins, which are made of long chains of amino acids. In the human body, peptides regulate the activity of many systems by interacting with target cells. Enzymes break proteins into peptides so they can exert their influence on systems and get them operating as they should. Some peptides have hormonal activity, others have immune activity; some inhibit growth factors that stimulate scar formation, some play a role in wound healing, and still others affect the pathology of skin conditions such as atopic dermatitis and eczema. Some peptides have demonstrated a remarkable anti-inflammatory effect. Peptides are as abundant and intricate as the stars in the heavens.

Whether peptides have benefit when applied topically to skin for wound healing, skin-barrier repair, or as disinfectants is difficult to ascertain because they generally cannot penetrate skin. At the same time they remain stable because they are too hydrophilic, or water-loving, an ironic fact since peptides can become unstable in water-based formulas (Sources: *IFSCC Magazine*, July 2004, page 153; and Biotechniques, July 2002, pages 190–192). But details like that have never bothered the cosmetics industry. Whether an ingredient really makes a difference doesn't enter into marketing or advertising campaigns. All that matters is that the ingredient is new and that the story about it sounds believable.

Further, because peptides are vulnerable to the presence of enzymes, when peptides are absorbed, the abundant enzymes present in skin can break the peptides down to the point where they have no effect at all. However, research is examining how different types of synthesized peptides can remain stable. Creating specific peptide chains in the lab and then attaching a fatty-acid component to them allows peptides to overcome being absorbed and remaining stable, their inherent limitations. Lab-engineered peptides appear to have the kind of efficacy and benefit that go beyond the skin's surface, but further conclusive, long-term research is essential to gain an understanding of what, if anything, is really taking place (Sources: *The Journal of Investigative Dermatology*, September 2005, pages 473–481; *Cosmetics & Toiletries*, June 2004, page 30; and *Pharmaceutical Research*, March 2004, pages 389–393). It is reasonable to assume that as synthetic peptide technology broadens, we will see more options for use in skin-care products promoting anti-aging properties—and, specifically, tissue regeneration (Source: *Cosmetics & Toiletries*, March 2003, pages 43–52).

Despite the fact that there is no published research showing that specific peptides in skin-care products can have superior or even improved results when applied topically, that doesn't stop the cosmetics companies from putting the stuff in their products, claiming, of course, that they can accomplish miraculous feats for skin. There are several of these ingredients but mainly what you will find are copper peptides, palmitoyl pentapeptide-3, acetyl hexapeptide-3, and neuropeptides. None of these have independent supporting evidence that they can perform as claimed, at least not from any source other than the companies selling the products. Often these studies are done with a single comparison, which is meaningless given that there are hundreds of options that could skew the results, if they were studied scientifically. But that isn't the way cosmetics research is done (Source: *International Journal of Cosmetic Science*, June 2005, pages 155–160).

For these specialized peptides to exert a benefit beyond that of a water-binding agent, three criteria must be met: the peptides must be stable in their base formula, they must be paired with a carrier that enhances absorption into the skin, and they must be able to reach their target cell groups without breaking down. Oops, I nearly forgot, they must be safe to use! Achieving these goals is no easy feat. Cosmetics companies would love for you to believe they have figured this out, but that is not the case any more than we have a cure for cancer. But this is definitely a promising area in skin care that once developed will have significant potential in the realm of anti-aging skin-care ingredients. For now, peptides have potential benefit as cell-communicating ingredients and most of those used in skin-care products offer value as water-binding agents.

(Sources: *Journal of Cosmetic Dermatology*, June 2008, pages 143–148; *Journal of Cosmetic Science*, January–February 2008, pages 59–69; *Journal of Investigative Dermatology*, May 2005, pages 450–455; *New England Journal of Medicine*, January 2003, pages 361–363; *International Journal of Cosmetic Science*, December 2001, pages 207–218; and *Proceedings of the National Academy of Sciences*, January 2000, 371–376.)

ACETYL HEXAPEPTIDE-3

One of my favorite examples of how the cosmetics industry takes an ingredient and either misleads or exaggerates to the point of fabricating information about it is acetyl hexapeptide-3. This synthetically derived peptide is used primarily in skin-care products claiming to have a muscle-relaxing effect similar to Botox injections. Typically, the claims have to do with this peptide being able to calm muscle contractions, specifically those involved in making facial expressions, thus reducing the appearance of expression lines. The company selling this ingredient (trade name Argireline) is Centerchem (www.centerchem. com). According to their Web site, "Argireline works through a unique mechanism which relaxes facial tension leading to a reduction in superficial facial lines and wrinkles with regular use. Argireline has been shown to moderate excessive catecholamines release." The truth of this claim about the effects of topical application of Argireline is based only on information from Centerchem; there is no published research substantiating any use of Argireline topically on skin.

Catecholamines are compounds in the body that serve as neurotransmitters, including epinephrine, adrenaline, and dopamine. Epinephrine prepares the body to handle emergencies such as cold, fatigue, and shock. A deficiency of dopamine in the brain is responsible for the symptoms of Parkinson's disease. These actions are not something you want a cosmetic to inhibit or reduce.

If acetyl hexapeptide-3 really worked to relax facial muscles, it would work all over the face (assuming you're using the products as directed). If all the muscles in your face were relaxed you'd have sagging, not youthful, skin, not to mention that it also would affect your hand (you apply it with your fingers after all), which would prevent you from picking up a cup or holding the steering wheel of your car. Despite all the fear about Botox that is disseminated by companies featuring this peptide in their "works like Botox" products, there is considerably more efficacy, usage, and safety documentation available for Botox.

Despite the claims made for acetyl hexapeptide-3, there is actually a clinical study showing this ingredient does not work in any way like Botox in reducing wrinkles (Source: *International Journal of Cosmetic Science*, October 2002).

It is also interesting to note that Botox itself, when applied topically on skin, has no impact—either on the skin or the muscles—in any way, shape, or form! (Source: *Cosmetic Dermatology*, July 2005, pages 521–524.)

ANTI-IRRITANTS

Anti-irritants make up another vital aspect of any skin-care formulation. Regardless of the source, irritation is a problem for all skin types, yet it is almost impossible to avoid. Whether it is from the sun, oxidative damage from pollution, the environment, or from the skin-care products a person uses, irritation can be a constant assault on the skin. Ironically, even such necessary ingredients as sunscreen agents, preservatives, exfoliants, and cleansing agents can cause irritation. Other ingredients, like fragrance, menthol, and sensitizing plant extracts, are primary irritants and are almost always void of genuine benefits for skin, so using them is a negative, at least if you're serious about creating and maintaining healthy skin.

Anti-irritants are incredibly helpful because they allow skin healing time. They can also reduce the problems caused by oxidative and other sources of external damage. Anti-irritants include substances such as allantoin, aloe, bisabolol, burdock root, chamomile extract, glycyrrhetinic acid, grape extract, green tea, licorice root, vitamin C, white willow, willow bark, willowherb, and many, many more. Their benefit to skin should be strongly considered, because this is that rare case where too much of a good thing is better!

Skin is Permeable

Can skin-care ingredients be absorbed into skin? There is no question that they can. Of course it's a bit of a paradox that while the skin is designed to keep substances out of the body it can also let other substances in. State-of-the-art skin-care formulations are designed to both stay on the surface and be absorbed beyond the surface to exert beneficial influences on the support systems underneath.

What all skin types need is a combination of ingredients that stay on the surface (technically in the layer called the stratum corneum), as well as penetrate to protect and supplement the lower layers of skin. The right combination includes emollients and antioxidants that stay on the surface, antioxidants and skin-identical ingredients that can penetrate a bit further into the epidermis, and antioxidants and cell-communicating ingredients that can move deeper yet and influence the development of cells in the healthiest manner possible. When you deliver an abundance of these multifaceted substances to skin it is getting the best the cosmetics industry has to offer.

Which substances can penetrate the skin? That is determined by the molecular weight of the substance. Skin's barrier (the stratum corneum or corneal layer) is able to defend against the diffusion of many molecules, but not the ones that are small enough to pass through its otherwise impenetrable layers. This is referred to as the Dalton Rule, which set a standard molecular/atomic weight for any given substance. Larger molecules measuring over 500 Dalton cannot pass the stratum corneum, but if they're under 500 Dalton they sail through. An example of a substance that can sail through the skin is nicotine, as in nicotine patches. In contrast, insulin's Dalton weight is so high that cannot be absorbed into skin at all, thus diabetics must obtain insulin via shots rather than just sticking a patch on skin.

(Sources: *Journal of Biomechanics*, April 2008, pages 788–796; *Journal of Cosmetic Dermatology*, June 2007, pages 75–82; and *Skin Pharmacology and Skin Physiology*, February 2006, pages 106–121.)

There Is No Single Miracle Ingredient

All of the factors above, antioxidants, skin-identical ingredients, and cell-communicating ingredients, are leading elements that contribute to making a state-of-the-art moisturizer. And there are many brilliant formulations in stable packaging that include these substances. It is now far easier than before for a consumer to purchase a truly exceptional product for their skin type, regardless of the name on the label.

Contrary to what the cosmetics industry at large would like you to believe, a state-of-the-art moisturizer does not rely on a single star ingredient to enhance skin's appearance or function, or to improve the appearance of wrinkles. Month after month, consumers are faced with new ingredients, each claiming superiority over any number of predecessors. Everything from vitamin C and collagen to some exotic plant from a distant forest or exotic location, or perhaps a newly derived molecule, is advertised as being the answer for your skin. Yet the majority of these have no substantiated, non-company-funded research to prove these assertions. And even when there is research showing the ingredient can be effective for skin, that doesn't make it better or more essential than other ingredients. This constant yet ever-changing list of "best" ingredients may keep things interesting for cosmetics marketing departments and the media, but it rarely helps the consumer determine what is needed to maintain healthy, radiant skin.

Think about it like your diet. While broccoli or grapes may be incredibly healthy to eat, if you only ate grapes you would soon become malnourished and your body would suffer. Skin lives in the same way. Skin is a complex structural organ requiring many substances to function in a younger and healthier manner. And by that I mean in the way it did before it became damaged by the sun—remember the backside test of aging.

WHAT ARE SERUMS, TREATMENTS, ANTI-WRINKLE PRODUCTS, ETCETERA FOR?

These are strictly marketing terms, nothing more. They do not tell you anything about what the product can do for your skin. Serums are not specially enhanced in any way, anti-wrinkle products do not get rid of wrinkles or offer any additional benefit for skin, anti-gravity products don't lift skin, and on and on. They are all moisturizers with deceptive, meaningless names. As long as a product is well formulated with a variety of great ingredients you will achieve the best results. Everything else is seductive marketing mumbo jumbo, and the reason thousands of "anti-wrinkle" products line the shelves is that they tell us what we want to hear, even when none of them can perform to the extent their label promises.

TAKING CARE OF DRY SKIN

Those with truly dry skin (not caused by irritating or drying skin-care products) know that, over and above antioxidants, skin-identical ingredients, and cell-communicating ingredients, which can conquer most moisturizing needs, additional help is required to help skin feel normal or younger. Emollients are necessary to provide dry skin with the one thing it's missing, the ability to keep moisture in skin. Emollients are ingredients like plant oils, mineral oil, shea butter, cocoa butter, petrolatum, and fatty acids (animal oils, including emu, mink, and lanolin, the latter probably the one ingredient that is most like our own skin's oil). More technical-sounding emollient ingredients like triglycerides, benzoates, myristates, palmitates, and stearates are generally waxy in texture and appearance but provide most moisturizers with their elegant texture and feel. All of these are exceptionally beneficial for dry to very dry skin and easily recognizable on an ingredient list.

Overall, emollients create the fundamental base and texture of a moisturizer and impart a creamy, smooth feel on the skin. Silicones (appearing on the label in terms ending in "siloxane") are another interesting group of lubricants for skin. They have the most exquisite, silky texture and an incredible ability to prevent dehydration without suffocating the skin. All of these ingredients spread over the skin to create a thin, imperceptible layer, recreating the benefits of our own oil production, preventing evaporation, and giving dry skin the lubrication it is missing.

FOR THOSE WITH NORMAL TO OILY SKIN OR MINIMAL DRYNESS

You may be wondering what to use if you don't have dry skin but still want to give your normal or oily skin such all-important ingredients as antioxidants, skin-identical ingredients, and cell-communicating ingredients. Products (moisturizers) in cream, balm, thick lotion, or ointment form are bound to be problematic if you have any degree of oiliness. Even many lighter-weight lotions can be too emollient for someone with oily skin. What works instead is to look for water-based or very light fluid or serum-type products that are loaded with antioxidants, skin identical ingredients, and cell communicating ingredients. These include well-formulated toners—which are all I use because of my oily skin. Using products with a light, fluid texture will give your skin what it needs without layering on emollients, thickeners, or other heavier ingredients that are fundamental for dealing with dry skin but often spell trouble for combination or oily skin.

If you have combination skin but suffer from very dry areas, you will want to be sure the cleanser and toner you are using are not the cause of your dry skin, owing to the irritation and dehydration many formulations can cause. If the dryness is not from the products you are using, you may have no choice but to address the dryness with a more emollient moisturizer. The key is to only apply it to the dry areas and make sure it doesn't migrate to oily zones.

What about sunscreen? Great question, because this is a daily essential for every skin type! Because most sunscreen formulations apply and perform best when formulated in lotion- or cream-based emulsions, this can be a tricky area to navigate for someone with oily skin or oily areas. The good news is that silicone technology has made it possible to create ultralight sunscreens that allow the active ingredients to remain suspended and spread easily (and uniformly) over skin. They aren't as prevalent as standard sunscreen creams and lotions, but such products are available from most of the major skin-care companies. You can also opt to use a well-formulated toner and then wear a foundation with sunscreen. That way you get the benefit of the antioxidants, skin-identical ingredients, and cell-communicating ingredients as well as sunscreen without layering products that feel heavy or too emollient on your skin.

(Sources: *Current Molecular Medicine*, March 2005, pages 171–177; *Dermatology*, February 2005, pages 128–134; *Skin Research and Technology*, November 2003, pages 306–311; *Journal of the American Academy of Dermatology*, March 2003, pages 352–358; *Applied Spectroscopy*, July 1998, pages 1001–1007; and *Skin Pharmacology and Applied Skin Physiology*, November–December 1999, pages 344–351.)

DRY UNDERNEATH AND OILY ON TOP

Several things can cause the combination of a layer of dry, flaky skin combined with oily skin. More often than not this is caused by using the wrong combination of skin-care products. An emollient, wipe-off cleanser, followed by a toner that is too emollient for your skin type, and then an unnecessarily emollient moisturizer can prevent the lower layer of skin from exfoliating, creating a thick, dry, flaky lower layer and a greasy layer on top.

Conversely, if you have oily skin, using a drying cleanser followed by a toner with irritating or drying ingredients, and then applying an emollient moisturizer can create the same condition. The drying toner and cleanser can cause the skin to be dry and flaky, while the emollient moisturizer adds to your own excess oil production, aggravating it and making the skin look both oily and dehydrated.

The condition of dry skin underneath and oily skin on top rarely requires additional skin-care products. Instead, taking a completely different approach and eliminating overly drying or overly emollient products can help a great deal.

It is also possible that the dry layer covered by an oily layer could be a result of psoriasis, rosacea, seborrhea, or eczema. See the chapters dealing with those special skin problems and consult a dermatologist for an exam, if necessary.

DRY PATCHES OF SKIN

Skin can develop dry patches for many reasons. Makeup left on overnight can cause irritant or allergic reactions; but there are also drying skin-care products, dermatitis, eczema, and heavy moisturizers that can cause a buildup of dead skin cells. Any and all of these can contribute to dry patches of skin. The best advice is to avoid drying skin-care products and to use only the lightest-weight moisturizer for dry skin areas.

If the dry patches are chronic or itchy, they can be a form of topical dermatitis or eczema and may require treatment by a dermatologist. If you've done your best to eliminate the cause of the problem and the problem persists, one of the best ways to calm down the appearance of dry patches is with an over-the-counter cortisone cream. Lanacort and Cortaid are 1% hydrocortisone creams meant for dry patches of skin, for short-term use only. It is amazing how effective they can be. If the problem lingers, consult a dermatologist for topical prescription options, but for many people over-the-counter hydrocortisone is all it takes.

WHAT ABOUT EYE CREAMS?

Most women believe that eye creams are specially formulated for the skin around the eye area. Although the eye area does tend to be more prone to allergic or sensitizing reactions and often shows wrinkles before other areas of the face, it turns out the product formulations for eye creams don't differ from those for face products. There is no evidence, research, or documentation validating the claim that eye creams have special formulations that set them apart from other facial moisturizers. There is also no research indicating what ingredients should be used around the eye but not on the face or vice versa.

Aside from the actual lack of research, I have also never interviewed a dermatologist, cosmetic chemist, cosmetic ingredient manufacturer, or opthalmologist who has ever identified what moisturizer-type ingredients the eye area needs or doesn't need in comparison to the face. On occasion one of these "experts" might say that they eye is more sensitive and therefore doesn't need ingredients that cause irritation, which is just utter nonsense—the face doesn't need irritating ingredients either! What is problematic for the eye area is problematic for the face.

It only takes a quick look at the ingredient labels of any moisturizer or eye moisturizer to see that they don't differ except for the higher price and the tiny containers the eye creams come in. Eye creams are a great way to waste money on a skin-care product that is truly unnecessary.

The only time you might want to use a different product around the eyes is if the skin there happens to indeed be different from the skin on the rest of the face. For example, if your face is normal to oily and doesn't require a moisturizer except occasionally on the cheeks or around the eyes, then an emollient, well-formulated moisturizer of any kind will work beautifully—you do not need to seek out a special eye cream! If you are using a well-formulated face moisturizer (anti-wrinkle cream or whatever the name is on the label), it can and should be used around the eye area.

Ironically, one of the drawbacks of many so-called eye creams is that they rarely contain sunscreen. For daytime, that makes most eye creams a serious problem for the health of skin. You could believe that you were doing something special for your eyes, but you would actually be putting them at risk of sun damage and wrinkling by using an eye cream without sunscreen. This is another example of the way cosmetics marketing and misleading information can waste your money and hurt your skin.

IS THERE A DIFFERENCE BETWEEN A DAYTIME VERSUS NIGHTTIME MOISTURIZER?

Putting aside the claims, hype, and misleading information you may have heard, the only real difference between a daytime and nighttime moisturizer is that the daytime version should contain a well-formulated sunscreen. A popular myth told repeatedly by cosmetics salespeople echoes the notion that skin is doing some kind of special repairing at night that it isn't doing during the day. Even if that were true, and there is no research indicating it is, exactly what those ingredients are supposed to be has never been identified in any medical or scientific journal.

Skin is struggling to heal and repair itself 24 hours a day. It is not doing anything different at night than it is doing the day except taking a rest from the assault of sun exposure. And therein lies the only difference between a daytime and nighttime moisturizer. For daytime wear, unless your foundation contains an effective sunscreen, it is essential that your moisturizer features a well-formulated, broad-spectrum sunscreen rated SPF 15 or higher. Well-formulated means it must contains the UVA-protecting ingredients of titanium dioxide, zinc oxide, avobenzone (also called butyl methoxydibenzoylmethane), Tinosorb or ecamsule (Mexoryl). As for moisturizing in general, your skin needs all the state-of-the-art ingredients I described in this chapter—antioxidants, skin-identical ingredients, and cell-communicating ingredients—regardless of the time of day.

CHAPTER 9
EVERY SKIN TYPE CAN BENEFIT FROM EXFOLIATING

Perhaps no other part of a daily skin-care regime can have more immediate impact than gently exfoliating skin. Though there are several different ways to exfoliate skin, by far the most effective and well-researched options are alpha hydroxy acids (abbreviated to AHAs) and beta hydroxy acid (abbreviated to BHA). The benefits of using a well-formulated AHA or BHA can be apparent almost immediately, or at the very least within a few days of use. Best of all, your skin will continue to improve over time with ongoing use.

SKIN SHOULD EXFOLIATE NATURALLY...

...on its own, but it doesn't. The top dead layer of normal skin (the stratum corneum) sheds on a regular basis (millions and millions of skin cells every few minutes). This shedding process relates to the physiology of skin, and the way skin cells grow and function. New skin cells are produced in the lower layers of skin (the stratum basal layer); they then move to the surface, changing shape as they go, eventually dying and forming the outer, protective layer of skin (sometimes referred to as the horny layer). These dead skin cells on the surface are eventually shed as newer cells from the lower layers travel to the surface and push them off, continually creating new "dead" layers of skin.

When we are young, skin cells are regenerated and turn over very quickly, about once a week for children. As we age, the rate of skin-cell renewal changes, with the time ranging from about every three weeks through our teens and 20s, and then slowing as we age with the rate varying depending on how healthy the skin is (it's quicker with skin that hasn't been sun damaged or lost estrogen).

Sun damage and stages of menopause both reduce the ability of skin cells to reproduce in a healthy, normal manner. Beyond being smart about sun protection, considering various options of hormone replacement therapy, using skin-care products laden with antioxidants, skin-identical ingredients, and cell-communicating ingredients, or using a prescription retinoid such as tretinoin, there isn't much else that you can do to help improve cell production aside from exfoliation.

WHAT HAPPENS WHEN YOU EXFOLIATE

Sun damage causes the outer layer of skin to become thick and the lower layer of skin (which holds support structures such as collagen and elastin) to become thin and inflexible. In addition to affecting the regeneration of skin cells in the lower layers of skin, the shedding process on the surface can also become inefficient, causing a buildup of skin cells on the outer layers. Sun damage, loss of estrogen, dry skin, oily skin, and disorders such as psoriasis or rosacea can all affect how smoothly this natural exfoliation process takes place. When normal or healthy exfoliation doesn't happen because of these reasons, skin can become rough, scaly, thickened, discolored, and look more lined.

Different forms of exfoliation help to remove the built-up outer layer of skin to uncover a more normal, younger-looking layer hiding beneath. The most effective skin-care options for helping skin with this essential function are a well-formulated (meaning pH-correct) alpha hydroxy acid (AHA; the ingredient shown on the label would be glycolic acid, lactic acid, or gluconoalactone), or beta hydroxy acid (BHA; appearing on the label as salicylic acid). Although salicylic acid is the only BHA option, there are a variety of AHAs. The five major types of AHAs that show up in skin-care products are glycolic, lactic, malic, citric, and tartaric acids. Of these, the most commonly used and most effective AHAs are glycolic and lactic acids. Both of these have the ability to penetrate the skin, plus they have the most accumulated research on their functionality and benefit for skin.

AHAs and BHA are available from several cosmetics brands. Using these types of products on a routine basis (which for some may mean once or twice daily, and for others every other day or just twice per week) will make a remarkable difference in your skin's appearance, not to mention its healthy functioning.

WHY EXFOLIATE

What happens when we help the outer layer of skin function more normally? Your face can truly look younger! The best analogy I can think of is to compare it to the heels of your feet. Before you get a pedicure the built-up, dead layers of skin on your heels look dry, rough, discolored, and scaly, and lines are pronounced. Once that layer is removed, and it can be removed fairly aggressively without damaging anything, your heels look much better. Moreover, once you apply moisturizer, which can now be absorbed better because it hasn't been blocked by the presence of overproduced skin cells, Voila! You have "younger"-looking feet. The wrinkles are gone, the thick scaly appearance is gone, the dryness is gone, and your heels look beautiful. I'm not suggesting we should be that aggressive from the neck up or on most parts of the body, but the same benefits you gain when exfoliating skin on your feet hold true for the face. You just have to be gentler than you are with your heels!

Enhancing skin's exfoliation process and smoothing its texture aren't the only benefits of using an AHA or BHA product. Not only do these products make skin feel and look smoother, but a good deal of impressive research has shown they also provide protection from UV damage (provided you're routinely using a well-formulated sunscreen) and sun-induced tumor development. Even better, they do this while delivering a noticeable improvement in skin structure, and providing significant barrier repair function and collagen stimulation.

(Sources: *Experimental Dermatology*, January 2005, pages 34–40; *Experimental Dermatology*, April 2003, Supplemental, pages 57–63; *Cancer Letters*, December 2002, pages 125–135; *Molecular Carcinogenesis*, July 2001, pages 152–160; and *Dermatologic Surgery*, May 2001, page 429.)

All of these enhancements and the skin is neither compromised nor hindered in any way—now that's exciting! (Source: *Archives of Dermatologic Research*, June 1997, pages 404–409).

Those struggling with acne need to know that exfoliation of facial skin can also unclog pores by keeping dead skin cells from blocking the pore opening so sebum (oil) can flow more normally, which helps reduce blemishes and blackheads; exfoliation also allows antibacterial agents to penetrate to where the bacteria causing acne are hiding.

(Sources: *Archives of Dermatologic Research*, April 2008, Supplemental, pages S31–S38; *Journal of Cosmetic Dermatology*, March 2007, pages 59–65; *Skin Pharmacology and Physiology*, May 2006, pages 283–289; *Journal of Cosmetic Science*, March–April 2006, pages 203–204; *European Journal of Dermatology*, March–April 2002, pages 154–156; *Food and Chemical Toxicology*, November 1999, pages 1105–1111; and *Journal of the American Academy of Dermatology*, September 1996, pages 388–391.)

AHAS VERSUS BHA

The primary difference between AHAs and BHA is that AHAs are water-soluble, while BHA is lipid-(oil) soluble. This unique property of BHA allows it to penetrate the oil in the pores and exfoliate accumulated skin cells inside the pore's follicle lining that can clog them. BHA is best used where blackheads and blemishes are the issue, and AHAs are best for sun-damaged, thickened, dry skin where breakouts are not a problem. (Sources: *Expert Opinion in Pharmacotherapy*, April 2008, pages 955–971; *Seminars in Cutaneous Medicine and Surgery*, September 2008, pages 170–176; and *Global Cosmetic Industry*, November 2000, pages 56–57.)

What glycolic, lactic, and salicylic acids do is "unglue" the outer layer of dead skin cells, allowing healthier cells to come to the surface. You can expect almost immediate benefits from regular use of an AHA or BHA product, such as improved skin texture and color, unclogged pores, and moisturizers being better absorbed by the skin. Sun damage in particular causes the top layer of skin to become thicker, creating a dull, rough appearance on the surface of skin. Fortunately, both AHAs and BHA affect the top layers of skin, and they help to improve the appearance of sun-damaged, dry, and/or thickened skin. (Sources: *Free Radical Biology and Medicine*, May 17, 2008; *International Journal Cosmetic Science*, February 2005, pages 17–34; *Dermatologic Surgery*, May 1998, pages 573–577; and *Archives of Dermatologic Research*, June 1997, pages 404–409.)

SCRUBS VERSUS AHAS AND BHA

Hands-down, using a well-formulated AHA or BHA product is preferred to routine use of a topical scrub. Because AHAs and BHA work through chemical processes, they can penetrate the superficial layers of skin and produce better results than cosmetic scrubs, which work only on the very outermost exposed surface of the skin. And the damaged, built-up layers of skin are not just those you see on the very surface.

Scrubs can only deal with the very top, superficial layer of skin, although those products that have a rough, coarse, uneven texture can cause skin damage by tearing into the skin as it sands away at the surface, causing tiny tears that damage the skin's barrier and cause more problems than they help. If you do want to use a manual scrub, be sure it feels smooth and even on the skin or you will be inadvertently hurting your skin. Or, instead of a scrub, you can simply use a gentle washcloth with your daily cleanser, which works just as well to exfoliate the surface of skin as any cosmetic scrub you can buy.

There is no risk that AHAs and BHA will cause you to lose too much skin. Technically, there is a drop-off rate, meaning that the AHA and BHA will exfoliate only the dead or damaged surface skin and leave the healthy skin alone. This is the main reason why you will see a drop-off in performance when using an AHA or BHA product. The dramatic results when you begin exfoliating (when the thickened, discolored layers of skin are being removed) seem much more impressive than the results from continued use. This is to be expected. Still, it's important to note that continued use of an AHA or BHA product is required in order to maintain skin's smooth, even-toned, healthy appearance.

HOW DO YOU CHOOSE WHICH EXFOLIANT IS BEST FOR YOU?

As a rule, AHAs are best for normal to dry, sun-damaged skin because they only exfoliate on the very surface of skin rather than penetrating inside the pore. AHAs have research showing they improve collagen production and increase skin's moisture-binding ability. My 8% Alpha Hydroxy Acid Gel is a great option for all skin types and can be worn under a moisturizer without feeling heavy or layered with product. I've listed other well-formulated AHA products on my subscription-based Web site, www.Beautypedia.com.

BHA also exfoliates on the surface of skin but has extra properties that make it better for normal to oily or combination skin—and especially blemish- prone skin. Salicylic acid can exfoliate inside the pore and it has anti-inflammatory and mild antibacterial benefits as well.

First-time users of a BHA product can begin with a 1% concentration of salicylic acid; those with oily to very oily skin and stubborn blackheads or blemishes should begin with a 2% concentration. Once you know the concentration you want to try, the only thing left to decide is whether you want a gel, liquid (2% strength only), or lotion texture.

Generally, if you have normal to oily skin with moderate breakouts a gel is a great place to start. If you have very oily skin with moderate to severe breakouts a liquid without alcohol or irritating plant extracts is a great option. If you have normal to combination skin lotions are a wonderful option. Which one to choose? That depends on your personal preference and experimenting to see what works best for you. I offer several BHA options in my line (more than any other cosmetic line I've ever reviewed) and provide a list of the best BHA products on my Beautypedia Web site.

HOW DO YOU USE AHAS OR BHA?

You can apply an AHA or BHA product once or twice a day. Also, depending on your skin's sensitivity, you can apply either of these around the eye area, making sure to keep them off the eyelid and away from the eye itself. Apply the AHA or BHA product after the face is cleansed and after your toner has dried (if you are using one). Once the AHA or BHA has been absorbed, you can apply any other product, such as additional moisturizer, serum, eye cream (if you simply must use one), sunscreen, and/or foundation. Whether or not you use a moisturizer with an AHA or BHA product totally depends on what type of skin you have, how it reacts to the AHA or BHA product, and what kind of base the AHA or BHA you're using comes in. Some AHAs and BHA come in moisturizing bases so an extra product isn't required. Important Note: The skin needs only one good exfoliant, and that's it. Overexfoliating will further irritate the skin, and the long-term effects of that are unknown.

Some people experience a tingling or slight stinging sensation when they use AHA or BHA products with appropriate concentrations and pH. Some people have had minor to severe flaking and redness. Minor, short-term reactions can also occur, given the nature of AHAs and BHA. However, long-term irritation, redness, flaking, or patches of dermatitis are not healthy for the skin, and if any of these symptoms occur you should reduce the frequency of application or consider a gentler (less concentrated) product. Observe your skin. If it gets very dry and flaky, use an additional moisturizer for a period of time until the skin calms down and gets used to the new level of exfoliation. If it gets red and irritated, use the product less frequently, though still regularly (perhaps once a day, or two or three times a week). If it still gets very dry and irritated, consider stopping altogether. Severe irritation is not the goal or the desired result. For various reasons, some people's skin cannot tolerate any AHA or BHA products without acting up.

WHAT ABOUT CLEANSERS WITH AHAS OR BHA INGREDIENTS?

I never recommend cleansers that contain AHAs or BHA, for several reasons. First, if they are in a water-soluble cleanser, you run the risk of possible contact with the eyes, which can cause irritation. Second, AHAs and BHA work on the skin or the pores when they have been absorbed. When they are in a cleanser, they get rinsed down the drain before they can work. Some companies shockingly recommend leaving the cleanser on the face for several minutes so the AHAs or BHA can be absorbed into the skin, but that means the detergent cleansing agents would be left on the skin for longer than necessary, and that absolutely can cause unwanted irritation. Cleansing the face gently is imperative for everyone who wants to have healthy skin. (Sources: *Skin Research and Technology*, February 2005, pages 53–60; and *Dermatology*, March 1997, pages 258–262.)

pH SENSITIVE AHA AND BHA

Without getting too technical, pH is a measurement referring to how acidic or alkaline a product is. The pH scale is numbered 1-14, with 1 being the most acidic and 14 being the most alkaline. Tap water is right in the middle of the scale, with an average pH of 7, which is considered pH-neutral. Given that AHAs and BHA exfoliate skin due to their acidic component, pH is critical to their performing as claimed or not offering much, if any, benefit to skin.

AHAs work best at concentrations of 5% to 10% with a pH of 3 to 4, and their effectiveness diminishes as you go above a pH of 4.5. BHA works best at concentrations of between 1% and 2%, and at an optimal pH of 3, diminishing in effectiveness as you go past a pH of 4. Both AHAs and BHA lose their effectiveness as a product's pH goes up or the concentration of the ingredient goes down. (Sources: *Dermatologic Surgery*, February 2005, pages 149–154; and *Cosmetic Dermatology*, October 2001, pages 15–18.)

If the cosmetics industry isn't forthcoming about the necessary percentages and pH for a BHA or AHA product (and most companies aren't), how can you tell if it provides decent or effective exfoliation? Consumers can't, not unless they are shopping with pH measuring paper in hand, which is exactly how I rate exfoliants when I review products for my book *Don't Go To The Cosmetics Counter Without Me*, 7th Edition, and on my Web site at Beautypedia.com.

As a general rule, it is best if the AHA ingredient is either second or third on the ingredient list, making it likely that the product contains a 5% or higher concentration of AHAs. For salicylic acid, because only a 2% to 0.5% concentration is required, it is fine if this ingredient is located toward the middle or end of the ingredient list.

It is interesting to note that—at any pH—AHAs provide the added benefit of helping to keep water in the skin at the same time that exfoliation is taking place. This is due to the way they affect skin cells, which adds increased protection. AHAs can also increase the production of ceramides in the skin, which help keep it moist and healthy (Source: *Dry Skin and Moisturizers: Chemistry and Function*, edited by Marie Loden and Howard Maibach, 2000, page 237).

While BHA penetrates deeper into the pore than AHAs, it can be less irritating than AHAs. This is due to BHA's chemical relation to aspirin. Aspirin (acetylsalicylic acid) has anti-inflammatory properties and so, on the skin, BHA (salicylic acid), which is derived from aspirin, retains some of its same anti-inflammatory benefits.

One more advantage that the BHA salicylic acid has for those struggling with acne it that it's also mildly antibacterial. When an effective BHA product is combined with a potent topical disinfectant containing benzoyl peroxide, the 1-2 punch against bacteria improves your odds for successfully managing breakouts (Source: Steinberg, David C., *Preservatives for Cosmetics*, 2nd Edition, Allured Publishing, pages 39-40).

AHA IMPOSTORS

There are AHA sound-alikes, including sugarcane extract, mixed fruit acids, fruit extracts, milk extract, and citrus extract. You may think you've purchased a more natural AHA product when you see these less-technical names, but that isn't the case. Although glycolic acid is derived from sugarcane, and lactic acid from milk, that doesn't mean that sugarcane extract or milk extract are the same as glycolic or lactic acid, even though they do share these acids' water-binding properties, in much the same way as salicylic acid shares the anti-inflammatory properties of its close relation, aspirin.

Unless you see glycolic, lactic, malic, tartaric, or citric acid on the ingredient list, the exfoliation picture will be all too vague and meaningless, making it impossible to determine what you are really buying. My advice is to be very suspicious of any product that claims an association with AHAs but contains a variety of ingredients that are only sound-alikes.

BHA IMPOSTORS

Products boasting that they contain a natural source of salicylic acid (BHA) usually add willow bark. Willow bark contains salicin, a substance that when taken orally is converted by the digestion process to salicylic acid. That means the process of converting willow bark to salicylic acid requires the presence of enzymes to turn the salicin into salicylic acid. The claim that willow bark, especially in the tiny amount used in cosmetics, can mimic the effectiveness of salicylic acid on skin is in all likelihood impossible. However, willow bark may indeed have some anti-inflammatory benefits for skin because, in this form, it appears to retain more of its aspirin-like composition.

WHAT ABOUT HIGHER CONCENTRATIONS OF AHAS?

Removing the outer layer of skin can be taken too far. But that's not because of any danger to the skin, it's just that too much skin irritation can cause its own problems. Higher concentrations (above 10%) of AHAs may be too much for skin and the FDA agrees with this assessment (Source: www.fda.gov). Without more evidence showing a benefit from higher concentrations, I feel that you can achieve great results without any unwanted side effects when you stick with AHA products containing no more than 10% AHAs, or BHA products with no more than 2% salicylic acid. Further, the positive results women and men perceive with higher concentrations of AHAs may come from the swelling and edema these products cause. That may diminish the appearance of wrinkles and make the skin feel smoother, but it is most likely not best for the long-term health of the skin due to the increased amount of constant irritation.

CAN YOU EXFOLIATE TOO OFTEN?

What about exfoliating too often? In terms of overdoing it, yes, you can, and then your skin will respond with irritation and inflammation and that isn't good for skin. But does exfoliating skin hinder or harm cell production? Some of my readers have asked me about something known as the Hayflick Limit. The Hayflick Limit is a phenomenon that explains how many times skin cells will be reproduced. There seems to be a preset genetic determination of the number of times a skin cell will be regenerated. This turnover limit only applies what happens in the lower layer of skin where skin cells are produced (the basal layer). What happens on the surface in regard to exfoliation doesn't affect the number of times new skin cells are created. Exfoliation is strictly about the dead surface layer of skin and that doesn't get anywhere near the lower layers where new skin cells are being reproduced. Besides, removing the top layers of skin doesn't cause new skin cells to be formed; the two functions are not related. So you don't need to worry about damaging new skin cells by using topical exfoliants. You do want to be careful to avoid exfoliants that are too strong or too abrasive because of the irritation and inflammation such products cause. They can harm skin more than help it, but that still doesn't affect cell regeneration or speed up the Hayflick Limit.

You may have heard or read that some cosmetics companies are proclaiming that people should stop exfoliating their skin. The reasoning is that by doing so you hold on to your epidermal (surface) cells longer, which creates a more youthful look. There is no reason to preserve our epidermal cells (the outer layers of skin); after all, they die and shed normally! Routine exfoliation just helps them do it in a healthier, more normal manner. What they are confused about is the notion of wanting to preserve the basal layer of skin where skin cells are regenerated, yet that is not in any way related to exfoliation on the surface of skin. If there is research showing that exfoliation changes cell regeneration I have never seen it. What I have seen is lots of research showing that exfoliation is incredibly beneficial for skin. There is even research showing that glycolic acid can reduce skin cancer occurrences, which is astounding.

For the health and appearance of your skin, exfoliation is a key component. It is necessary for most skin types and is as basic as a gentle cleanser, sunscreen, and the need for skin to get topically applied antioxidants and cell-communicating ingredients!

(Sources: *International Journal of Cosmetic Science*, June 2008, pages 175–182; *Phytotherapy Research*, November 2006, pages 921–934; *Journal of Cosmetic Dermatology*, September 2006, pages 246–253; *Aesthetic and Plastic Surgery*, May–June 2006, pages 356–362; *Journal of Dermatology*, January 2006, pages 16–22; *Cosmetic Science*, September–October 2002, pages 269–282; *Molecular Carcinogenesis*, July 2001, pages 152–160; and *British Journal of Dermatology*, February 2001, pages 267–273.)

POLYHYDROXY ACIDS

The search for an effective form of AHA or an extra ingredient that can enhance performance and reduce irritation has been a popular topic of discussion among cosmetics formulators. Gluconolactone is a type of polyhydroxy acid that NeoStrata (the company that developed and patented this ingredient) believes serves both ends: It is supposed to be just as effective as AHAs but also less irritating.

Gluconolactone (PHA) is similar to AHAs. The significant difference between the two is that gluconolactone has a larger molecular structure, which limits its penetration into the skin, resulting in a reduction of irritating side effects in some skin types. Is gluconolactone better for your skin than AHAs? Research indicates that AHA and PHA perform identically, with AHA having a slight edge for improving the appearance of skin and PHA having less risk of irritation (Source: *Cutis*, February 2003, pages S14–S17).

EXFOLIATING OILY SKIN

All skin types can benefit from exfoliating but those who have oily or blemish-prone skin, or clogged pores can benefit significantly. Blackheads or blemishes can occur if the oil gland produces too much sebum. Sebum is a soft wax that should liquefy when it reaches the surface of the pore, spreading a thin, imperceptible protective layer over the skin. But when too much sebum is produced, the liquefying process can get backed up. Add to that problem a tendency for skin cells that should be naturally sloughing off to instead fall inside the pore lining and get stuck. The more skin cells that build up in the oil gland, the more oil will be held back from flowing easily out of the pore (the pore is the exit path for oil), and the result can be a blackhead or, when the right bacteria that cause inflammation are present, an acne lesion.

Often with oily skin, cells that should be shedding on a regular, daily basis are being held back. One thing that keeps cells from sloughing off is that self-same oil (sebum). The oil works as an adhesive, preventing the shedding skin cells from going where they are supposed to go—off the face. One way to keep pores from getting clogged is to help skin cells shed as freely as possible so they don't get trapped inside the pore. The more you keep skin cells exfoliating in a normal manner, the less cell debris can fill up the pore.

Another issue for oily skin with clogged pores is that the oil gland itself has a skin lining (epithelial lining). For some reason, this lining inside the pore can become thickened or misshapen and choke off and block the flow of oil out of the pore. Using exfoliants that can exfoliate the lining of the pore, thus restoring a more natural shape, can encourage a normal flow of oil and eliminate clogged pores.

EXFOLIATING DRY SKIN

The reasons for exfoliating dry skin are different from the ones for treating oily, blemish-prone skin, though the objective is the same: removing dead skin cells that are not shedding normally. Skin can be dry for many reasons, including lack of moisture, a buildup of dead skin cells that don't easily shed, and abnormal skin cells that adhere together in a way that prevents normal exfoliation and normal moisture retention. (Dry-looking skin can also be caused by moisturizers that are too emollient and hold dead skin cells in place, preventing healthy shedding. When this happens, the surface of the skin feels "greasy" or moist, and the underlying layer feels dry.) When you help dry skin shed dried-up, dead skin cells, it can make room for plumper (moisture-filled), less-dry skin cells to come to the surface, which can lend a fresher look to the skin. This also allows moisturizers to more easily penetrate the skin because there are fewer dried-up skin cells in the way to block absorption. Exfoliating helps the dead, surface-skin cells shed at a more normal rate, making room for the lower layers of newer skin cells. And for dry skin it is also helpful to efficiently remove dead skin cells to reduce the chance of pores becoming clogged and creating blackheads and whiteheads.

EXFOLIATING SUN-DAMAGED SKIN

One of the primary manifestations of sun-damaged skin is that the outer layer of skin becomes thickened, similar to a callous. This thickened layer is your skin's response to the damage caused by unprotected exposure to ultraviolet radiation from the sun. While this thickened layer provides a minimal amount of sun protection (it is thought to protect with the equivalent of an SPF of 2), it ends up creating far more problems than advantages. As you have read in Chapter Seven on sun protection, an SPF of 2 is truly meaningless and useless for skin. This thickened outer layer of the skin produced by sun damage causes skin to look dull and more wrinkled than it really is; it also adds a yellowish or gray tint to skin and reduces the ability of good skin-care ingredients to penetrate. Using effective topical exfoliants to remove this thickened, unattractive outer layer of skin can help skin feel smoother, look less wrinkled, have a healthier, more normal skin color, and reduce the chance of clogged pores. (Removing this layer of unhealthy skin does make the skin more sun sensitive, the way it was before it became sun damaged. Though it is always imperative to use a sunscreen, it is even more so if you are regularly using an exfoliant of any kind.)

CHAPTER 10
SKIN-CARE PLANNING:
GOING OVER THE BASICS

IS SKIN CARE ROCKET SCIENCE?

As I look over the material and research I've accumulated, from magazine articles and books on botanicals and herbal ingredients to medical and scientific journals, as well as from interviews with dermatologists, oncologists, and cosmetics chemists, I am amazed at the depth of information available on skin and skin care. It is also mind-boggling to realize how many thousands of products you can choose from when it comes to everything from cleaning the face, to protecting skin from the sun, moisturizing, fighting blemishes, or treating a large number of skin problems. You wouldn't think that taking care of your skin could be so complicated or shrouded in such controversy, but the truth is, it is very complicated. It is rocket science!

Despite being such a small part of the whole body, the face has the lion's share of topical problems, far more than those that take place from the neck down. Acne, wrinkles, sagging, sunburn, blackheads, dryness, rosacea, eczema, psoriasis, seborrhea, dry patches, swelling, and allergies, not to mention the impact of our concepts of beauty, are most evident on the face. There is a lot of money to be made if a cosmetics company can get a consumer to believe that their product(s) will make her more beautiful and do something to tackle one or more of those facial dilemmas. If a company can make the stuff sound utterly unique for the skin, even when it isn't, the sales figures rise astronomically.

As complicated and emotional as skin care can be, the actual skin-care routines can be streamlined and concise. Yet the details in each category are tricky because there is a lot you have to unlearn and then relearn. By now you have an overview of what works (such as being gentle, using sun protection, exfoliating, and what antioxidants, skin-identical ingredients, and cell-communicating ingredients do). You also know what doesn't (such as one special ingredient, jar packaging, eye creams, exaggerated claims, certain natural or exotic ingredients, and all essential oils) when it comes to cosmetics claims and various skin-care ingredients.

If you've gotten this far in the book (and haven't skipped chapters) you are also aware of how the cosmetics industry may be damaging your skin and what current research is revealing about optimal skin care. The next step is to arrange all these data in a way that helps you find an effective skin-care routine so you can stop wasting money on useless products that may be hurting your skin.

GOING OVER THE BASICS

Cleaning the skin, removing makeup, toning, exfoliating, and applying sunscreen, moisturizer, and facial masks are the general basic categories for taking care of your skin. This section reviews how those steps work, why they are important, and how the industry distorts their purpose or makes it difficult to know what to choose.

CLEANING THE SKIN

No other aspect of skin care is quite as basic as this one. Cleaning the face sets the stage for everything else that will take place on the skin. More so than any other part of your skin-care routine, it is essential that the cleansing products you use be gentle. Over-cleaning or using cleansers that are too drying or that strip the skin are major causes of irritation, dry patches, and redness. Not cleaning the skin well enough can clog pores or leave a residue on the face that can prevent skin cells from sloughing off. Using a cleanser that leaves a greasy film on the face can clog pores and prevent moisturizers from being able to be absorbed and do their job. It is essential to get this step right, and that means thoroughly, but gently, cleaning the face.

(Sources: *Dermatologic Therapy*, September–October 2008, pages 416–421; *Cutis*, July 2006, pages S34–S40; *SKINmed*, May–June 2005, pages 183–185; *Clinical Dermatology*, September–October 2004, pages 360–366; and December 2001, pages 12–19.)

Generally, most skin-care routines start with using a makeup remover. Although that can work effectively, it is an option, not a requirement. My preference is to recommend that all skin types start with using a gentle, water-soluble cleanser. I've already explained how important being gentle is, but just to reiterate: Irritating and inflaming the skin triggers a cascading chain reaction that can include increased oil production, flaky dry skin, depletion of collagen, and other factors that "age" skin.

But why start with a cleanser as opposed to an eye-makeup/facial-makeup remover? You can begin with an eye or makeup remover, which is indeed an option. However, wiping at the face is a problem because tugging on the skin damages the elastin fibers in skin, increasing the potential for sagging, especially around the eyes. The less you pull the better your skin will hold up in the long run. Washing your face with a water-soluble cleanser reduces pulling (the water cuts friction), and most if not all of the makeup is rinsed down the drain. Then if you still need a makeup remover it would only be for touch-up, causing minimal pulling. So a gentle, water-soluble cleanser is a great place to start!

WHAT IS THE BEST CLEANSER?

Using the right cleanser makes all the difference in the world because it determines how your skin is going to react to everything else you put on it. Greasing up your skin with a wipe-off, cold cream–type cleanser can clog pores and leave a film on the skin, which means all the other products you put on will be sitting on top of that instead of being easily absorbed. Trying to degrease the skin with a drying toner after using this kind of greasy cleanser to remove makeup can cause irritation and a range of other problems. Using a cleanser that is overly drying in the hopes of treating oily skin or blemishes absolutely won't work. The irritation and barrier damage to skin impede healing, increase acne-causing bacteria in skin, and increase oil production because irritation stimulates oil production. Using a gentle, water-soluble cleanser is the best option for the entire face, and this is true for all skin types. (Sources: *Skin Research and Technology*, February 2005, pages 53–60; and *Dermatologic Therapy*, January 2004, pages 16–25.)

Most of us are familiar with the three primary categories of cleansers available: wipe-off cleansers (including cold creams and creamy makeup removers), soaps of all kinds (including bar cleansers, which technically are not soap), and water-soluble cleansers (creamy, lotion, or shampoo-like cleansers that rinse off).

What differentiates a good water-soluble cleanser from a poor one? Three basic qualities:
1. It washes off makeup without leaving the face dry (like soaps) or greasy (like cold cream), or drying skin, as liquid cleansers can sometimes do;
2. It contains no obvious fragrance (even though the fragrance ingredients would quickly rinse off the face, any potential for needless irritation should be avoided), or abrasive, scrublike particles (scrubs should be used carefully and judiciously, not as part of cleaning the skin twice a day); and
3. It matches your skin type, meaning it should be more emollient for dry skin and provide more thorough cleansing (not drying and irritating) for oily/combination skin.

Some cleansers on the market are labeled "water soluble," but in actuality they need to be wiped off with a wet washcloth. If the cleanser must be wiped off with a tissue or washcloth, it need not be a problem but it would only be an option for someone with dry skin.

Water-soluble cleansers are not only the gentlest way to clean the face, they are also the most efficient. Everything is done at the sink. Imagine splashing your face generously with (tepid) water, then massaging a water-soluble cleanser on evenly over your face, including the eyes, and then rinsing it off with more water, preferably with your hands. Once the face is rinsed, it shouldn't feel greasy or dry.

Expensive water-soluble cleansers are truly a waste of money. First there is nothing in a cleanser that warrants the price difference. There are only so many ingredients that can clean the face and remove makeup. Second, when cleansers do contain some bells and whistles to make you think you're getting something special, those ingredients would just be rinsed down the drain without ever getting a chance to be absorbed and provide a benefit on the skin.

In my book *Don't Go to the Cosmetics Counter Without Me*, 7th Edition, and on my Web site, www.Beautypedia.com, I provide a complete summary of the best water-soluble cleansers for each skin type.

Summary: Use only water-soluble cleansers that rinse off completely when water is splashed on the face, leaving the face with a clean, soft feeling that is neither dry nor greasy. Creamy, water-soluble cleansers are an option for dry skin.

Basic directions: Wash your hands first and then splash the face generously, including the eyes, with tepid water (not hot or cold). Once the face is soaking wet, take your cleanser and massage it generously all over the face, including the eyelids. Rinse very well. If traces of makeup are left behind, or if you have very oily skin, you may need to repeat this step. Use a gentle washcloth if you are wearing heavy makeup, ultra-matte foundations, or other hard-to-remove makeup, or want an alternative to using a scrub.

WHAT ABOUT CLEANSERS WITH "ACTIVE" INGREDIENTS?

More and more products of all kinds in the cosmetics industry, from eye shadows to concealers, foundations, and cleansers, are proclaiming that they contain active ingredients or specialty ingredients that can fight free-radical damage, acne, wrinkles, skin discolorations, and even sun damage. Since we have to clean our face twice a day, the notion of having a cleanser, or any product, with a dual purpose sounds like it would be the best of both worlds. Ingredients such as exfoliants (AHAs and BHA), anti-acne help (benzoyl peroxide), and antioxidants (such as vitamins and myriad plant extracts) are being added along with claims that they are providing benefits beyond just cleansing.

There are many problems with this concept. First, the ingredients would be rinsed down the drain in a rinse-off product or wiped away with a wipe-off product. The extras just don't stay around long enough to positively impact skin. More problematic is the inclusion of ingredients you don't want to get in your eye when splashing, such as AHAs (glycolic acid) or benzoyl peroxide. While there is research showing that benzoyl peroxide in cleansers can be beneficial, the risk to the eyes isn't the best, and a leave-on product would be far more effective. One more downside to active ingredients in cleansers is that plant extracts and vitamins don't remain stable when exposed to water. Even when these ingredients are encapsulated there are limitations to the cleansing process that hinders their effectiveness.

SUNSCREEN IN CLEANSERS

The topic of sunscreens in cleansers is a unique discussion. If a cleanser has active sunscreen ingredients, that means it needs to remain on the skin after you are done washing and rinsing in the shower or bath. Assuming the product includes UVA-protecting ingredients, is applying sunscreen as simple and convenient as washing your face or body? The answer is yes. Any product labeled with an SPF is regulated by the FDA and has to meet the testing standards for all SPF products, which these specialized cleansers do. But in terms of practical use they have some significant caveats and concerns you need to consider.

What remains unclear, beyond what it takes for a product to get approved for an SPF rating, is what happens during its actual use. For example, even using a typical SPF has limitations if you don't apply it liberally, or if you apply other products over it that dilute its potency. Both these conditions would be especially true of cleansers with sunscreen. What happens when additional skin-care products are applied over these sunscreen actives after you get out of the shower? Does the sunscreen diminish if you apply an exfoliant, moisturizer, and/or makeup on top of the actives adhering to your skin? Or what happens if you vigorously dry your skin with a towel? There is a strong possibility that you would indeed be reducing the SPF protection. The sunscreen chemist I spoke with concerning this issue told me that simply manipulating sunscreen ingredients so they adhere to skin doesn't mean they're impervious to being rubbed off once other products are applied afterward, or with a towel when you get out of the shower. Because of these potential unanswered limitations, I cautiously recommend that you *not* rely only on a cleanser with sunscreen for your sun protection.

WHAT ABOUT BAR SOAP?

For many reasons it is best to avoid bar soap, especially from the neck up, but it can also be helpful to avoid it from the neck down. Although this is particularly true if you have problems with dry skin or breakouts, there are issues with using most bar soaps or bar cleansers no matter what type of skin you have.

Some people believe that the tight sensation they feel after washing with soap means their face is clean; tight like you almost can't open your mouth without feeling your skin stretch. The thinking is that the more squeaky-clean your face feels, the better off you are. Yet the feeling you associate with being clean is nothing more than irritated, dried-out, and stressed skin. The difficulty with asking someone to break a soap habit is that soap really does clean the skin thoroughly. Unfortunately, it cleans too thoroughly, and ends up causing irritation and all the associated skin problems that come with irritating the skin (Source: *Skin Research and Technology*, July 2001, pages 49–55).

The major issue with bar soap is its high alkaline content (meaning it has a high pH). "The increase of the skin pH irritates the physiological protective 'acid mantle', changes the composition of the cutaneous bacterial flora and the activity of enzymes in the upper epidermis, which have an acid pH optimum" (Source: *Dermatology*, March 1997, pages 258–262). That technical description basically explains that skin's normal pH is about 5.5, while most bar soaps have a pH of around 8 to 10, which negatively impacts the surface of skin by causing irritation and increasing the presence of bacteria in the skin. There is definitely research showing that washing with a cleanser that has a pH of 7 or higher, which is true for many bar soaps and bar cleansers, increases the presence of bacteria significantly when compared to using a cleanser with a pH of 5.5. (Sources: *Clinics in Dermatology*, January–February 1996, pages 23–27; and *Dermatology*, 1995, volume 191, issue 4, pages 276–280.)

What about specialty soaps that come in clear bars, have nonsoap-sounding names, or contain creams and emollients that appear to have none of the properties of regular soap? Bar cleansers (and technically they're not soap) often have a lower pH and are therefore far less irritating to skin. However, the ingredients that keep the bar cleanser in its bar form can theoretically absorb into skin and clog pores. There is also no convenient way for a consumer to test each particular bar to be sure the pH is compatible with skin. Further, many of the so-called gentle bar cleansers I've reviewed contain fairly drying, irritating, and potentially pore-clogging ingredients. So much for specialty soaps being different! Worse yet, the soaps designed for oily or acned skin contain even harsher ingredients. Soaps designed for dry and sensitive skin often contain beneficial ingredients such as glycerin, petrolatum (mineral oil), or vegetable oil, and while they might make the face feel somewhat less stiff after you rinse, and reduce the irritation potential, the skin still doesn't need the ingredients that hold the soap in its bar shape. (Sources: *International Journal of Cosmetic Science*, August 2008, pages 277–283; and *International Journal of Dermatology*, August 2002, pages 494–499.)

Here's a rundown of some basic categories of soaps. Remember, just because a product is advertised as soap doesn't mean it is.

Castile soaps use olive oil instead of animal fat, but the cleansing agent, sodium hydroxide, is still fairly irritating to the skin.

Transparent soaps look milder or less drying because of their unclouded, clear appearance, but many contain harsh cleansing ingredients, can still have an alkaline pH, and the ingredients that give the bar its shape can clog pores.

Acne soaps often contain very irritating ingredients in addition to harsh cleansers that, especially when combined with other acne treatments, can super-irritate the skin. There is no reason to overclean the skin. Breakouts have nothing to do with how clean your skin is! A study in *Infection* (March–April 1995, pages 89–93) demonstrated that "in the group using soap the mean number of inflammatory [acne] lesions increased…. Symptoms or signs of irritation were seen in 40.4% of individuals…." Furthermore, if the acne cleanser contains antibacterial agents, the benefit would be washed down the drain, though there is research showing the cleansers containing benzoyl peroxide can have benefit but they were not in soap form (Source: *Journal of Drugs in Dermatology*, May 2006, pages 442-445).

Cosmetic soaps or bar cleansers are sold at the cosmetics counters for far more money than they are worth. Although these are advertised as being gentle or specially formulated, they are no better than or different from what you can buy at the drugstore. The irritating and pore-clogging ingredients are still included regardless of the price or claim.

Superfatted soaps contain extra oils and fats that supposedly make them gentler for the face. Basis soap is one of the most popular superfatted specialty soaps. However, the extra glycerin, petrolatum, or beeswax in these soaps won't prevent irritation and can cause breakouts.

Oatmeal soaps are supposed to be better at absorbing oil and soothing sensitive skin than other soaps or bar cleansers. There are studies demonstrating that oatmeal can have anti-irritant properties. How that translates into a bar cleanser is unknown, but the benefits are probably nonexistent given the amount of time the oatmeal is actually on the skin and the presence of other irritating ingredients. Plus, the oatmeal particles are fairly large and end up usually being more abrasive on skin, and that isn't gentle in the least.

"Natural" soaps are those that contain vitamins, fruits, vegetables, plants, flowers, herbs, aloe, and specialty oils; these ingredients are gimmicks and serve no purpose when it comes to cleansing the face. They don't nourish the skin or provide any other health benefit—that is sheer marketing whimsy and nothing more. Plus, the cleansing agents and the ingredients that keep the soap in bar form are the same as in any other bar cleanser.

Beauty bars and *Syndet* cleansers such as Dove are about 50% sodium cocoyl isethionate (a form of coconut oil) and, although it is not as irritating as other cleansing agents found in soaps, it is still potentially irritating and drying, especially in such a high concentration. Dove claims to be moisturizing, and it does contain emollients to help soften the effect of the cleansing agent. If the manufacturers left out the drying and irritating ingredients altogether, they wouldn't need to add emollients to counteract them. Also, the ingredients that help the bar keep its shape can clog pores. Dove is a better bet than most bar cleansers but can still create an uphill battle for getting the skin you want (Source: *Cutis*, May 2006, pages 317–324).

EYE-MAKEUP REMOVERS

Eye-makeup removers are extremely helpful but you need to use them carefully. Repeated pulling at the skin can be problematic because it stretches skin and damages the skin's elastin fibers. Elastin is a stretchable, elastic protein found in skin tissue that is responsible for the flexible, resilient nature of healthy skin. When skin is being pulled and yanked, elastin's orderly arrangement can change. Regardless of the direction you pull—up, down, or sideways—if you see the skin move, you are tugging on the skin's elastic fibers and helping the skin to sag sooner than it would otherwise. No matter how gently it's done, this pulling distends the tissue more than enough to stretch it. Watch closely in the mirror the next time you start wiping off your makeup, particularly eye makeup. If it takes that much pulling to remove your makeup, consider what I am about to suggest concerning how to get your makeup off.

The process is pretty straightforward if your makeup is water soluble. Because so many water-soluble cleansers use mild ingredients that don't affect the eyes any differently than makeup removers do, they can easily remove all of your makeup, including eye makeup. When you use water with a gentle face cleanser that slips over the face and is easily rinsed off, it decreases friction and minimizes any pulling. Then if there are any traces of makeup left behind you can use your gentle makeup remover to get them, which will require far less pulling and tugging. If you are used to wiping off makeup, it can take a while to get used to washing it off, but it is the most effective and least problematic way to remove eye makeup.

The exception to this rule is when you are using waterproof or water-resistant makeup, waterproof mascara, very heavy or thick foundations, or ultra-matte or transfer-resistant foundations. In these instances, it is necessary to use a gentle, wipe-off makeup remover to help get all your makeup off before using the cleanser, and to be as delicate as possible in doing that.

REMOVING ALL YOUR MAKEUP IS ESSENTIAL

If you want a basic remedy for potentially eliminating or at the very least reducing puffy or irritated skin around the eyes, here it is: Be sure to remove every last trace of eye makeup before you go to bed. You would be surprised how much makeup can be left behind if you aren't careful. A dermatologist I often consult with mentioned that when she is looking at her patients' skin under a magnifying glass she is always dismayed to see how much makeup is crusted into the lines around the eyes. Not a pretty picture. If you wear foundation, concealer, eyeshadows, eye pencils, and mascara, you must be sure it is all off every night. Going to sleep wearing makeup causes irritation, whether it's left on skin or gets directly into the eye. It can also clog pores when left on the face overnight, preventing skin from shedding skin cells in a normal manner. If you're noticing a bumpy texture or reddened skin on the eyelid or under the eye, it may be because you're not removing all of your eye makeup.

WASHCLOTHS VERSUS SCRUBS

Using a washcloth every night to help get your makeup off or for exfoliation can be just as effective, if not more so, than using a scrub you purchase. Scrubs are an option when they are gentle (overly abrasive scrubs can be irritating and damaging to the skin's vital protective surface), but why use a second product when you only need one? Plus you wouldn't want to use a scrub product over the eye area and risk getting those particles in the eye. To be certain that you are getting all your makeup off and gently exfoliating at the same time, using a washcloth in conjunction with a gentle, water-soluble cleanser is a great option. The goal is to always remove your makeup thoroughly every night, since leaving any amount of makeup on all night long can cause irritation, breakouts, or dryness. One more thing: be sure to use a clean washcloth every time. Re-using a damp washcloth will transfer unhelpful bacteria to skin, even if you thoroughly rinse before re-using.

WATER TEMPERATURE IS IMPORTANT!

While it is of vital importance to pay attention to the right type of cleanser, it is also important to pay attention to the temperature of the water you use. For the most part, splashing water on the face is one of the most nonirritating things you can do to your skin (though on rare occasions there are people with serious atopic dermatitis who find water irritating to the skin). Although water is the gentlest part of cleaning the face, it is gentle only when the water is tepid. Hot water can burn and irritate the skin, and cold water will shock and irritate it. Because the goal is always to be gentle to reduce irritation, redness, and swelling, and to prevent any negative impact on the skin's immune response, using tepid water is essential. (Sources: *Advances in Skin & Wound Care*, 2000, volume 13, pages 127–128; and *Acta Dermato-Venereologica*, July 1996, pages 274–276.)

Water is also frictionless, a beneficial quality that is another very important reason to choose it. When you splash your face with tepid water, your hands glide over the face, letting you avoid pulling and tugging at the skin. That means you can remove makeup without stretching the skin tissue, making it overall a better way to treat skin.

WHAT DO TONERS TONE?

In reality, toners—also referred to as astringents, clarifiers, refiners, fresheners, and tonics—don't tone anything. At least not by the dictionary definition of "tone," which refers to the "normal firmness of a tissue or an organ." The term "toner" is a caprice invented by the cosmetics industry and, therefore, it can mean anything they want it to. I have heard that toners do everything from balance the skin and close pores to deep-clean and prepare the skin for other products. They do none of that. In fact, toners of any kind do not close pores, they do not deep-clean pores, and they do not reduce oil production. If toners could do any of that, given the repeated daily use of these items by most women, who would have a visible pore left on their face?

There are no ingredients in toners that can firm skin and return it to its normal state. What well-formulated toners can do is help reduce inflammation, add antioxidants, skin-identical ingredients, and cell-communicating ingredients to skin, soothe skin after cleansing, help remove any last traces of makeup, and impart some lightweight moisturizing ingredients to skin. All of those things can have a beautiful, significant impact on the appearance of your skin and can make a huge difference, but you still haven't "toned" anything.

Regrettably, not all toners are created equal, and many are terribly formulated, especially those containing alcohol, meaning they have a real capacity to cause irritation, redness, and dryness. No matter what toners are called (astringent, freshener, pore cleanser, clarifying lotion, witch hazel, and so on), and whether they are inexpensive or expensive—if they contain irritants they are bad for skin.

When toners don't contain irritants they can still fall flat when they are poorly formulated and lack any real beneficial ingredients for skin (such as antioxidants, skin-identical ingredients, or cell-communicating ingredients). Your toner should not only be free of irritants but it should also be filled with state-of-the-art ingredients for your skin.

It is best if the toner is fragrance-free, but those are hard to find. In my book *Don't Go to the Cosmetics Counter Without Me* and on my Web site at www.Beautypedia.com, I provide a complete list of the best toners for each skin type. I am also pleased to state that all of the toners in my Paula's Choice line meet the standards outlined above for what a state-of-the-art toner needs to be effective for skin.

Summary: Many irritant-free toners are a fine alternative as an extra cleansing step after cleaning the skin with a water-soluble cleanser. Toners won't close pores and they won't deep-clean, but depending on the formulation they can leave the face feeling soft and smooth, remove the last traces of makeup or oil, reduce or eliminate irritation, provide antioxidant protection, soothe the skin, and lightly moisturize skin. For some skin types, a toner can be the only moisturizer you need to use (especially during summer).

Basic directions: After cleansing the face, soak a large cotton ball with the toner and gently stroke it over the face and neck.

ALCOHOL IS ALWAYS A PROBLEM FOR SKIN

Fortunately, the use of alcohol in toners has definitely decreased over the past several years. However, it still shows up, especially in astringents and toners aimed at those with oily or acne-prone skin. If you were under the impression that alcohol is somehow helpful for acne you would be mistaken. There is no research showing that to be the case. For alcohol to be effective in disinfecting skin and killing acne-causing bacteria, it would need to be 60% to 70% pure alcohol. Most astringents with alcohol are only in the 20% range. Even at a 40% level you would not get an effective disinfectant, although you would get an effective irritant that kills skin cells and causes free-radical damage. Further, the irritation and dryness alcohol causes depletes the skin's intercellular matrix and protective outer barrier. Not only does that damage the skin's ability to heal, but at the same time it increases the presence of bacteria in the skin. In the long run, all of that can only make breakouts worse (Source: *Archives of Dermatological Research*, 1995, volume 287, issue 2, pages 214–218).

Note: Do not be confused by cosmetics that contain ingredients that sound like alcohol but are not. For example, cetyl alcohol, stearyl, or other alcohol esters are not the type of alcohol I'm warning you about. Remember to check the ingredient list; if it says "sd alcohol" followed by a number, or uses the terms "ethanol" or "isopropyl alcohol" on the label, those are the kinds to avoid. The exception to this is when this type if alcohol makes up only a tiny percentage of a product's contents. When that's the case, the risk of irritation and dryness is, in all likelihood, impossible.

Aside from alcohol, other irritating ingredients found in toner-type products include acetone (that's nail-polish remover), citrus (lemon, grapefruit, and orange juice are incredibly irritating to the skin because of their high acid content), camphor, mint, peppermint, menthol, volatile plant extracts, fragrance (or essential oils, which are nothing more than fragrance additives), and witch hazel. All of these ingredients can hurt the skin because of irritation or skin sensitivity, and should be avoided.

If a toner does contain irritants, all that irritation does to a pore is temporarily cause it to swell, which can make the pore look smaller for maybe a few minutes. Toners that contain alcohol can remove the surface oil from the skin, but if you've cleansed the skin properly there should be no excess surface oil left. You can't get inside the pore with a toner to deep-clean it without causing damage (if you could, we would all have spotless, empty pores), so toners surely don't work in that capacity. Most of all, toners do not reduce oil production. Oil production is controlled primarily by hormonal activity (Source: *Medical Electron Microscopy*, March 2001, pages 29–40).

If anything, the irritation caused by alcohol and other irritating ingredients can stimulate oil production by triggering neurogenic inflammation in the pore, thus producing more oil. I will discuss this concept more in Chapter Fifteen, *Solutions for Acne* (Sources: *Archives of Dermatologic Research*, July 2008, pages 311–316; *Dermatology*, January 2003, pages 17–23; and *Medical Electron Microscopy*, March 2001, pages 29–40.)

EXFOLIANTS

All skin types can benefit from exfoliation. The issue is not whether to exfoliate, but which type you should use and how often. The chief options are alpha hydroxy acids (AHAs), beta hydroxy acid (BHA), and topical scrubs, with the latter being the least effective and least beneficial by comparison. I discuss the process of exfoliation and the various types of exfoliants available (and how to use them) in Chapter Nine, *Every Skin Type Can Benefit from Exfoliating*. I list the best exfoliants for all skin types in my book *Don't Go to the Cosmetics Counter Without Me*, 7th Edition, and on my Web site, www.Beautypedia.com.

RETINOIDS (RETINOL, RETIN-A, DIFFERIN, AND TAZORAC)

Retinoids are an important topic to discuss when it comes to skin care. Retinoids are a general term referring to a vast range of ingredients derived from vitamin A (retinol is the technical name for vitamin A). Retinol is a cosmetic ingredient while other retinoids such as tretinoin (the general term is all-trans retinoic acid or just retinoic acid) or adapalene (the active ingredient in Differin) are prescription-only topical ingredients. Prescription-only, topically applied retinoids are significant for skin because they can positively affect the way cells are formed deep in the dermis.

If you have sun-damaged, dry, wrinkled, or acne-prone skin, you should become familiar with the prescription-only product names Retin-A, Renova, Differin, Avita, and Tazorac, which all contain different forms of retinoids. The active ingredient in Retin-A, Avita, and Renova is tretinoin; Differin uses adapalene; and Tazorac uses tazorotene. In fact, both Renova and Tazorac have been approved by the FDA for the treatment of wrinkles.

Retinol is a cosmetic ingredient, and when it is absorbed into skin it can become the more active form of all-trans retinoic acid, making it a cosmetic alternative to prescription options. Different forms of retinol, in descending order of potency in cosmetics, are retinol, retinylaldehyde (also referred to as retinal), retinyl palmitate, retinyl propionate, and retinyl acetate.

(Sources: *Clinics in Dermatology*, November–December 2008, pages 633–635; *American Journal of Clinical Dermatology*, November 2008, pages 369–381; *Journal of Drugs in Dermatology*, July 2008, pages S2–S6; *Harvard Women's Health Watch*, September 2007, pages 6–7; *Archives of Dermatology*, May 2007, pages 606–612; *Clinical Interventions in Aging*, 2006, volume 1, issue 4, pages 327–348; *Dermatologic Surgery*, June 2004, pages 864–866; *Archives of Dermatology*, November 2002, pages 1486–1493; *Clinical and Experimental Dermatology*, October 2001, pages 613–618; and www.fda.gov.)

Note that retinoids are not exfoliants, though many people think that's what they do. Exfoliants such as AHAs and BHA primarily affect the top layers of skin, improving its appearance, integrity, and protection potential. They also help improve the function of the pore. In contrast, retinoids affect the lower layers of skin (dermis), where new skin cells are produced. Retinoids actually communicate with a skin cell as it is being formed, telling it to develop normally instead of developing as a sun-damaged or genetically malformed skin cell.

Why the confusion about the effect retinoids can have on the skin? Primarily it's due to the fact that products containing retinoids, and even the milder form retinol, can cause irritation and inflammation, resulting in the skin becoming flaky and dry. This flaking and dryness is not exfoliation, nor is it a desirable or advantageous result. If retinoids cause your skin to be consistently dry and flaky, it is a problem and you should probably avoid products that contain it, reduce how often you use them, or consider a retinoid product with a lesser potency.

Despite the valuable effect retinoids can have for skin, don't expect them to "erase" wrinkles. That's because, while the improvement is impressive and the improvement in the overall function of skin cells is notable, it is neither dramatic nor superior to surgery or medical cosmetic corrective procedures. However, if skin cells can be produced with a healthier form and shape, the skin's surface will have a smoother appearance, skin cells will do their job of turning over in a more normal fashion, the protective outer layer of skin will remain intact, enhancing the skin's healing response, and on and on. In essence, the skin will behave and look the way it did (to some extent) before it was damaged by the sun.

Regardless of these positive effects, retinoids will be useless, and the skin will be prone to more damage, if you do not wear a sunscreen as well. Not a wrinkle cream in the world, even one approved by the FDA, can have positive results if you don't use an effective sunscreen; without that, you are just adding to damage you already have accumulated.

What retinoids, AHA, and BHA products have in common is that once you stop using them, your skin will revert to the way it was before. These products will not produce permanent change. The smooth exterior lasts only as long as you use them. Yet when used together, long-term, they are a formidable weapon in the battle against wrinkles and blemishes.

SUNSCREEN

Regardless of the time of year, where you live, the color of your skin, or the amount of time you spend in the sun, sunscreen should be an essential part of your morning skin-care routine. It takes only a few minutes in the sun—the time it takes to walk to your car or to your office—for sun damage to begin. Over time this can cause serious wrinkling, even if you don't tan on a regular basis. For detailed information on sunscreen, refer to Chapter Seven, *Sun Sense And Sensibility.*

MOISTURIZERS
(THEY AREN'T WHAT YOU THINK THEY ARE)

I wish I could find another word for this step but I haven't, and it would probably only complicate matters anyway. In reality, not everyone needs a "moisturizer" but everyone needs to add antioxidants, skin-identical ingredients, and cell-communicating ingredients to their skin every day to maintain and achieve as much as possible the skin they want. The standard term for this final skin-care step is moisturizer, but as I explained in Chapter Eight, this step is not about giving skin moisture, and it isn't about applying a lotion or cream. It's not about anti-wrinkle products or treatments or serums, or lifting products either. This final step is about giving skin the substances it needs to repair itself, heal, create healthy skin cells, make healthy collagen and elastin, and improve the skin's immune response. Those ingredients fall into the three categories of antioxidants, skin-identical ingredients, and cell-communicating ingredients. Regardless of the product's name or its texture, choosing a product loaded with these elements is vital for making any skin function more normally and look as young and healthy as possible.

All skin types require antioxidants, skin-identical ingredients, and cell-communicating ingredients. As long as a product in this general category is well formulated and includes an array of those key ingredients (antioxidants, skin-identical ingredients, and cell-communicating ingredients) the only thing you need to think about is the texture, because aside from that the name on the product's label is irrelevant and, more often than not, deceptive marketing mumbo jumbo.

Among products that are well-formulated, the only thing that differentiates all "moisturizers" and anti-wrinkle or similar products from one another is the texture. If you have dry to very dry skin you need a product with these state-of-the-art ingredients that come in a cream form, if you have normal to dry skin a lotion will work well. If you have normal to slightly dry skin or combination skin a lightweight lotion or serum is your best choice. If you have oily or blemish-prone skin a gel or liquid toner is an excellent form but you may also want to consider a mattifying serum (not to be confused with foundation primers, which typically do not have impressive formulas in terms of providing the types of ingredients outlined above).

FACIAL MASKS

If there is one truly optional step in skin care, masks are it. Whatever miraculous properties may be attributed to masks, no research supports the assertions of benefit attributed to the special muds, minerals, vitamins, or plant life these products contain. These exotic components range from seaweed to volcanic earth, unusual muds, enzymes, vitamins, and just about anything else you can think of, all associated with a fantastic jumble of characteristics to make the products seem life-altering for your skin. Cellulite is smoothed, wrinkles are eliminated, and acne is cured all with the application of a facial mask! I would offer to sell you a bridge if you believe any of this, but there aren't enough bridges in the world to accommodate the number of women taken in by these claims.

For an example of the insanity regarding facial masks and mud-mask spa treatments, consider the preposterous claims revolving around moor mud. Depending on the Web site, the multitude of claims made for this substance range from curing vaginitis to healing arthritis, acne, and wrinkles. Based on the fact that it was used by the Romans in 120 B.C. (at least that was the information proffered by several spas offering moor-mud treatments), the association with ancient medicine must have value. (Though I doubt any of the people proposing these claims would want to get sick in ancient Rome.) Here are the qualities another spa attributed to their moor mud: "As biological beings, the atoms in the human body have an intrinsic affinity for like atoms in nature, so whether moor products are taken internally or externally, the body automatically extracts the substance it needs to reestablish order and harmony." First, if that were accurate then there would be no risk of poisonous substances in nature, and that simply is not true. Moor mud refers to wet earth with a limited ability to grow plant life because of the acidic nature of the soil.

Other claims for masks say they offer the benefit of detoxifying properties. Again, there is no research showing this to be the case, but the world of spa treatments and cosmetics is all about outlandish claims, not proof. To begin with, what exactly are these toxins that need to be eliminated from our bodies, and that supposedly cause so many skin problems? Where is the information or data indicating exactly what toxins need to be removed from the body and how is this taking place? If it is possible to "detox" by the application of a facial mask, what biological or physiological process is taking place to allow that to happen? Are the toxins being leached through skin? Drained out of the body in some fashion? This all adds up to magic along with some murky smoke and mirrors. It isn't based on a shred of reality.

Despite the litany of bogus claims ascribed to facial masks, they can still have a benefit for some skin types. Someone with dry skin may find an emollient facial mask soothing and relaxing. Someone with oily skin may find a facial mask with oil-absorbing properties beneficial. Perhaps that's hard to believe, but it really is that uncomplicated!

Facial masks, by their very design, are meant to be used occasionally. In that way they are much like dieting or exercising—when it's done occasionally little gain can be derived. Meanwhile the skin's need for antioxidants or anti-irritant protection, skin barrier repair, or (for someone with breakouts) the need for disinfecting or oil absorption is a daily one, and it's not solved by a once-a-week fix.

CHAPTER 11
SOLUTIONS FOR WRINKLES

THE BASICS

TWICE A DAY: Gentle cleanser (preferably fragrance free with no coloring agents added)
Recommended cleansers: CeraVe Hydrating Cleanser; Clinique Liquid Facial Soap, Mild Formula; Paula's Choice One Step Face Cleanser for Normal to Dry Skin; Kiehl's Ultra-Moisturizing Cleansing Cream; Neutrogena Extra Gentle Cleanser.

NIGHTTIME: Makeup remover (preferably fragrance free with no coloring agents added)
Recommended makeup removers: Mary Kay Oil-Free Eye Makeup Remover; Nivea Visage Eye Makeup Remover; Paula's Choice Gentle Touch Makeup Remover; DHC Eye Makeup Remover; Sephora FACE Waterproof Eye Makeup Remover.

TWICE A DAY: Toner formulated with antioxidants, skin-identical ingredients, and cell-communicating ingredients
Recommended toners: MD Formulations Moisture Defense Antioxidant Spray; Paula's Choice Moisture Boost Hydrating Toner; Paula's Choice Skin Recovery Toner; Bioelements Calmitude Hydrating Solution.

ONCE OR TWICE A DAY: Exfoliate with an AHA or BHA product
Recommended AHA exfoliants: Neutrogena Healthy Skin Face Lotion Night; Paula's Choice 8% Alpha Hydroxy Acid Gel; Peter Thomas Roth Glycolic Acid 10% Moisturizer.
Recommended BHA exfoliants: Paula's Choice 1% Beta Hydroxy Acid Lotion; Paula's Choice 2% Beta Hydroxy Acid Lotion; Bare Escentuals bareVitamins Skin Rev-er Upper.

DAYTIME: Sunscreen with SPF 15 or greater that preferably also contains antioxidants, skin-identical ingredients, and cell-communicating ingredients
Recommended daytime moisturizer with sunscreen: Avon Ageless Results Renewing Day Cream SPF 15; Olay Regenerist Enhancing Lotion with UV Protection SPF 15; Paula's Choice Skin Recovery Daily Moisturizing Lotion with Antioxidants & SPF 15; Dr. Denese New York SPF 30 Neck Defense Day Cream UVA/UVB; Good Skin All Bright Moisturizing Sunscreen SPF 30.

NIGHTTIME: Moisturizer or product in a texture suitable for your skin type with antioxidants, cell-communicating ingredients, and skin-identical ingredients
Recommended moisturizers: Good Skin All Calm Moisture Lotion; Olay Total Effects 7-in-1 Anti-Aging Moisturizer, Mature Skin Therapy; Paula's Choice Hydrating Treatment Cream; Paula's Choice Skin Recovery Moisturizer; Clinique Super Rescue Antioxidant Night Moisturizer (three versions available).

DAYTIME OR NIGHTTIME OPTIONAL CHOICE: Specialty treatment such as tretinoin, retinol, or a serum/gel with extra antioxidants, skin-identical ingredients, and cell-communicating ingredients.

Note: For specific product choices for your skin type from my product line please visit www.paulaschoice.com; for products for your skin type from other product lines please visit www.beautypedia.com.

DRY SKIN DOESN'T CAUSE WRINKLES

Dry skin's enduring association with wrinkles is as inseparable in the mind of the consumer as love and marriage. Nonetheless, the simple truth is dry skin and wrinkles are not related in the least. I know that statement may be hard to accept because we're so conditioned by advertising and product claims to think otherwise, but believing the myth can hurt your skin by inducing you to concentrate on treating your dry skin or loading up on moisturizers hoping it will get rid of wrinkles. It just doesn't work that way.

Abundant research has made it perfectly clear that wrinkles and dry skin are not related in terms of cause and effect. Extensive studies and analysis have shown dry skin is frequently a by-product or result of other assaults on skin that are really the cause of wrinkles. In other words, dry skin is primarily a symptom of other factors causing wrinkles.

If dry skin doesn't cause wrinkles, what does? Wrinkles are permanent lines etched into skin from environmental causes (sun damage and pollution) and internal causes (genetic changes, muscle movement, estrogen loss, and fat depletion). Nowhere, outside of ads and product claims, is dry skin ever mentioned as a cause of wrinkles. (Sources: *Current Molecular Medicine*, March 2005, pages 171–177; *Fertility Sterility*, August 2005, pages 289–290; *Cutis*, February 2005, Supplemental, pages 5–8; *Rejuvenation Research*, Fall 2004, pages 175–185; *Journal of Dermatology*, August 2004, pages 603–609; and *Contact Dermatitis*, September 2002, pages 139–146.)

The dilemma is that, in fact, dry skin does look more wrinkled and—here's the crux of the confusion—wrinkled skin looks better with a good moisturizer on it. That's how we get sucked into this myth about wrinkles and dry skin. A woman with oily skin has her own built-in moisturizer (that's basically what moisturizers are: oils or oil-like ingredients and water), which helps her skin look smoother without the aid of a moisturizer. That's also why women with oily skin can look less wrinkled. A woman with dry skin will notice it makes her wrinkles look more prominent, and this effect is softened and improved after a moisturizer is applied. The skin's own oil doesn't forestall or in any way change wrinkles, but keeping them lubricated (the same principle as applying a moisturizer) makes wrinkles look better temporarily.

Sun damage is by far the most notable cause of wrinkling, a fact easily proven by something I refer to as the backside test of aging. In other words, compare the areas of your skin that rarely, if ever, see the sun with the parts of your body exposed to the sun on a daily basis. Those areas of skin with minimal sun exposure (such as your backside) are rarely if ever dry, and they also have minimal to no signs of wrinkles or aging. Instead they will have far more of the firmness, elasticity, and color of "younger" skin because they have not been subjected to years of cumulative exposure to sunlight. Most people who have never, or rarely, exposed their bare backside to the sun will find a radical difference between it and those parts of the body that have been exposed to the sun. What you will notice is crepey skin on the face and hands, some loss of elasticity, lines, furrows, some skin discoloration (usually darkening, redness, or ashiness), and signs of new freckling. However, the skin on your bottom will be smooth, evenly toned (no freckling or discoloration), and (unless there has been a fluctuation in weight, in which case the backside may be out of shape and saggy), it will be elastic and without lines, crow's feet, crepiness, or any sign of wrinkles. These differences become more prominent the older you are and the more sun exposure you've experienced.

As discouraging as this information may be, the good news is that today many state-of-the-art ingredients can go further than just making wrinkles and dry skin look better temporarily.

The truth is, moisturizing the skin does not have any long-term effect on wrinkles. That doesn't mean moisturizers can't make wrinkles less apparent, because they absolutely do, but the notion that these soothing creams, lotions, gels, and serums can do anything to erase wrinkles or stop aging in its tracks is wishful thinking fostered by constant reinforcement from the cosmetics industry—the same reinforcement that plays on a woman's (and, increasingly, a man's) insecurities about looking older because of their wrinkles.

Another important distinction between dry skin and wrinkles is that when the outer layer of skin becomes dry or irritated the surface can literally crack, and something referred to as "fine lines" can appear. These "fine lines" are not the same as permanent lines caused by intrinsic (genetic aging) or extrinsic (sun damage) factors. This type of dry-skin damage can "look" wrinkled, which is why the elusive term "fine lines" is used. That also explains why the cosmetics industry uses the term fine lines, because those are just what moisturizers can easily correct. Fine lines (better described as nonpermanent lines) nicely disappear with almost all moisturizers; on the other hand, permanent lines don't go away no matter how much moisturizer you put on them. Extremely dry skin can also crack and chafe if it isn't moisturized, causing a parched appearance and a tight, irritated feeling, which is why dry skin feels so uncomfortable.

Keep in mind that part of what makes the skin feel parched and dry is that the skin's intercellular matrix is deteriorating due to sun damage and age. The intercellular matrix is the cement within the skin that keeps skin cells together, helps prevent individual skin cells from losing water, and fights off environmental stresses that damage skin. It is actually the intercellular matrix that gives skin a good deal of its surface texture and feel. Using products that restore the skin's matrix is what great skin-care is all about. Water (as in moisture) doesn't help that part of the skin's health at all; what will help are antioxidants, skin-identical ingredients, and cell-communicating ingredients, along with anything we can do to protect skin from the sun.

WHY "ANTI-WRINKLE" CREAMS *CAN'T* WORK BETTER THAN BOTOX

Or why can't any skin-care product work better than dermal fillers? Or laser resurfacing? Or chemical peels? Or face-lifts? Or eye lifts? Because no skin-care product can address the complex physiological processes that cause wrinkles. Even a specific medical cosmetic corrective procedure or surgery cannot address all the issues that cause the face to look older. Here are some of the factors we face that the cosmetics industry can't fix.

Sun damage! The one thing the cosmetics industry can address to some extent is sun protection. Even so, the total damage caused by pervasive, recurring, cumulative, unprotected, or inadequate sun protection over the years adds up to severe damage that cannot be changed by a skin-care product. And there are limitations even with medical cosmetic corrective procedures. (Sources: *Archives of Dermatological Research*, January 2006, pages 294–302; *British Journal of Dermatology*, December 2005, Supplemental, pages 37–46; *Journal of Dermatology*, August 2004, pages 603–609; and *Journal of Investigative Dermatology*, September 2003, pages 578–586.)

Fat depletion and movement in the face. The fat pads of the cheek, forehead, and jaw move down and in on the face as the skin becomes less supple and firm, and the fat content also becomes depleted and deteriorates over time. Overall, a thinner face will be more wrinkled than a fuller face. Women who tend to gain weight and have it show on their face have fewer wrinkles than women who don't. Products that claim they contain fat that can be absorbed into and build back the fat in your skin—if that were possible—would be something that could make skin look younger. But the cosmetics industry isn't going to lie about that. Instead they lie about collagen in a product being able to build up collagen in your skin. What company is going to sell you the notion it can make your face fatter? So that's one lie they won't tell you though theoretically it could really help. (Sources: *Journal of Drugs in Dermatology*, November–December 2006, pages 959–964; *Dermatologic Surgery*, August 2006, pages 1058–1069; *Annals of Plastic Surgery*, March 2004, pages 234–239; and *Dermatologic Surgery*, October 2003, pages 1019–1026.)

Loss of estrogen due to perimenopause and eventually menopause. Estrogen produces healthier skin cells and collagen, and resilient elastin. As we lose estrogen our skin is less and less able to maintain these options. (Sources: *Climacteric Journal of the International Menopause Society*, August 2007, pages 289–297; *Journal of the American Academy of Dermatology*, October 2005, pages 555–568; and *Experimental Dermatology*, February 2005, page 156.)

Genetics. The genes you inherit may hinder or help a great deal, but they too are only part of the picture given environmental influences and the other factors listed here. (Sources: *Current Problems in Dermatology*, 2007, volume 35, pages 28–38; and *Journal of Investigative Dermatology*, February 2006, pages 277–282.)

Bone loss. As the skeletal support structure of the face loses density and bulk, it provides less architectural support for skin so the skin becomes draped in a sagging manner instead of how it looked when we were younger. (Sources: *Facial Plastic Surgery Clinics of North America*, May 2007, pages 221–228; *Skin Therapy Letter*, April 2006, pages 1–3; and *Journal of the American Academy of Dermatology*, February 1998, pages 248–255.)

Cell senescence. As we age, skin cells eventually lose the capacity to divide and re-create themselves. The result is thin, inelastic, dry skin and impaired skin function in general. This process is known as the "Hayflick phenomenon," named after Dr. Leonard Hayflick, who identified the condition in 1965; it has also been called genetically programmed cell death.

(Sources: *Dermatology*, August 2007, pages 352–360; *Molecular Biology Reports*, September 2006, pages 181–186; and Cell Cycle, September 2004, pages 1127–1129.)

Smoking. Smoking tobacco is the most preventable cause of skin aging. In addition to having a strong association with a number of systemic diseases, the effects of smoking are to blame for exacerbating or causing many dermatological conditions, including poor wound healing, premature skin aging, squamous cell carcinoma, melanoma, oral cancer, acne, psoriasis, and hair loss. People who smoke for a number of years tend to develop an unhealthy yellowish hue to their complexion. Even if you haven't been a smoker for very long the damage still takes place very quickly and insidiously. A large panel study conducted in 2008 showed that facial wrinkling, while not yet visible, can be seen under a microscope in smokers as young as 20 years old. (Sources: *International Journal of Dermatology*, October 2008, pages 1086–1087; *Journal of Dermatological Science*, December 2007, pages 169–175; *Archives of Dermatology*, December 2007, pages 1543–1546; and *Journal of Investigative Dermatology*, April 2003, pages 548–554.) If you smoke, please do whatever it takes to quit, regardless of your age or how long you've smoked. Your body will thank you in numerous healthy ways.

Facial expressions. Facial movement causes wrinkles. If you do facial exercises to reduce the appearance of wrinkles imagining that you're building up the muscles underneath you would only be making matters worse. Repetitive facial movements such as smiling, frowning, and raising your eyebrows actually lead to more fine lines and wrinkles in those areas. Each time we use a facial muscle, a groove forms beneath the surface of the skin, which is why we see lines form with each facial expression. As skin ages and loses its elasticity and collagen content, the skin stops springing back to its line-free state, and these grooves become permanently etched on the face. Botox works because it paralyzes muscle movement where it is injected, preventing these creases from taking place. (Sources: *Clinics in Dermatology*, March–April 2008, pages 182–191; and *Oral and Maxillofacial Surgery Clinics of North America*, February 2005, pages 1–15.)

Gravity. Gravity constantly pulls on our bodies, and its effect on our skin becomes more pronounced as we age. By the age of 50 the elastin content in our skin can no longer take the strain: the nose droops, ears elongate, eyelids fall, jowls form, and the upper lip can disappear while the lower lip becomes more pronounced.

Regardless of the claim in the label, no cosmetic or skin-care product can address all of these physiological issues and problems. A combination of products and medical treatments can achieve a great deal of success against these issues, but to imagine that a single miracle cream or ingredient can do this all by itself is just not reality.

HOW SKIN AGES AND WRINKLES

How the skin ages and wrinkles is a very complicated process that involves an almost limitless range of physiological occurrences. There isn't any single cause that can be addressed with a cosmetic to erase or minimize the inevitable, because the "aging" process itself is so complex and intricate. Skin, all by itself, ages in many identifiable ways. Adding one plant extract or a vitamin to the skin won't address what is needed to deal with the myriad issues that need to be confronted to slow down the aging process. A long series of extrinsic factors (sun damage, pollution, free-radical damage, smoking) and intrinsic factors (genetically predetermined cell cessation, chronological aging, hormone depletion, immune suppression) combine and culminate in what we define as aged skin.

CELLULAR RENEWAL AND REPAIR

Cellular renewal and repair are well-established marketing terms used by the cosmetics industry to sell skin-care products. Having the ability to generate healthy cell growth (in other words, the way that younger skin cells reproduce) is a claim many antiwrinkle and antiaging moisturizers make.

This idea of stimulating healthy cell growth definitely has some basis in scientific research, as I point out throughout this book. But the cosmetics industry distorts the concept of cellular renewal, turning it into a great deal of misinformation represented by overpriced products. Here are the facts about what it is possible to do for skin, regardless of the price tag on the product you are buying.

Essentially, any skin-care product that can protect skin from environmental stress (antioxidants and sunscreen), reinforce the epidermis (skin-identical ingredients), and help produce healthier skin cells (cell-communicating ingredients) can help encourage healthy cell production, generate healthier collagen and elastin, improve the skin's immune response, and prevent cellular damage. When you add exfoliants to this mix to remove the unhealthy buildup of dead skin cells on the surface, you have a strategy that can truly make skin look as young as is possible, at least from the world of skin care.

Inasmuch as many things can help skin with cellular renewal and repair, that is still not the panacea the cosmetics industry makes it out to be. Even if women used every product being sold for anti-aging and fighting wrinkles, they could never deliver any of the extreme changes extolled on the labels.

SUNSCREEN, TRETINOIN, AND EXFOLIANTS —A VERY GOOD PLACE TO START

One of the fundamental characteristics of sun-damaged skin is that the outer layer becomes thickened and yellow and the underlying layer, where new skin cells are produced, becomes damaged, generating abnormal cell growth and hypermelanin production. The abnormal cell growth also results in malformed elastin, collagen deterioration, and distorted circulation of the blood and lymph systems. Regular use of sunscreen can slow this damage, allow for some improvement, and prevent further destruction. But topical tretinoin has been shown to partially reverse the clinical and histological (structural) changes induced by the combination of sunlight exposure and chronological aging. A formulation of tretinoin in an emollient cream (as in Renova, Avita, Tazorac, or generic tretinoin) has been extensively investigated in multicenter double-blind trials, and has been shown to produce significant improvement within four to six months of daily use when used as part of a regimen including sun protection and moisturizer.

Alpha-hydroxy acids (AHAs) have also been widely used for therapy of photodamaged skin, and these compounds have been reported to normalize hyperkeratinization (over-thickened skin) and to increase viable epidermal thickness and dermal glycosaminoglycans content. In other words, AHAs have a postive effect on the surface and lower layers of skin. To sum this all up, recent work has substantially described how the aging process affects the skin and has demonstrated that many of the unwanted changes can be improved by topical therapy.

Add sunscreen to the mix and a "moisturizer" in a texture for your skin type that is loaded with antioxidants, skin-identical ingredients, and cell-communicating ingredients and you have the best combination possible to fight wrinkles.

(Sources: *Cutis*, August 2001, pages 135–142; *Journal of the European Academy of Dermatology and Venereology*, July 2000, pages 280–284; *American Journal of Clinical Dermatology*, March-April 2000, pages 81–88; *Journal of Cell Physiology*, October 1999, pages 14–23; *Skin Pharmacology and Applied Skin Physiology*, May-June 1999, pages 111–119; *British Journal of Dermatology*, December 1996, pages 867–875.)

CHAPTER 12
SOLUTIONS FOR PERIMENOPAUSE & MENOPAUSE

THE BASICS

There are no special cosmetic skin-care products that can affect skin that is experiencing perimenopausal or menopausal symptoms, so you need to follow the skin-care routine for your skin type or special concerns. Consider talking to your physician about hormone replacement therapy, a topical hormone cream or lotion, or alternative hormone replacement therapy.

Note: The issue of hormone loss is an extremely complex and controversial medical issue it is essential to discuss treatment options with your physician. There is no panacea, either natural or otherwise, and the pros and cons of any treatments need to be evaluated rationally. Do not be misled by headlines or Web sites that present one-sided information, because the research about all the potential treatments is not conclusive in any way. Each one has its negatives and positives that must be personally evaluated before a decision is made. The information below will give you a cursory overview so you can begin the process of evaluating whether to incorporate this into an overall anti-aging program, or decide if you want to consider a particular option as a skin-improvement approach.

WHEN YOUR BODY MAKES LESS ESTROGEN

It has been said that menopause starts the day you get your first menstrual cycle. I don't know if that's a hopeful comment or a depressing one, but any way you slice it a woman will have periods for about 30 to 40 years after they first begin, and then they'll stop. There is still a great deal of research that needs to be done on all the issues surrounding perimenopause (referring to the symptoms taking place in the years before the onset of menopause as estrogen production begins to fall off), menopause (the actual cessation of the menstrual cycle), and postmenopause (the years after your period has stopped). What is known for certain is that when the body has less estrogen available changes in the appearance of skin, hair, bone, and other physical manifestations begin to take place.

Perimenopause and menopause are brought about by the body's changes in hormone production. The irksome side effects of menopause are caused primarily by the imbalance between a woman's female hormones (estrogen and progesterone, which become depleted) and her male hormones (like androgens such as testosterone). Because the male hormones decline more slowly, there are proportionately more of them, so they have a stronger impact. This imbalance, for example, can affect hair growth.

When estrogen levels decrease, many women experience an increase in androgen production, resulting in varying amounts of dark hair growth on the face—particularly around the chin and moustache area above the lip. Ironically, while the hair on your face may get darker, the hair on your head will have reduced growth and you may experience some balding; even the individual hairs actually become smaller in diameter.

The diminishing levels and eventual loss of estrogen and progesterone also affect skin negatively. Aside from experiencing problems caused by sun damage, perimenopausal and menopausal women will have thinner, looser, and less elastic skin, reduced production of collagen, cessation of oil gland function, impeded wound healing, and dry skin. Other parts of the body are also influenced by the diminishing amount of female hormones; the vaginal lining becomes thin and can burn and itch, and the breasts' mammary tissue is replaced with more fat tissue, which can cause sagging.

To make matters even more frustrating, perimenopause and menopause can also bring hot flashes, flushes, night sweats and/or cold flashes, a clammy feeling, intermittent rapid heartbeat, irritability, mood swings, trouble sleeping, heavier periods, flooding, loss of libido, itchy skin, and more brittle nails, just to name a few.

As complex and multifaceted as this all sounds, there are actually some fairly exciting options for addressing the side effects of perimenopause and menopause, and these include both alternative herbal options and conventional Western medical choices. For the purpose of this section I'm going to highlight a few of the current options as they affect skin, but it is also important to find a doctor or medical expert who is practiced and proficient on the complexities of this topic.

Warning: Please avoid the Web sites, companies, alternative health practitioners, or physicians who do not offer a balanced approach to this issue. Medical options are not evil or dangerous, as many alternative-based professionals or companies assert, and herbal alternatives are not as ineffective or as unproven as many medical doctors assert. Both approaches play a role in mitigating some of the more annoying (as well as intolerable) symptoms of perimenopause and menopause, and both have their pitfalls.

(Sources: *Journal of the European Menopause and Andropause Society*, November 2008, pages 227–232, and July 2001, pages 43–55; *Epidemiology Biomarkers & Prevention* 16, December 2007, pages 2524–2525; *Journal of Biomaterials and Science Polymer Edition*, 2008; volume 19, issue 8, pages 1097–1099; *Endocrine Pathophysiology*, author C. B. Niewoehner, published by Hayes Barton Press, 2004; and *Journal of Clinical Dermatology*, 2001, volume 2, issue 3, pages 143–150.)

HORMONES FOR WRINKLES AND HEALING

Estrogen appears to aid in the prevention of the skin's aging in several ways. Topical and systemic estrogen therapy can increase the skin collagen content and therefore maintain skin thickness. In addition, estrogen maintains skin moisture by increasing ceramides and hyaluronic acid in the skin and by maintaining the stratum corneum's barrier function. Sebum levels are higher in postmenopausal women receiving hormone replacement therapy. The wrinkling of skin may also be lessened with estrogen as a result of the effects of the hormone on the elastic fibers and collagen. And aside from of its influence on skin aging, it has been suggested that estrogen increases wound healing by regulating the levels of cytokines, proteins that generate an immune response. In fact, topical estrogen has been found to accelerate and improve wound healing in elderly men and women.

Benefits from taking hormones are dose dependent and are also affected by whether you start taking the hormones during perimenopause or postmenopause. There are compelling reasons to consider hormonal treatment as part of a battle plan for wrinkles. It is a multifaceted, controversial issue, with possible risks you need to consider. The following information will provide an overview to help you create a dialogue with your physician to evaluate all the options available to you.

(Sources: *Journal of the American Academy of Dermatology*, September 2008, pages 391–404; *British Medical Journal*, May 2008, pages 1227–1231; *Clinical Interventions in Aging*, 2007, volume 2, issue 3, pages 283–297; and *International Journal of Cosmetic Science*, October 2006, pages 335–341.)

HORMONE REPLACEMENT THERAPY

Hormone Replacement Therapy (HRT) or Estrogen Replacement Therapy (ERT) describes prescription-only treatments that give your body estrogen and/or progesterone. HRT, taken in pills or via skin patches, has been shown to restore some amount of the skin's support tissue and elastic quality. A number of studies have demonstrated that ERT and HRT can increase the thickness and elasticity of skin as well as lessen the appearance of skin's "aging." Estrogen appears to aid in the prevention of skin aging in several ways, including an increase in collagen production, improving barrier function, and creating healthy skin cells; it can also increase wound healing, and improve skin elasticity.

(Sources: *Skin Research and Technology*, May 2001, page 95; *Maturitas European Menopause and Andropause Society*, May 2000, pages 107–117; and *American Journal of Clinical Dermatology*, 2001, volume 2, issue 3, pages 143–150.)

There are serious risks associated with ERT and HRT and there are controversies regarding their effects on heart disease, osteoporosis, and breast cancer. But there seems to be little opposition to the notion that they ease hot flashes, night sweats, mood swings, and vaginal thinning while improving the appearance of skin experiencing perimenopause. It is essential to weigh the pros and cons of ERT and HRT to decide if they are the right direction for you.

Around the age of 40 you can consider getting a baseline estrogen count to determine what normal is for you. That way you can monitor the changes and balancing effect that varying combinations of supplements are having on your body.

(Sources: *Climateric Journal of the International Menopause Society*, August 2007, pages 289–297; and *Experimental Dermatology*, February 2006, pages 83–94.)

TOPICAL APPLICATION OF PROGESTERONE AND ESTROGEN

There are a lot of believers in "natural estrogen" and "natural progesterone" creams and lotions. Particularly for progesterone, the Internet is replete with advocates and believers who are convincing in their rhetoric, describing it as the fountain of youth. It's important to point out that while natural progesterone applied to the skin is absolutely an option for perimenopausal and menopausal symptoms and improvement in the appearance of skin, the versions you buy at health food stores or over the Internet are not regulated in any way by the FDA, and so they are, in actuality, merely cosmetics. That means any cosmetics company can put progesterone or estrogen into whatever products they want to and make outrageous claims for them.

Having said that, there is research showing that topical application of 2% progesterone creams can have benefit for improving the appearance of skin, reducing wrinkles, and increasing elasticity. The same is true for topical application of estrogen. For both estrogen and progesterone, applying patches or creams with these actives appears to greatly reduce the risk associated with oral medications. Objective research about topically applied estrogen and progesterone is limited and should be discussed with your physician before you consider this route.

(Sources: *Maturitas European Menopause and Andropause Society*, May 2007, pages 77–80; *British Journal of Dermatology*, September 2005, pages 626–632; *Journal of Clinical Pharmacology*, June 2005, pages 614–619; *Menopause*, March 2005, pages 232–237; and *Drugs in Aging*, 2004, volume 21, issue 13, pages 865–883.)

SKIN-CARE OPTIONS

I would love to say that there are traditional or state-of-the-art skin-care products out there that positively address the changes that occur in perimenopausal and menopausal skin, but there aren't. There is simply no information available to suggest that applying soy extract, black cohosh, or evening primrose oil to skin can mitigate any of the changes taking place in the epidermis and dermis, and definitely not in comparison to taking those substances orally. None of those substances are a problem if they show up in skin-care products, but their benefits are most likely not any different from those of other anti-inflammatory and antioxidant cosmetic ingredients.

The truth is that the real basics for skin care continue to apply to perimenopausal and menopausal women alike: sun protection, treating the skin type you have (not all menopausal women have dry skin, wrinkles, skin discolorations, or skin disorders), considering using Retin-A or Renova, and using gentle skin-care products. If you have dry skin, use an emollient moisturizer laden with antioxidants, skin-identical ingredients, and cell-communicating ingredients. The use of hydroquinone or arbutin-based skin-lightening products is another important option. But there are no cosmetics you can apply to skin that can alter the actual condition of your skin caused by the depletion of hormones.

Pharmaceutical options, such as over-the-counter products containing USP progesterone or prescription-only estrogen creams, can be applied topically and there is some research showing they can have benefit for skin. But here again you need to discuss this with your physician because these products are not without warnings and potential risks.

AHAS AND BHA FOR POSTMENOPAUSAL WOMEN

What about the use of effective AHAs and BHA for menopausal women? Does exfoliating help all skin types? For the most part the answer to this question is yes. Removing built-up layers of dead skin cells gently and without abrading skin (as can happen with scrubs) can be incredibly effective for all ages. How often to exfoliate depends more on the condition of your skin than anything else, including how old you are. Once you're past age of 70 skin can become so thin it can literally tear when gently scratched or rubbed. This thinning is a result of many factors but primarily it is brought about by a combination of estrogen loss, genetic aging, and sun damage. All of these things cause the skin cells to produce "less skin" as well as less healthy skin. In terms of genetic aging, skin cells seem to have a preprogrammed mechanism that slows down skin-cell turnover, and sun damage causes a buildup of dead skin cells on the surface of skin. AHAs and BHA help the outer layer of skin to shed more normally by removing built-up dead skin cells. For some women in their 70s, 80s, and 90s with extremely fragile skin that may be problematic (they may indeed need the dead skin cells to stick around on the surface for as long as possible). It would thus be important to experiment with frequency to see how the skin responds. Perhaps instead of using the AHA or BHA product every day you should only use it every other day or every few days to get the best results. If AHAs and BHA can be tolerated in some fashion there is a great deal of benefit to be achieved in removing dead skin cells at the surface, as that absolutely helps improve the appearance of skin and allows healthier skin cells to come to the surface. It has also been shown that AHAs and BHA can stimulate the production of collagen, which also has benefit.

SUPPLEMENTS FOR HORMONAL CHANGES

The following information is from www.drweil.com. Dr. Andrew Weil is the author of many books on alternative and medical remedies and treatments for an immense range of health concerns. These are his suggestions for oral supplements or dietary additions to treat perimenopausal or menopausal symptoms.

Soy foods. The isoflavones in soy foods help balance hormone levels and have some estrogenic activity. There is ongoing research about the safety and efficacy of isolated soy isoflavone supplements. Although the initial results look promising, many physicians currently recommend using natural soy foods rather than supplements. Choose from tofu, soy milk, roasted soy nuts, or tempeh.

Flaxseed. Substances called lignins in flaxseed are important modulators of hormone metabolism. Grind flaxseed daily in a coffee grinder at home and use 1 to 2 tablespoons a day.

Dong quai. Dong quai (*Angelica sinensis*) is known both in China and the West for its ability to support and maintain the natural balance of female hormones. It does not have estrogenic activity. This is one of the herbs for menopause that should not be taken if a woman is experiencing heavy bleeding.

Black cohosh *(Cumicifuga racemosa)*. One of the best-studied traditional herbs for meno-pause, black cohosh is used to help alleviate some symptoms of menopause, including hot flashes. Black cohosh seems to work by supporting and maintaining hormonal levels, which may lessen the severity of hot flashes. Many women report that the herb works well but it isn't effective for everyone. While any therapy that influences hormonal actions should be a concern, black cohosh does not appear to have estrogenic activity and thus may be safe for women with a personal or family history of breast cancer.

Vitamin E. A daily dose of 400 IUs of natural vitamin E (as mixed tocopherols and tocotrienols) can help alleviate symptoms of hot flashes in some menopausal women.

B vitamins. This group of water-soluble vitamins may help women deal with the stress of menopausal symptoms.

Evening primrose oil or black currant oil. These are sources of gamma-linolenic acid (GLA), an essential fatty acid that can help influence prostaglandin synthesis and help moderate menopausal symptoms.

CHAPTER 13
SOLUTIONS FOR SKIN LIGHTENING

THE BASICS

TWICE A DAY: Gentle cleanser (preferably fragrance free with no coloring agents added)
    Recommended cleansers: Clinique Liquid Facial Soap, Mild Formula; Paula's Choice One Step Face Cleanser for Normal to Dry Skin; Paula's Choice One Step Cleanser for Normal to Oily/Combination Skin; Kiehl's Ultra-Moisturizing Cleansing Cream; Neutrogena Extra Gentle Cleanser.

NIGHTTIME: Makeup remover (preferably fragrance free with no coloring agents added)
    Recommended makeup removers: Mary Kay Oil-Free Eye Makeup Remover; Nivea Visage Eye Makeup Remover; Paula's Choice Gentle Touch Makeup Remover; DHC Eye Makeup Remover; Sephora FACE Waterproof Eye Makeup Remover.

TWICE A DAY: Toner formulated with antioxidants, skin-identical ingredients, and cell-communicating ingredients
    Recommended toners: MD Formulations Moisture Defense Antioxidant Spray; Paula's Choice Moisture Boost Hydrating Toner; Paula's Choice Healthy Skin Refreshing Toner; M.A.C. Lightful Softening Lotion.

ONCE OR TWICE A DAY: Exfoliate with an AHA or BHA product
    Recommended AHA exfoliants: Neutrogena Healthy Skin Face Lotion Night; Paula's Choice 8% Alpha Hydroxy Acid Gel; Murad Night Reform Treatment.
    Recommended BHA exfoliants: Paula's Choice 1% Beta Hydroxy Acid Lotion; Paula's Choice 2% Beta Hydroxy Acid Lotion; Estee Lauder Fruition Multi-Action Complex.

ONCE OR TWICE A DAY: Skin-lightening product containing a melanin-inhibiting ingredient such as hydroquinone, vitamin C, arbutin, or azelaic acid
    Recommended skin lightening products: Alpha Hydrox Spot Light Targeted Skin Lightener; Mary Kay TimeWise Even Complexion Essence; Dermalogica ChromaWhite TRx Extreme C; Paula's Choice Clearly Remarkable Skin Lightening Lotion; Paula's Choice Clearly Remarkable Skin Lightening Gel.

DAYTIME: Sunscreen with SPF 15 or greater that preferably also contains antioxidants, skin-identical ingredients, and cell-communicating ingredients
    Recommended daytime moisturizer with sunscreen: Clinique City Block Sheer Oil-Free Daily Face Protector SPF 25; MD Formulations Moisture Defense Antioxidant Moisturizer SPF 20; Paula's Choice Skin Recovery Daily Moisturizing Lotion with Antioxidants & SPF 15; Paula's Choice Pure Mineral Sunscreen SPF 15; DDF Moisturizing Photo-Age Protection SPF 30.

NIGHTTIME: Moisturizer or product in a texture suitable for your skin type with antioxidants, cell-communicating ingredients, and skin-identical ingredients
> **Recommended moisturizers:** Olay Total Effects 7-in-1 Anti-Aging Moisturizer, Mature Skin Therapy; Paula's Choice Hydrating Treatment Cream; Paula's Choice Skin HydraLight Moisture-Infusing Lotion; Clinique Super Rescue Antioxidant Night Moisturizer (three versions available); BeautiControl Cell Block-C Intensive Brightening Elixir.

DAYTIME OR NIGHTTIME OPTIONAL CHOICE: Specialty treatment such as tretinoin, retinol, or a serum/gel with extra antioxidants, skin-identical ingredients, and cell-communicating ingredients

Note: For specific product choices for your skin type from my product line please visit www.paulaschoice.com; for products for your skin type from other product lines please visit www.beautypedia.com.

SKIN LIGHTENING

Brown spots on skin are called hyperpigmentation, chloasma, or melasma, and can appear for several reasons. One repercussion of sun damage is areas of skin discoloration known as solar lentigenes, more popularly called liver spots, sun spots, or age spots. They are definitely not associated with the liver, but they often have everything to do with unprotected sun exposure. On lighter skin types, solar lentigenes emerge as small brown patches of freckling that grow over time. On women with darker skin tones, they appear as small patches of ashen-gray skin that tend to enlarge over time.

Brown or ashen patches of skin can also occur due to birth-control pills, pregnancy, or estrogen replacement therapy. In those instances, the discoloration is referred to as pregnancy masking or hormone masking.

Regardless of the source, the issue is the same: site-specific, increased melanin production, or hyperpigmentation. Melanin is the pigment or coloring agent of skin. It is created by melanin synthesis, a complex process controlled partly by an enzyme called tyrosinase.

There are many products and ingredients to choose from when trying to reduce skin discolorations. When it comes to selecting treatment for these areas, the most important thing to realize is that it takes experimenting to find what works for you. Hydroquinone and sunscreen are the two options that have the most research and proof of efficacy, and certainly nothing is as important as sunscreen, but that doesn't diminish other choices depending on your preferences or experience.

Another important factor to consider is the depth of the discolored pigment within the skin. If the discoloration is superficial then topical agents along with sunscreen can make a significant impact. If the discolorations are large, deeper, and more evident, then more penetrating medical procedures such as laser removal, IPL treatments (intense pulsed light), and chemical peels should be a consideration.

It is also important to keep in mind that even if you do have a medical procedure to remove or reduce the appearance of skin discolorations you would still need to maintain sun protection to keep them from coming back (and to discourage new ones from appearing).

That would mean diligent use of a sunscreen along with other topical, melanin-inhibiting products such as hydroquinone in 2% to 4% concentrations, a prescription retinoid such as tretinoin, azelaic acid in 15% to 20% concentrations, or products containing arbutin and vitamin C.

COSMETIC INDUSTRY HYPE

Skin-lightening products abound in the cosmetics industry. Their promise—of making skin lighter or lightening and removing brown skin discolorations—shows up worldwide, but most notably in Asian and Middle Eastern countries where the beautiful darker skin colors are apparently considered less aesthetically appealing than lighter skin tones. The names of the products in this arena are compelling, and of course the all-natural versions boast of plant extracts that can do the job and are better than prescription formulas. As you have probably come to expect from the cosmetics industry, when it comes to what the products and ingredients can actually do the claims are misleading and often downright deceptive. Almost all of the products offered are enclosed in far prettier packaging and adorned with far more beguiling names than most other cosmetic products, but are filled with formulations that barely live up to even a fraction of the illusion they present.

Even if somehow there was a plant extract or miracle formulation, none of that explains why the suggested routines also include a special cleanser, toner, treatment, moisturizer, or sunscreen. It all adds up to a waste of money and endless disappointment. In my book *Don't Go To The Cosmetics Counter Without Me* and on my Web site at www.Beautypedia.com, I review most of these products and explain at length which ones work, which ones barely have any impact, and which ones are a complete waste of money.

The information that follows gives you an overview of what research shows does work to improve brown skin discolorations. Reality isn't as sexy as fantasy, but the actual results and cost savings have their own rewards. Wasting money is not pretty, nor is using discoloration-reducing products that have little to no hope of causing visible improvement.

SUNSCREEN

Perhaps no other aspect of skin care can prevent, reduce, and potentially eliminate sun-induced and hormonal skin discolorations than the diligent use of a sunscreen. No other aspect of controlling or reducing skin discolorations is as important as the use of sunscreen, SPF 15 or greater with the UVA-protecting ingredients avobenzone (butyl methoxydibenzyl-methane), ecamsule, Tinosorb, titanium dioxide, or zinc oxide. Using any other product or medical treatment without also using a sunscreen is a waste of time and money. Sun exposure is one of the primary, fundamental causes of hypermelanin production and exacerbates excess melanin production from hormonal triggers such as pregnancy. Before you consider any other treatment for skin discolorations, sunscreen is unconditionally the first and most practical step. See, I told you the reality wasn't going to be as fun as the fantasy!

(Sources: *Journal of the European Academy of Dermatology and Venereology*, July 2007, pages 738–742; *Journal of the American Academy of Dermatology*, December 2006, pages

1048–1065; *Skin Therapy Letter*, November 2006, pages 1–6; and *British Journal of Dermatology*, December 1996, pages 867–875.)

HYDROQUINONE

Hydroquinone is a strong inhibitor of melanin production that has long been established as the most effective ingredient for reducing and potentially eliminating melasma (Source: *Journal of Dermatological Science*, August, 2001, Supplemental, pages 68–75). In different concentrations it inhibits or prevents skin from making the substance responsible for skin color. Hydroquinone does not bleach the skin, which is why calling it a "bleaching agent" is a misnomer; it can't remove pigment from the skin cell. But blocking the skin's ability to synthesize melanin absolutely can reduce and eliminate the brown discolorations, whether they are caused by sun damage or hormonal influences. Over-the-counter hydroquinone products can contain 0.5% to 2% concentrations while 4% concentrations of hydroquinone (and sometimes higher) are available only from physicians.

Even though hydroquinone, applied topically, has proven to be the most effective ingredient for skin lightening and has been available without a prescription for more than 50 years in the United States, some concerns have been raised about its safety. Yet research indicates skin reactions are rare and minor, or a result of using extremely high concentrations of hydroquinone, or of using hydroquinone products that have been adulterated with dangerous ingredients.

Hydroquinone-based products were banned in South Africa years ago where problems were most frequently seen. However, hydroquinone products in South Africa and other countries are notorious for containing mercury and glucocorticoids, among other caustic and illegal contaminants, which were believed by many to be the cause of the disorders experienced (Sources: *International Journal of Dermatology*, February 2005, pages 112–115; and *British Journal of Dermatology*, March 2003, pages 493–500).

There is abundant research showing hydroquinone to be safe and extremely effective. (Sources: *Cutis*, April 2008, pages 356–371 and August 2006, pages S6–S19; *Journal of Cosmetic Laser Therapy*, September 2006, pages 121–127; *American Journal of Clinical Dermatology*, July 2006, pages 223–230; and *Journal of the American Academy of Dermatology*, May 2006, pages S272–S281.)

Interestingly, hydroquinone happens to be a potent antioxidant (Source: *Journal of Natural Products*, November 2002, pages 1605–1611).

Questions concerning hydroquinone in terms of it being a carcinogen have also been addressed in the research. Problematic incidences have been shown when hydroquinone was fed or injected into rats in large doses, though with topical use there has been no research showing it to be mutagenic on humans or animals (Source: *Critical Reviews in Toxicology*, November 2007, pages 887–914). In fact, there is even research showing that workers who handle pure hydroquinone actually have lower incidences of cancer than the population as a whole (Source: *Critical Reviews in Toxicology*, May 1999, pages 283–330).

Dr. Susan Taylor, founding director of the Skin of Color Center in New York City and assistant professor of dermatology at Columbia University stated, "Hydroquinone is the gold standard for treating pigmentation disorders and has been for many years. I consider it to be very safe and effective" (Source: *Pittsburgh Post-Gazette*, Wednesday, September 6, 2006).

Tri-Luma Cream ($101 for 1.05 ounce) is a prescription-only medication containing fluocinolone acetonide 0.01% (a form of cortisone), hydroquinone 4%, and tretinoin 0.05% for skin lightening. There is a good deal of research showing this combination to be a triple-threat for skin discolorations. Even though it is pricey, in comparison to many skin-lightening products available at cosmetics counters and spas this one is a bargain. It also has research showing it works. (Source: *British Journal of Dermatology*, September 2008, pages 697–703.)

Whether or not you consider using hydroquinone in a skin-care product is up to you. What is abundantly clear is that hydroquinone is a well-researched ingredient, incredibly effective for its intended purpose, and that no other ingredient can begin to compare with its effectiveness.

Hydroquinone can be an unstable ingredient in cosmetic formulations. Upon exposure to air or sunlight it can turn a strange shade of brown. It is thus essential when you are considering a hydroquinone product to be sure it is packaged in a non-transparent container that doesn't let light in and that minimizes the amount of air exposure. Hydroquinone products packaged in jars are not recommended because once opened they quickly become ineffective.

(Sources: *Journal of Drugs in Dermatology*, September–October 2005, pages 592–597; *Journal of Dermatological Science*, August 2001, pages S68–S75; *Critical Reviews in Toxicology*, May 1999, pages 283–330; *Journal of Cosmetic Science*, May–June 1998, pages 208–290; and *Dermatological Surgery*, May 1996, pages 443–447.)

TRETINOIN AND RETINOL

A great deal of research shows that the use of tretinoin, a derivative of vitamin A found in the prescription-only topical creams such as Renova or Retin-A, is effective in treating skin discolorations. However, the response to treatment is less marked than with other topical treatments such as hydroquinone or azelaic acid.

Results can also take far longer with tretinoin than with other treatments, requiring at least six months or more before improvement is seen. As such, tretinoin is generally not recommended as the only treatment option for skin discoloration, but is used in combination with other effective topicals. Even though tretinoin can be disappointing for immediate skin-lightening improvement, that should in no way diminish the critical role it plays in the overall improvement in skin from the standpoint of cell production, collagen production, elasticity, skin texture, and dermal thickness. That's why tretinoin, in combination with more effective skin-lightening treatments, makes a powerful contribution in the battle against sun-damaged and aged skin.

(Sources: *Journal of the Academy of Dermatology*, December 2006, pages 1048–1065; *Skin Therapy Letter*, November 2006, pages 1–6; and *International Journal of Dermatology*, April 1998, pages 286–292.)

Retinol, which is the entire vitamin A molecule, has some research showing it to be effective in reducing the appearance of skin discolorations. (Source: *Bioscience, Biotechnology, and Biochemistry*, October 2008, pages 2589–2597.) I recommend several moisturizers and serums with retinol in my book *Don't Go to the Cosmetics Counter Without Me*, 7th Edition and on my Web site, www.Beautypedia.com.

AHAS AND BHA AND CHEMICAL PEELS

AHA and BHA products, in concentrations for AHAs between 4% to 10% and BHA in concentrations of 1% to 2%, can be effective by not only accelerating cell turnover of the top layers of skin but also by directly inhibiting melanin formation. That makes them a formidable asset in reducing or eliminating the appearance of brown discolorations. (Source: *Experimental Dermatology*, January 2003, pages S43–S50.)

As part of a skin-care routine, in combination with other treatments such as kojic acid, hydroquinone, azelaic acid, and laser resurfacing, AHAs or BHA can be very effective for improving the overall appearance of sun-damaged skin, inhibiting melanin production, increasing cell turnover, and helping other skin-lightening ingredients penetrate the skin better.

Physicians and aestheticians can apply AHA, BHA, or trichloroacetic acid peels in varying concentrations to improve the appearance of skin discolorations as well. (Sources: *Journal of Dermatology*, January 2007, pages 25–30; and *Dermatologic Clinics*, July 2005, pages 353–362.)

Although AHA and BHA peels are popular procedures, cryotherapy is an inexpensive procedure in which the brown skin discoloration is burned from the skin, usually with liquid nitrogen. This has been shown to have better efficacy than peels, but although cryotherapy was more likely to produce substantial lightening it was more painful and took more time to heal. (Source: *Journal of the European Academy of Dermatology and Venereology*, March 2008, pages 316–319.)

KOJIC ACID

A by-product of the fermentation process of malting rice for use in the manufacture of sake, Japanese rice wine, kojic acid definitely has convincing research, both in vitro and in vivo and in animal studies, showing that it is effective for inhibiting melanin production. (Sources: *Cellular Signaling*, September 2002, pages 779–785; *Biological and Pharmaceutical Bulletin*, August 2002, pages 1045–1048; *Analytical Biochemistry*, June 2002, pages 260–268; *American Journal of Clinical Dermatology*, September–October 2000, pages 261–268; and *Archives of Pharmacal Research*, August 2001, pages 307–311.)

However, kojic acid in concentrations high enough to make a difference can be irritating, and far more irritating than the more effective hydroquinone. (Source: *Skin Lightening and Depigmenting Agents*, emedicine.com, July 2008.)

So why don't more products claiming to lighten skin contain kojic acid? Kojic acid is an extremely unstable ingredient in cosmetic formulations. Upon exposure to air or sunlight it turns a strange shade of brown and loses its efficacy. Many cosmetics companies use kojic dipalmitate as an alternative because it is far more stable in formulations. However, there is no research showing that kojic dipalmitate is as effective as kojic acid, though it is a good antioxidant.

AZELAIC ACID

Azelaic acid is a derivative of grains such as wheat, rye, and barley, yet while it has a natural origin it is created from oleochemicals (chemicals derived from oils or fats). It is considered very effective when applied topically in a cream formulation at a 15% to 20% concentration, and should be considered for a number of skin conditions. For the most part, azelaic acid is recommended as an option for acne or rosacea, but there is also some research showing it to be effective for the treatment of skin discolorations. Azelaic acid in concentrations of 15% and 20% is available by prescription only. Twenty percent azelaic acid is available by prescription only in Azelex and 15% azelaic acid is found in the prescription-only Finacea. (Sources: *Journal of Dermatology*, January 2007, pages 25–30; *Cutis*, February 2006, pages 22–24; and *Medical Hypotheses*, March 1999, pages 221–226.) Concentrations lower than 15% (usually less than 1%) show up in cosmetic skin-care products. When combined with other "actives" ranging from retinol to AHAs and vitamin C it can be another option when you begin experimenting to find what works for you.

ARBUTIN

Arbutin is a hydroquinone derivative isolated from the leaves of the bearberry shrub, cranberry, blueberry, and most types of pears, and serves a similar purpose. Because of arbutin's hydroquinone content it can have melanin-inhibiting properties (Source: *Journal of Pharmacology and Experimental Therapeutics*, February 1996, pages 765–769). Although the research describing arbutin's effectiveness is persuasive (even if most of the research has been done on animals, in vitro, or by companies selling products using the ingredient), concentration protocols have not been established. That means we just don't know how much arbutin it takes to have an effect in lightening the skin. Moreover, most cosmetics companies don't list the word "arbutin" on their products because there are patents controlling its use in skin-care products for skin lightening and it is extremely expensive. To get around this problem many cosmetics companies use plant extracts that contain arbutin, such as bearberry, but the amounts of those used in most skin-care products are exceptionally small and the likelihood of seeing benefit is anyone's guess. (Sources: *British Journal of Dermatology*, December 2008, pages 1267–1274; and *Journal of Cosmetic Science*, July–August 2006, pages 291–308). That's why many products containing tiny amounts of plant sources of arbutin have names like "brightening" or "illuminating" rather than "whitening" or "lightening."

OTHER ALTERNATIVES

Plant-derived or natural-oriented skin-care ingredients send out a definite siren song to consumers. Anyone developing "natural" alternatives to hydroquinone has an eager audience ready and willing to give them a try. To that end the number of new ingredients that are cropping up is seemingly endless. The following are a few of the ingredients, with their Latin or technical name, that might show up in a skin-care product claiming to inhibit melanin production.

Paper mulberry (*Broussonetia kazinoke*); Mitracarpe (*Mitracarpus scaber,* an extract of bearberry); Bearberry (*Arctostaphylos uva-ursi*); Yellow dock (*Rumex crispus* or *Rumex occidentalis*); glutathione; leukocyte extract (a form of peptide); *Aspergillus orizae* (a fungus); Licorice root (*Glycyrrhiza glabra*); and the following Chinese plant extracts: Yohimbe (*Pausinystalia yohimbe*); Cang Zhu (*Atractylodes lancea*), Bai Xian Pi (*Dictamnus dasycarpus* root-bark); Hu Zhang (*Polygonum cuspidatum* or giant knotweed rhizome); Gao Ben (*Ligusticum* rhizome or Chinese lovage root); Chuanxiong (*Rhizoma ligustici*); and Fangfeng (*Radix sileris* also *Radix ledebouriella*).

Whether these ingredients can have much impact on skin discolorations is anyone's guess, though they may indeed have anti-inflammatory and antioxidant properties. Theoretically any antioxidant can have overall benefit in improving the way skin cells react to the environment, particularly in regard to sun exposure. Reducing the effect of UV radiation on the skin is a significant benefit for inhibiting melanin production. However, the research about these ingredients is extremely limited and mostly done by the ingredient manufacturers. Even when the research has been independent it did not compare the ingredients to others, so how much more or less effective these may or may not be has not been evaluated.

(Sources: *Journal of Investigate Dermatology*, Symposium Proceedings, April 2008, pages 20–24; *Chinese Journal of Integrated Medicine*, September 2007, pages 219–223; *Phytotherapy Research*, November 2006, pages 921–934; and *Household and Personal Products Industry Magazine*, April 2001.)

VITAMIN C

Vitamin C is considered a stable and effective antioxidant for skin. For skin lightening, several studies have shown it can have benefit for inhibiting melanin production. What complicates the issue of vitamin C is that the vitamin has many forms, and these are used in skin-care products in a wide variety of concentrations. Some of the options may be magnesium ascorbyl phosphate, L-ascorbic acid, ascorbyl glucosamine, and ascorbic acid. While the amount of research isn't definitive the vitamin offers other benefits along with its skin-lightening ability. Still, there are very few studies showing any of these to have benefit for inhibiting melanin production and the tests that do exist used concentrations far greater than what shows up in most skin-care products. Generally the amount of vitamin C in these studies ranged from 5% to 10%, while most skin-care products containing vitamin C use less than a 1% concentration. (Source: *International Journal of Dermatology*, August 2004, pages 604–607.)

LASER AND LIGHT TREATMENTS

Pigment deep in the dermis does not respond well to topical agents. Resurfacing procedures such as chemical peels and liquid nitrogen can be helpful but recurrences often happen too quickly for patient satisfaction. As a result, intense pulsed light devices (IPL) and laser treatments have far outpaced these other procedures. While IPLs and laser treatments may significantly help rid skin of brown discolorations the treatments are expensive, the results are not consistent, and problems can occasionally occur. Of course, without strict use of a sunscreen with UVA-protecting ingredients the discolorations almost always come back. Moreover, laser treatments of this kind have been a problem for those with darker skin tones, though new research indicates that specific lasers now pose only rare incidences of unwanted side effects.

After taking all of the pros and cons into consideration, it's clear that when laser and light treatments do work they can make a marked difference in the appearance of the face, arms, hands, and chest, which are the areas of the body most prone to hyperpigmentation. The results can be startling, and completely eliminate any appearance of the problem. (Source: *Journal of the American Academy of Dermatology*, May 2008, pages 719–737.)

LASER

LASER (**l**ight **a**mplification by **s**timulated **e**mission of **r**adiation) light is emitted in a single, high-intensity beam of coherent energy. This light source is absorbed by water, hemoglobin, and melanin in the skin. The absorption of this energy destroys the melanin and prevents its regrowth. The wavelength of the particular type of laser dictates the depth of laser penetration and the amount of melanin that can be targeted.

Based on the absorption spectrum of melanin, the Q-switched ruby laser (694 nm) and the Q-switched Nd:Yag laser (1064 nm) are the lasers of choice for the treatment of brown discolorations. In a randomized controlled trial of 27 patients with solar lentigines on the back of the hand, the best treatment was with the Q-switched Nd:Yag laser compared with a krypton laser, 532-nm diode pumped laser, or liquid nitrogen. (Source: *Lasers in Surgery and Medicine*, February 2006, pages 94–97.)

The Q-switched ruby laser treatment is a safe procedure for the treatment of solar lentigines even in dark-skinned individuals. In addition to concentrating on melanin content alone, considering other factors in the patient's background is required for minimizing side effects, especially postinflammatory hyperpigmentation in darker skin. (Source: *Dermatologic Surgery*, November 2008, pages 1465–1468.) Never go for a laser treatment without a discussion of pros and cons with the physician.

Adverse effects from laser treatment include discomfort, redness, mild swelling, and postinflammatory hyperpigmentation. Patients should always have a test spot performed before a full treatment.

INTENSE PULSED LIGHT

An offshoot of laser treatment is intense pulsed light (IPL), in which high-intensity pulses of a broad wavelength (515–1200 nm) of light deliver it to the skin, targeting the cells containing melanin. IPL has been shown to work well for greatly improving or ridding the skin of brown discolorations. (Source: *Annals of Plastic Surgery*, November 2007, pages 479–483.)

FRACTIONAL PHOTOTHERMOLYSIS

Fractional photothermolysis (Fraxel) is a recent development in laser technology. It was approved by the U.S. Food and Drug Administration for the treatment of dyspigmentation in 2005. Fraxel works by causing thermal damage to microscopic zones of the epidermis and dermis. With a single Fraxel treatment, an estimated 15% to 20% of the skin undergoes laser resurfacing, while the surrounding normal skin is thought to help in the healing process. Based on the fraction of skin that experiences thermal damage, the skin experiences less short-term downtime, and with four to six treatments can give the same improvement as would be seen in ablative laser resurfacing. This technology has been shown to provide significant clinical improvement in brown discolorations as well as improvement in sun damage and scarring. (Source: *Seminars in Cutaneous Medicine and Surgery*, March 2008, pages 63–71.)

COMBINATION TREATMENTS

Diligent and consistent use of sunscreen with the UVA-protecting ingredients of avobenzone (buytl methoxydibenzyl methane), Tinosorb, Mexoryl SX (ecamsule), titanium dioxide, or zinc oxide, is the first line of defense when tackling skin discolorations. Many researchers feel that 2% to 4% hydroquinone lotions can be more effective when combined with Retin-A or Renova, and AHAs or BHA, along with other plant extracts, vitamins, and/or azelaic acid. It is also extremely helpful to consider chemical peels or laser treatments to remove or lighten skin discolorations; you can then use topicals to maintain the improvement. (Sources: *Journal of Cosmetic Dermatology*, April 2004, pages 76–87; and *Cosmetic Dermatology*, August 2001, pages 13–16.)

Chapter 14
Solutions for Dry Skin

The Basics

TWICE A DAY: Gentle cleanser
   Recommended cleansers: The Body Shop Aloe Calming Facial Cleanser, for Sensitive Skin; Kiehl's Ultra Moisturizing Cleansing Cream; Paula's Choice Skin Recovery Cleanser for Normal to Very Dry Skin; CeraVe Hydrating Cleanser; DHC Cleansing Milk.

NIGHTTIME: Makeup remover
   Recommended makeup removers: Mary Kay Oil-Free Eye Makeup Remover; Paula's Choice Gentle Touch Makeup Remover; DHC Eye Makeup Remover; Elizabeth Arden All Gone Eye and Lip Makeup Remover; Physician's Formula Eye Makeup Remover Lotion for Normal to Dry Skin.

TWICE A DAY: Toner (optional)
   Recommended toners: MD Formulations Moisture Defense Antioxidant Spray; Paula's Choice Moisture Boost Hydrating Toner; Paula's Choice Skin Recovery Toner; Bioelements Calmitude Hydrating Solution.

ONCE OR TWICE A DAY: Exfoliate
   Recommended AHA exfoliants: Neutrogena Healthy Skin Face Lotion Night; Paula's Choice 8% Alpha Hydroxy Acid Gel; Peter Thomas Roth Glycolic Acid 10% Moisturizer.
   Recommended BHA exfoliants: Paula's Choice 1% Beta Hydroxy Acid Lotion; Paula's Choice 2% Beta Hydroxy Acid Lotion; Jan Marini Factor-A Plus Mask.

DAYTIME: Sunscreen with antioxidants
   Recommended daytime moisturizer with sunscreen: Good Skin All Bright Moisturizing Sunscreen SPF 30; Mary Kay TimeWise Day Solution Sunscreen SPF 25; Elizabeth Arden Extreme Conditioning Cream SPF 15; Paula's Choice Skin Recovery Daily Moisturizing Lotion SPF 15.

NIGHTTIME: Emollient-rich moisturizer with antioxidants, cell-communicating ingredients, and skin-identical ingredients
   Recommended moisturizers: M.A.C. Strobe Cream, Osmotics TriCeram, Paula's Choice Hydrating Treatment Cream, Paula's Choice Skin Recovery Moisturizer; SkinMedica Rejuvenative Moisturizer.

NIGHTTIME: Specialty treatment such as tretinoin (Renova), a retinol product, or a serum with extra antioxidants

   Note: For specific product choices for your skin type from my product line please visit www.paulaschoice.com; for products for your skin type from other product lines please visit www.Beautypedia.com.

REPAIRING THE PROBLEM

To prevent or eliminate dry skin, the goal is to maintain the health of the skin's intercellular matrix. Moisture loss is definitely a symptom of dry skin, but simply giving the skin moisture won't repair the intercellular matrix because no matter how much water you give it there is no way for it to stay put. What is far more significant is to give the skin the substances lacking in the skin's epidermis—called the intercellular matrix—that holds skin cells together and allows the skin to function as it should, namely keeping hold of it's water content. Substances like glycerin, lecithin, cholesterol, ceramides, hyaluronic acid, and many, many more, allow the surface of skin to behave in a somewhat younger way, similar to how it did before sun damage began causing problems. Just compare the parts of your body that haven't seen the sun very much with the parts that have and you'll get a good idea of what the problem really is. For most of us, the parts of our bodies not exposed to the sun don't look or act like dry skin.

Without question, moisturizers play a significant role for dry skin. The number of products aimed at this problem is staggering, and they go by all kinds of names. The key thing is to ignore the names and pay more attention to the texture: the more emollient it is, the better it is for dry skin. Fortunately, almost all moisturizers and anti-wrinkle products, by whatever name, are wonderfully able to take care of most dry skin conditions.

UNDERSTANDING DRY SKIN—IT ISN'T ABOUT WATER

Ironically, dry skin does not seem to be about a lack of moisture. The studies that have compared the water content of dry skin to normal or oily skin don't seem to find a statistically significant difference in moisture content between them (Source: *Journal of Cosmetic Chemistry*, September/October 1993, page 249). As mentioned in the earlier discussion of moisturizers, too much water can be a problem because it can disrupt the skin's intercellular matrix, where the substances that keep skin cells bonded to each other are, ensuring that the outer layer of skin is intact and smooth.

What is thought to be taking place in dry skin is that the intercellular matrix has somehow become impaired or damaged, and that creates water loss. It's not that the skin doesn't have enough water, but rather it doesn't have the ability to prevent water loss, or to keep the right amount of water in the skin cell. When the intercellular matrix is disrupted, it impairs the integrity or health of the skin and the skin inevitably becomes dry, literally torn and ruptured.

There are some genetic factors that create this weakened or ineffective outer layer of skin, but some of the things we do to our skin cause dryness as well. Perhaps the biggest offense is the use of drying skin-care products such as soaps, harsh cleansers, or products with drying or irritating ingredients. All of these disrupt the outer layer of the skin, destroying the intercellular matrix and causing dry skin. In skin-care products, the ingredients that are the worst culprits are alcohol, witch hazel, fragrance, camphor, menthol, citrus, and peppermint.

Weather and the way we heat and cool our homes, cars, and workplaces are also problematic for creating or worsening dry skin. Constant exposure to arid environments, as well as to air blasting from drying heaters or air conditioners, also destroys or impairs the skin's outer layer and intercellular matrix. Adding a humidifier to your home can make a world of difference in preventing external factors like this from causing dry skin to occur in the first place.

Unprotected sun exposure is another factor that damages the outer layer of skin. Sun damage causes abnormal cell production, resulting in a malformed outer layer of skin. In this situation skin cells adhere poorly to each other, and the result is that the surface of new skin being formed is continually unhealthy and unable to provide reliable protection. Removing the damaged outer layer of skin can also make a world of difference in the health and appearance of the skin's surface. AHAs, BHA, and cosmetic skin-resurfacing procedures handle this problem beautifully. Tretinoin is also helpful for its role in improving cell production.

Perimenopause and menopause also factor into the causes of dry skin. Estrogen helps maintain skin's moisture content by increasing mucopolysaccharides and hyaluronic acid in the skin, helping to maintain the function of the skin's outer layer. Loss of estrogen also reduces the lipid content of skin, which eliminates the skin's natural protection against dryness.

TOO MUCH WATER CAN BE A PROBLEM

While companies love to boast about how much water their products can put in your skin, it turns out that may not be a good thing because too much water is particularly hard on dry skin. Overhydration can indeed be a problem, and products that brag about increasing water content in skin cells by 180% can be doing more harm than good. This contention isn't new, and was supported in an article in *Cosmetics & Toiletries* magazine (May 2000, page 18). The article reviewed a book by Loden and Maibach called *Dry Skin and Moisturizers, Chemistry and Function.* One of the points in this book that impressed the reviewer was the fact that "prolonged water contact is not innocuous. Intense dermatitis can occur simply by prolonged water exposure…. Water alone also disrupts the SC [stratum corneum—the outer, surface layer of skin]…." Their studies show that water can directly disrupt the barrier lipids [the substances that protect the surface of skin and are similar to how skin is disrupted when washed with strong cleansers]. That means water can break down the stuff that binds skin cells together, actually degrading skin in the same way that strong cleansing agents can. (Note: *Cosmetics & Toiletries* magazine is a cosmetics industry journal read by cosmetics executives, formulators, and packaging companies.)

Another article, in *Contact Dermatitis* (December 1999, pages 311–314), stated that "Water is a skin irritant, which deserves attention because of its [pervasiveness]…. In occupational dermatology, the importance of water as a skin irritant is especially appreciated. The irritancy of water has been demonstrated by occlusion experiments; occlusion with either closed chambers or water-soaked patches has been shown to produce clinical and histopathological inflammation. Functional damage, as revealed by increased transepidermal water loss, has also been shown…. However, much remains to be done to clarify the risk factors and mechanisms of water-induced irritation."

What this means is that those with dry skin should avoid soaking in a tub or taking long showers. Water is great, but it can be overdone and end up causing more problems than it helps.

DRINKING WATER

Wouldn't it be great for those with dry skin if just drinking eight or more glasses of water a day could prevent or change dry skin? Drinking water is definitely important for the health of the body but that doesn't translate to getting rid of dry skin. If drinking water were all it took to eliminate dry skin, no one would have dry skin! Attempting to overdrink is always accompanied by an almost immediate need to go to the bathroom, where the excess water is quickly eliminated. So even if the extra water could be delivered to skin cells it would never have the chance to get there.

PRACTICAL GUIDELINES FOR DRY SKIN

Dry skin does show improvement and feels vastly better when a well-formulated moisturizer and gentle cleansing products are used, and dry air is kept off the skin. Here are some practical recommendations for helping your skin never have a dry day again:

- If you can add a humidifier in your home, bedroom, or workplace, do so. You can also fill your bathtub with water and let it sit. This will fill the air with much needed moisture in the winter. It is surprising how beneficial this can be for skin.
- Use gentle cleansers from head to toe. Harsh or drying soaps or cleansers of any kind will either create dry skin or make matters worse.
- Avoid immersing your skin in water for long periods of time. This includes taking long showers.
- At night, apply an effective AHA or BHA product. This is great for dry feet, legs, and arms, as well as the face! You may have to experiment to find out how frequently to apply these types of products, but it is essential to exfoliate the outer layer to get rid of the unhealthy buildup of dry, sun-damaged skin.
- In the morning it is essential to apply an emollient moisturizer with an SPF 15 or greater that has the UVA-protecting ingredients avobenzone (butyl methoxydibenzylmethane), Tinosorb, Mexoryl SX (ecamsule), titanium dioxide, or zinc oxide.
- At night an emollient moisturizer that's made with plant oils, skin-identical ingredients, antioxidants, and cell-communicating ingredients can help a great deal.
- For very dry skin, apply a layer of olive oil or other plant oils, such as safflower, almond, or canola, over your nighttime moisturizer as an extra treatment.

CHAPTER 15
SOLUTIONS FOR ACNE

THE BASICS

TWICE A DAY: Gentle cleanser (irritating and drying products hurt the skin's ability to heal, stimulate oil production, and increase acne-causing bacteria in the skin)

Recommended cleansers: Clean & Clear Foaming Facial Cleanser, Sensitive Skin; Neutrogena One Step Gentle Cleanser; Jan Marini Bioglycolic Bioclean; Paula's Choice One Step Face Cleanser for Normal to Oily/Combination Skin; Paula's Choice Skin Balancing Cleanser.

NIGHTTIME: Makeup remover

Recommended makeup removers: Mary Kay Oil-Free Eye Makeup Remover; Nivea Visage Eye Makeup Remover; Paula's Choice Gentle Touch Makeup Remover; DHC Eye Makeup Remover; Sephora FACE Waterproof Eye Makeup Remover.

TWICE A DAY: Toner (optional)

Recommended toners: MD Formulations Moisture Defense Antioxidant Spray; Paula's Choice Moisture Healthy Skin Refreshing Toner; Paula's Choice Skin Balancing Toner; Pevonia Botanica Sensitive Skin Lotion.

ONCE OR TWICE A DAY: Exfoliate with a BHA (salicylic acid) gel or liquid that does not contain irritating ingredients such as alcohol or menthol

Recommended BHA exfoliants: Paula's Choice 1% Beta Hydroxy Acid Gel; Paula's Choice 2% Beta Hydroxy Acid Gel; Paula's Choice 2% Beta Hydroxy Acid Liquid; Neutrogena Oil-Free Acne Stress Control 3-in-1 Hydrating Acne Treatment; Cosmedicine Speedy Recovery Acne Treatment Daytime Blemish Lotion SPF 15.

ONCE OR TWICE DAY: Use an over-the-counter or prescription antibacterial product (preferably a gel, liquid, or serum)

Recommended antibacterial products: Clinique Acne Solutions Emergency Gel Lotion; Stridex Power Pads; Serious Skin Care Clearz-It Acne Medication;Paula's Choice Blemish Fighting Solution; Paula's Choice Extra Strength Blemish Fighting Solution.

ONCE OR TWICE A DAY: Use a retinoid, such as Differen, Retin-A, Renova, Tazorac, Avita, Aberela, or Atralin, among others (or their generic versions)

DAYTIME: Sunscreen in a foundation or pressed powder to reduce the number of products applied to skin

Recommended foundations with sunscreen: Boots No7 Stay Perfect Foundation SPF 15; L'Oreal True Match Super-Blendable Makeup SPF 17; Revlon ColorStay Active Light Makeup SPF 25; Shiseido Sun Protection Liquid Foundation SPF 42; Paula's Choice Best Face Forward Foundation SPF 15.

Recommended pressed powders with sunscreen: Chanel Purete Mat Shine Control Powder SPF 15; Avon Anew Beauty Age-Transforming Pressed Powder SPF 15; Prescriptives Flawless Skin Total Protection Powder SPF 15; Shiseido Pureness Matifying Compact Oil-Free SPF 16; Paula's Choice Healthy Finish Pressed Powder SPF 15.

NIGHTTIME: **Over dry areas such as the eye, cheeks, or forehead, use a moisturizer in gel or lotion form with antioxidants, cell-communicating ingredients, and skin-identical ingredients**

Recommended moisturizers: Clinique Super Rescue Antioxidant Night Moisturizer, for Combination Oily to Oily Skin; MD Formulations Moisture Defense Antioxidant Hydrating Gel; Prescriptives Super Line Preventor Extreme; Paula's Choice Skin Balancing Moisture Gel; Paula's Choice HydraLight Moisture-Infusing Lotion.

Note: For specific product choices for your skin type from my product line please visit www.paulaschoice.com; for products for your skin type from other product lines please visit www.Beautypedia.com.

BUSTING ACNE MYTHS

There's no way around it: One of the most worrisome and prevalent skin-care problems many women suffer through at some point in their lives is some degree of acne. Whether it's blackheads, whiteheads (milia—hard white bumps that do not contain pus and are not swollen or red), papules (inflamed, red, raised bumps that do not contain pus), or pustules (inflamed, red, raised bumps that contain pus), blemishes are commonplace skin imperfections. "Acne affects approximately 95% of the population at some point during their lifetime." This common disorder can range from mild to severe forms, can sometimes cause extensive scarring, and typically occurs between the ages of 11 and 50 (Source: *Journal of Reproductive Medicine*, September 2008, pages 742–752).

Regardless of your age, gender, skin color, or ethnicity, what causes acne is the same across the board (Source: *British Journal of Dermatology*, May 2000, pages 885–892). As a result there are certain basics for fighting breakouts that are essential if you are going to have any chance of winning the battle. To create a plan of action—and it does take an organized plan of action and experimentation—it is essential to let go of all the persistent and pervasive but inaccurate information concerning blemishes and instead learn what really can help your skin. You can't choose wisely if you don't know what you're fighting against! If you don't understand all your options and don't focus on what can work and what can't, you will end up making the condition worse than it was to begin with, or find temporary relief only to have the problems show up time and time again.

First and foremost, you need to get over four major myths about treating breakouts—because they will not only fail to prevent or eliminate a blemish, but they can also cause a whole range of additional skin problems.

The first myth is the notion that you can dry up a blemish. Water is the only thing you can "dry up," and a blemish has nothing to do with being wet. Skin cells, however, do contain water, and when you dry up the skin you are really drying up the water in the skin cell. Drying up skin impairs the intercellular matrix (skin's protective barrier), which can increase the presence of bacteria in the pore and cause flaking and a tight, dry feeling. None of that stops breakouts, but it can lead to irritation and add another predicament to your skin-care woes. What's true is that blemishes are aggravated by oil production, which needs to be reduced and/or absorbed. Absorbing oil on the skin or in the pore is a radically different process from drying up skin. When you "dry" a blemish, all you're doing is reducing its water content via drying or very absorbent ingredients. That will make the blemish appear smaller, but it slows healing and exaggerates flaking, which really doesn't make things look better.

The second myth is that blemishes are caused by dirty skin. Unfortunately, this mistaken belief causes harsh overcleaning of the face with soaps and strong detergent cleansers. That only increases the risk of irritation and dryness, while doing nothing to prevent blemishes. Not only that, the ingredients in bar cleansers and soaps that keep them in a hard bar form can clog pores and actually cause breakouts. The truth is that gentle cleansing and overall gentle skin care are critical to getting breakouts under control (Source: *Cutis*, December 2001, Supplemental, pages 12–19).

The third myth is that you can spot-treat blemishes. You can reduce the redness and swelling of a blemish with a salicylic acid (BHA)–based product or with a benzoyl peroxide–based product, but treating acne that way is a bad idea. For most types of blemishes (other than those created by an immediate reaction to a cosmetic or some other topical irritant or sensitizing reaction), by the time it shows up on the surface of the skin it has been at least two to three weeks in the making. It takes time for conditions in the pore to create a blemish. Dealing with only the blemishes you see means you would be ignoring the blemishes that are in the process of forming.

The fourth myth is that ingredients like alcohol, menthol, peppermint, eucalyptus, or lemon have any benefit for acne. If anything, those ingredients not only are damaging to the skin's barrier, thus inhibiting healing, but they also generate irritation and irritation can cause an increase in oil production. This is because stress-sensing nerve endings in the skin increase oil production in the sebaceous (oil) gland. (Sources: *Clinical Dermatology*, September–October 2004, pages 360–366; and *Dermatology*, January 2003, pages 17–23.) All skin types need to avoid unnecessary irritants, but this rule is even more dire when acne is present.

WHAT CAUSES BLEMISHES?

At the heart of the matter acne is an inflammatory disorder. Interaction between a whole series of physical triggers creates redness and swelling that ends in the eruption of a blemish. Understanding how to stop this sequence of events from taking place, along with reducing inflammation, will let you begin to create a successful skin-care routine. (Source: *Expert Opinions in Pharmacotherapy*, April 2008, pages 955–971.)

The five major factors (and one minor one) that contribute to the formation of blemishes are:

1. Hormonal activity (primarily androgens, male hormones)
2. Overproduction of oil by the sebaceous (oil) gland (the oil gland is an important formation site of active androgens, which control oil production)

3. Irregular or excessive shedding of dead skin cells, both on the surface of skin and inside the pore
4. Buildup of bacteria in the pore
5. Irritation
6. Sensitizing reactions to cosmetics, specific foods (rarely), or medicines.

Fundamentally, this is how a blemish occurs: Inside an oil gland a type of bacteria called *Propionibacterium acnes* (or *P. acnes*) finds a perfect environment for growth. Dead skin cells and excess oil in the oil gland provide just the kind of conditions that *P. acnes* needs to thrive. As *P. acnes* settles in, thanks to an abundant supply of sebum, it reproduces, which causes irritation and inflammation. That's why most blemishes are red and swollen. (Source: *Cutis*, January 2008, pages 81–86.)

Each hair follicle grows from a sebaceous (oil) gland that secretes an oily, firm wax called sebum. The structure that the oil gland and hair follicle share is called the pilosebaceous duct or unit, more popularly referred to as a pore. When things are going well, the sebum smoothly leaves the pore and imperceptibly melts on the skin's surface, helping to keep the skin surface moist and smooth. When things aren't going well, as when the pore becomes plugged with sebum and dead skin cells and bacteria run amok, a blemish is the outcome. Surplus sebum is generated primarily by hormonal activity. (Source: *Journal of the American Academy of Dermatology*, December 2001, pages 957–960.) When too much oil is produced, it can become mixed with dead skin cells from the skin's surface, with poorly sloughed skin cells from the pore's lining, and with small pieces of hair debris from the follicle. This combination of sebum, dead skin cells, and small pieces of hair can clog the pathway out of the hair follicle/oil gland, creating quite a backup. Now you've got problems. (Source: *International Journal of Cosmetic Science*, June 2004, pages 129–138.)

When your body produces too much oil, and dead skin cells on the surface of skin or inside the pore aren't shed normally, they can join together in blocking the exit from a pore. All the excess oil and dead skin cells solidify as a soft, white substance that plugs the pore. If the surface of the pore is covered by skin, it is called a whitehead (milia). If the pore is open, without any skin covering, the top of the plug is exposed to air and darkens from the oxidation, causing a blackhead.

Whiteheads and blackheads become pimples when *P. acnes* begins growing inside the plug, causing irritation and inflammation. Finally the inflammation and excess oil cause the wall of the oil gland to rupture, spilling the contents (oil, cell debris, bacteria, and all) into the surrounding skin tissue. The body's immune system then responds, sending lymph to the inflamed area to help with repair (and causing swelling), and you now have a pimple.

Now that you know what causes the problem the all-important question is, what can you do to control these symptoms? Can you slow down oil production? How do the skin cells build up and clog the pore, and how do you stop that from happening? How do you kill and inhibit the bacteria that cause the inflammation and redness?

WHY ME?

Why my skin? Why another blemish or blackhead? Why can't I have smooth, poreless skin? Why me? Believe me, I know this feeling.

Why do you suddenly, at the age of 28 or 48, have blemishes? Why haven't you out-grown the blemishes and oily skin that have plagued you since you were 14, and that at age 35 are worse than ever? Why, at 40, do you have incessant blackheads and breakouts that won't go away no matter what you do, and you've done everything? Why do you still have acne when you're 18 and have tried oral antibiotics, Retin-A, sulfur masks, topical antibiotics, and every cosmetic skin-care routine imaginable? These are great questions and I understand them well.

Regardless of how old you are, breakouts and oily skin are upsetting, and anyone can be a victim! The main culprits in all these scenarios are hormones, because hormones are what affect oil production, and because their levels fluctuate at different times of life.

Breaking out is definitely most prevalent during adolescence. Statistics suggest that three out of four teenagers have problems with breakouts and various forms of acne. That isn't surprising when you consider that adolescence is a time of colossal hormonal changes that stimulate sebaceous (oil) glands and increase sebum production, which in turn increases the chances for breakouts. But acne can happen at any age. More than 40% of all women will experience some form of acne. (Sources: *Journal of Pediatric and Adolescent Gynecology*, August 2008, pages 171–176; and *Journal of European Dermatology and Venereology*, November 2001, pages 541–545.)

Anything that can raise hormone levels—stress, the menstrual cycle, pregnancy, birth-control pills, or certain medications such as corticosteroids, and lithium—can act as a trigger. Specific foods are not responsible for breakouts, but an individual can have allergies to specific foods which may result in blemishes. There is also speculation that foods with hormone additives (specifically poultry and beef), iodine in food (shellfish), or fluoride in toothpaste may aggravate blemishes.

There's no question that hormone activity is the main thing responsible for oily skin and breakouts. When hormones gush, blemishes can flare, but hormones alone are not enough to create this annoying skin malady. For some unknown reason(s), something goes wrong in the oil gland, blocking the natural flow of oil. Theories about what causes acne generally focus on a genetic predisposition that creates either a defective oil gland, a malfunctioning pore lining that doesn't shed properly, or oil (sebum) that itself is in some way abnormal (too thick or irritating to the skin). In real life, you have to address most, if not all, of these issues if you want to reduce the chances of breakouts.

There are many theories about why some people have more severe cases of acne than others. Some suggest that it's increased levels of male hormones, while others say that a genetic abnormality of the oil gland is the culprit. Hypersensitivity to *P. acnes* may also account for the great variation in the severity of acne (Source: *Dermatology*, 1998, volume 196, issue 1, pages 80–81). There is even research showing that the actual fatty-acid components of the oil gland may be responsible. Most likely it's a combination of all these factors that causes the differences between those with mild or severe breakouts, and so the best approach is to deal with them one by one and through experimentation eliminate the sources of the problem.

YOU CAN'T ZAP ZITS

As I mentioned above you can reduce the redness and swelling of a blemish with a salicylic acid (BHA)–based product or with a benzoyl peroxide–based product, but treating acne that way is a bad idea. Myriad products promise clear skin, and several pledge to zap zits, dry up blemishes, and drink up oil. The commercials and ads sound convincing, but a closer look reveals that many of these products really can't zap zits or dry up oil (you can never really dry up oil), and, if anything, can make matters worse. Spot-treating only the blemish you see doesn't prevent other blemishes from forming. It takes consistency (regularly exfoliating, disinfecting, absorbing oil, hormonal balance) to stop breakouts. Further, many of these products that assure you they can zap zits contain drying, irritating, or sensitizing ingredients that actually make matters worse.

If you just pay attention to what you see on the surface without taking into consideration what is occurring underneath, you can't help heal the skin, reduce breakouts, or prevent scarring. Finding solutions that address each problem—hormonal activity, oil production, exfoliating the skin (and the pore), and killing the bacteria that cause the infection—is the only course of action that makes sense. Focusing on that single lesion without keeping the entire picture in mind can result in more breakouts, increased risk of scarring, and additional skin problems such as redness, surfaced capillaries, irritation, and dry skin.

OR CAN YOU ZAP ZITS?

ThermaClear and Zeno are two handheld devices sold as being able to really zap zits. Let me start with the warnings for these two machines right from the beginning and then I'll get to the details:

Don't use these devices if:

- You have acne or blemishes that tend to scar or you get red marks that take awhile to heal. These devices may make acne scarring worse by overheating the epidermis, inhibiting skin's ability to heal.
- You have acne that tends to be red and inflamed. The heat, in some cases, can make the inflammation worse.
- If you have more than ten lesions at a time. In this case the Zeno/Thermaclear won't be cost- or time-efficient and there are better options to consider.

Now, for those of you who haven't heard of the Thermaclear ($145) or Zeno ($89–$200, depending on which Zeno you choose), both of these devices use heat to combat the bacteria that contribute to acne. They are sold as being best for mild to moderate acne involving individual pimples, not full-blown breakouts all over the face, and certainly not for cystic or nodular acne. These devices are truly limited but that won't stop lots of people from giving them a try despite the hefty price tag for what amounts to a simple heat-emitting machine.

Both devices are battery-operated and make similar claims. Of course, both describe themselves as being unique and different from each other, but for all intents and purposes they work the same way. What is different is the cost factor. Each hand-held device uses a tip that needs to be discarded and replaced. The Thermaclear device uses a chrome tip that you can use for a year before it needs to be replaced for a cost of $19.95.

With Zeno, the tip provides a fixed number of treatments before it must be replaced (and sets of replacement tips aren't cheap: they range from $19–$25). How many treatments you get depends on which Zeno device you choose. For example, the Zeno Mini offers 45 treatments (that's 45 individual pimple treatments, one pimple is treated by one tip, a single tip does not do a full face of treatments), and the Zeno MD offers 150 treatments (that's a 150 individual blemishes that can be treated). Clearly the Zeno device is the pricier option both initially and long term, and the more acne lesions you have, the more you'll spend.

It is good news that neither company positions their device as a one-stop treatment for mild, intermittent breakouts. Yet consumers more often than not ignore these details and will try a new option without using other products to combat acne. (Biore Pore Strips come to mind; no matter how many warnings were on the box, most women I've spoken to over the years had no idea they were there.)

Instructions for using both devices are very similar: you wait for the device to charge and when it's ready (indicated by colored lights on both devices) you place the treatment tip directly on a blemish and a controlled heat pulse is generated. You have to hold the device on the blemish for two and a half minutes and (according to the Web site for Zeno) after that "you can clear up a pimple in two hours."

When you place the tip against a blemish, without pressure, a heat "burst" occurs and it happens quickly. There is no risk of "burning" skin when used as directed, but it definitely heats skin. With either device, you must wait several seconds for it to recharge before treating another pimple. Twice a day is the recommended usage, and depending on how many pimples you are trying to treat that can take a lot of time. This is supposed to be less expensive and faster than seeing a dermatologist or using over-the-counter treatments such as benzoyl peroxide or salicylic acid. Does that sound possible or true to anyone? It certainly doesn't to me, and the research doesn't support that notion either.

One other claim made for Thermaclear that will likely catch the eye of many consumers is that their device is FDA-cleared—which, on the surface, conveys some type of special status. It isn't special or a stamp of approval for acne treatment in the least. All heat-emitting devices such as Thermaclear are classified as Class II laser instruments. Just to keep this in perspective, another example of a Class II laser product is the common laser pointer, like the ones used in a classroom or business meeting setting. Doesn't sound too fancy or high-tech now, does it? A Class II light-emitting device does not require a prescription or medical supervision, which is why these devices can be sold without restrictions.

So how does heat possibly affect a pimple? The theory is that the type of heat energy these devices produce when in close contact with a pimple has an oxidizing effect on porphyrins. Porphyrins are naturally occurring substances that are part of a cell's protoplasm (fluid structure). It seems that acne-causing bacteria are able to synthesize and store large amounts of porphyrins. When porphyrins are exposed to heat and light energy, they reach an excited state and a chemical reaction that forms an extra oxygen molecule happens. In much the same way benzoyl peroxide works on acne lesions, the extra oxygen kills acne-causing bacteria, thus reducing the size and severity of a pimple (Sources: *Journal of Cosmetic and Laser Therapy*, June 2005, pages 63–68, and June 2004, pages 91–95).

What's not as clear (pun intended) is whether or not Thermaclear and Zeno devices deliver enough power with each pulse of light to significantly impact acne. There are no published, peer-reviewed studies proving either device to be effective (some published studies have used other devices that are available to physicians, not the general public). Instead, each company has done clinical trials whose results are impressive. But would you expect anything less? Considering the marketing and cost of these devices, the companies certainly aren't going to go on record with clinical trials showing their treatments were average to poor or that they paled in comparison to what doctor-administered light treatments can accomplish.

It's even more telling that none of the clinical trials compared these heat-emitting devices to a sensible anti-acne skin-care routine, or to spot-treating a blemish with salicylic acid or benzoyl peroxide, options that might possibly have superior results.

The Thermaclear Web site mentions that their clinical trials showed the device can be used with benzoyl peroxide, which is nice, but that still doesn't tell you if the benzoyl peroxide worked or would work better than the Thermaclear. No mention was made of other anti-acne active ingredients such as salicylic acid, glycolic acid, or prescription vitamin A products. All in all, the information about these devices is limited, with great-sounding claims and little real scientific evidence in support of the assertions.

As for Zeno, they claim that none of the in-office heat/light-emitting devices (namely Thermage or Intense Pulsed Light) used to treat acne have been shown to be as effective as Zeno. That's a misleading, absurd claim, because thus far a comparison study has not been done. Moreover, the minimal research that exists for treating acne with light and heat energy has been about long-term results for the entire face, not spot treating when a zit pops up.

If you decide to try either device, I recommend purchasing them from Sephora because they have an excellent return policy should you find Thermaclear or Zeno is not for you. And make no mistake: Neither Zeno nor Thermaclear should replace a reliable anti-acne skin-care routine or trump the advice given to you by a dermatologist working with you to get your acne under control.

Is there a legitimate reason to invest in these devices and are they really a great adjunct to an anti-acne routine, or are they a waste of money? The quick answer is that both devices may help for their intended purpose, but I would never recommend either as a stand-alone treatment, neither for efficacy or cost.

WHAT YOU CAN DO

Effective blemish treatment works by reducing oil production, eliminating skin-cell buildup on the surface of skin and in the pore, and killing the bacteria, *P. acnes*, that caused the inflammation in the first place. That's why the best course of action for blemishes is twofold, both topical (what you put on the skin, whether it's an over-the-counter or a prescription option) and systemic (prescription oral medication that addresses the issue of oil production and bacterial growth).

TOPICAL OPTIONS

- Clean the skin gently with a water-soluble cleanser that doesn't contain ingredients that can clog pores or irritate the skin. This helps reduce further irritation and redness, and reduces oil production triggered by nerve endings on the skin's surface, which would make matters worse.
- Remove dead skin cells and encourage healthy skin-cell turnover, both from the skin's surface and inside the pore, to help skin shed more normally.
- Absorb or reduce excess oil to reduce the main cause of clogged and enlarged pores.
- Kill the bacteria (*P. acnes*) that are causing the eruption, inflammation, redness, and swelling.
- Topical retinoids (Retin-A, Tazorac, Avita, generic tretinoin, Differin) to normalize cell function, allowing the pore to function normally.
- Laser treatments.

SYSTEMIC OPTIONS

- Oral antibiotics to eliminate bacterial growth.
- Birth-control pills and hormone blockers to control oil production.
- Accutane, the only prescription medication capable of curing acne.

EXPERIMENT

You need to experiment to discover exactly how to put these various steps together in a combination that works for you. Unfortunately, there isn't one absolutely right way. It is essential to try different options until you find what suits your skin type and your specific condition. If you are consistent and avoid veering from your special battle plan, you stand a pretty good chance of winning a good part of the war against blemishes and blackheads. But the battle plan must deal with all of a blemish's causes.

WHAT YOU SHOULDN'T DO

Don't use harsh or irritating skin-care products. Throughout this book I discuss the need for gentle cleansing for all skin types. This concept is particularly difficult for someone with oily or blemished skin to believe, despite the research backing it up, because the desire to really clean the skin is almost irresistible. Yet a paper published in the *Proceedings of the Fourth International Symposium on Cosmetic Efficacy* (May 10–12, 1999, entitled "The Effects of Cleansing in an Acne Treatment Regimen") concluded that 52% of the time a hydrating face wash gave better results in reducing comedones, papules, and pustules when used with benzoyl peroxide. By comparison, this type of gentle cleanser was more effective than either soap or a benzoyl peroxide cleanser alone.

What is most frustrating is that many of the blemish products on the market actually make breakouts worse or cause more skin problems than you started out with. Products designed to tackle acne often contain ingredients like harsh surfactants and overly abrasive scrub particles, as well as alcohol, menthol, peppermint, camphor, and eucalyptus, lemon, or grapefruit oils. All of these ingredients are extremely irritating, and the resulting irritation can impair the skin's ability to heal or to fight bacteria as well as trigger oil production.

What makes all these standard, harmful "blemish-fighting" ingredients worse is that they don't reduce any of the factors causing breakouts. They can't disinfect, reduce oil production, affect hormonal activity, or help exfoliation. Instead, they kill more skin cells than necessary, which can further clog pores, produce dry skin, cause irritation, and make skin redder. A blemish by definition is already irritated, red, and swollen, so it doesn't make any sense to use ingredients that will make it even more irritated, red, and swollen.

Skin-care products with irritating ingredients, such as facial masks, astringents, toners, and facial scrubs (which also contain waxes), are a big no-no. These can all hurt the skin, and that can aggravate acne. If a product irritates the skin, if it tingles or burns, it is not helping. And not only does irritation stimulate oil production, promote redness, increase swelling, and dry out the skin, it can also add small, rashlike pimples to the breakouts you're already trying to deal with.

Bar soaps and bar cleansers are often recommended for acne, yet all of them contain ingredients that can clog pores. Soaps contain tallow, and bar cleansers contain other heavy, wax-based thickening agents that can clog pores. Shockingly, high-pH soaps and cleansers (those with a pH of 8 or higher) can actually increase the presence of bacteria in the pore! All this makes matters much worse inside the pore, again greatly increasing the risk of breakouts.

Oversqueezing, picking, digging, scraping, or poking at pimples may be hard to resist, and you may think it speeds healing, but in fact it sets you up for more problems. Creating scabs and constantly reinjuring the lesion just increases the chances of scarring. There is nothing wrong with gentle squeezing to remove a blemish's contents, but unless you are extremely careful you will create more problems than you started with.

Many women think they can use hot compresses to bring pimples to a head. Actually, hot compresses severely damage skin by burning it; the heat causes more redness and swelling; and the whole process can also rupture the pore, increasing the possibility of more breakouts. The same is true of steaming the face or using hot water. Hot water burns the skin, impairing the skin's ability to heal and fight bacteria. Tepid water is what you need to help soothe the skin and calm things down. Use tepid water and a gentle, water-soluble cleanser on the face, and do not wipe off makeup. Wiping and rubbing will make the irritation worse, and can also make the skin sag and cause wrinkles.

Be careful that the breakouts you're struggling with aren't a result of hair products getting on the face. Hairspray, mousse, hair gel, and other styling products contain polymers (plastic-like, film-forming ingredients) that can clog pores and cause pimples. Be especially careful if you routinely use pomades or styling waxes.

Don't smoke. A study in the *British Journal of Dermatology* (July 2001, pages 100–104) concluded, "According to multiple logistic regression analyses acne prevalence was significantly higher in active smokers (40.8%…) as compared with non-smokers (25.2%). A significant linear relationship between acne prevalence and number of cigarettes smoked daily was obtained…. In addition, a significant dose-dependent relationship between acne severity and daily cigarette consumption was shown by linear regression analysis…. Smoking is a clinically important contributory factor to acne prevalence and severity."

WHEN TO SEE A DERMATOLOGIST

Some women run to see a dermatologist the second they see a blemish. Others put it off well past the time when over-the-counter options have stopped working, even when their breakouts are still rampant. Though there are many options for dealing successfully with breakouts outside the realm of prescription medications, if your acne is severe or chronic it may indeed be best to seek medical attention. Dermatologists have a host of options in their arsenal that can be more effective than over-the-counter products in reducing sebum production, creating healthy skin-cell turnover, and fighting bacterial infection.

Most prescription-only options such as the tretinoins (Retin-A, Tazorac, Avita, generic tretinoin), Differin (technically adapalene), and azelaic acid (trade name Azelex), plus topical antibiotics, oral antibiotics, and hormone blockers, have no nonprescription counterparts. Dermatologists also have one option that can be an absolute cure for acne and breakouts. That option is Accutane, the only medication that has a chance of curing acne as opposed to just keeping it under control. All of these options are discussed in this chapter.

Nonetheless, it is completely acceptable to start with the options available over the counter or from some cosmetics lines. Research indicates that the first line of defense against blemishes is from over-the-counter products. Some of these are similar to what a doctor would prescribe, such as salicylic acid products to exfoliate and benzoyl peroxide products to disinfect. (Sources: *Dermatologic Clinics*, January 2009, pages 17–24; and *Lancet*, December 2004, pages 2188–2195.)

To make sure you have the best chance that these products will work, it is essential that they be well formulated and that they don't contain any irritating ingredients. If after a period of time you find those options don't work or aren't working as well as you would like, you can always make an appointment with a dermatologist.

WHAT ABOUT DIET?

There is little, if any, scientific evidence that diet affects acne, although specific food allergies certainly can be a contributing factor. But that depends on what you personally are allergic to: not everyone has the same food allergies. Likewise, drinking soda pop, not exercising, popping vitamins, and eating healthy or unhealthy foods will neither help nor hurt acne. Lots of Olympic-caliber athletes have acne-prone skin, and lots of people who don't exercise and are overweight have a flawless complexion. However, if certain foods—such as nuts, shellfish (because of their iodine content), milk products, or wheat—seem to make your acne worse, it is best to avoid them. Try omitting them one by one to see if it makes a long-term difference in your skin. (Source: *Journal of the American Academy of Dermatology*, September 2008, pages 534–535.)

TOOTHPASTE FOR ACNE? NOT

Incidentally, fluoride in toothpaste may be the source of breakouts around the mouth. The research for this is very old, with a couple of studies published in the 1970s and even the 1950s. That is not exactly current information, but if you tend to have acne just around your mouth, it is simple enough to try nonfluoride toothpaste for awhile and see if things improve. If your acne is indeed triggered by fluoride, consult your dentist about alternative cavity-prevention treatments. (Source: *Archives of Dermatology*, 1975, volume 11, page 793.)

OIL-FREE IS A BAD JOKE

But the joke is on us, because while "oil-free" is a meaningless claim, it may mislead consumers into buying products that can actually clog pores. There are plenty of ingredients that don't sound like oils but that can absolutely aggravate breakouts. On the other hand, not all oils clog pores. Meanwhile, many cosmetics (anything that is in a lotion or cream form) contain waxlike thickening agents that may clog pores. When any product looks like a cream or a lotion (as opposed to a fluid), the ingredients that give it that consistency may clog pores. Despite the problems these ingredients can cause, they show up in lots and lots of so-called "oil-free" products.

Above and beyond the products that claim to be oil-free, label after label promises that the product is "noncomedogenic" or "nonacnegenic." Most of us have bought products with this assurance, only to find that they did cause breakouts. I wish I could say otherwise, but the truth is you can't trust any product that makes the claim that it's not comedogenic because there is no approved or regulated standard for that assertion. What many women already know from experience is that trying to guess how their skin will react based on a product's promises, especially when it comes to blemishes, is truly a lost cause—or at the very least a difficult problem with no easy, slam-dunk answers.

WILL IT MAKE ME BREAK OUT?

So if you can't trust the terms "oil-free," "non-comedogenic," or "nonacnegenic," how do you know if a product will cause problems? Why does it seem so impossible to find products that won't cause breakouts? The simple answer is that it's because most ingredients used in cosmetics can cause breakouts, depending on your skin type.

There is evidence that some specific ingredients can trigger breakouts, but there are no absolutes. I wish there were, but there aren't. Several Web sites that showcase lists of comedogenic ingredients have caused quite a stir for many women. The major source of information for these data appears to be Dr. Fulton's *Step by Step Program for Clearing*

Acne, published in 1983 by Harper & Row (though credit is not given on any Web site, it is the exact same information presented in the book). At the time—and 1983 is a long time ago—Fulton's research on the causes of breakouts was unprecedented. Fulton applied cosmetic ingredients to rabbits' ears and waited to see what happened. As promising as this research was, it has never been repeated, and is rarely cited in later research, except when it suits a company's marketing agenda. There are many reasons why lists of this kind are unreliable. (Source: *Journal of the American Academy of Dermatology*, March 2006, pages 507–512.)

First, the methodology involved pure concentrations of the ingredient, not the concentrations that are used in actual cosmetic formulations, which are usually only a fractional percentage. It also didn't address the issues of usage and application. For example, the exposure risks of specific ingredients are very different for a cleanser, which is left on the skin for a few seconds, and a lotion or liquid that is left on the skin for hours. Beyond this, the research didn't look at the host of plant extracts or sunscreens in cosmetics that were introduced during the early '80s. To call this list out of date and inconclusive would be an understatement! (Source: *Cutaneous and Ocular Toxicology*, 2007, volume 26, issue 4, pages 287–292.)

Another point is that lists of this kind can't account for the thousands and thousands of cosmetic ingredients being used in skin-care and makeup products today! A lot of them are emollients, waxy thickening agents, or irritants that can cause skin problems. Whether they do or not, however, is completely dependent on the amount used and the nature of the individual ingredient (some ingredients cause problems in far smaller amounts than other ingredients, while others cause problems in various combinations). A comprehensive list would not only be impossible, it would also be nothing more than guesswork.

There are no easy answers for this one, but you can understand that trying to research, categorize, classify, and make absolute conclusions about thousands of ingredients with an infinite number of possible combinations is just not humanly possible. So, what's a woman to do when trying to fend off blemishes and still use skin-care and makeup products? The easiest and most reliable quality for a consumer to consider is the consistency of the product. The thicker the product, meaning those with a high, thick, or creamy viscosity, the more likely it is to cause problems. That means you can feel safer with a gel or serum, since these have a low or watery viscosity.

What about greasiness? It is safe to assume that a product with any plant or mineral oils on the ingredient list, especially if they are listed high up on the ingredient list, can make the skin feel greasy. Greasiness doesn't necessarily trigger breakouts, but it definitely doesn't help skin exfoliate and it won't feel great on oily or combination skin.

Finally, it makes more sense to watch out for irritating ingredients than so-called pore-clogging ingredients. It doesn't take much alcohol, menthol, peppermint, balm mint, eucalyptus, camphor, lemon, grapefruit, or lime to cause a negative skin reaction that can impede the skin's healing process by stimulating bacteria production—and that won't help heal blemishes.

BLEMISH-FIGHTING BASICS

Each of the following products and product categories reflects state-of-the-art treatments for blemishes, acne, and blackheads. How to put them all together is addressed above in "The Basics" section.

All of the products described below address each of the factors that cause pimples. These are the best options for reducing oil production, disinfecting the skin, improving exfoliation, and for controlling hormonal activity, and are a potential cure for blemishes. Finding the combination that works for you is the first goal, and then you must focus on hitting all the steps and carrying them out consistently.

Gentle cleansing is the first place to start. I've already elaborated on the need for gentle cleansing, but let me say it one more time for added emphasis. Using a water-soluble cleanser gently cleans your skin without stimulating the oil glands, increasing redness, or creating dryness. This step is standard for any skin-care routine because it makes an instant difference in the appearance and feel of the skin, and it is essential for reducing breakouts. Once you stop using drying, irritating, pore-clogging soaps or bar cleansers, and you realize how nice your skin feels when it is no longer dry and irritated, you will never go back to the old way again. Just be certain the water-soluble cleanser you select doesn't contain irritating ingredients and won't dry out the skin. Using cleansers that contain exfoliating agents, topical disinfectants, or oil-absorbing ingredients is not the best option because the active ingredients would be washed away before they had a chance to have an effect on skin. Save these ingredients for another step.

Killing acne-causing bacteria comes next. There aren't many options for disinfecting the skin. Alcohol (when used in the right concentrations) and sulfur can be good disinfectants, but they are too drying and irritating, causing more problems than they help, and that can generate more breakouts. Plant-derived disinfectants such as tea tree oil (melaleuca) are an option but there are no products currently being sold that contain a high enough concentration to reliably kill bacteria. Benzoyl peroxide is still the best over-the-counter disinfectant to consider, and is available over-the-counter in 2.5%, 5%, and 10% concentrations.

If benzoyl peroxide isn't effective, a topical antibiotic or a topical antibiotic combined with benzoyl peroxide prescribed by a doctor are excellent options. If you are seeing a physician, one of typical treatments they might choose is to prescribe an oral antibiotic to kill stubborn, blemish-causing bacteria from the inside. However, an oral antibiotic should be a last resort because of systemic problems and problems with resistant bacteria. Oral antibiotics can indeed kill blemish-causing bacteria, but they also kill good bacteria in the body, causing yeast infections and stomach problems. In addition, *P. acnes* in your body can develop resistant strains in a short period of time, making the antibiotic you're taking ineffective, and then you have to move on to the next one, which reduces your choices of antibiotics should you need them for a serious illness.

Exfoliate! Because blemishes occur inside the pore and involve oil production, an effective 1% to 2% salicylic acid (beta hydroxy acid—BHA) product is a crucial over-the-counter starting point for exfoliating the skin. Salicylic acid is lipid soluble, which means it can exfoliate through oil, so it can get inside the pore and exfoliate the pore's cell lining and improve its shape, plus it is extremely gentle. I recommend using BHA in a gel, liquid, or extremely light lotion formula because these formulas are unlikely to contain waxy thickening agents or emollients that can clog pores. Alpha hydroxy acids (AHAs) can be helpful for surface exfoliation, but they can't affect the pore lining, and it's essential to do that to deal with one of the root causes of a blemish.

Scrubs are an option for extra exfoliation, but because they typically come in thick formulations and those ingredients can clog pores, a washcloth with your gentle cleanser can provide the same benefit without any problematic added ingredients.

Improving cell production with retinoids is also very helpful. Tretinoins or other vitamin A prescription derivates, as found in Differin, are prescription options for generating healthy cell growth that can change the shape of the pore, allowing for normal oil flow. This improvement can eliminate the environment that allows the blemish to develop.

Absorbing or controlling excess oil is another consideration. Clay masks are an option for absorbing oil as long as they contain no irritating ingredients. Using milk of magnesia as a facial mask is a simple and effective way to absorb oil. Birth-control pills and hormone blockers can also equalize hormones, reducing or eliminating the source of excess oil production.

When all else fails, meaning your breakouts persist after you've tried these over-the-counter and prescription options, then you can still try photodynamic therapy or Accutane. Accutane is the only medication that can essentially cure acne and is essentially the last option in any experiment to deal with acne because of its serious side effects especially if a woman becomes pregnant while using it.

EXFOLIANTS: BHA VERSUS AHA

Referred to as beta hydroxy acid (BHA), salicylic acid can be a judicious starting point in the treatment of breakouts for all skin types. This is a multifunctional ingredient that addresses many of the systemic causes of blemishes (Source: *Seminars in Dermatology*, December 1990, pages 305–308), and it is exceedingly effective when combined with benzoyl peroxide (Source: *Skin Pharmacology and Physiology*, May 2006, pages 283–289). For decades dermatologists have been prescribing salicylic acid because it is such an effective keratolytic (exfoliant). Yet, in addition to salicylic acid's incredibly helpful exfoliating properties, it can do even more. Salicylic acid is a derivative of aspirin (both are salicylates—aspirin's technical name is acetyl salicylic acid) and so it also functions as an anti-inflammatory (Sources: *Seminars in Cutaneous Medicine and Surgery*, September 2008, pages 170–176; and *Archives of Dermatology*, November 2000, pages 1390–1395). Combining exfoliation with reduced irritation has many advantages for skin, especially for someone struggling with breakouts. Diminishing or eliminating the redness and swelling blemishes cause can help skin heal, prevent scarring, and decrease the chance of further breakouts.

Preventing pores from becoming clogged is a requisite key to preventing blemishes. One way to achieve this is to improve the shape of the pore lining. The lining of a pore is made of skin cells (epithelial tissue) that can become thick and misshapen, preventing the natural flow of oil out of the pore. To act on the pore lining it is necessary to exfoliate inside the pore, dislodging excess skin cells. Exfoliants such as alpha hydroxy acids (AHAs) or mechanical scrubs have limitations for blemish-prone skin due to their inability to penetrate inside the pore. AHAs are water-soluble and can't get through the oil. Mechanical scrubs have particle sizes that are too large for them to have any effect below the surface of skin, though they can make the surface smoother. Salicylic acid is the perfect answer. It is an effective exfoliant, it is lipid soluble (so it effortlessly penetrates into the pore), and it is an anti-inflammatory so it can actually reduce irritation, swelling, and redness.

Another notable aspect of salicylic acid for breakouts is that it has antimicrobial properties (Sources: *Preservatives for Cosmetics*, by David Steinberg, Allured Publishing, 1996; Health Canada Monograph Category IV, *Antiseptic Cleansers*). That means it can be effective in killing the bacteria that cause acne. Together, all these properties mean salicylic acid is one of the more multifunctional ingredients in combating the causes of acne.

As wonderful as this sounds, salicylic acid is a tricky product to buy. The concentration must be at least 0.5%, but 1% to 2% is far more effective. Additionally, the formula's pH is a critical factor. For salicylic acid to work as an exfoliant on skin, it must be in a formulation with a pH of 3 to 4; if it isn't, it loses its ability to exfoliate skin (Source: *Cosmetic Dermatology*, October 2001, pages 65–72). Plus the product must not contain any irritating ingredients. Well-formulated salicylic acid products do exist, and once you've found the right one, it can be a successful part of your battle plan to fight blemishes.

(Other sources: *Journal of the European Academy of Dermatology and Venereology*, May 2008, pages 629–631; *Dermatology*, January 2003, pages 68–73; and *European Journal of Dermatology*, July–August 2002, pages 64–50.)

OVER-THE-COUNTER ANTIBACTERIAL OPTIONS

Benzoyl peroxide, which was briefly discussed above, is considered the most effective over-the-counter choice for a topical antibacterial agent in the treatment of blemishes. (Sources: *Dermatologic Clinics*, January 2009, pages 33–42; and *Skin Pharmacology and Applied Skin Physiology*, September–October 2000, pages 292–296.) The amount of research demonstrating the effectiveness of benzoyl peroxide is exhaustive and conclusive. Benzoyl peroxide's main attributes are its ability to penetrate into the pore that holds the hair follicle to reach the bacteria and prevent them from creating inflammation, in essence destroying their ability to cause breakouts. Benzoyl peroxide has a low risk of irritation, and it also doesn't have potential to create the problem of bacterial resistance that some prescription topical antibacterials (antibiotics) do. (Sources: *British Journal of Dermatology*, August 2008, pages 480–481; and *Dermatology Therapy*, March–April 2008, pages 86–95.)

Benzoyl peroxide solutions range from 2.5% to 10%. For the sake of your skin, start with the less potent concentrations. A 2.5% benzoyl peroxide product is much less irritating than a 5% or 10% concentration, and it can be just as effective. It completely depends on how stubborn the strain of bacteria in your pores happens to be.

Despite benzoyl peroxide's superior disinfecting and penetrating properties, some bacteria just won't give up easily, and in those situations a different weapon may be necessary. That's when you should consider prescription topical disinfectants (topical antibiotics).

PRESCRIPTION ANTIBACTERIALS

If your skin doesn't respond to benzoyl peroxide in the various over-the-counter higher strengths or in combination with a well-formulated BHA (salicylic acid), the next step is a prescription topical antibacterial, meaning some type of antibiotic, in a liquid, lotion, or gel form. Topical antibiotics have limitations. They can have difficulty penetrating the hair follicle, and long-term use can lead to antibiotic-resistant strains of bacteria. Erythromycin, tetracycline, and clindamycin are the most popular topical antibiotics.

You can use these antibiotics alone, but a good deal of research points to the greater benefit of combining these with benzoyl peroxide to create a potent and effective treatment. Studies indicate that when topical clindamycin or erythromycin are combined with benzoyl peroxide, both have demonstrated clinical efficacy in the treatment of acne. When used in tandem, they promise greater efficacy than either individual agent alone, through their antibacterial and anti-inflammatory complementary effects. Together they have an earlier onset of action, are significantly more effective against inflamed and total lesions, and are better tolerated, which should improve usage. (Sources: *Dermatology Clinics*, January 2009, pages 25–31; *British Journal of Dermatology*, January 2008, pages 122–129; *Journal of Cutaneous Medical Surgery*, January 2001, pages 37–42; and *American Journal of Clinical Dermatology*, 2001, volume 2, issue 4, pages 263–266.)

Warning: Do not apply benzoyl peroxide and a retinoid (such as Retin-A, Renova, Tazorac, Avita, generic tretinoin) at the same time. Benzoyl peroxide inactivates retinoids (Source: *British Journal of Dermatology*, September 1998, page 8). The exception to this is Differin (adapalene), which is compatible with benzoyl peroxide.

DAPSONE: THE LATEST ANTIBACTERIAL OPTION

Dapsone is a topical disinfectant gel available by prescription in 5% strength. The brand name for the anti-acne drug is Aczone, and it is made by Allergan (of Botox fame). Dapsone is a drug that comes from the sulfone family of drugs. Its relation to sulfur explains its antibacterial action.

Double-blind, large-scale studies examining dapsone's effectiveness on adolescent acne have shown that it is well-tolerated and brought about "clinically meaningful" improvements in acne lesion count after 12 weeks, with improvements continuing with ongoing usage. Side effects were similar to that of the "vehicle gel," which was not identified in the studies.

Although Aczone is an option for inflammatory acne and research on its efficacy is positive, what's lacking are critical comparative studies with other known, established anti-acne drugs (both prescription and over-the-counter). I wouldn't consider Aczone unless you have tried benzoyl peroxide, retinoids, and salicylic acid, all of which have a large body of research proving their efficacy and safety. If those actives haven't produced satisfactory results, talk to your physician about Aczone/dapsone.

Sources: *Cutis*, February 2008, pages 171–178 and November 2007, pages 400–410; *Journal of Drugs in Dermatology*, October 2007, pages 981–987; and *Journal of the American Academy of Dermatology*, March 2007, pages e1-e10).

TEA TREE OIL VERSUS BENZOYL PEROXIDE

Tea tree oil has some interesting research demonstrating it to be an effective antimicrobial agent. The *Journal of Applied Microbiology* (January 2000, pages 170–175) stated that "The essential oil of *Melaleuca alternifolia* (tea tree) exhibits broad-spectrum antimicrobial activity. Its mode of action against the Gram-negative bacterium *Escherichia coli* AG100, the Gram-positive bacterium *Staphylococcus aureus* NCTC 8325, and the yeast *Candida albicans* has been investigated using a range of methods…. The ability of tea tree oil to disrupt the permeability barrier of cell membrane structures and the accompanying loss of chemiosmotic control is the most likely source of its lethal action at minimum inhibitory levels." In addition, "In a randomized, placebo-controlled pilot study of tea tree oil in the treatment of herpes cold sores, tea tree oil was found to have [a] similar degree of activity as 5% acyclovir" (Source: *Journal of Antimicrobial Chemotherapy*, May 2001, page 450). For acne there is also some published information showing it to be effective as a topical disinfectant for killing the bacteria that can cause pimples (Source: *Letters in Applied Microbiology*, October 1995, pages 242–245). But there is also a medical review of tea tree oil challenging the viability of these studies (Source: *Journal of Antimicrobial Chemotherapy*, February 2003, pages 241–246).

However, the crux of the matter for any potential efficacy in a commercial product is, how much tea tree oil is needed to have an effect? *The Medical Journal of Australia* (October 1990, pages 455–458) compared the efficacy of tea tree oil to the efficacy of benzoyl peroxide for the treatment of acne. A study of 119 patients using 5% tea tree oil in a gel base versus 5% benzoyl peroxide lotion was discussed. There were 61 patients in the benzoyl peroxide group and 58 in the tea tree oil group. The conclusion was that "both treatments were effective in reducing the number of inflamed lesions throughout the trial, with a significantly better result for benzoyl peroxide when compared to the tea tree oil. Skin oiliness was lessened significantly in the benzoyl peroxide group versus the tea tree oil group." However, while the reduction of breakouts was greater for the benzoyl peroxide group, the side effects of dryness, stinging, and burning were also greater—"79% of the benzoyl peroxide group versus 49% of the tea tree oil group."

Given these results, a 2.5% strength benzoyl peroxide solution would be better to start with to see if it is effective, rather than starting with the more potent and somewhat more irritating 5% or 10% concentrations. However, if you were interested in using a 5% strength tea tree oil solution to see if that would be effective, at this time I know of no products stating how much tea tree oil they contain. It appears that almost all tea tree oil products on the market contain little more than a 1% concentration, if that, which is probably not enough to be of much help for breakouts.

TRETINOIN FOR BLEMISHES

Retinoid is the general category name for any and all forms of vitamin A. Tretinoin is a form of vitamin A and, therefore, comes under the general heading of retinoids. The best-known products that contain tretinoins are Retin-A, Renova, Retin-A Micro, Tazorac, Avita, and generic tretinoin. These are all basic treatments for blemishes because they change the way skin cells are formed in the layers of skin as well as in the pore. If skin cells have an abnormal shape, they tend to stick together and shed poorly, often getting backed up in the pore. Tretinoin can transform cell production by improving shedding and by unclogging pores, thereby producing a significant reduction in inflammatory lesions. Topical tretinoins and antibacterial agents have complementary actions and they work well together, but their application must be separated, at least if the antibacterial agent you're using is benzoyl peroxide. Benzoyl peroxide can render tretinoin ineffective when the two are applied together. The solution is to use benzoyl peroxide in the morning and your tretinoin product at night. Tretinoins are not able to kill *P. acnes*, the bacteria that cause the breakouts, but an antibacterial agent can. Meanwhile, tretinoins can improve and restore the shape of the pore, opening a clear pathway for the antibacterial agent so it can be more active. (Sources: *American Journal of Clinical Dermatology*, June 2008, pages 369–381; *Clinical Therapy*, June 2007, pages 1086–1097; and *Journal of the European Academy of Dermatology and Venereology*, December 2001, page 43.)

One of the major drawbacks to the use of tretinoin is the irritation it can cause. For some people this can be so severe as to prevent its use. But there are alternatives. There is a great deal of research showing that adapalene (brand name Differin), another retinoid but different from tretinoin, can be just as effective as tretinoin but without the irritation (see the following section on Differin).

Meanwhile, remember that using any tretinoin product can make the skin more vulnerable to sun damage and sunburn. It is essential to wear an SPF 15 sunscreen that contains the UVA-protecting ingredients avobenzone (butyl methoxydibenzylmethane), Mexoryl SX (ecamsule), Tinosorb, titanium dioxide, or zinc oxide as the active ingredient. Zinc oxide and titanium dioxide are occlusive and can possibly clog pores, and synthetic sunscreen ingredients can be sensitizing for some skin types, so it may take experimentation to find the right sunscreen that works best for your skin type.

DIFFERIN

Where does Differin fit into this picture? Differin (also called adapalene) is a retinoid, a form of vitamin A that has been shown in clinical studies to be less irritating than tretinoin. According to a study published in the March 1996 *Journal of the American Academy of Dermatology*, Differin was also significantly more effective in reducing blemishes and was better tolerated than tretinoin gel. Other more recent studies have come to the same conclusion, which is that, by several measures, adapalene cream and gel were less irritating upon multiple dosing than various tretinoin creams and gels. (Sources: *International Journal of Dermatology*, October 2000, pages 784–788; and *Journal of Cutaneous Medical Surgery*, October 1999, pages 298–301.)

It seems that Differin has a radarlike ability to positively affect the skin-cell lining of the pores, substantially improving exfoliation and helping to prevent blockage. Moreover, for those with oily skin, the original Differin comes in a lightweight gel formula that is barely felt on the skin. It contains little more than water and cellulose, a sheer thickening agent. Differin is also available in a cream base for those with dry skin and blemishes.

Should you consider Differin? If you have tried Retin-A or other tretinoins and had difficulty dealing with the irritation, or if you just want to see if Differin can work better for you (which it may), then it is certainly an option. Unlike tretinoin products, Differin is not inactivated by benzoyl peroxide, which means you can apply both at the same time.

AZELAIC ACID

Azelaic acid 15% gel was approved for the treatment of rosacea in the U.S. in 2008, but has also been approved for the treatment of acne in many European countries, where it has demonstrated success. Two randomized, multicenter, controlled clinical trials compared the effects of azelaic acid 15% gel with those of topical benzoyl peroxide 5% or topical clindamycin 1%, all using a twice-daily dosing regimen. The primary endpoint in the intent-to-treat analysis was a reduction in inflammatory papules and pustules. Azelaic acid resulted in a 70% to 71% median reduction of facial papules and pustules compared with a 77% reduction with benzoyl peroxide 5% gel and a 63% reduction with clindamycin. Azelaic acid 15% gel was well-tolerated. In addition, a one-year European observational study conducted by dermatologists in private practice evaluated the safety and efficacy of azelaic acid 15% gel used as monotherapy or in combination with other agents in more than 1200 patients with acne. Most physicians (81.9%) described an improvement in patients' symptoms after an average of 34.6 days, and 93.9% of physicians reported patient improvement after an average of 73.1 days. Both physicians and patients assessed azelaic acid 15% gel to be effective, with 74% of patients being "very satisfied" at the end of therapy. Azelaic acid 15% gel was considered "well-tolerated" or "very well-tolerated" by 95.7% of patients. (Sources: *Journal of Drugs in Dermatology*, January 2008, pages 13–16; and *Journal of the American Academy of Dermatology*, August 2000, Supplemental, pages 47–50.)

ORAL ANTIBIOTICS

If topical exfoliants, retinoids, and antibacterial agents don't provide satisfactory results, an oral antibiotic prescribed by a doctor may be an option to kill stubborn, blemish-causing bacteria. Several studies have shown that oral antibiotics, used in conjunction with topical tretinoins or topical exfoliants, can control or reduce many acne conditions. (Sources: *Cutis*, August 2008, pages S5–S12; and *International Journal of Dermatology*, January 2000, pages 45–50.)

As effective as oral antibiotics can be, they should be a near-last resort, not a first line of attack. Oral antibiotics can produce some unacceptable long-term health problems. Some dermatologists tend to give the negative side effects of oral antibiotics short shrift and prescribe them as if they were nothing more than candy for their acne patients. Oral antibiotics are anything but candy. They kill the good bacteria in the body along with the bad, and that can result in chronic vaginal yeast infections as well as stomach problems. A more worrisome side effect is that the acne-causing bacteria can become immune to the oral antibiotic. According to an article in the *American Journal of Clinical Dermatology* (2001, volume 2, issue 3, pages 135–141), "The main cause for concern following the use of systemic antibiotics is the emergence of antibiotic-resistant strains of *P. acnes.*" Similarly, a paper presented at the General Meeting of the American Society for Microbiology in May 2001 (www.asmusa.org/memonly/abstracts/AbstractView.asp?AbstractID=47544) stated that "antibiotic treatment in patients with severe acne causes development of anti-biotic resistance…. The prevalence of antibiotic resistance to tetracycline, erythromycin, clindamycin and trimethoprim-sulphamethoxazole…" was found after two to six months. "When patients with acne are treated with antibiotics, the risk of development of antibiotic resistance should be realized. The use of antibiotics to treat acne should be restricted and other regimens should be tested."

This means that if you have been taking an oral antibiotic to treat your acne for longer than six months it can stop being effective. It also explains the situation that leaves many women puzzled, since initially the antibiotic they were taking gave incredible results, but then became ineffective. (Source: *Seminars in Cutaneous Medicine and Surgery*, September 2008, pages 183–187.)

An even more serious argument against taking oral antibiotics was discussed in the *American Journal of Clinical Dermatology* (July–August 2000, pages 201–209), which stated: "At a time when there is global concern that antibiotic resistance rates in common bacterial pathogens may threaten our future ability to control bacterial infections, practices which promote the spread of antibiotic-resistant bacteria must be fully justified."

The decision to use oral antibiotics should not be taken lightly. The course of action you take should be discussed at length with and monitored by both you and your dermatologist.

NIACINAMIDE AND NICOTINIC ACID FOR ACNE

Niacinamide and nicotinic acid are derivatives of vitamin B3. There is a handful of studies showing they can be helpful for improving the appearance of acne, most likely for their anti-inflammatory capacity. Many cosmetics companies are beginning to include these two ingredients in the products they're aiming at blemish-prone skin as well as in "anti-wrinkle" products. Especially when they're part of a great skin-care routine that also includes either an over-the-counter benzoyl peroxide antibacterial and salicylic acid exfoliant, or a prescription topical antibiotic with benzoyl peroxide, they contribute to a powerful combination of products to combat the events taking place in skin that is fomenting acne.

(Sources: *Journal of Cosmetic Laser Therapy*, June 2006, pages 96–101; and *Journal of Cosmetic Dermatology*, April 2004, pages 88–93.)

BIRTH-CONTROL PILLS FOR ACNE?

Oral contraceptives (OCs) can reduce acne lesions, in part by decreasing androgens (male hormones) as well as by increasing estrogen levels in the body, both of which are important factors in what causes blemishes. OCs should not be the first-line therapy or monotherapy for acne, but they can serve as a good alternative for those with mild to moderate acne.

If you are a woman (sorry, guys) looking for a way to reduce breakouts, you might want to discuss your skin problems with your gynecologist instead of your dermatologist. The FDA has approved low-dosage birth-control pills (Ortho Tri-Cyclen and generic norgestimate/ethinyl estradiol) for use in the treatment of acne. In Canada, Diane-35, a combination of cyproterone acetate and ethinyl estradiol is approved for the treatment of acne (Source: *Skin Therapy Letter*, 1999, volume 4, number 4). Depending on your lifestyle and medical history, you could solve two problems with one prescription.

How does the birth-control pill work on acne? Increased oil production can be caused by the body's androgen (male hormone) production, which can be highest just before menstruation starts. It appears that low-dosage birth-control pills can decrease the presence of excess androgens, thereby decreasing breakouts. They work particularly well when used in conjunction with other therapies such as topical antibacterial agents or tretinoins (Source: *Skin Therapy Letter*, February 2001, pages 1–3). For a lot of women this is no surprise. Many have noticed an improvement in their skin after they started taking birth-control pills.

According to a double-blind, placebo-controlled study published in *Fertility and Sterility* (September 2001, pages 461–468), other "low-dose birth-control pills can be an effective and safe treatment for moderate acne." The double-blind, placebo-controlled, randomized clinical trial found that the birth-control pill containing levonorgestrel (Alesse®) reduced acne.

Low-dose oral contraceptives also result in a low occurrence of estrogen-related side effects like nausea, headaches, and breast tenderness, in addition to low, if any, weight gain (Source: *Medscape* press release, September 7, 2001).

Is taking birth-control pills to control acne right for you? There are risks associated with taking birth-control pills, and these should be taken into account before you make a final decision. These risks include increased chances of heart attack, strokes, blood clots, and breast cancer (and these are compounded if you smoke), not to mention possible side effects such as vaginal bleeding, fluid retention, melasma (dark-brown skin patches), and depression. All of those potential side effects may not be a worthwhile trade-off for clear skin. However, if you're already considering or using the pill for birth control, this remedy may be worth looking into.

ACCUTANE: A PERSONAL SAGA

Looking back, my only regret is that I waited so long. I tried. I really tried. I patiently waited for my skin to clear up. Spent untold dollars on dermatologists and followed their instructions. Diligently wiped antibiotic lotions over my face and took oral antibiotics for years. I faithfully used Retin-A, and slathered on sulfur masks. I used facial masks to try and soak up oil during the day. For most of that time my skin did improve, but it never really stopped breaking out and I still had to put up with oily, incessantly greasy-looking skin. Besides, despite the improvement I saw from using antibiotics and the other treatments, I didn't want to stay on them forever. Adapting to the antibiotics was a risk I wasn't willing to continue taking. Who knew how much longer I would continue breaking out? It had been going on since I was 11, and by then I was 38.

I had known about Accutane for a long time. I knew it had some pretty serious, even dangerous, side effects, and that most dermatologists didn't prescribe it very often, and then only for the most serious cases. My acne and oily skin were serious to me, but not as bad as the pictures I had seen of the cystic acne cases that responded brilliantly to treatment with Accutane. Then, in 1990, a woman I worked with and two of her friends started taking Accutane. They not only lived through it, their skin looked flawless! More than flawless—radiant (at least in comparison to what it looked like before).

"Considered the biggest breakthrough in acne drug treatment over the last 20 years, Accutane is the only drug that has the potential to clear severe acne permanently after one course of treatment" (Sources: *FDA Consumer* magazine, March–April 2001; and www.fda. gov). It also has the most serious side effects and risks of any other cosmetic prescription treatment for acne.

WHAT IS ACCUTANE—A POSSIBLE CURE?

Accutane (its generic name is isotretinoin) is a drug derived from vitamin A, and it is taken orally. It essentially stops the oil production in your sebaceous glands (the oil-producing structures of the skin) and literally shrinks these glands to the size of a baby's. This prevents sebum (oil) from clogging the hair follicle, mixing with dead skin cells, rupturing the follicle wall, and creating pimples or cysts. Normal oil production resumes when treatment is completed and the sebaceous glands slowly begin to grow larger again, but never (or at least rarely) as large as they were before treatment.

"Because of its relatively rapid onset of action and its high efficacy with reducing more than 90% of the most severe inflammatory lesions, Accutane has a role as an effective treatment in patients with severe acne that is recalcitrant to other therapies" (Source: *Journal of the American Academy of Dermatology*, November 2001, Supplemental, pages 188–194).

In a large percentage of patients who complete a four- to six-month treatment with Accutane, acne is no longer considered to be clinically significant, though almost one-fifth of patients can have a recurrence of acne within the first two years (Source: *Journal of Drugs in Dermatology*, October 2008, pages 963–966). But generally the recurrence is milder than before treatment. Of course, a percentage of people still receive no benefit from taking Accutane, no matter how many treatments they take.

By the way, while dosage and duration depend on the severity of the patient's acne, the treatments generally last 16 weeks. If a second treatment is necessary, an eight-week rest period is required between treatments. Interestingly, acne continues to improve even after the course of treatment is completed, although doctors do not know exactly why.

"[Accutane] is the treatment of choice for severe nodulocystic acne. It represents the sole agent that effectively addresses all of the pathophysiological factors in the production of acne" (Source: *Seminars in Cutaneous Medical Surgery*, September 2001, pages 162–165).

ACCUTANE—RISKY STUFF

So what's the catch with this "miracle" drug and why don't doctors prescribe it to everyone? Accutane is controversial for many reasons, but principally because of its most insidious side effect: It has been proven to cause severe birth defects in nearly 90% of the babies born to women who were pregnant while taking it. Before physicians knew about this alarming hazard, and when it was first prescribed in France back in the 1970s before enough research had been conducted to establish its safety, more than 800 babies out of 1,000 were born seriously deformed. The only way to avoid this risk is to abstain from sex during treatment or, according to the information provided with every prescription, to use a minimum of two forms of birth control. If you are taking a birth-control pill, you still need to use a condom or diaphragm. You will need to discuss with your physician how long to continue using the extra birth-control precautions after you are done taking Accutane.

If you aren't pregnant or are not trying to conceive, are there still risks? Absolutely. Commonly reported, although temporary, side effects of Accutane include dry skin and lips, mild nosebleeds (your nose can get really dry for the first few days), hair loss (I lost a small amount of hair that grew back when I finished the four months of treatment), aches and pains, itching, rash, fragile skin, increased sensitivity to the sun, headaches (mild to severe—mine were fairly mild), and peeling palms and hands.

A study in the *Journal of Cutaneous Medical Surgery* (April 2000, pages 66–70) followed 124 people through their course of treatment with Accutane. "The majority of patients experienced persistent dryness of lips. Dry eyes affected 40% of patients; this continued throughout treatment in 25%. Contact lens wearers were more likely to develop conjunctivitis. Lower back pain was reported early in about 30% of patients and fewer than 10% of patients would develop it later in the course of treatment. Joint pain was noted in 16.5% of patients at the first visit and there was little change with ongoing treatment. Hair loss was experienced in a small percentage but was rarely noted on more than one occasion. Headaches occurred in less than 10% and were occasionally severe, but most often intermittent and recorded at a single visit. Depression occurred in 4% of patients and tended to persist throughout the treatment. All these patients completed the full course of treatment." The study concluded: "patients treated with [Accutane] experienced a predictable series of side effects. Some occurred fleetingly, but several persisted for the duration of treatment."

More serious, although much less common, side effects include nausea, vomiting, blurred vision, changes in mood, depression (discussed later in this chapter), severe stomach pain, diarrhea, decreased night vision, bowel problems, persistent dryness of eyes, calcium deposits in tendons (doctors don't know yet whether this is significant), an increase in cholesterol levels, and yellowing of the skin.

Understandably, many people, doctors included, are scared off by these side effects, above and beyond the risk to pregnant women. That's why dermatologists recommend Accutane only to patients with chronic acne (large, recurring cysts or blemishes that can permanently distort the shape and appearance of the skin), or sometimes to people with less-severe acne that has not responded successfully to other forms of treatment. Many doctors won't prescribe Accutane at all.

Although the high risk of birth defects and the other side effects should be taken seriously, it seems a shame that Accutane has been kept away from many acne patients. It is the most effective, short-term drug for acne available today. All other acne treatments require ongoing, tenacious adherence to the program and they don't offer a cure. The public is largely misinformed about Accutane's potential dangers as well as its potential benefit. Many doctors believe that if it weren't for the proven risk of birth defects, Accutane would be prescribed almost as frequently as antibiotics. Not surprisingly, it is prescribed much more frequently to men. (Source: *British Journal of Clinical Pharmacology*, January 2009, pages 137–138.)

Given what I have learned, I wish somebody had told me about Accutane twenty years ago! It would have saved me a lot of time, money, and heartache. Although oral and topical antibiotics, exfoliants, gentle cleansing, staying away from products that aggravate breakouts, and using facial masks to absorb excess oil can work successfully for lots of people, for many people these questions remain: "When will I outgrow acne? How long will I have to struggle with the pain of breakouts?" Sadly, there is no telling if you're ever going to outgrow it. People who don't outgrow it, and lots of women don't, are looking at years of applying topical solutions and taking oral antibiotics that sometimes work well and sometimes don't. A short-term course of Accutane, following all precautions and being aware of side effects, is a seemingly small price to pay to avoid decades of stubborn acne.

ACCUTANE PREGNANCY WARNINGS IGNORED

Despite warnings and information regarding Accutane's detrimental effect on fetuses, women are still becoming pregnant while taking it. According to an August 17, 2001, FDA press release, the Centers for Disease Control and Prevention (CDC) reported "that despite prevention efforts some women who take Accutane, a prescription medication given for severe acne and known to cause birth defects, still become pregnant while on this medication." The CDC also reported that a symbol intended to remind women that they must not get pregnant while taking these medications is commonly misinterpreted. The two studies, "Continued Occurrence of Accutane-exposed Pregnancies" and "Interpretations of a Teratogen Warning Symbol," were published in *Teratology* (2001, volume 64, issue 3, pages 142–147 and 148–153). (Teratogen refers to a substance or process that causes developmental malformations and birth defects.) Both of these studies indicate that there are serious problems related to women either not understanding or not being fully informed about the risks of becoming pregnant while taking Accutane.

The press release went on to say that "Since 1988, the CDC and the Food and Drug Administration (FDA) have worked closely to help educate health care providers and women of reproductive age who may be prescribed Accutane. The devastating birth defects caused by Accutane include: brain defects, heart defects, and facial defects such as babies born without ears." Women who want to take Accutane are supposed to have two negative pregnancy tests before beginning the medication, use two forms of effective birth control during treatment, and have repeat pregnancy tests every month during the course of medication. It turns out that many women do not follow these recommendations. Moreover, many doctors do not inform their patients that this is required, despite the fact that more women are taking Accutane for their acne than ever before.

In response, the FDA has established new restrictions designed to prevent women from becoming pregnant while they are taking Accutane. According to the FDA, the new requirements for being allowed to take Accutane, and for a doctor's ability to prescribe the drug, will include mandatory monthly pregnancy tests. Pharmacists will be allowed to fill only a one-month supply at a time, requiring proof of a negative pregnancy test from the patient. Physicians will have to place an "Accutane Qualification Sticker" on their prescriptions to establish that the patient has had a negative pregnancy test.

You can find more information about the CDC's work on Accutane and birth defects at www.cdc.gov/ncbddd/bd/accutane.htm. For more information about the FDA's review of Accutane and birth defects, please see www.fda.gov/cder/drug/infopage/accutane/default.htm.

DEPRESSION FROM ACCUTANE

According to an article in the *Journal of the American Academy of Dermatology* (October 2001, pages 515–519), "The Food and Drug Administration (FDA) has received reports of depression and suicide in patients treated with [Accutane].… [F]rom 1982 to May 2000 the FDA received reports of 37 US patients treated with [Accutane] who committed suicide; 110 who were hospitalized for depression, suicidal ideation, or suicide attempt; and 284 with nonhospitalized depression, for a total of 431 patients. Factors suggesting a possible association between [Accutane] and depression include a [limited time] association between use of the drug and depression.… Compared with all drugs in the FDA's Adverse Event Reporting System database to June 2000, [Accutane] ranked within the top 10 for number of reports of depression and suicide attempt."

In contrast to this report, a paper presented at the 59th Annual Meeting of the American Academy of Dermatology (March 27, 2001, Washington, DC) stated that "Up to the current time, a rate of 12 suicides per 8 million isotretinoin-treated patients has been documented. Half of these patients were on concomitant [other] medications. A small number of patients have reported that depression subsided when isotretinoin was withdrawn and recurred with treatment resumption. In the United States, 64 suicides occurred between 1991 and 1999 in patients who at one time took isotretinoin. Thirty occurred during treatment, 24 after treatment was stopped (6 months to 10 years), and 10 occurred in patients whose treatment status was unknown.

"These numbers must be compared with general suicide statistics in the United States. In total, 30,000 suicides occur per year (in the general population, the rate is 11.4 per

100,000). Eighty percent are males. Suicide is the third leading cause of death in the 15- to 24-year age group (6000 per year). So when isotretinoin patients are observed, the 64 total suicides must be compared with an expected suicide rate of more than 10 times that number (670). These data suggest that in these patients the suicides were likely due to factors other than isotretinoin treatment. The isotretinoin suicide rate of 1.8 per 100,000 is well below that of the general population, as noted above. In addition, in the isotretinoin patients, there was no alteration in the typical US pattern of suicide in terms of gender distribution, relationship to depression, underlying psychiatric disorders, or lack of warning signs (typical of youth suicide)."

Further research confirming that Accutane is not associated with depression concluded that there was no increase in depressive and anxiety symptoms in the isotretinoin treatment group compared to that in the topical [acne medication] group. Instead, successful treatment of acne seems to improve both depressive and anxiety symptoms as well as improving quality of life. (Sources: *International Journal of Dermatology*, January 2009, pages 41–46; and *Archives of Dermatology*, May 2005, pages 557–560.)

Despite the controversy, Hoffman-La Roche, the makers of Accutane, is adding a warning about depression to the product information insert. Hoffman-La Roche is also removing copy from their ads that suggests Accutane can relieve the "psychological trauma" and "emotional suffering" associated with acne. The lengthy package insert for Accutane did include warnings about depression but not about possible suicide or psychosis.

As is true with any medication, all the pros and cons must be considered before starting treatment. If you or the teen you are responsible for already have a history of depression, then the potential for exacerbated depression must be taken into account and discussed with your physician.

HANDLING THE SIDE EFFECTS OF ACCUTANE

How do you deal with some of the side effects when taking Accutane? It helps to be prepared. If you take Accutane, stay out of the sun! This drug makes the skin photosensitive even if you are wearing sunscreen (and you must wear sunscreen). Any prolonged sun exposure can cause severe redness and fever. Treat dry areas of the face with a moisturizer. If your nose becomes dry, apply a thin layer of petroleum jelly (Vaseline) on the skin inside the nose, and do it frequently. That will make a big difference. Do not use any skin-care products that can cause irritation or dryness. Avoid bar soaps, washcloths, AHA and BHA products, scrubs, hot water, and facial masks. If you are using tretinoin, Differin, azelaic acid, or topical antibiotics, I suggest you stop using them unless your doctor recommends that you continue. Dry eyes can be treated with artificial teardrops; do not use products like Visine that simply constrict blood flow and can dry out the eyes even more. Headaches and body aches are eased quite nicely with ibuprofen. Be sure to drink plenty of water. If you have any concerns, discuss them at once with your physician.

Pay attention to your mood. If you find yourself feeling excessively depressed, hostile, angry, or have even a fleeting thought of suicide speak to your doctor immediately. It is also essential for your doctor to monitor your blood. Cholesterol can shoot up dangerously high and liver function must be monitored. It is extremely important that you stay in close contact with your physician during the entire time you are taking Accutane.

HORMONE BLOCKERS FOR ACNE?

Using a testosterone-blocking drug to reduce the hormone levels responsible for activating oil production is controversial; it's also an approach to treating acne and oily skin that is not very well-researched. The most frequently prescribed hormone blocker is known as spironolactone (brand name Aldactone). It is an option only for women, however, because without testosterone men start to develop female characteristics such as enlarged breasts and softer skin. But because testosterone can be one of the primary causes of acne, curtailing its presence in the body may have positive results—namely, acne clears up and oil production slows.

What kind of results can you expect? A study described in the *Journal of the American Academy of Dermatology* (September 2000, pages 498–502) looked at "85 women with acne treated consecutively with spironolactone…. Results: Clearing of acne occurred in 33% of patients treated with low doses of spironolactone; 33% had marked improvement, 27.4% showed partial improvement, and 7% showed no improvement. The treatment regimen was well tolerated, with 57.5% reporting no adverse effects." Another study, reported in the *Archives of Dermatology* (September 1998, volume 134, number 9), reviewed "38 patients: 4 with severe acne (with cystic lesions), 32 with moderate acne, and 2 with mild acne. Improvement in acne, defined as a lessening in severity of acne classification, was observed in 32 (97%) of 33 patients who continued to follow up while receiving therapy. Of the 32 patients with improvement in their acne, all 4 patients with severe acne improved to moderate acne, 26 of 27 patients with moderate acne improved to mild acne and in 2 the acne disappeared, and both patients with mild acne experienced complete resolution. One patient had no improvement in her acne."

While those statistics aren't exciting, they may be of interest for women who have not responded well to other treatments. But the side effects of Aldactone are as daunting as those for Accutane. The list of adverse effects includes abdominal cramping, nausea, diarrhea, headache, reduced sexual drive (libido), dry mouth, excessive thirst, unusual tiredness, unusual muscle weakness, skin rash, deepening of voice, irregular or no menstrual periods, and slowed heart rate, plus enlarged breasts in men, and breast tenderness in women.

Moreover, hormone blockers require long-term use to effectively treat acne. When you stop taking them, the testosterone returns and so can the acne. Because hormone blockers require repetitive, continuous use, at least for treating acne, I strongly recommend trying Accutane before trying hormone blockers. Although Accutane's side effects can be more serious than those of the hormone-blocking drugs, use of Accutane is very short term, involving only a few months, and it can be a permanent cure.

ORAL SUPPLEMENTS FOR ACNE?

Very little, if any, research points to vitamins, herbs, or minerals of any kind or in any combination as having an effect on breakouts. What little research does exist shows zinc to be a valid option to consider. A handful of studies have compared oral antibiotics to zinc, with zinc showing some benefit. A study reported in *Dermatology* (2001, volume, 203, issue 2, page 40) evaluated "the place of zinc gluconate in relation to antibiotics in the treatment of acne. Zinc was compared to minocycline [an antibiotic] in a multicenter randomized double-blind trial. 332 patients received either 30 milligrams elemental zinc or 100 milligrams minocycline over 3 months. The primary endpoint was defined as the percentage of the clinical success rate on day 90...." The study concluded that "Minocycline and zinc gluconate are both effective in the treatment of inflammatory acne, but minocycline has a superior effect evaluated to be 17% in our study."

In conjunction with other treatments, zinc may prove to have even better results. But zinc is not a benign supplement. High doses of zinc can be toxic. Avoid taking more than 100 mg of zinc per day from a supplement (Source: www.drweil.com). It is also recommended that you take a daily multivitamin, because increased levels of zinc mean that the body requires more copper and manganese. There is only a very fine line between safe and unsafe amounts of oral supplementation of zinc (Source: *Journal of Trace Elements in Medicine and Biology*, January 2006, pages 3–18).

Pantothenic acid (vitamin B5) is touted as being effective for acne. However, there is only one study supporting this notion and it dates from the early 1980s (Source: *International Journal of Dermatology*, 1981, volume 20, pages 278–285). There is no current research showing this to be an effective treatment.

Vitamin A is another oral supplement thought to be helpful for acne. In one study showing it to have a positive impact, the participants were given 300,000 IU per day. Considering that the usual recommended daily amount is 10,000 IU, the 300,000 IU dose is a large enough amount of vitamin A to be possibly toxic and is not recommended. At this time there is no reliable research pointing to any oral supplement other than zinc as being helpful in the treatment of acne.

PHOTODYNAMIC THERAPY

Photodynamic Therapy (PDT) is a procedure done in a doctor's office that involves topical application of 20% 5-aminolevulinic acid, a photosensitizing cream (ALA, under the tradename Levulan), in conjunction with light exposure. The ALA is applied to the skin and is then "activated" when you sit in front of a red or blue LED panel (light-emitting diode) or IPL (intense pulsed light), which explains the name photodynamic. The IPL is not related to UV light from the sun but the LED is; in fact, you could just go out in the sun to activate the ALA.

Initially Photodynamic Therapy was cleared by the FDA in 1999 for the treatment of actinic keratosis (AK), precancerous lesions found on the head and scalp. A year later, the BLU-U, Blue Light Photodynamic Therapy Illuminator, was also FDA approved for the treatment of AK.

Shortly after that, PDT started being looked at for treating acne. Today many physicians feel PDT is a very effective option for acne, especially for those who aren't having success with traditional topical treatments. It is thought to work by shrinking the skin's oil glands, which could significantly reduce the amount of oil within the pores, thereby reducing blemishes. ALA-PDT may also kill bacteria that cause acne breakouts and normalize the shedding of dead skin cells within the follicle. It also seems to improve the skin's overall texture, and holds promise in the repair of acne scarring.

A series of three to five one-hour treatments are usually performed, timed over a given period at two- to four-week intervals. The number of treatments recommended depends on the severity of acne. (Sources: *Journal of Cosmetic Dermatology*, September 2008, pages 180–188; *Journal of Drugs in Dermatology*, July 2008, pages 627–632; and *Lasers in Surgery and Medicine*, February 2007, pages 180–188.)

There is also research showing that having microdermabrasion before the procedure can enhance the effectiveness of the PDT, both by helping improve results and shortening the time needed to activate the ALA. (Source: *Journal of Drugs in Dermatology*, February 2007, pages 140–142.)

Initially the results of ALA-PDT for acne treatments seemed promising. However more recent studies have put those results in question, showing minimal success as well as uncomfortable side effects of burning and hyperpigmentation. The need for repeated treatments in the doctor's office and the cost doesn't make this a practical process, not to mention that topical treatments are still required to achieve and maintain improvement. Outcome can also vary based on skin color. (Sources: *British Journal of Dermatology*, December 2008, pages 1245–1266; *Acta Dermato-Venereologica*, July 2007, pages 325–329; and *Lasers in Surgery and Medicine*, January 2007, pages 1–6.) As a treatment, PDT needs to be evaluated rationally with your physician, who should present the pros and cons and not describe this treatment as only having benefits.

CHEMICAL PEELS

Many studies have shown chemical peels are useful adjuncts for the treatment of acne. But which type should you choose? Most physicians and aestheticians have a penchant for glycolic acid (AHA) or lactic acid (AHA) peels because of their popularity and well-marketed product lines often sold by physicians and aestheticians. Yet there is reason to consider a salicylic acid peel (BHA) over an AHA peel. The glycolic acid and salicylic acid peels are similarly effective, but research has shown the salicylic acid peel can have sustained effectiveness and fewer side effects (Source: *Dermatologic Surgery*, January 2008, pages 45–50).

Chemical peels do have shortcomings for treating acne. They are not cures, they must be done repeatedly, and they are expensive. Before choosing this option, all the other topical options should be exhausted.

MICRODERMABRASION

Trying to separate out the information about microdermabrasion is like trying to decide if you should get a new car. It looks really good from the outside and seems to do everything, plus the salesperson makes it sound like a great investment—but what are the risks (cost, insurance, safety)? And beyond that, are there better, more effective options? Microdermabrasion is heralded on the Internet as a panacea that will solve skin problems from acne to wrinkles, but the issue is not that simple, the results are not that miraculous, and there are other options to consider.

What makes microdermabrasion enticing and so prevalent is that everyone can do it—a facialist, aesthetician, or even someone your doctor hired as a receptionist in his or her office. The machine itself is a relatively inexpensive investment for a salon, spa, or medical practice, and for the most part it is exceptionally simple to use, which helps explain its popularity.

In essence microdermabrasion is merely a superficial scrubbing of the skin. Using aluminum oxide crystals or other abrasive substances, the machine blows these particles against the skin via a tube. The same tube is then utilized to vacuum the material off the skin almost simultaneously. Despite its widespread use and the accolades microdermabrasion receives on Web sites, research has not kept pace with the testimonials. There are few published studies, and those that do exist were for the most part paid for by the companies selling microdermabrasion machines. In general, microdermabrasion studies have been conducted only in small groups of patients. Protocols, units, and settings have differed. There remains a major disparity between the popularity of microdermabrasion and the amount of comprehensive scientific data documenting the efficacy of the procedure. Plus there are almost no studies comparing microdermabrasion to other acne treatments.

All in all, there is no compelling reason to try microdermabrasion, just as there is also no compelling reason not to give it a try. The cost isn't significant and the results will be evident after the first treatment, although multiple continuing treatments are required to maintain the benefits. However, as is true for chemical peels or laser and light devices used to treat acne, they aren't cures and they don't change the need for other topical treatments such as retinoids, exfoliants, or antibacterials.

(Sources: *Seminars in Cutaneous Medicine and Surgery*, September 2008, pages 212–220; *American Journal of Clinical Dermatology*, February 2005, pages 89–92, and July 2003, pages 467–471; and *Dermatologic Surgery*, September 2005, pages 1160–1165.)

SULFUR

Some facial masks, particularly masks that are part of a skin-care routine for acne, contain sulfur, which can have some benefit as a disinfectant for breakouts (Source: *American Journal of Clinical Dermatology*, June 2004, pages 459–462). However, it is an unnecessary (compared to other options) and fairly strong substance to use to disinfect the skin, especially when you leave it sitting on your face in a facial mask for a period of time. There are gentler ways to disinfect the skin. Sulfur has lost its status and to some extent has been abandoned as an option for treating breakouts since the 1980s, thanks to the other successful topical choices available.

REMOVING BLEMISHES

This isn't a pretty topic, but it is a fact of life and human nature that just leaving a blemish or blackhead alone is almost impossible. Fortunately, gently removing a blackhead or blemish with light-handed squeezing can actually help the skin. Removing the stuff inside a blackhead or especially a pimple relieves the pressure and reduces further damage. Yes, squeezing can be detrimental to the skin, but it's the way you squeeze that determines whether you inflict harm. If you oversqueeze, pinch the skin, scrape the skin with your nails, or press too hard, you are absolutely doing more damage than good. Gentle is the operative word and, when done right, squeezing with minimal pressure is the best (if not the only) way to clean out a blackhead or blemish.

Although I never recommend steaming the face (heat can overstimulate oil production, cause spider veins to surface, and create irritation), a tepid to slightly warm compress over the face can help soften the blackhead or blemish, making it easier to remove. First, wash your face with a water-soluble cleanser, pat the skin dry, then place a slightly warm, wet cloth over your face for approximately 10 to 15 minutes. Once that's done, pat the skin dry again. Using a tissue over each finger to keep you from slipping and tearing the skin, apply even, soft pressure to the sides of the blemish area, gently pressing down and then up around the lesion. Do this once or twice only. If nothing happens, that means the blemish cannot be removed, and continuing will bruise the skin, risk making the infection or lesion worse, and cause scarring. Again, only use gentle pressure, protect your skin by using tissue around your fingers, and do not oversqueeze.

Be sure to use a salicylic acid or benzoyl peroxide solution after you're done to soothe the skin and reduce inflammation. Do not remove blackheads or blemishes more than once or twice a week or you can cause too much irritation.

PORE STRIPS?

Pore strips in all their varying incarnations are meant to remove blackheads. You place a piece of cloth with a sticky substance on it over your face, as you might do with a Band-Aid, wait a bit for it to dry, and then rip it off. Along with some amount of skin, blackheads are supposed to stick to the strip and come right out of your nose. There is nothing miraculous about these products, nor do they work all that well. The main ingredient on these strips is a hairspray-type substance. If the instructions are followed closely you can see some benefit in removing the very surface of a blackhead. In fact, you may at first be very impressed (or grossed out) with what comes off your nose.

Unfortunately, that leaves the majority of the problem deep in the pore. What has me most concerned about pore strips is they are accompanied by a strong warning not to use them over any area other than the intended area (nose, chin, or forehead) and not to use them over inflamed, swollen, sunburned, or excessively dry skin. It also states that if the strip is too painful to remove, you should wet it and then carefully remove it. What a warning!

Also, despite the warning on the package, I suspect most women will try these strips wherever they see breakouts. If I didn't know better, I know I would. The way these strips adhere, they can absolutely injure or tear skin. They are especially unsafe if you've been using Retin-A, Renova, Differin, AHAs, or BHA; having facial peels; taking Accutane; or if you have naturally thin skin or any skin disorder such as rosacea, psoriasis, or seborrhea.

YOU STILL NEED SUNSCREEN

There is no way around it: Even if you are battling blemishes, you still need to minimize sun damage by using an effective sunscreen. In fact, it's especially important because, as part of that battle, you should be exfoliating the skin, which can make it more susceptible to the sun's rays.

Unfortunately, the last thing someone with oily skin needs is another product on her skin. Most sunscreens, even those that claim to be oil-free, contain ingredients that can cause blemish flare-ups. The few sunscreens that are indeed lighter in weight tend to be alcohol-based, posing new problems because alcohol can be an irritant. Plus the sunscreen ingredients themselves can cause breakouts, particularly the so-called "nonchemical" sunscreens, which contain titanium dioxide or zinc oxide. Even though titanium dioxide and zinc oxide are superior sunscreen agents, doing their work with little to no risk of irritation, they are occlusive and can clog pores. Other types of synthetic sunscreen ingredients can cause irritation and also result in breakouts. So you're between a rock and a hard place. Yet you still need sunscreen. In my opinion, the best option in this situation is to wear a foundation with a reliable SPF (preferably SPF 15) that uses either avobenzone, titanium dioxide, or zinc oxide as one of the active ingredients. Finding a foundation with sunscreen that contains avobenzone is difficult because it is rarely used in makeup. That's because of the risk of eye irritation should a person apply the foundation around the eyes or on the eyelid (a practice many engage in, and rightly so). So you'll mostly find foundations with titanium dioxide as the active ingredient, and these are worth experimenting with to see how your blemishes respond. Many people with acne find that titanium dioxide in foundations with sunscreen is not a problem.

More good news: a foundation that contains sunscreen is less of a problem than moisturizers when it comes to causing breakouts, regardless of the ingredients. Foundations are designed to stay on top of the skin, rather than be absorbed. Additionally, going for this option means using one product instead of two, if you were going to wear a foundation anyway. The fewer products you put on your skin, the better, and this is doubly true for someone afflicted with breakouts or oily skin. And please, if you do choose to wear a foundation that contains sunscreen, don't forget that the other parts of your body that are exposed to sun during the day need sunscreen, too.

The bottom line: It takes experimentation and diligence to find a comfortable sunscreen for any skin type, but even more so for someone with oily skin and a tendency toward breakouts.

CHAPTER 16
SOLUTIONS FOR BLACKHEADS

THE BASICS

TWICE A DAY: Gentle cleanser

Recommended cleansers: Clean & Clear Foaming Facial Cleanser, Sensitive Skin; Neutrogena One Step Gentle Cleanser; Jan Marini Bioglycolic Bioclean; Paula's Choice One Step Face Cleanser for Normal to Oily/Combination Skin; Paula's Choice Skin Balancing Cleanser.

NIGHTTIME: Makeup remover

Recommended makeup removers*: Mary Kay Oil-Free Eye Makeup Remover; Nivea Visage Eye Makeup Remover; Paula's Choice Gentle Touch Makeup Remover; DHC Eye Makeup Remover; Sephora FACE Waterproof Eye Makeup Remover.

TWICE A DAY: Toner loaded with antioxidants, skin-identical ingredients, and cell-communicating ingredients

Recommended toners: MD Formulations Moisture Defense Antioxidant Spray; Paula's Choice Moisture Healthy Skin Refreshing Toner; Paula's Choice Skin Balancing Toner; Clinique Mild Clarifying Lotion.

ONCE OR TWICE A DAY: Exfoliate with a BHA (salicylic acid) gel or liquid that does not contain irritating ingredients such as alcohol or menthol

Recommended BHA exfoliants: Paula's Choice 1% Beta Hydroxy Acid Gel; Paula's Choice 2% Beta Hydroxy Acid Gel; Paula's Choice 2% Beta Hydroxy Acid Liquid; Neutrogena Oil-Free Acne Stress Control 3-in-1 Hydrating Acne Treatment; Bare Escentuals bareVitamins Skin Rev-er Upper; Cosmedicine Speedy Recovery Acne Treatment Daytime Blemish Lotion SPF 15.

ONCE OR TWICE A DAY: Use a retinoid, (either Differen, Retin-A, Renova, Tazorac, Avita, Aberela, Atralin, among others, or their generic versions)

DAYTIME: Sunscreen in foundation or pressed powder to reduce the number of products applied to skin

Recommended foundations with sunscreen: Boots No7 Stay Perfect Foundation SPF 15; L'Oreal True Match Super-Blendable Makeup SPF 17; Revlon ColorStay Active Light Makeup SPF 25; Shiseido Sun Protection Liquid Foundation SPF 42; Paula's Choice Best Face Forward Foundation SPF 15.

Recommended pressed powders with sunscreen: Chanel Purete Mat Shine Control Powder SPF 15; Avon Anew Beauty Age-Transforming Pressed Powder SPF 15; Prescriptives Flawless Skin Total Protection Powder SPF 15; Shiseido Pureness Matifying Compact Oil-Free SPF 16; Paula's Choice Healthy Finish Pressed Powder SPF 15.

NIGHTTIME: Over dry areas such as the eye, cheeks, or forehead, use a moisturizer in gel or lotion form with antioxidants, cell-communicating ingredients, and skin-identical ingredients

Recommended moisturizers: Clinique Super Rescue Antioxidant Night Moisturizer, for Combination Oily to Oily Skin; MD Formulations Moisture Defense Antioxidant Hydrating Gel; Prescriptives Super Line Preventor Extreme; Paula's Choice Skin Balancing Moisture Gel; Paula's Choice HydraLight Moisture-Infusing Lotion.

Note: For specific product choices for your skin type from my product line please visit www.paulaschoice.com; for products for your skin type from other product lines please visit www.Beautypedia.com.

STRUGGLING WITH BLACKHEADS AND LARGE PORES

In general, the process for dealing with blackheads and large pores is fairly similar to the way you deal with blemish-prone skin, although if pimples aren't present you don't need the topical antibiotics and antibacterial agents. Bacteria are not involved in the formation of blackheads.

I understand the frustration of battling blackheads. Insidious and glaring, blackheads make skin look mottled and unclean. The truth about blackheads (which are usually accompanied by oily skin) and whiteheads (usually accompanied by dry skin) is hard to accept. What is the truth? The truth is they are just hard to get rid of. It is hard to win the battle against clogged pores! However, because there are only a handful of options for dealing with this annoying skin malady, it's relatively simple to explain.

Pores that are functioning normally produce a normal amount of sebum (oil) and easily distribute the oil to the surface of skin. Hormones, almost exclusively, regulate the amount of sebum production. When a normal amount of oil is produced it moves effortlessly through the pore and out onto the surface of skin, where it melts into an imperceptible film that forms a protective barrier over the face.

Hormones can cause too much oil to be produced, or skin cells can block the exit path of the oil, or, when you have pores that are malformed, the oil in the pore can get clogged and then blackheads or whiteheads form. Further exacerbating these conditions is the buildup in the pore of skin-care or makeup products—mixed in with skin cells, these can get trapped in the sticky sebum sitting in the pore. When sebum and skin cells sit in a pore that is not covered over by skin, they are exposed to air, which causes the sebum and skin cells to oxidize and turn black. If the sebum and skin cells are sitting in a pore that is covered by skin, they are not exposed to air and remain clear, forming a slight white bump under the skin.

What's behind all this is primarily a genetic predisposition accompanied by the right conditions (mentioned above) randomly occurring in any one of the thousands of pores we have on our face. Not to mention unknown reactions to the over 50,000 cosmetic ingredients we may come in contact with from products we use.

Other than avoiding products that are too emollient (meaning thick or greasy creams), not using moisturizers when you don't need them, and not using drying or irritating products, the basic skin-care needs for dealing with whiteheads and blackheads are:

Gentle, water-soluble cleansers (and avoiding bar soap). The ingredients that keep bar soap in its bar form can clog pores, and irritation can cause skin cells to flake off before they're ready and accumulate in the pore. It's actually getting harder and harder to find a cleanser that isn't gentle. But be careful of cleansers that are too emollient and leave a greasy film on the skin, which can cause further problems.

Use salicylic acid in a gel or liquid with no extraneous irritating ingredients to exfoliate skin. Gently exfoliating skin can both remove the excess skin cells on the surface of the face (so they don't build up in the pore), and exfoliate inside the pore (to improve the shape of the pore, allowing a more even flow of oil through it). Keep in mind that the inside structure of the pore itself is lined with skin cells that can build up, creating a narrowed shape that doesn't allow natural oil flow. But don't get carried away with this step. Removing too many skin cells (overdoing it) can cause problems and hurt skin. Exfoliation is essential for both dry and oily skin when you are trying to eliminate blackheads or whiteheads. The only difference is that someone with dry skin will want an exfoliant that has a more moisturizing base. The best option for exfoliating skin both within the pore and on the surface of the skin is a salicylic acid (beta hydroxy acid—BHA) lotion, gel, or liquid. Salicylic acid can penetrate the pore to help improve the shape of the pore lining, allowing an unobstructed path of oil flow.

Absorbing excess oil. This step is more for those with oily skin. It's really not an option for those with whiteheads (milia) and dry skin, because with milia the problem has less to do with excess oil, and more to do with oil trapped in the pore. Clay masks are an option as long as they don't contain other ingredients that are irritating. Cosmetics companies also offer a handful of silicone-based oil-absorbing products meant to be worn under makeup; these get mixed reviews from women but are worth a trial run. A few of my personal favorites are OC Eight Professional Mattifying Gel, Clinique Pore Minimizer Instant Pefector, and Smashbox Anti-Shine or Compact Anti-Shine.

Improving cell production can help the pore function more normally. Effective products to consider for all skin types are the tretinoins (Retin-A, Tazorac, Avita, Renova), as well as Differin. These can be used by themselves or with a BHA product. Research has definitely established that Retin-A, Renova, and Differin have positive effects on the way pores function, and these products should be considered for very stubborn cases or when blackheads are accompanied by breakouts.

For those with oily-skin troubles, certain low-dose birth-control pills may be an option to reduce the hormone levels that create the excess oil that is at the root of the problem. And, when all else fails, Accutane can be considered. Be aware that many doctors are reluctant to prescribe Accutane for "merely" oily skin and blackheads.

Blackheads can be made to seem less noticeable with pore strips, but only when the instructions on the box are followed exactly and they are not overused. Pore strips do not affect pore function.

Facialists and aestheticians can extract blackheads without damaging skin, which is a helpful service when they know what they are doing.

For all skin types, AHA or BHA peels, microdermabrasion, and laser resurfacing can improve the appearance of blackheads and whiteheads; however, they don't necessarily improve pore functioning (which depends on the depth of the treatment); rather, they temporarily get rid of the surface problem, making your skin look better.

EMPTY, ENLARGED PORES?

Once a pore is emptied and the unsightly blackhead is removed, it can take a period of time for the pore to heal and close up. Maintaining the regimen of gentle cleansing, exfoliating, and absorbing oil can go a long way toward making this happen. If your skin can tolerate Retin-A, Renova, or Differin, these products can help promote healing by further improving cell production in the pore. However, even after all this, an empty, open, but permanently damaged pore can be an unattractive, leftover by-product of the original problem. If you have patiently adhered to all the "right" steps, there is very little else that can be done to change the damage. Time will tell if the effects of improving pore function can shrink a pore, but it does take time, and not everyone will have the same results. Microdermabrasion, AHA or BHA peels, and laser resurfacing can improve the appearance of pores, but these are considered temporary fixes and are not noted for actually changing or correcting the problem. Most likely the improvement is caused by the skin's swelling which makes the pores look smaller. Again, it is hard to determine success rates because no published results from long-term studies are available.

The struggle to cover up large pores is nothing less than maddening. The very nature of a depression in the skin makes it difficult, if not impossible, to keep the indentation from showing. Especially if your skin is still oily, and even if you use an extremely matte foundation, such as Revlon's regular ColorStay, Lancome's Teint Idole, or Estee Lauder's Double Wear, the oil can still cause some shifting, creating a look of pooled foundation in the pore.

I apologize for sounding dismal about this, but when there are limitations in the skin and in the world of makeup, searching for better options or alternatives can waste money and only increase your frustration. Here is a game plan to tackle the problem. It isn't foolproof and it won't work for everyone, but these are the best options available.

1. Avoid moisturizer over the open-pore areas of the face before applying makeup—even if you have dry skin. Any extra "slip" on the skin will cause makeup to pool in the pore. If the skin is dry and flaky, be more diligent in the evening about treating your skin. Then in the morning use a toner with skin-identical ingredients and anti-irritants to help soothe skin and reduce any dry feeling, yet not add anything that can make skin feel slippery. That means it is essential that your foundation contain your sunscreen, because an additional sunscreen under the foundation will almost certainly cause slippage.

2. Do use a matte or ultra-matte foundation. Even if you have dry skin, these stay on far better than other foundations, are somewhat impervious to oil production, and, therefore, prevent the foundation from slipping into the pore.

3. Consider wearing a tiny amount of milk of magnesia under your foundation over the open-pore area. This is a bit like applying spackle that has minimal to no movement. It can absorb oil at the same time and the foundation glides over it, creating an even surface. This works better under matte foundations than under ultra-matte foundations. You may also want to consider any of the oil-absorbing products mentioned in the "Struggling With Blackheads and Large Pores" section above.

4. For more stubborn problems, touch up your makeup several times during the day with oil-blotting papers. Then dust the face with a pressed powder designed to be worn as a foundation. Pressed powder foundations apply a slightly thicker layer of powder than normal pressed powders do, and can better hide the pore. But do this only with a brush; never use a sponge or pad to apply powder because they can place way too much product on the face, making things look cakey and thick.

CHAPTER 17
SOLUTIONS FOR ROSACEA

THE BASICS

Note: Please be aware that even with careful consideration and adherence to usage guidelines I cannot guarantee that the products recommended below will not cause problems for your rosacea-affected skin. Rosacea is a frustrating disorder that can cause skin to flare with little or no provocation, even from the most benign cosmetic ingredients.

TWICE A DAY: Gentle cleanser (irritating and drying products hurt the skin's ability to heal, stimulate oil production, and increase acne-causing bacteria in the skin)
  Recommended cleansers: CeraVe Hydrating Cleanser; Cetaphil Gentle Skin Cleanser; Clinique Liquid Facial Soap Extra Mild; Eucerin Redness Relief Soothing Cleanser; Paula's Choice Skin Recovery Cleanser for Normal to Very Dry Skin; Paula's Choice One Step Face Cleanser for Normal to Oily/Combination Skin.

NIGHTTIME: Makeup remover
  Recommended makeup removers: Neutrogena Oil-Free Eye Makeup Remover; Bobbi Brown Instant Long-Wear Makeup Remover; Clinique Take the Day Off Makeup Remover for Lids, Lashes, and Lips; Paula's Choice Gentle Touch Makeup Remover.

TWICE A DAY: Toner that includes antioxidants, skin-identical ingredients, and cell-communicating ingredients
  Recommended toners: Estee Lauder Verite Soothing Spray Toner; Bioelements Calmitude Hydrating Solution; Paula's Choice Moisture Boost Hydrating Toner; Paula's Choice Healthy Skin Refreshing Toner; Paula's Choice Skin Recovery Toner.

ONCE A DAY: Exfoliate with a BHA (salicylic acid) gel or liquid that does not contain irritating ingredients such as alcohol or menthol
  Recommended exfoliants: Clinique Mild Clarifying Lotion; Serious Skin Care Clarify Acne Medication Clarifying Treatment; Paula's Choice 1% Beta Hydroxy Acid Lotion; Paula's Choice 1% Beta Hydroxy Acid Gel.

ONCE OR TWICE DAY: Use a prescription antimicrobial gel, liquid, or serum, or azelaic acid

DAYTIME: Sunscreen in a foundation to reduce the number of products applied to skin
  Recommended foundations: L'Oreal True Match Super-Blendable Makeup; Maybelline New York Instant Age Rewind Custom Face Perfector Cream Compact Foundation SPF 18; Illuminare Ultimate All Day Foundation/Concealer Matte Finish Sunscreen Makeup SPF 21; Chanel Mat Lumiere Long Lasting Soft Matte Makeup SPF 15; Paula's Choice All Bases Covered Foundation SPF 15; Paula's Choice Barely There Sheer Matte Tint SPF 20.

NIGHTTIME: Over dry areas such as the eye, cheeks, or forehead, use a moisturizer in gel or lotion form with antioxidants, cell-communicating ingredients, and skin-identical ingredients

  Recommended moisturizers: Good Skin All Calm Moisture Lotion; Osmotics TriCeram; MD Formulations Moisture Defense Antioxidant Hydrating Gel; Clinique Super Rescue Antioxidant Night Moisturizer (three versions available depending on skin type); Paula's Choice Skin Recovery Moisturizer; Paula's Choice HydraLight Moisture-Infusing Lotion.

Note: For specific product choices for your skin type from my product line please visit www.paulaschoice.com; for products for your skin type from other product lines please visit www.beautypedia.com.

ANOTHER PROBLEM

As if the issues surrounding skin type (normal, oily, sun-damaged, blemish-prone), skin sensitivities, and allergic reactions weren't enough, a large percentage of the population deals with various strange medical conditions that primarily show up on the face adding to their skin-care concerns. These problems make selecting the appropriate skin-care routine extremely tricky. It becomes a challenge to find the right combination of products that will benefit the skin and not make matters worse. The most common skin disorders of the face are rosacea, eczema, psoriasis, and seborrhea.

Early identification goes a long way toward reducing the symptoms of these skin afflictions because it can help sufferers avoid buying products that are likely to exacerbate the condition. Except for eczema, these skin disorders require a dermatologist's care; they cannot be treated at the cosmetics counter or with over-the-counter products from the drugstore. Finding the right skin-care and makeup routines, and the products that work with each of these conditions is very important because products that contain problematic, irritating, or drying ingredients will absolutely make matters worse and can undo some of the benefits the medical treatments provide.

The National Rosacea Society, at www.rosacea.org, is an excellent source (though it does have paid advertisers) for detailed and ongoing information concerning treatment and research for rosacea.

ROSACEA

Rosacea is no fun. It is a stubborn skin disorder that is frustrating and extremely difficult to treat. Thought to afflict at least 30% to 50% of the Caucasian population, it is frequently misdiagnosed by dermatologists and physicians. Rosacea develops over a long period of time, starting with what at first seems like a tendency to blush easily, a ruddy complexion, or an extreme sensitivity to cosmetics. The distinctive redness or flushing, which appears in a characteristic butterfly pattern over the nose and cheeks, is likely to be the first indication that rosacea may be what your skin is struggling with. Though bothersome, the subtle initial redness is often ignored by women as being just a skin-tone or color problem and not a skin disorder.

Another challenge with identifying rosacea is that pustules (pimples) and papules (red raised bumps) that resemble acne are often present. That makes rosacea look like acne and that means it's often misdiagnosed. But, unlike most acne conditions, rosacea is rarely, if ever, accompanied by blackheads. The distinctive flushing and extreme skin sensitivity also differentiate rosacea from acne. The final toll on the face is the presence of flaky patches that may or may not be accompanied by either dry or oily skin, or possibly by both at the same time.

Rosacea can be extremely confusing for a woman because the dry, flaky skin responds minimally or not at all to moisturizers and the acnelike bumps and whiteheads respond minimally, or not at all, to typical acne treatments. Adding to the elusive nature of this disorder the skin is its extreme reactivity to outside influences. Flare-ups can be caused by sun exposure, heat, stress, sweating, exercise, and friction.

For men it can create a bulbous nose, typified by redness, lumpy swollen areas, and noticeable veining, called rhinophyma, as well as puffy cheeks (rhinophyma rarely occurs in women). In the past, the occurrence of rhinophyma was wrongly thought to be caused by drinking too much alcohol, but no amount of alcohol can change the appearance of the nose in this manner. (Sources: *Annals of Plastic Surgery*, July 2008, pages 114–120; and *Journal of Otolaryngology Head and Neck Surgery*, April 2008, pages 269–272.)

Even more confounding, when rosacea first develops it may appear, disappear, and then reappear a short time later. This fluctuation also makes diagnosis difficult. Yet, despite its evasive beginnings, the condition rarely reverses itself (meaning there is no cure), and it almost always becomes worse without treatment.

As rosacea progresses and changes, what usually happens over time is that the affected areas of the face don't return to their normal color and stay persistently red. Other symptoms, such as enlarged, surfaced blood vessels (called telangiectasia) start appearing; flaky patches, oily skin, increased skin sensitivity, and breakouts can become more visible, too.

TYPES OF ROSACEA

The National Rosacea Society Expert Committee on the Classification and Staging of Rosacea identified four types of rosacea (Source: *Journal of the American Academy of Dermatology*, April 2002, pages 584–587):

Papulopustular: Papules and pustules are often seen, with persistent facial redness and some swelling.

Phymatous: Thickening of the skin occurs with enlarged pores and surface nodules, and often rhinophyma is present.

Erythematotelangiectatic: Flushing and persistent redness is present with visible blood vessels (telangiectasias), along with swelling, stinging, and burning along the cheeks, chin, and forehead. The skin can also be dry.

Ocular: The white part of the eye (sclera) has a persistent sensation of burning, grittiness, dryness, and a feeling that something is in the eye, with visible blood vessels. Often sties, blepharitis (inflammation of the eyelid), and conjunctivitis (pink eye) are present and recurring. Most eye makeup increases this irritation to the point where it becomes very uncomfortable.

WHAT CAUSES ROSACEA?

Surprisingly, no one really knows what causes rosacea, but theories do exist and there those who champion one over the other. UV light is thought to be a culprit for causing rosacea. A genetic propensity for producing capillaries (angiogenesis) is another. There is also research suggesting that the vitamin D3 pathway may be deficient, creating an environment where rosacea symptoms can manifest more easily.

(Sources: *Experimental Dermatology*, August 2008, pages 633–699; *Cosmetic Dermatology*, April 2008, pages 224–232; *Archives of Dermatological Research*, March 2008, pages 125–131; and *Journal of Dermatological Treatment*, 2007, volume 18, issue 6, pages 326–328.)

One of the more popular theories being debated is whether the presence of a mite called *Demodex folliculorum* that is present in skin is responsible for the inflammatory aspect of rosacea. There is some evidence that this mite, which thrives on a large percentage of people, especially older people, is more prevalent in those with rosacea. But the research is hardly conclusive. (Sources: *British Journal of Dermatology*, September 2007, pages 474–481; *Cutis*, September 2004, pages S9–S12; and *Acta Dermato-Venereologica*, January 2002, pages 3–6.)

Other research indicates that unidentified and unknown microbes are creating the inflammatory response and other symptoms seen in rosacea. But whether it is an unknown microbe under the skin or the *Demodex folliculorum* mite, research shows that the active ingredient metronidazole may work to control the situation. Since it can kill both the mite and other microbes, you would be covering both issues with one medication. (Sources: *Journal of Drugs in Dermatology*, May 2007, pages 495–498; and *Advances in Therapy*, September–October 2001, pages 237–243.)

Despite the fact that a clear understanding of why rosacea happens is lacking, many cosmetics companies want you to believe their skin-care products can control different aspects of the disorder, especially with respect to the mite mentioned above. But there is no research showing that over-the-counter products control any aspect of rosacea other than mitigating redness and inflammation and not making it worse.

What this all adds up to is that no one answer is right or wrong. We simply don't know what is actually taking place, although it seems to be a complex interplay between physiological events taking place in the skin and how it responds to external influences. What is certain, regardless of the cause, is that if they are left untreated, rosacea symptoms will increase, resulting in chronic redness, swelling, breakouts, surfaced capillaries, and/or flaking skin.

ROSACEA OR ACNE?

For years rosacea was referred to as "acne rosacea." That only added to the confusion, because rosacea is not acne. Yet because the papules and pustules that can accompany rosacea look like acne, many doctors misdiagnose it and end up prescribing medications that make matters worse instead of better. The right medication is crucial for relieving the cause of the disorder. You and your doctor need to know exactly what you are dealing with to be sure you are receiving the right treatment. Understanding the difference between acne and acne rosacea can make a huge difference in the health of your skin.

ROSACEA CAN AFFECT THE EYES

Ocular rosacea refers to a condition where rosacea affects the eye and, according to an item in the March 2001 issue of *Cosmetic Dermatology*, it is significantly underdiagnosed and untreated. They note that "an estimated 13 million U.S. adults [with rosacea],... indicated they also experienced discomfort or redness of the eyes in varying degrees." Those with ocular rosacea most commonly experience irritation of the lids and eye, as well as sties and chronically red eyes. In rare cases, ocular rosacea can also affect the cornea. This condition can be treated, usually with soothing eye drops (but not Visine), along with oral or topical antibiotics, but it requires a dermatologic evaluation before any action is taken.

SOLUTIONS FOR ROSACEA

Rosacea is much like any other pervasive skin disorder, from breakouts to eczema, because there are no easy answers. Cosmetics companies looking for your money have a penchant for claiming that their line has the answer to your problems, yet these products—such as exfoliants, anti-irritants, antifungal ingredients, antioxidants, and so on—often have no relation to the needs of someone struggling with rosacea. But for most women looking for the magic bullet the hope that the next product can make a difference is just too tempting. In reality, even well-formulated products, meaning primarily those that are free of topical skin irritants, can be a problem for rosacea.

So where do you begin when you're dealing with rosacea? Because rosacea is so often misdiagnosed, the place to start is with a dermatologist who has experience with this disorder. Next come skin-care considerations, to be sure the products you are using aren't making matters worse, and then lifestyle considerations, because what you do can trigger flare-ups. As is true for all skin types and skin disorders, it takes experimenting to find what works for you. What is crucial for everyone but especially for those with rosacea is to follow the skin-care basics of being gentle in every part of their routine. Finally, using leave-on products that are loaded with antioxidants, skin-identical ingredients, and cell-communicating ingredients to normalize the skin as much as possible is the best place to start.

GENTLE SKIN-CARE PRODUCTS

Redness, irritation, and skin sensitivities are part and parcel of rosacea. Anything that exacerbates inflammation in the skin will cause more problems. Gentle cleansers, a soothing toner with anti-irritants, plus application of antioxidants, skin-identical ingredients, and cell-communicating ingredients in a lightweight base at night, and a sunscreen during the day are the basics.

The National Rosacea Society (www.rosacea.org) surveyed 1,000 of its members who identified alcohol, witch hazel, fragrance, menthol, peppermint, and eucalyptus as contributing to flare-ups. It isn't always easy to identify those substances on a label when they are listed under their chemical or Latin names, as the FDA requires for ingredient labels. Moreover, there are many fragrant components and lots of other potentially irritating skin-care ingredients in many products. Even if you've been diligent in checking your products, you can still run into problems because it is often hard to determine what is causing your own specific flare-ups. Yet as difficult as it is to pinpoint exactly what ingredients may trigger rosacea, the ones listed in Chapter Six, *Skin's Enemy: Irritation and Inflammation*, as being problematic for irritation give you a good idea about what to avoid. Keep in mind that not everyone responds the same way to any of these ingredients. But avoiding these as much as possible will, at the very least, start you in the right direction to reduce the redness and dry flaky skin. (Sources: *Cosmetic Dermatology*, July 2008, pages 383–386; *Dermatologic Therapy*, 2004, volume 17, pages S26–S34; and *Cutis*, December 2001, pages S12–S19.)

SALICYLIC ACID

I feel strongly that anecdotal information is correct when it points to the benefits of using a gentle toner or moisturizer that contains 1% to 2% salicylic acid (BHA) in a base with a pH of 3 to 4 for rosacea as well as other skin types. Salicylic acid is an exfoliant that helps to remove the built-up layers of dry, flaky skin on the face caused by sun damage or skin disorders Further, because salicylic acid is related to aspirin (both are salicylates), it can also have anti-inflammatory properties on the skin, reducing redness and swelling. There are those on the Internet who disagree with my conclusion about this, but supportive research is lacking in either direction. For that reason, because it takes experimenting to find out what works, I encourage you to give this step a try.

ANTIOXIDANTS

Rosacea is a common, chronic, light-sensitive, inflammatory skin disease of unknown origin. Some research has shown that higher peroxide levels (a measure of free-radical damage), and lower levels of antioxidants in skin may trigger rosacea or at the very least make it worse. Using products that restore antioxidants to the skin, along with barrier-repair ingredients (skin-identical ingredients) as explained in Chapter Six, *Skin's Enemy: Irritation and Inflammation*, can go a long way to help any skin type, including rosacea (Source: *Journal of the American Academy of Dermatology*, November 2008, pages 36-41).

TOPICAL ANTIMICROBIAL TREATMENTS

As stated above, no one really knows what causes rosacea, though one of the possibilities is that the presence of a microbe under the skin causes the symptoms. Killing off the microbe seems to be the most helpful way to improve the appearance of skin and, if caught early enough, keep matters from getting worse. Only a handful of topical prescription treatments exist that can combat the microbe(s) responsible for rosacea. The success of these topical medications, when combined with an oral antibiotic, can be significant. Nevertheless, when you are considering an oral antibiotic you must take into account the risk of microbe resistance taking place after prolonged use (meaning that after period of time the antibiotic will no longer be effective). If that happens, that specific oral antibiotic will no longer be effective to help with other types of infections you may encounter, limiting your options if you get sick.

The most popular topical treatment is metronidazole, under the trade names MetroGel, MetroLotion, or MetroCream. It has been well studied and has shown impressive results. It is particularly effective when paired with an oral antibiotic such as doxycycline. Daily maintenance with topical metronidazole can absolutely decrease relapses and allow for longer intervals between flare-ups.

Another topical option is to use a prescription medication that combines benzoyl peroxide with erythromycin (an antibiotic), the same one that is more typically recommended for those with acne. There is some research showing it can be as or more effective than topical metronidazole. (Sources: *Journal of the American Academy of Dermatology*, January 2007, pages 107–115; *Cutis*, January 2007, pages 73–80; and *Journal of Dermatology*, August 2004, pages 610–617.)

AZELAIC ACID

In December of 2002 the FDA approved azelaic acid as a topical prescription treatment for mild to moderate rosacea. Azelaic acid, in concentrations of either 15% or 20%, is an interesting, versatile ingredient that is prescribed not only for rosacea but also for acne and brown skin discolorations. It can have some irritating side effects similar to an AHA, but they are typically mild and transient. Overall, azelaic acid is considered a very effective and safe therapy for rosacea. On average, twice-daily application of azelaic acid has shown results in reducing the rosacea symptoms of redness, flaking, and papules that are similar to once-daily application when using metronidazole. One study demonstrated that azelaic acid was as effective as metronidazole but was tolerated better by patients. (Sources: *Journal of the European Academy of Dermatology and Venereology*, January 2009, pages 22–28; *International Journal of Dermatology*, May 2007, pages 533–538; and *Cutis*, April 2006, pages S3–S11.)

ORAL ANTIBIOTICS

Oral antibiotics have long been used to successfully treat rosacea, but because there is growing concern about prolonged treatment causing bacterial resistance—both for the individual taking the medication and the population as a whole—it has taken a back seat to other options. Yet oral antibiotics truly make a difference in the appearance of rosacea, and the frustration about what to prescribe has confounded the medical world. In May 2006, the FDA approved doxycycline (Oracea™) as the first oral prescription therapy for the treatment of rosacea. This antibiotic is prescribed at a level where it does not cause bacterial resistance, but can still make a significant improvement in the appearance of rosacea symptoms.

(Sources: *International Journal of Dermatology*, March 2008, pages 284–288; *Journal of Drugs in Dermatology*, January 2006, pages 16–21; *Cutis*, April 2005, pages S19–S24; Skin Therapy Letter, "Oral Therapy for the Treatment of Rosacea," www.skincareguide.com.)

RENOVA OR DIFFERIN

Having to explore and experiment is one of the most troublesome aspects of dealing with rosacea because no single treatment or protocol works for everyone. With that in mind, retinoids can be worth a try even though there isn't much research supporting their use. Both Renova (active ingredient tretinoin) and Differin (adapalene) would be two of the more typical options that can be prescribed. If you decide to go this route, pay attention to the way your skin is reacting, and discontinue use if it becomes more red and irritated than when you started. (Source: *Journal of Drugs in Dermatology*, October 2006, pages 921–922.)

LIFESTYLE CONSIDERATIONS

Several lifestyle factors can make rosacea worse, although these are not the same for everyone because people have different reactions to the same ingredients or external elements. These catalysts can include hot liquids, spicy foods, exposure to extreme temperatures (including cooking over a hot stove), alcohol consumption, sunlight, stress, saunas, hot tubs, smoking, rubbing or massaging the skin, irritating cosmetics, and anything else that overstimulates the skin and blood vessels.

LASERS AND LIGHT-EMITTING DEVICES

One of the more expensive ways to treat a selection of rosacea-related problems is with various lasers, including PDL (pulsed dye laser) or light emitting devices (IPL—Intense Pulsed Light). Lasers and IPLs are most successful at reducing and even possibly eliminating dilated blood vessels, persistent redness, swelling, enlarged pores, and skin thickening. What makes these options expensive is that repeated treatments are needed, and often insurance doesn't cover the cost. The cost of each treatment session can range from $300 to $700, though some clinics offer package deals make individual treatments less expensive. While some people will see dramatic results, that isn't true for everyone, because not everyone gets the same level of improvement or any improvement at all. It is important to keep in mind that none of this is a cure, and that continued success would require using topical and/or oral methods to keep the condition at bay.

(Sources: *British Journal of Dermatology*, September 2008, pages 628–632; *Lasers in Surgery and Medicine*, April 2008, pages 233–299; *Journal of Cosmetic Dermatology*, December 2005, pages 262–266; *Dermatologic Surgery*, October 2005, pages 1285–1289; and *Cutis*, March 2005, pages 22–26.)

CHAPTER 18
SOLUTIONS FOR PSORIASIS

THE BASICS

TWICE A DAY: Gentle cleanser

    Recommended cleansers: CeraVe Hydrating Cleanser; Cetaphil Gentle Skin Cleanser; Clinique Liquid Facial Soap Extra Mild; Eucerin Redness Relief Soothing Cleanser; Paula's Choice Skin Recovery Cleanser for Normal to Very Dry Skin; Paula's Choice One Step Face Cleanser for Normal to Oily/Combination Skin.

TWICE A DAY: Toner with antioxidants, skin-identical identical ingredients, cell-communicating ingredients

    Recommended toners: Pevonia Botanica Sensitive Skin Lotion; MD Formulations Moisture Defense Antioxidant Spray; Paula's Choice Moisture Boost Hydrating Toner; Paula's Choice Healthy Skin Refreshing Toner.

ONCE A DAY: Use a BHA (salicylic acid) lotion, liquid, or gel

    Recommended BHA products: Clinique Mild Clarifying Lotion; Serious Skin Care Clarify Acne Medication Clarifying Treatment; Paula's Choice 1% Beta Hydroxy Acid Lotion; Paula's Choice 1% Beta Hydroxy Acid Gel; Paula's Choice 2% Beta Hydroxy Acid Liquid; Paula's Choice 2% Beta Hydroxy Acid Gel.

ONCE OR TWICE A DAY: A medicated topical cream, lotion, or gel with active ingredients designed for treating psoriasis

DAYTIME: Sunscreen either in foundation or a moisturizer

    Recommended daytime moisturizers with sunscreen: Olay Regenerist Enhancing Lotion with UV Protection SPF 15; Estee Lauder DayWear Plus Multi Protection Anti-Oxidant Lotion SPF 15, for Oily Skin; Neutrogena Age Shield Sunblock SPF 30; Paula's Choice Skin Balancing Daily Mattifying Lotion with SPF 15 & Antioxidants; Paula's Choice Skin Recovery Daily Moisturizing Lotion with SPF 15 & Antioxidants.

    Recommended foundations with sunscreen: L'Oreal True Match Super-Blendable Makeup SPF 17; Maybelline New York Instant Age Rewind Custom Face Perfector Cream Compact Foundation SPF 18; Prescriptives Flawless Skin Total Protection Makeup SPF 15; Paula's Choice All Bases Covered Foundation SPF 15; Paula's Choice Best Face Forward Foundation SPF 15.

NIGHTTIME: Moisturizer with antioxidants, skin-identical identical ingredients, cell-communicating ingredients

    Recommended Moisturizers: Clinique Super Rescue Antioxidant Night Moisturizer (three versions available depending on skin type); SkinMedica Rejuvenative Moisturizer; Paula's Choice Hydrating Treatment Cream; Paula's Choice Skin Balancing Moisture Gel.

THE HEARTBREAK OF PSORIASIS

Though dramatic, the heartbreak of psoriasis was a phrase used for years to describe this chronic skin condition. Psoriasis is identified by the presence of thickened, scaly areas of skin sometimes accompanied by papules (small, solid, often-inflamed bumps that, unlike pimples, do not contain pus or sebum). These bumps are usually slightly elevated above the skin surface, sharply distinguishable from normal skin, and can be red to reddish brown in color. Dotted over the various parts of the face and body, the lesions are usually covered with small whitish silver scales that stick to the cystlike swelling; if scraped off, the skin may bleed. The extent of the disease varies from a few tiny patches to generalized involvement of most of the skin from head to toe. More typically, just the elbows, knees, scalp, and chest are involved.

It is thought that psoriasis affects over 7 million people in the United States alone, but for most people it tends to be mild and aesthetically unappealing rather than a serious health concern, which is probably why fewer than 2 million people seek medical treatment for it (Source: *OTC Journal Newsletter*, October 15, 2001, online at www.otcjournal.com/profiles/astr/20011015-1.html).

WHAT CAUSES PSORIASIS?

What makes psoriasis so frustrating is that no one knows for certain exactly what causes the problem, although recent studies suggest it may be related to an immune system problem. Referred to as an immune-mediated disorder, it triggers inflammation and sets off a trigger that causes the skin to make too many cells at breakneck speed. Many feel this theory holds the most water because immunosuppressant medications can reduce or eliminate psoriatic lesions.

Psoriasis is the recurring, persistent growth of too many skin cells that are not able to shed properly, accompanied by red, oozing patches of skin. A normal skin cell matures in 28 to 45 days, while a psoriatic skin cell takes only 3 to 6 days. Both men and women can get psoriasis at any age, so it isn't unusual to start noticing red, swollen, flaky bumps on your skin late in life. (Source: *British Journal of Nursing*, March 2008, pages 284– 290.)

What's particularly confounding to those with psoriasis is the randomness of the disorder. For no rhyme or reason lesions come and go, severity is arbitrary, and duration is anyone's guess. Stress, skin irritation, injury, and health problems such as flus and viruses have been reported to precede a recurrence. Climate may also play a factor, with dry, cold weather triggering recurrences and sunny warm weather improving it or even causing remission. Too much alcohol, smoking, and obesity may also play a role but no one is sure why.

TYPES OF PSORIASIS

Psoriasis appears in several forms. The scaly, papule kind called plaque psoriasis is the most common. Other forms include guttate psoriasis, typified by small, dotlike lesions all over the body; pustular psoriasis, with weeping lesions and intense scaling; and erythrodermic psoriasis, characterized by severe sloughing and inflammation of the skin. Psoriasis can range from mild to moderate to severe and disabling.

Sadly, there is no cure for psoriasis, but there are many different treatments, both topical and systemic, that can be added to your skin-care routine to obtain optimal results. Experimenting with a variety of options is essential to find the treatment that works for you, but all of them require a doctor's attention.

NAIL PSORIASIS

Even though flaky, red lesions on the surface of skin are the most obvious manifestations of psoriasis, over 50% of the time the nails can also be affected. Manifesting in a variety of ways, psoriasis of the nails can include pitting, lifting of the nail away from the nail bed, white discolorations, and ridges. Although there have been important advances in the treatment of psoriasis as it pertains to the skin, options for dealing with the way it affects the nail are barely researched. While a number of treatment alternatives currently exist for nail disease, the general gross lack of clear evidence regarding these choices often makes it difficult to select the most efficient, safe, and optimal treatments. Even though the current literature has shown some support for the use of topical, oral, and combination therapies for nail psoriasis, the available results aren't sufficient to make one regimen stand out. That means experimenting is the way to go and find what works for you. (Source: *Journal of the American Academy of Dermatology*, July 2007, pages 1–27.)

SKIN CARE

As with all skin types, treating the skin gently and not using skin-care products containing irritants that cause inflammation is extremely important. It is even more important for those with psoriasis; because this skin condition is an inflammatory condition, reducing inflammation becomes even more critical. Gentle cleansers, products that help soothe skin, not scrubbing the skin, and avoiding anything that dries the skin and disrupts the skin's barrier are essential as a starting point. Protecting the skin's barrier with emollients, antioxidants, skin-identical ingredients, and cell-communicating ingredients (retinol) can allow skin to heal and help maintain the natural defense healthy skin can provide. In essence you need to follow the skin-care routine for your skin type in terms of dryness or oiliness as recommended in this book. Following those steps will help you create a healthy starting point for the other medications your doctor may select for you.

As a rule, the best place to start is with treatments that pose the least risk and have the least side effects. Topical prescription creams and lotions are the preferred way to begin as they generally are the most benign and can be extremely helpful. If that treatment doesn't work the next step would be sun exposure or exposure to sun lamps. Due to its immune-suppressing and skin cell-damaging effects, ultraviolet radiation can control psoriasis. If that fails, oral medications or injections are the final approach. A curve ball in treatment is that the body can become resistant to the medications and lesions can start showing up again after a long period of remission, requiring a new round of experimenting to find what works.

TRIAL AND ERROR

The options for treatment are complex and varied. It is a grab bag of choices, each offering their own pros and cons with varying degrees of success based on each individual's experience. And new drugs are being researched and added to the list of options all the time. For example, three new drugs were approved by the FDA in 2008 (Taclonex Scalp, the Xtrac Velocity light-emitting device, and an oral medication called Humira with the active ingredient being adalimumab).

Of the various therapies available to treat psoriasis, it is generally best to start with those that have the least-serious side effects, such as topical steroids (cortisone creams), coal-tar creams or shampoos, or sulfur-based creams and shampoos, along with careful exposure to sunshine. If those methods are not successful, you can proceed to the more serious treatments involving oral medications. More often than not, successful treatment requires a combination of methods.

All of the treatments, both topical and oral, are often used in varying combinations for the best results. Frequently, several combination treatments are used in rotation to reduce the potentially harmful side effects of each one or the decrease in or lack of effectiveness.

Discovering whether any of these will work for you, alone or in combination, takes patience and a systematic, ongoing review and evaluation of how your skin and health are doing. Successful treatment, as is true with all chronic skin disorders, requires diligent adherence to the regimen and a realistic understanding of what you can and can't expect.

It is also important to be aware of the consequences of the varying treatment levels. For example, continued long-term use of topical cortisone creams can cause skin thinning, stretch marks, and built-up resistance to the cortisone medication itself, so that it actually becomes an ineffective treatment. Exposure to sunlight without adequate protection (particularly from UVA radiation) can cause skin cancer. Oral steroids can have serious withdrawal effects, including increased bouts of psoriasis. Accutane causes birth defects if a woman becomes pregnant while taking it. Several systemic psoriatic treatments can cause liver problems, nausea, and severe irritation. Each option has its own set of pros and cons that need to be researched and discussed at length with your physician.

For more information on the current status of available treatment, visit the Web site for the National Psoriasis Foundation (NPF) at www.psoriasis.org/.

THE SUN

Natural sunlight can significantly improve, or even clear, psoriasis. Ultraviolet (UV) light from the sun suppresses the skin's immune response and damages the production of skin cells, slowing their overproduction and reducing scaling. Daily, short, nonburning exposure to sunlight clears or improves psoriasis in many people. Therefore, sunlight may be included among initial treatments for the disease (Source: National Institutes of Health, Department of Health and Human Services, *Questions and Answers about Psoriasis*, January 2002, online at www.niams.nih.gov/hi/topics/psoriasis/psoriafs.htm).

Regular daily doses of sunlight, taken in short exposures with adequate sun protection, are strongly recommended. Sun protection is vital not only to prevent sunburn, which may make psoriasis worse, but also to reduce skin damage from the sun's UV radiation. This outdoor approach to treating psoriasis is often referred to as climatotherapy or phototherapy. Some people travel to Florida, Hawaii, the Caribbean, or the Dead Sea in Israel (where special clinics offer treatment solariums and supervised medical assistance) to use swimming in sulfur or mineral baths along with natural sunlight. In some countries, medical plans actually cover trips to these types of sunny climates and mineral spas for subscribers with psoriasis.

When you can't get to sunshine, medically supervised administration of light via UVB lamps may be used to minimize widespread or localized areas of stubborn and unmanageable psoriasis lesions. UVB light is also used when topical treatments have failed, or in combination with topical treatments. The short-term risks of using controlled UVB exposure to treat psoriasis are minimal, and long-term studies of large numbers of patients treated with UVB have not demonstrated an increased risk of skin cancer, suggesting that this treatment may be safer than sunlight. (Sunlight has both UVA and UVB radiation; UVA causes skin cancer, while UVB mainly triggers sunburn.) UVB treatments are considered one of the most effective therapies for moderate to severe psoriasis, with the least amount of risk. There are even sources of UVB light therapy, called narrow-band UVB, that give off only the part of the UV spectrum band that is most helpful for psoriasis and that reduce the risk of wide-band UVB light.

PRESCRIPTION ONLY TREATMENTS FOR PSORIASIS

COAL TAR

Coal tar is a very old and very effective remedy with a great deal of research showing its success for many forms of psoriasis. Coal tar is a topical medication available both over the counter and by prescription; the difference between the two options is in the potency and amount of coal tar the medication contains. Coal tar inhibits certain skin substances that trigger cell proliferation, thus reducing the appearance of psoriasis. Enhanced benefit can be seen when coal tar is combined with UV light exposure. Referred to as the Goeckerman regimen, it involves the dermal application of a crude coal tar (polycyclic aromatic hydrocarbon) and exposure to ultraviolet radiation. Coal tar can be combined with other psoriasis medications like topical steroids. (Source: *International Journal of Dermatology*, August 2008, pages 800–805.)

Because coal tar can make the skin more sensitive to UV light, extreme caution is advised when you combine coal tar use with UV therapy (or exposure to the sun) to avoid getting a severe burn or causing significant skin damage. Other downsides to coal tar are the irritation it can cause, the unpleasant smell, and its tendency to stain clothes.

ANTHRALIN

Much like coal tar, anthralin (also called dithranol) is a topical prescription medication that has been used to treat psoriasis for decades. Though anthralin's action on skin is not clear, it appears to inhibit cell proliferation. It has few serious side effects but can irritate or burn the normal-appearing skin surrounding psoriatic lesions. Anthralin also stains anything it comes into contact with. It is prescribed in a range of concentrations, but the most effective form is a hard paste that is very difficult to apply, requiring a great deal of patience; also, it can't be used over inflamed lesions, and must not get on the face. There are a variety of regimens for its use, but the negative side effects and cumbersome and time-consuming application process often make it a less-than-desirable option.

VITAMIN D3

Calcipotriol, which also goes by the name calcipotriene, is a form of vitamin D3 that has a good deal of published research about its pharmacology, efficacy, tolerability, and use in treating psoriasis. In cream or ointment form (trade name Daivonex/Dovonex), calcipotriol by itself is as effective as other therapies such as betamethasone valerate cream or coal tar. It is used twice a day. (Sources: *Journal of Dermatologic Treatment*, June 2006, pages 327–337; and *American Journal of Clinical Dermatology*, 2001, volume 2, issue 2, pages 95–120.)

Vitamin D3 is not the same compound as the vitamin D found in most commercial vitamin supplements. Calcipotriene action inhibits cell proliferation and enhances cell differentiation in the skin of patients with psoriasis, but also appears to have effects on immunologic markers that are thought to play a role in the cause of psoriasis.

Calcipotriene is generally well tolerated in short- and long-term studies in adult patients, with the major side effect being irritation. In addition, calcipotriene ointment has proven beneficial in combination with other topical, phototherapy, or systemic antipsoriatic treatments, reducing the dosage and/or duration of some of these treatments and potentially improving their benefit/risk ratio. Calcipotriene ointment is valuable as a first- or second-line therapy option for the management of mild to moderate psoriasis and also in combination with other antipsoriatic agents for more severe psoriasis. Other forms of vitamin D3 creams include calcitriol and tacalitol.

TOPICAL STEROIDS/CORTISONE

Prescription topical corticosteroids (steroids/cortisone creams utilizing an active ingredient such as desoximetasone) have been used for years as the first-step approach in the treatment of psoriasis. Cortisones reduce inflammation, itching, and potentially reduce cell buildup. Brands differ in potency, and the more powerful the drug, the higher the risk of more severe side effects, which include burning, irritation, dryness, acne, thinning of the skin, dilated blood vessels, and loss of skin color. Less potent drugs should be used for mild to moderate psoriasis, saving the high-potency drugs for more severe conditions. An effective regimen uses high-potency cortisones, such as halobetasol (Ultravate), daily until the psoriasis plaque flattens out, after which they are applied only on the weekends.

Another high-potency corticosteroid, mometasone (Elocon), needs to be administered only once a day and is as effective—or more effective—than other corticosteroids while having a lower risk of severe side effects. These very potent drugs carry a small risk of causing hormonal problems for a period of time after the drug has been withdrawn. The larger the area treated with corticosteriods, the higher the risk, especially if the area is covered by heavy material or is bandaged. Also, in most cases, resistance to these drugs eventually develops; and the disease can recur after treatment is stopped (Source: http://my.webmd.com/content/article/1680.51881).

Low- to mid-potency topical steroids are good for short-term treatment, limited to a 2–4 week duration. It is recommended that their use be of limited duration to minimize the risks associated with topical steroids, such as collagen depletion and skin thinning. Topical steroids are more effective than calcipotriene (calcipotriol, or vitamin D3), pimecrolimus, and tacrolimus, but those treatments are associated with fewer long-term risks and are therefore recommended for long-term therapy when possible, perhaps when alternated with cortisones. Another negative of using cortisone is that with continued use it becomes less and less effective. (Sources: *Journal of the American Academy of Dermatology*, January 2009, pages 120–124; and *Journal of the European Academy of Dermatology and Venerology*, July 2008, pages 859–870.)

RETINOIDS

Topical retinoids such as Tazorac (active ingredient tazarotene) have been shown to have a positive effect on psoriasis (Source: *Cutis*, January 1999, pages 41–48), particularly in combination with other treatments (Source: *International Journal of Dermatology*, January 2001, pages 64–66). Tazarotene is a synthetic acetylenic retinoid. Some research has shown it to be more effective than tretinoin (Renova and Retin-A). A positive feature of tazarotene is its ability to maintain clinical response after discontinuation of treatment. Side effects can include irritation, burning, and flaking skin (Source: *Journal of the European Academy of Dermatology and Venereology*, July 2008, pages 859–870). Retinoids improve cell development and mitigate the damage caused by topical cortisones when used as a combination or alternating treatment.

SALICYLIC ACID (BHA)

Salicylic acid (beta hydroxy acid) in strengths of 1.8% to 3% is approved by the FDA as an over-the-counter treatment for psoriasis. Because BHA is a keratolytic, it can "unglue" skin cells and increase exfoliation, thereby removing the scaly buildup of psoriatic lesions. Sometimes simply using a well-formulated BHA product can be enough to keep psoriasis under control. It is also helpful when combined with other therapies, because by removing overproduced layers of skin BHA allows other topical medications to better penetrate skin. Finally, because of salicylic acid's chemical relationship to aspirin, it has anti-inflammatory properties and can reduce the redness and inflammation associated with psoriasis. (Sources: *Clinical Dermatology*, July–August 2008, pages 380–386; and *Journal of the American Academy of Dermatology*, February 2006, pages 266–271.)

Salicylic acid is available in many forms, such as gels, lotions, creams, and liquids, and it is often combined with other topical medications to enhance their effectiveness. (Source: www.psoriasis.org). The primary concern in choosing a well-formulated salicylic-acid product is to be sure the concentration is stated clearly on the product, and that the pH of the product is no higher than 3.5.

ARGAN OIL

Derived from the argan tree, argan oil has been used for the treatment of psoriasis and has a relatively popular following. However, there is no research showing it to have any benefit over and above being an emollient, which would be true of any plant oil.

METHOTREXATE

Methotrexate is a systemic anti-cancer drug that can reduce the overproduction of cells, which is helpful in the treatment of psoriasis. However, it has conflicting research concerning its effectiveness despite its use during the last three decades. The long-term adverse effects of methotrexate are well known. The most frequent adverse effects that occur during methotrexate therapy are abnormal liver function test results, nausea, and gastric complaints. The most feared adverse effects are liver damage and the suppression of bone marrow activity. However, liver problems associated with methotrexate are related to a high cumulative dose. This means that rotating types of therapy, or using methotrexate intermittently instead of continuously, can reduce the risk. Most people tolerate low-dose methotrexate therapy relatively well, provided they work closely with their physician and watch carefully for adverse effects and drug interactions during treatment. (Sources: *Clinical Rheumatology*, 2001, volume 20, issue 6, pages 406–410; and *American Journal of Clinical Dermatology*, January–February 2000, pages 27–39.)

In the area of new options for psoriasis, methotrexate has been shown to be less beneficial than adalimumab, etanercept, efalizumab, and infliximab, but because it the least expensive it can still be a good option to start with if systemic therapy is being considered. (Sources: *British Journal of Dermatology*, 2008, www.BJD.org; and *Clinical Experimental Dermatology*, August 2008, pages 551–554.)

CYCLOSPORIN

Under the trade name Neoral, cyclosporin is a strong immune-suppressant drug and a primary medication used to prevent the rejection of transplanted organs such as the liver, kidneys, and heart. In skin diseases, cyclosporin acts by reducing inflammation in the skin and also reducing cell proliferation by blocking immune factors that may be generating the problem. Studies have shown cyclosporin to be effective and well tolerated in short-term treatment of severe psoriasis (Source: *American Journal of Clinical Dermatology*, 2001, volume 2, issue 1, pages 41–47), though not as effective as newer options such as etanercept or infliximab.

Cyclosporin is a serious medication. Temporary side effects of cyclosporin can include headaches, gingivitis, joint pain, gout, body-hair growth, tremors, high blood pressure, kidney problems, and fatigue. Of serious concern is the National Toxicology Program's *Eighth Report on Carcinogens* (1998), which warns that cyclosporin is "known to be a human carcinogen based on studies in humans." All of these factors must be weighed and carefully assessed before deciding on this course of treatment.

ORAL FORMS OF VITAMIN A (RETINOIDS)

Etretinate (trade name Tegison), **acitretin** (Soriatane), and **isotretinoin** (Accutane) are retinoids. Etretinate and acitretin are similar to isotretinoin, except that etretinate and acitretin are approved by the FDA only for use in the treatment of psoriasis, while isotretinoin is also approved by the FDA for use in treating acne. How oral retinoids work in the treatment of psoriasis is not completely understood, although they are thought to block the overproduction of skin cells. The substantial amount of data on the clinical effectiveness of these treatments, either alone or in combination with other therapies such as sunlight or etanarcept, makes them great options. (Sources: *Seminars in Cutaneous Medicine and Surgery*, September 2008, pages 197–206; *British Journal of Dermatology*, June 2008, pages 1345–1249; and *European Journal of Dermatology*, November–October 2000, pages 517–521.)

While none of these retinoids are to be used when a woman is pregnant, the risks associated with usage are considered serious and extremely problematic even for women who are not pregnant. All systemic retinoids have the strong potential to cause major fetal abnormalities, including neurological and skeletal deformities. For the patient, its use may potentially cause liver and cholesterol problems, which are just a few of the side effects. It is essential that effective contraception be used for at least one month before and throughout treatment. However, because etretinate can remain in the blood for up to three years after treatment, birth control must be continued for an indefinite period of time following therapy. It has not yet been determined how long it is necessary to wait before becoming pregnant after you stop taking etretinate to ensure that none of the drug remains in your system (Source: www.fda.gov/cber/bldmem/072893.txt). As a result of the risks associated with etretinate, particularly the length of time it can stay in the system, acitretin and isotretinoin are considered safer choices, and are just as effective for severe psoriasis (Source: *Journal of the American Academy of Dermatology*, November 2001, pages S150–S157).

Severe fetal abnormalities do occur if a woman is or becomes pregnant while taking either acitretin or isotretinoin (Accutane), but because these drugs don't remain in the system for long after you are finished with treatment, no long waiting period is required before becoming pregnant. Specifics regarding how long to wait after treatment before considering having a baby should be discussed with your physician.

ETANERCEPT AND INFLIXIMAB

Etanercept (trade name Enbrel) and infliximab (trade name Remicade) are antitumor medications that are used in the treatment of psoriasis. Both have research showing them to be helpful, with less-serious side effects than other oral medications, and they can be used in combination with topical therapies. (Sources: *Health Technology Assessments*, September 2006, pages 13–26; and *British Journal of Dermatology*, January 2002, pages 118–121.)

5-FLUOROURACIL

Also known as fumaric acid esters under the brand name Efudex, this is a chemotherapy drug. When applied topically, it is considered one of the primary options for the treatment of psoriasis affecting the nails. It can also be taken orally for severe psoriatic symptoms. (Sources: *Clinical Dermatology*, September–October 2008, pages 522–526; *British Journal of Dermatology*, September 2005, pages 549–551, and April 2004, pages 741–746; and *Cutis*, July 1998, pages 27–28.)

ELIDEL

Elidel is the trade name for the topically applied, prescription-only cream containing pimecrolimus. It is one of a new generation of nonsteroidal medications recommended for psoriasis. The first drug of this class was Protopic, which contains the active ingredient tacrolimus. (Source: *Journal of the American Academy of Dermatology*, February 2002, pages 228–241.)

No one is quite sure why Elidel works on certain types of dermatitis, and it is not a cure (Source: www.fda.gov/cder/foi/label/2001/021302lbl.pdf). It is intended for long-term use, but only for short or intermittent periods. That means you can start using it when symptoms show up and stop using it when the symptoms go away. When symptoms recur, you start once again, and you can keep up with that pattern of application forever.

A concern about using a treatment that lowers the immune response is the need to avoid sunlight, because the body will be less able to defend against UVR (ultraviolet radiation) damage. Other common side effects may include headache, flu, sore throat, and fever. If you have had warts, herpes, or shingles in the past, Elidel can trigger recurrences.

Despite the serious side effects, there is no question that research shows this drug to be successful in treating atopic dermatitis and psoriasis. And the sooner you use it when symptoms occur, the quicker and better your skin will respond. (Sources: *International Journal of Clinical Practice*, May 2003, pages 319–327; *Journal of Allergy and Clinical Immunology*, May 2003, pages 1153–1168, and August 2002, pages 277–284; and *Journal of Investigative Dermatology*, October 2002, pages 876–887.)

COMBINATION THERAPY

The most typical combination therapy for psoriasis is something called **PUVA**. PUVA involves the use of a prescription medication called Psoralen and exposure to ultraviolet light A (UVA)—hence the initials PUVA. It is also called "photochemotherapy" because Psoralen functions similar to other types of chemotherapy used for cancer treatment. It is considered extremely effective and patients can remain clear of lesions for about three months. (Source: *International Journal of Immunopathological Pharmacology*, April–June 2008, pages 481–484.)

The drug Psoralen, which can be taken orally as a pill or applied topically to the skin, makes the skin more sensitive and receptive to UV radiation, which the entire body is exposed to. To avoid exposing the entire body to UV light the 308 nanometer excimer laser can be used. Either combination suppresses the growth of abnormal skin cells. The good news is that PUVA can eliminate or dramatically reduce psoriatic lesions for the majority of people who use it, and there is evidence it can provide extended remissions. The bad news is that Psoralen and UVA light are phototoxic and carcinogenic. (Sources: *European Journal of Dermatology*, January February 2008, pages 55–60; and *Journal of Dermatology*, July 2007, pages 435–440.)

Getting rid of psoriasis can mean a lot, but putting your skin at risk for premature aging and some skin cancers may be trading one problem for another. This risk should be taken into consideration when considering this treatment. (Sources: *Journal of Investigative Dermatology*, March 2005, pages 505–513, and June 2002, pages 1038–1043; www.psoriasis. org; *Biochemical Pharmacology*, January 2002, pages 31–39; and *Cutis*, November 2001, pages 345–347.)

CHAPTER 19

SOLUTIONS FOR SEBORRHEA AND ECZEMA

THE BASICS

TWICE A DAY: Gentle cleanser
   Recommended cleansers: CeraVe Hydrating Cleanser; Cetaphil Gentle Skin Cleanser; Clinique Liquid Facial Soap Extra Mild; Eucerin Redness Relief Soothing Cleanser; Paula's Choice Skin Recovery Cleanser for Normal to Very Dry Skin; Paula's Choice One Step Face Cleanser for Normal to Oily/Combination Skin.

TWICE A DAY: Toner with antioxidants, skin-identical identical ingredients, cell-communicating ingredients
   Recommended toners: Pevonia Botanica Sensitive Skin Lotion; MD Formulations Moisture Defense Antioxidant Spray; Paula's Choice Moisture Boost Hydrating Toner; Paula's Choice Healthy Skin Refreshing Toner.

ONCE A DAY: Use a BHA (salicylic acid) lotion, liquid, or gel
   Recommended BHA products: Clinique Mild Clarifying Lotion; Serious Skin Care Clarify Acne Medication Clarifying Treatment; Paula's Choice 1% Beta Hydroxy Acid Lotion; Paula's Choice 1% Beta Hydroxy Acid Gel; Paula's Choice 2% Beta Hydroxy Acid Liquid; Paula's Choice 2% Beta Hydroxy Acid Gel.

ONCE OR TWICE A DAY: A medicated topical cream, lotion, or gel with active ingredients designed for treating seborrhea and/or eczema

DAYTIME: Sunscreen either in foundation or a moisturizer
   Recommended daytime moisturizers with sunscreen: Olay Regenerist Enhancing Lotion with UV Protection SPF 15; Estee Lauder DayWear Plus Multi Protection Anti-Oxidant Lotion SPF 15, for Oily Skin; Neutrogena Age Shield Sunblock SPF 30; Paula's Choice Skin Balancing Daily Mattifying Lotion with SPF 15 & Antioxidants; Paula's Choice Skin Recovery Daily Moisturizing Lotion with SPF 15 & Antioxidants.
   Recommended foundations with sunscreen: L'Oreal True Match Super-Blendable Makeup SPF 17; Maybelline New York Instant Age Rewind Custom Face Perfector Cream Compact Foundation SPF 18; Prescriptives Flawless Skin Total Protection Makeup SPF 15; Paula's Choice All Bases Covered Foundation SPF 15; Paula's Choice Best Face Forward Foundation SPF 15.

NIGHTTIME: Moisturizer with antioxidants, skin-identical identical ingredients, cell-communicating ingredients
   Recommended moisturizers for eczema: Osmotics TriCeram; CeraVe Moisturizing Cream; Clinique Super Rescue Antioxidant Night Moisturizer for Very Dry to Dry Skin; Paula's Choice Skin Recovery Moisturizer; Paula's Choice Hydrating Treatment Cream.

SEBORRHEA

Seborrhea is a skin disease of the sebaceous (oil) glands marked by an increased secretion of sebum (oil) or a thickened sebum discharge. It can resemble acne and blackheads. One of the differences between acne and seborrhea is that in seborrhea the increased oil production is often accompanied by a scaly, thickened skin, especially on the scalp, and the oil itself can have a strange, viscous texture. However, in seborrhea—and sometimes in acne—the sebum (a firm, waxlike substance in the pore that liquefies into oil on the surface of the skin) in the sebaceous gland accumulates, causing the gland to become swollen and filled to the brim. When this overproduced sebum is covered over by skin, it forms a small, firm mound called a whitehead. When the sebum is exposed to air (not covered by skin) and the duct fills with dead skin cells, the sebum turns dark from oxidation and the blemish becomes a blackhead. The size of the eruption, the texture of the oil, and the flaky skin are what differentiate seborrhea from acne.

Seborrhea can show up wherever there are lots of oil glands. The scalp, sides of the nose, eyebrows, eyelids, behind the ears, and the middle of the chest are the areas most commonly affected. Other areas, such as the navel and the skin folds under the arms, breasts, groin, and buttocks, may also be involved. The swelling, breakouts, and accompanying yellowish, greasy-appearing scales make this skin disorder hard to miss.

Seborrhea is identified by excessive yellowing, thickened scaling, accompanied by excessive oiliness, and is possibly triggered by a yeast organism (yeast is a type of fungus) present in the hair follicle (Source: *British Journal of Dermatology*, March 2001, pages 549–556). Seborrhea can occur at any age, but typically it is seen in infants, when it is called "cradle cap." Because yeast, or some other form of fungus, likely triggers seborrhea, antimicrobial agents capable of targeting this type of organism have been shown to have a high success rate.

Prescription medications for the treatment of seborrhea include ciclopiroxolamine 1% in a cream base. This is an antifungal that has been shown to be effective in a well-controlled study (Source: *British Journal of Dermatology*, May 2001, pages 1033–1037). Topical metronidazole (Noritate, MetroLotion, MetroGel, and MetroCream) can also have significant positive results, and are very effective in the treatment of seborrhea (Source: *Journal of Family Practice*, June 2001, volume 50, issue 6). An oral medication, terbinafine, has been identified as beneficial in the treatment of seborrhea as well (Source: *British Journal of Dermatology*, April 2001, pages 854–857).

Several over-the-counter topical treatments for seborrhea include zinc pyrithione 1% (Dandrex, Zincon, Head and Shoulders, Denorex), coal-tar preparations (DHS, Neutrogena T-Gel, Ionil T, Tegrin, Esorex), ketaconazole (Nizoral), selenium sulfide 1% (Selsun Blue), and selenium sulfide 2.5% (Selsun). A very good fragrance-free moisturizer with zinc pyrithione is DermaZinc Cream; it is available from www.dermadoctor.com.

As in the treatment of psoriasis, UV light therapy can be of benefit for those who suffer from seborrhea, but it carries the same risks mentioned above for psoriasis. Topical steroids are often of limited use because they can cause thinning of the skin.

Treating seborrhea takes patience and experimenting to find what works for you. All of these medications, either alone or in combination, are options for achieving the best results.

ECZEMA (ATOPIC DERMATITIS)

On a personal note, I suffered from eczema for many years. At one point in my life almost 80% of my body was affected, and the resulting itching and scratching, sores, irritation, and discomfort were more awful than I can put into words. For years I struggled with medications and a varying assortment of cortisone creams and bar soaps, from Basis to Aveeno, until the day my dermatologist found the right cortisone strength and I started to stay away from topical irritants. Then my skin finally settled down—but the problem didn't go away until much later in life.

Eczema is a general term representing a range of irritated, rash, inflamed skin problems. It also goes by the name contact dermatitis, atopic dermatitis, irritant dermatitis, and allergic dermatitis. By any name, approximately 10% to 20% of the world population is affected by this chronic, relapsing, and very itchy rash at some point during childhood and into adulthood, although it tends to get better as you get older.

Without question eczema is a difficult, uncomfortable, often painful skin disorder. When you have it, you generally know it by the cracked, abraded, blistered, crusted, weepy, reddened, patchy, dry skin surface, accompanied by persistent, almost unbearable itching and the tendency for everything you touch to make matters worse. A simple act like washing your hands, applying eye makeup, or wearing scratchy material can instigate a flare-up that feels interminable.

Almost anything can trigger eczema, and sometimes nothing at all can precede a bout of oppressive itching, scratching, and rashes. Wool (from clothing to carpets), shampoos, hair dyes, nail polish, jewelry, plants, undergarments (elastic waistbands and spandex bras are special villains), deodorant, tight socks, nylons, pet allergies, excessive heat or air conditioning (which increases dry and itchy skin), bathing too often (which leaches moisture out of the skin), using harsh or mild soaps, hot water, vigorous rubbing or massaging, chlorinated water, salt water, and even sweat (this triggered my eczema almost instantaneously) are all possible offenders. In the world of cosmetics, preservatives, irritants (such as peppermint, menthol, alcohol, camphor, eucalyptus, fragrance, and essential oils), bath salts, bubble bath, scrubs, AHAs, BHA, and loofahs are all potent eczema triggers.

Despite this daunting list, everyone is different, and what irritates your skin might not irritate someone else's. There is no exact science to discovering what causes your skin to react; rather, it is a process of paying attention to what you come into contact with, seeing what makes things worse for your skin, and then eliminating or avoiding those things at all costs.

Generally, an impaired surface skin barrier condition, such as dry skin or irritated skin, is more prone to the sensation of itching and chapping, so a state-of-the-art skin-care routine as explained in this book is essential for finding a reliable way to deal with the rashes and itching. Gentle cleansers, along with gentle toners and moisturizers loaded with antioxidants and skin-identical ingredients, are essential. It is also important to keep bathing time short, avoid bath salts or bubble baths, use lukewarm to warm water (avoid hot water most of all, and that includes jacuzzis), and avoid bar soaps of any kind (they all contain potential irritants). Using fragrance-free, gentle liquid cleansers that also contain moisturizing agents, and applying and reapplying moisturizers quickly afterward, can help a lot.

Unquestionably, well-formulated moisturizers minimize dryness and are a mainstay in treating mild to chronic eczema. It is believed that regular and frequent use of emollient moisturizers can reduce the amount of topical steroids needed in the maintenance treatment of eczema. The more emollient the cream the better, and when fatty acids are included in the formula it's particularly helpful. Fatty acids are ingredients such as triglycerides, oleic acid, linoleic acid, evening primrose oil, borage oil, fish oil, flaxseed oil, coconut oil, and palm oil (Source: *Skin Pharmacology and Applied Skin Physiology*, March 2002, pages 100–104). While using a moisturizer twice daily is considered adequate, it is essential to keep a moisturizer with you at all times so that you can reapply it every time you wash your hands. During the day it is essential that you apply an emollient moisturizer with an SPF 15 or greater that contains UVA-protecting ingredients on exposed areas of your body. In the case of eczema, because of the risk of irritation and skin sensitivity, the UVA-protecting ingredients should be only titanium dioxide and zinc oxide, with no avobenzone or other synthetic sunscreen agents of any kind. Synthetic sunscreen agents have a potential to cause skin irritation, and skin afflicted with eczema is much more prone to reacting to irritants, even those (like AHAs or BHA) that traditionally offer skin more benefits than problems.

For years, topical corticosteroids (cortisone) have been the drug of choice for treating eczema. These products are available in a vast range of strengths and molecular structures that allow for varying skin penetration and potency. The risks associated with prolonged use of a potent corticosteroid are that it may result in skin deterioration and adaptation (that means it stops having an effect on the skin). Because of these risks, newer nonsteroidal treatments for eczema have been formulated and have been approved by the FDA. However, if these newer treatments are not effective for you, concerns about skin breakdown (which happens with any long-term cortisone use) and adaptation should not limit your use of a good, potent steroid. It is still a valid way to get control of the eczema. As much as possible, try to minimize the frequency of cortisone application, using it only as necessary to keep the irritation abated. But don't cut back too far because there is a point of no return where if you don't use enough your skin becomes an itchy, rashy mess.

SOLUTIONS FOR ECZEMA—ATOPIC DERMATITIS

One of the more typical treatments for eczema is Protopic, containing the active ingredient tacrolimus in a 0.1% and 0.03% concentration ointment for adults and a 0.03% concentration ointment for children two years of age and older. It is a nonsteroidal (meaning not cortisone) ointment indicated for patients with moderate to severe eczema and for whom standard eczema therapies such as cortisone creams have not worked or are not considered healthy. Plus, with repeated use, cortisone can cause thinning of the skin and prematurely age skin. Another version of this same class of active ingredients is pimecrolimus, and some research has shown it to be as effective as tacrolimus in the treatment of eczema. (Sources: *Journal of Drugs in Dermatology*, December 2008, pages 1153–1158; *Clinical Experimen-*

tal Dermatology, November 2008, pages 685–688; and *Cochrane Database System Review*, "Topical Pimecrolimus for Eczema," October 2007, 17(4): CD005500.)

What makes tacrolimus and pimecrolimus unique is that they have been used primarily orally to prevent transplant rejections due to their action as immunomodulators. In other words, by suppressing the immune system they prevent the body from rejecting a transplanted organ. They are thought to work the same way topically in some cases of moderate to severe dermatitis because of their effect in preventing the skin's own immune reaction from causing red, itchy, inflamed rashes. (In other words, in this form of eczema, it's as if the person's own immune system is attacking the skin, causing the itching, blistering, and irritation.) By stopping this immune reaction, they eliminate the problem.

Both of these topical medications can increase sun sensitivity, so sun protection is vital (but you already know that sun protection is vital each day regardless of what else you put on your skin).

Another interesting study on eczema, presented in the *Archives of Dermatology* (January 2001, pages 42–43), reported research in Japan that demonstrated that two-thirds of the patients with eczema improved after a month of drinking a liter of oolong tea daily. According to the study "118 patients … were asked to maintain their dermatological treatment. However, they were also instructed to drink oolong tea made from a 10-gram teabag placed in 1000 milliliters of boiling water and steeped for 5 minutes. After 1 month of treatment 74 (63%) of the 118 patients showed marked to moderate improvement of their condition. A good response to treatment was still observed in 64 patients (54%) at 6 months." The study concluded that "The therapeutic efficacy of oolong tea may well be the result of the antiallergic properties of tea polyphenols." While the study didn't look at the effect of tea drinking if the topical treatments were stopped, the patients did receive some benefit. So by combining topical treatments (moisturizers and possibly Protopic) with some oolong tea, perhaps the positive effects of both will add up, and those with eczema can breathe a sigh of relief.

CHAPTER 20
SOLUTIONS FOR CELLULITE

Technically called gynoid lipodystrophy, cellulite is a pervasive aesthetic problem. Regrettably, most of us (meaning women) have it to one degree or another. According to statistics, and this is really shocking, cellulite shows up on the thighs of more than 85% of females past the age of 18 regardless of ancestry, although it is more common for Caucasian and Asian women. To make matters worse, for women, cellulite represents stored, hard-to-metabolize fat that doesn't easily respond to exercise or weight loss. Ironically, weight isn't part of the problem. Rather, any amount of fat (and we all need some of it in our bodies) can show up as cellulite on women's thighs. Even weight loss isn't a solution, since for some women that can result in improvement while for others it can make matters worse. (Sources: *Plastic and Reconstructive Surgery*, August 2006, pages 510–516; and *Cosmetics & Toiletries magazine*, October 2004, page 49.)

Despite being a completely benign condition, much the way wrinkles are, cellulite is a major beauty concern of women worldwide, and its presence is surrounded with corresponding myths and deceptions that take the place of fact and reason. This means the cosmetics industry and lots of doctors and aestheticians want to sell you products or provide treatments (particularly expensive ones) claiming to slim, trim, tone, and de-bump your thighs.

Everything from loofahs, miracle ingredients, special washcloths, herbal supplements, vitamins, minerals, bath liquids, rubberized pants, brushes, rollers, body wraps, and toning lotions to electrical muscle stimulation, vibrating machines, inflatable hip-high pressurized boots, hormone or enzyme injections, and massage have been claimed to be successful cellulite treatments. If any of this worked you would assume by now no one would have cellulite, and that isn't the case in the least.

As the anti-cellulite market increases, research regarding the efficacy of these options remains at a bare minimum and is often obscured by self-serving studies from those who peddle these cures. Sadly, the lure of these supposed remedies is hard to fend off, because fighting cellulite is an uphill battle. For lots of women the mere hope or illusion that something may work is a powerful temptation, and that weakness is something the cosmetics industry counts on and exploits to the max. (Source: *Journal of Cosmetic Science*, November 2005, pages 379–393.)

REALITY ONLY HURTS A LITTLE

Trying to navigate and smooth out cellulite fact from fiction isn't easy but there is a small amount of good news: there are options that may make a difference. The bad news is that even the treatments that have some potential of working (and I say potential of working very carefully) rarely live up to the claims asserted, but improvement as opposed to merely wasting your money is definitely a turn for the better. A great way to start is to straighten out some popular myths about cellulite.

Men don't get cellulite. To some extent that's true, only about 5% of men have cellulite. Physiologically, women are far more prone to accumulating fat on the thighs and hips, while men gain weight in the abdominal area. Plus, for women, the connective tissue beneath the skin has more stretch and is vulnerable to disruption, which is the perfect environment for developing cellulite. Some men do get cellulite—just not as many as women, statistically. (Source: *Journal of Cosmetic Science*, March–April 2005, pages 105–120.)

Drinking water doesn't change fat or cellulite. If water could change skin structure and reduce fat I assure you no one would have cellulite, or would be overweight for that matter. Drinking water probably is beneficial (although there is really no research showing how much is healthy versus unhealthy) but there is no research showing that water consumption will impact fat anywhere on your body, let alone the dimples on your thighs.

Arguments for high water intake are generally based on the assumption that because our bodies consist mostly of water (50% to 70% of body weight, about 42 liters) and our blood, muscles, brain, and bones are made up mainly of water (85%, 80%, 75%, and 25%, respectively), we therefore need at least eight 8-ounce glasses of water each day. But assumptions aren't science, and this one is based on a non sequitur; it's like arguing that since our cars run on gasoline they always need a full tank to run efficiently. (Source: *American Journal of Physiology – Regulatory, Integrative, and Comparative Physiology*, November 2002, pages 993–1004.)

Water retention doesn't cause cellulite. It's ironic that low water intake is considered a possible cause of cellulite, and the polar opposite—retaining too much water—is thought to be a factor as well. There is lots of speculation around how water retention can affect cellulite, but there is no actual research supporting this notion. Further, fat cells actually contain only about 10% water, so claiming to eliminate excess water won't make a difference and any measurable result would be transient at best. It is true that water retention can make you look bloated and feel like you've gained weight, but water itself doesn't impact fat or the appearance of cellulite. (Source: *Journal of Strength and Conditioning Research*, November 2003, pages 817–821.)

There's no specialized diet that can specifically address cellulite. Eating healthy is always a good thing for your entire body. However, because weight in and of itself is not a cause of cellulite, dieting won't change the skin structure of your thighs, which is what causes the dimpled contours to show. For some people, cellulite is made worse by the accumulation of extra fat. In those cases, weight reduction may decrease the total area and depth of cellulite but it is unlikely to get rid of it altogether. (Source: *Clinical Dermatology*, July–August 2004, pages 303–309.)

Cellulite is not different from fat on the rest of the body. Theories abound about how cellulite differs from regular body fat. However, few studies show how cellulite clumps differently than other fat on your body. Overall, most researchers feel cellulite is just fat, plain and simple. Besides, even if cellulite is different in how it congregates, what you can and can't do about fat on any part of the body remains the same. (Source: www.quackwatch.org/01QuackeryRelatedTopics/cellulite.html.)

Exercise isn't a cure for cellulite. Exercise helps almost every system in the human body, but it won't necessarily impact the appearance of cellulite. Exercise doesn't improve skin structure and it can't affect localized areas of fat. In other words, you can't spot-reduce fat accumulation in a specific area. (Source: *British Journal of Plastic Surgery*, April 2004, pages 222–227.)

Toxins don't cause cellulite and trying to detox isn't helpful in the least. For consumers, detoxifying the body has taken on the meaning of purging it of pollutants or any other problem substances, whether from the environment or in the foods we eat. In terms of the way this concept has been mass-marketed, there is little research showing credible efficacy as to whether detoxification of the body is even possible. However, "detoxifying" the body, as it is used in the scientific community, describes the process of reducing cellular damage, primarily by means of antioxidants or enzymes that prevent certain abnormal or undesirable cell functions from taking place. There is no doubt this is helpful for the body. Whether or not this reduces cellulite is completely unknown, because skin structure and fat accumulation are not caused by toxins in the environment. Furthermore, there are no studies showing that toxins of any kind prevent fat from being broken down. (Sources: *Journal of Endotoxin Research*, April 2005, pages 69–84; and *Journal of Biochemistry and Molecular Biology*, May 2003, pages 258–264.)

WHAT CAUSES CELLULITE

There are three leading theories about cellulite formation:
1. Women have a unique, genetically determined skin structure on their thighs, which causes fat pockets to form (which would explain why only 5% of males have cellulite while more than 85% of females have cellulite).
2. The connective tissue layers on the thigh are too weak or thin to maintain a smooth appearance, allowing fat contours to show through. (This would also account for why men have less cellulite, since the skin structure on their thighs has a higher percentage of collagen.)
3. Vascular changes and possible inflammatory conditions may be to blame. (Sources: *Journal of Cosmetic Laser Therapy*, December 2004, pages 181–185; *Journal of Applied Physiology*, April 2002, pages 1611–1618; and *Skin Research and Technology*, May 2, 2002, pages 118–124.)

There isn't much you can do about genetics, but the hope to do something about the other causes— skin structure, fat concentration, and vascular changes—is the sphere of skin care and medicine. Most cellulite products come in the form of lotions and creams with a vast array of either exotic-sounding or lab-synthesized ingredients. And beyond topical products there are devices such as endermologie and microdermabrasion, along with medical treatments such as nonablative lasers and mesotherapy.

FAT-BUSTING LOTIONS, CREAMS, AND EXTRACTS GALORE

As far as skin-care products for the body are concerned, the litany of options is mesmerizing. Yet there is almost no uniformity between formulas. It would appear, if the claims are to be believed, that a wide variety of unrelated plant extracts can deflate or break down fat and/or restructure skin. Looking at the research, however, most articles suggest there is little hope that anything rubbed on the skin can change fat deposits or radically improve the appearance of cellulite.

The hope that botanicals have the answer is odd, since not a single study points to what concentration of an ingredient needs to be in a formulation, what physiochemical characteristics particular to each active ingredient need to be present, or whether these ingredients can retain any standardized properties between batches. (Sources: *Dermatologic Surgery*, July 2005, pages 866–872; and *The European Journal of Dermatology*, December 2000, pages 596–603.)

All sorts of ingredients are used in body products that claim they can get rid of cellulite. But if you look at the list of options, or peruse a cosmetics counter with all the products extolling their anti-cellulite prowess, it would be hard to imagine why anyone has one dimple left on their legs! Here are few of the plant extracts that show up in anti-cellulite products:

AGRIMONIA EUPATORIA LEAF EXTRACT

Research shows this plant extract inhibits the hepatitis B virus and has antioxidant properties. Whether or not it has a benefit when applied topically is not known. There is no research showing it to be effective for cellulite. (Sources: *Phytotherapy Research*, April 2005, pages 355–358; and *Journal of Ethnopharmacology*, January 2005, pages 145–150.)

AMINOPHYLLINE AND THEOPHYLLINE

Aminophylline and theophylline are medicines used to prevent and treat wheezing and other breathing difficulties caused by lung diseases such as asthma. These pharmaceutical ingredients are found in prescription bronchodilators—medications designed to open blocked air passageways in lungs—and also found in some cellulite lotions and creams. Aminophylline in particular gained notoriety as an ingredient in cellulite creams as a result of a study published in *Obesity Research* (November 1995, Supplemental, pages 561S–568S). However, the validity of this research was called into question because one of its authors was marketing an aminophylline cream being sold at the time, and thus was not considered an objective investigator. Also, the number of participants in the study was small, and most also were dieting and exercising at the same time they were applying the aminophylline cream. (Source: *Annals of Pharmacotherapy*, March 1996, pages 292–293.)

Doubt about aminophylline's value was also revealed in research published in *Plastic and Reconstructive Surgery* (September 1999, pages 1110–1114), which described a double-blind study that compared the effectiveness of three different treatments for cellulite on three separate groups of women. One investigated the twice-daily application of aminophylline cream compared with a placebo; another the twice-weekly treatment using endermologie (a machine rolled over the skin's surface, which has been claimed to get rid of cellulite) on one leg and nothing on the other; and a third combining endermologie on both legs with the same cream regimen used by the first group. "No statistical difference existed in measurements between legs for any of the treatment groups.... [Even] The best subjective assessment, by the patients themselves, revealed that only 3 of 35 aminophylline-treated legs and 10 of 35 [e]ndermologie-treated legs [felt] their cellulite appearance improved."

What keeps aminophylline in the spotlight is that there is research showing it to be lipolytic (meaning it can break down fat cells) when it is place in a petri dish containing fat cells in a laboratory setting. (Source: *Journal of Plastic and Reconstructive Aesthetic Surgery*, November 2008, pages 1321-1324) However, there is no other research showing these ingredients to be successful when injected into people wanting to get rid of some fat cells; add to that the risk of absorption causing bronchial involvement when it is applied topically or injected remains unclear.

ATRACTYLOYDES LANCEA ROOT EXTRACT

Also known as Chinese Thistle Daisy, this root extract is used in Chinese and Japanese alternative medicine for angiogenesis (the formation of new blood vessels) in type-2 diabetes because it contains beta-eudesmol. Some of its other components have been shown to have anti-inflammatory properties as well. Whether this effect can be of benefit when the entire extract is applied topically is unknown. (Sources: *Yajugaku Zasshi, The Pharmaceutical Society of Japan*, March 2006, pages 133–143; *European Journal of Pharmacology*, April 2005, pages 105–115; and *Planta Medica*, July 2001, pages 437–442.)

BUPLEURUM FALCATUM EXTRACT

Bupleurum is a plant used in Chinese medicine for a variety of ailments ranging from the common cold to liver problems. Some research has shown this extract to have anti-tumor, anti-inflammatory, and antioxidant properties. Whether or not these benefits can be delivered to skin in a lotion or cream is unknown. (Sources: www.naturaldatabase.com; *British Journal of Pharmacology*, December 2000, pages 1285–1293; *Planta Medica*, June 1998, pages 404–407; and *Life Sciences*, August 1998, pages 1147–1156.)

CAFFEINE

Since 1971 when the first Starbucks opened in my hometown of Seattle, I have been a coffee lover. And over the years I've developed a passion for Grande and Venti iced lattes. I would be thrilled to learn that this has somehow helped my thighs, but alas this is far from the case. Separate from my own anecdotal experience, caffeine is one of the more typical ingredients showing up in cellulite creams and lotions. There are two reasons for this. The first is caffeine's distant relationship to aminophylline. Aminophylline is a modified form of theophylline (Source: Yale New Haven Health Library, Alternative/Complementary Medicine, www.yalenewhavenhealth.org), and the fact that coffee contains theophylline (Source: *Progress in Neurobiology*, December 2002, pages 377–392). There is no research to prove or disprove that theophylline can affect cellulite. However, researchers have disproved aminophyilline's impact on cellulite. The second reason caffeine may show up in cellulite products stems from research showing it to have benefit for weight loss. But that's only when you drink it, not when you rub it on your thighs.

There are only two studies showing caffeine to have benefit for reducing cellulite. One was conducted by Johnson & Johnson, which owns the RoC brand, which sells cellulite creams that contain caffeine. The other was conducted by cosmetic ingredient manufacturers that sell anti-cellulite compounds (Source: *Journal of Cosmetic Science*, July–August 2002, pages 209–218). There is no other independent research to show that caffeine provides any benefit for treating cellulite.

Caffeine does have potential as an antioxidant, so it isn't a wasted ingredient in skincare products. It's just not one that can reduce the appearance of cellulite. (Sources: *BMC Complementary and Alternative Medicine*, March 2006, www.biomedcentral.com/1472–6882/6/9; *Bioscience, Biotechnology, and Biochemistry*, November 2005, pages 2219–2223; *Obesity Research*, July 2005, pages 1195–1204; and *Sports Medicine*, November 2001, pages 785–807.)

CARNITINE

This is a naturally occurring amino acid, and deficiencies of this small but essential component can result in muscle loss and a multitude of other problems. Research abounds for carnitine, especially acetyl-L-carnitine, which is considered to have more bioavailabilty in terms of its effect on aging and brain function. But how this amino acid affects skin when applied topically is unknown (Source: www.naturaldatabase.com).

ESCIN

Derived from horse chestnut (*Aesculus hippocastanum*), this ingredient has been prescribed as an oral supplement to reduce some symptoms of chronic vein insufficiency, such as varicose veins, pain, tiredness, tension, swelling in the legs, itching, and edema. However, because horse chestnut contains significant amounts of the toxin esculin, it can be lethal, and other experts recommend not using it. When applied topically, however, there is research showing that a gel containing 2% escin can improve circulation. Results from another study showed a reduction in inflammation in sports injuries when escin was combined with heparin (a mucopolysaccharide used as an anti-clotting medication), and a form of salicylic acid (diethylammonium salicylate). Escin is also a potent antioxidant. As a skin-care ingredient escin clearly has a place, but as for improving cellulite that's another story. While it may seem logical that blood flow and cellulite are related, the research just isn't there to support the notion, or your thighs. Plus, cellulite products contain far less of this ingredient than the amount used in the studies. (Sources: *British Journal of Sports Medicine*, 36 June 2002, pages 183–188; *Angiology*, March 2000, pages 197–205; www. naturaldatabase.com; *International Journal of Cosmetic Science*, December 1999, page 437; and *Archives of Dermatology*, November 1998, pages 1356–1360.)

AHAS AND BHA

Some cellulite creams have included glycolic or lactic acid (AHAs) or scrubs in an effort to somehow exfoliate away bumpy skin texture on the thighs. Theoretically, AHAs come the closest to having the potential for reducing the appearance of cellulite. If cellulite is a problem with skin structure, applying ingredients that help to improve it should make a difference. There are a number of studies demonstrating the effectiveness of AHAs for stimulating collagen synthesis and improving the overall structure of skin. What is important to recognize is that if AHAs can help, you don't need something labeled as a "cellulite cream." Any well-formulated AHA gel, lotion, or cream will work. (Sources: *Journal of Dermatology*, January 2006, pages 16–22; *Plastic and Reconstructive Surgery*, April 2005, pages 1156–1162; *Experimental Dermatology*, December 2003, pages 57–63; and *American Journal of Clinical Dermatology*, November–December 2000, pages 369–374.)

In terms of scrubs, there is absolutely no research showing that these have any impact on cellulite. You can't rub away cellulite or break up fat by rubbing, massaging, scrubbing, or abrading your skin. If anything overzealous scrubbing of the skin damages the skin's barrier, thereby depleting its structure and core strength, which doesn't help reduce the appearance of cellulite but can technically make matters worse.

GINKGO BILOBA LEAF EXTRACT

Research shows this potent antioxidant helps improve blood flow. Whether or not blood flow changes anything about cellulite is unknown. (Sources: *Medical Hypotheses*, March 2006, pages 1152–1156; *Journal of Burn Care and Rehabilitation*, November–December 2005, pages 515–524; *Journal of Pharmaceutical and Biomedical Analysis*, February 2005, pages 287–295; and *Planta Medica*, November 2004, pages 1052–1057.)

HESPERIDIN

Hesperidin is a flavonoid found in various plants such as citruses and evening primrose oil. It has potential as a potent antioxidant (as in reducing the effects of sun damage), and in the prevention of some cancers. It is also taken orally to improve circulation and to strengthen capillaries. There is no published research showing that it combats cellulite. (Sources: *Photochemistry and Photobiology*, September 2003, pages 256–261; *Phytotherapy Research*, December 2001, pages 655–669; and *Anticancer Research*, July–August 1999, pages 3237–3241.)

MALVA SYLVESTRIS EXTRACT

From a plant also known as Blue Mallow Flower, this extract may have some anti-inflammatory and soothing properties for the skin, as well as some potential antioxidant benefits. Its effects on cellulite are unknown. (Sources: www.naturaldatebase.com; *International Journal of Food Sciences and Nutrition*, February 2004, pages 67–74; and *Journal of Ethnopharmacology*, January 2004, pages 135–143.)

PANAX GINSENG ROOT EXTRACT

This root extract may have potent antioxidant properties (with anti-cancer potential) and may promote wound healing. Whether or not it can have an impact on cellulite is unknown. (Sources: *Journal of Agricultural and Food Chemistry*, April 2006, pages 2558–2562; *Phytotherapy Research*, January 2005, pages 65–71; *Archives of Pharmacal Research*, February 2002, pages 71–76; and *Cancer Letters*, March 2000, pages 41–48.)

PAULLINIA CUPANA SEED EXTRACT

Also called guarana, the primary use of this extract in herbal supplements and beverages is as a stimulant. In animal studies using mice, it has been shown to affect fat metabolism. There is also research showing that repeated use of guarana can result in persistent increases in heart rate and blood pressure as well as unfavorable actions on glucose and potassium homeostasis. Such effects could be detrimental in persons with hypertension, atherosclerosis, or glucose intolerance—conditions that are strongly associated with obesity. Guarana is sometimes used in cellulite products because of its theophylline and caffeine components. Research has shown it can be absorbed into the skin. Whether or not topical application can affect fat metabolism or have other associated health risks in humans is not known. (Sources: *Food and Chemical Toxicology*, June 2006, pages 862–867; *International Journal of Pharmaceutics*, April 2006; www.sciencedirect.com/; *Clinical Nutrition*, December 2005, pages 1019–1028; and *Clinical Pharmacology & Therapeutics*, June 2005, pages 560–571.)

PISUM SATIVUM

That's the Latin name for the garden pea, and while the plant does have antioxidant activity there is no research showing it can reduce cellulite. (Source: *Phytotherapy Research*, October 2003, pages 987–1000.)

PLECTRANTHUS BARBATUS EXTRACT

Also known as Forskolin or *Coleus barbatus*, this herb has information showing it to have cardiovascular and bronchial benefits. There is a small amount of research demonstrating Forskolin can stimulate lipolysis in these cells and that it also inhibits glucose uptake by fat cells when taken as a supplement. However, there is no information showing this effect on fat cells when applied topically. (Sources: www.naturaldatabase.com; and Memorial Sloan Kettering Cancer Center, *About Herbs*, www.mskcc.org/mskcc/html/11570.cfm.)

PORPHYRIDIUM CRUENTUM EXTRACT

This extract is derived from a type of red algae. There is research showing that components of red algae contain the omega-3 fatty acid eicosapentaenoic acid, the omega-6 fatty acid arachidonic acid, and other skin-friendly ingredients such as polysaccharides. Whether the entire red algae extract provides benefit on skin is not known. (Sources: *Bioseparation*, September 2000, pages 299–306; and *Free Radical Biology and Medicine*, February 1996, pages 241–249.)

RETINOIDS

If the layers of connective tissue beneath the skin on the thighs are indeed the main cause of cellulite (along with excess or poorly formed fat deposits), then improving skin structure should, theoretically, make a difference. There is growing evidence proving this to be the case. Retinol (the entire vitamin A molecule) or the prescription derivative tretinoin found in Renova or Retin-A, make up a group of ingredients known to help improve skin structure. When it comes to cellulite there are limited studies showing tretinoin to have benefit, though even then only a small improvement, but theoretically it should help and it's absolutely better than most other topical alternatives.

Of all the ingredients to look for in a cosmetic cellulite product, retinol should be at the top of the list. However, most cellulite products contain (at best) teeny amounts of retinol, and are often in packaging that won't keep this air-sensitive ingredient stable. One other point: Johnson & Johnson has a study showing the combination of retinol, caffeine, and ruscogenine can reduce the appearance of cellulite. Of course J&J-owned company RoC sells cellulite products with that combination of ingredients. (Sources: *Journal of Cosmetic Science*, July–August 2001, pages 199–210; *American Journal of Clinical Dermatology*, November–December 2000, pages 369–374; and *Journal of the European Academy of Dermatology & Venereology*, July 2000, page 251.)

RUSCOGENINE

An extract from the plant Butcher's Broom, ruscogenine has some research showing it to be effective when taken orally for improving the function of veins and capillaries. Whether or not it has benefit topically for cellulite isn't supported by independent research. (Sources: www.naturaldatabase.com; and *Journal of Alternative and Complementary Medicine*, June 2000, pages 539–549.)

SANTALUM ALBUM SEED EXTRACT

This is the Latin name for sandalwood extract, which is used in cosmetics as a fragrance. It can have antioxidant properties, and there is research showing it minimizes herpes breakouts. It also can be a skin irritant or sensitizer. Its effect on cellulite is unknown. (Sources: *Journal of Ethnopharmacology*, July 2000, pages 23–43; and *European Journal of Cancer Prevention*, August 1997, pages 399–401.)

TERMINALIA SERICEA EXTRACT

This extract has anti-inflammatory and antibacterial properties, but there is no research showing it to have any effect on the appearance of cellulite. (Sources: *Journal of Ethnopharmacology*, February 2005, pages 43–47; and *European Journal of Pharmaceutics and Biopharmaceutics*, March 2003, pages 191–198.)

ULVA LACTUCA EXTRACT

An extract from the plant known as Sea Lettuce, this has some anti-inflammatory and anti-oxidant properties for skin (Source: *Phytotherapy Research*, December 2000, pages 641–643). However, there is no research showing it to have any benefit for cellulite reduction.

UNCARIA TOMENTOSA EXTRACT

Also known as Cat's Claw, the plant has some research showing it to be an effective anti-inflammatory and antioxidant. There is also some evidence it may have cardiovascular effects by dilating peripheral blood vessels. It may also kill cancer cells without affecting normal cells (Sources: www.naturaldatabase.com; and *Journal of Ethnopharmacology*, February 2000, pages 115–126). Conversely, there is research showing it may increase the viability of some cancer cells (Source: *Pediatric Blood and Cancer*, January 2006, pages 94–98). Research showing it to have antioxidant or DNA-repairing benefits when applied topically has been presented by the Lauder Corporation (Source: *Phytotherapy Research*, March 2006, pages 178–183).

VISNAGA VERA EXTRACT

The extract from the plant *Ammi visnaga*, also known as khella, when taken orally, has caused some concern that it may cause nausea, dizziness, constipation, headache, itching, and insomnia. Khella may cause liver problems for some people. There is also some concern that it might cause photosensitivity since it contains khellin and furocoumarin. (Source: www.naturaldatabase.com.) It has no known benefit for cellulite reduction.

MESOTHERAPY

Mesotherapy is a procedure that has been claimed to dissolve fat from the repeated injection (and I mean lots and lots of injections) of various substances into the fat layers of skin. Mesotherapy actually got its start 50 years ago in France through the work of a physician who was trying to find a cure for deafness (Source: *Dermatological Times*, December 1, 2004). From there it gained notoriety in the United States after singer Roberta Flack appeared on ABC's 20/20 claiming mesotherapy helped her lose 40 pounds (although she said she also dieted and exercised, but what stood out for lots of people was the part that didn't involve diet and exercise).

Some of the substances being injected are homeopathic and some are pharmaceutical. Strangely, there isn't necessarily any consistency, and the cocktail of ingredients can vary from practitioner to practitioner. The fact that the material being injected isn't consistent and that not everyone discloses exactly what they are using makes this treatment very hard to evaluate. The most typically used substance in mesotherapy is phosphatidylcholine, but it can also be combined with deoxycholate. A handful of studies have shown that this can successfully reduce fat when injected into the skin, with one study demonstrating this for the undereye area. Theoretically, the reduction of subcutaneous fat may be caused by inflammatory-mediated cell death and resorption.

However, mesotherapy isn't without risk. Side effects included burning, erythema, and swelling at the injection site. In a few of the reliable studies that do exist, results are at best mixed with only about 50% of patients feeling they maintained improvement, 20% experienced some fading, and 30% had no benefit at all. Of course there is no way to no what other treatments, diet, or exercise these people used during the same period. There is concern that larger studies evaluating long-term safety and efficacy of phosphatidylcholine for cosmetic purposes are needed. Until further studies are performed, patients considering mesotherapy for cellulite must be aware that the substances currently being injected to treat this cosmetically undesirable situation have not been thoroughly evaluated for safety or efficacy.

Finding out if this would work for you would not be inexpensive. Mesotherapy costs $300–$500 for each treatment and about 10 to 15 sessions are recommended, so it ends up being more expensive than liposuction.

(Sources: *Dermatological Surgery*, April 2008, pages 529–542; *Journal of Cosmetic Dermatology*, December 2007, pages 250–257; *Journal of Cosmetic Laser Therapy*, December 2005, pages 147–154, and March 2005, pages 17–19; *Morbidity and Mortality Weekly Report*, November 2005, pages 1127–1130; *Aesthetic Plastic Surgery*, July–August 2003, pages 315–318; and *Plastic and Reconstructive Surgery*, July 2003, pages 162–170.)

ENDERMOLOGIE

Searching on the Internet, you would think endermologie was nothing less than a cure for cellulite. Physicians, spas, salons, and just about anybody else with the money to buy one of these machines want you to believe in their exaggerated, over-the-top claims. Endermologie is based on the unproven and illogical theory that deep massage can improve blood and lymph flow, which will thereby reduce cellulite. If you can massage cellulite away, why not roll it away? Of course you can't massage cellulite away, but it doesn't hurt to try, and, in a nutshell, that's the business of endermologie.

Developed in France in the 1980s, the FDA approved this high-powered, hand-held massage tool in 1998. It consists of two motorized rollers with a suction device; these are moved over the skin somewhat like a mix between an old-time wet-clothes wringer and a vacuum cleaner. (And just because the French invented this device doesn't mean they have solved their cellulite problems. European women are confounded by cellulite too, even though they tend not to have the weight problems Americans do. But remember, weight and cellulite are not directly related.)

While claims abound, legally those advertising endermologie treatment are only permitted to promote it for "temporarily improving the appearance of cellulite." Of course, somehow the word "temporarily" never is seen in the ads or Web sites promoting this device. Finding out if this works is time consuming and pricey. Anywhere from 10 to 20 treatments are recommended plus one or two maintenance visits per month are required to preserve any results. There is no typical cost, and depending on where you go prices can range from $75 to $200 per session.

In attempting to portray endermologie as a serious, effective treatment for cellulite, it is often presented as being FDA-approved as a Class I Medical Device, and therefore approved by the FDA for its intended purpose. While endermologie machines are indeed Class 1 Medical Devices, this has no meaning in terms of efficacy. Class I status is a designation indicating there is "minimal potential for harm to the user." No other aspect of the machine is approved or sanctioned by the FDA. According to the FDA (www.fda.gov), "Class I Medical Devices are subject to the least regulatory control…. Foreign establishments … are not [even] required to register their product with the FDA…. Examples of Class I devices include elastic bandages, examination gloves, and hand-held surgical instruments." The FDA attributes no efficacy value to endermologie machines. Whether these devices are harmful depends on how they are operated, meaning how aggressively they're used.

Despite the FDA's lack of recognition (and some warning letters admonishing those making false claims), you will often see lists of "studies" claiming to prove endermologie's effectiveness. Yet, some of these "studies" were neither published nor peer-reviewed. Rather, they were lectures presented worldwide at various medical conferences. These types of presentations are not studies. The information presented is one sided, and, more often than not, paid for by the company that owns the device, with the presenter receiving financial compensation for the endorsement. Such presentations are not held to the same scientific standard as published, peer-reviewed research. What you will certainly not see listed are the published studies indicating that endermologie doesn't work. (Sources: *Journal of Cosmetic and Laser Therapy*, December 2004, pages 181–185; *Plastic Reconstructive Surgery*, September 1999, pages 1110–1114; and *Aesthetic Plastic Surgery*, March 1998, pages 145–153.)

Regardless of conflicting evidence, endermologie and similar machines, such as ESC's Silhouette SilkLight Subdermal Tissue Massage System, are here to stay. It is an easy procedure to offer to clients and, for the most part, it seems to make women happy. Whether this is only psychological doesn't seem to matter. In the long run, complications are few and far between, so the only real downside is the potential waste of money, which doesn't stop those in the pursuit of perfection.

NON-ABLATIVE LASERS, LIGHT SYSTEMS, AND RADIO FREQUENCY

Intense pulsed light (IPL) is a consideration in the treatment of cellulite. The rationale for the use of IPL is based on the idea that it builds collagen, creating a thicker dermis, like that more typically seen in men—and men have less cellulite than women. Lasers may very well be the next generation in the world of cellulite therapies, but a lot more research is needed before this evolving treatment proves itself to be effective and worth the money. Ever since the FDA approved TriActive Laserdermology (Cynosure Inc, Chelmsford, MA) as a Class II medical device that "temporarily reduces the appearance of cellulite," lots of companies have wanted in on the action. TriActive combines a diode laser (at a wavelength of 810 nanometers) with localized cooling, suction, and mechanical massage (sort of a cross between a laser and an endermologie machine). In fact, much of the published research has been paid for or conducted by the companies manufacturing or selling these lasers (Source: *Journal of Drugs in Dermatology*, April 2008, pages 341–345).

Treatment protocols vary, but generally the process is done three times a week for two weeks followed by biweekly treatments for five weeks. A Class II medical device status indicates this laser can be sold and used without physician supervision, which means a growing number of salons and spas are advertising its success and changing the FDA classification of "temporarily reduces" to a more alluring "reduces" cellulite. (Sources: www.fda.gov/cdrh/pdf3/k030876.pdf; Securities and Exchange Commission Information, www.secinfo.com/dsvRx.z4y6.htm; and *Journal of Cosmetic and Laser Therapy*, June 2005, pages 81–85, and June 2004, pages 181–185.)

Another device approved by the FDA is the VelaSmooth system (Syneron Inc., Richmond Hill, Ontario, Canada), also called LipoLite. It combines near-infrared light at a wavelength of 700 nanometers, continuous wave radiofrequency, and mechanical suction. Twice-weekly treatments for a total of eight to ten sessions have been recommended. Each session usually costs around $200 or more. One of the only studies demonstrating this machine's efficacy included 20 women, and 18 of the 20 personally thought they saw improvement, yet the actual measurements only showed a 0.3-inch reduction in thigh circumference. Other research has been even more lackluster, or the studies were all questionable based on extreme bias, small panels, and no histological evaluation. These are hardly sweeping results by any standard, making it clear that larger-scale, more professional studies are needed, especially before you decide to spend $1,000 or more to see if these kinds of machines can get you what you want, namely smoother thighs, not a lighter wallet. (Sources: *Journal of Cosmetic Laser Therapy*, March 2007, pages 15–20, and December 2004, pages 187–190.)

Which to choose? Great question—but there's really no answer. Physicians always attest to the superiority of the machines they are using (but that changes as soon as they buy or rent a new one). In actuality, studies show most of these medical procedures have fairly equal results with no single machine having an edge over the other. (Source: *Lasers in Surgery and Medicine*, December 2006, pages 908–912.)

ELECTRICAL MUSCLE STIMULATORS AND IONTOPHORESIS DEVICES

According to www.quackwatch.com, "Muscle stimulators are a legitimate medical device approved for certain conditions—to relax muscle spasms, increase blood circulation, prevent blood clots, and rehabilitate muscle function after a stroke. But many health spas and figure-enhancing salons claim that muscle stimulators can remove wrinkles, perform face lifts, reduce breast size, reduce a 'beer belly,' and remove cellulite. Iontophoresis devices are prescription devices that use direct electric current to introduce ions of soluble salts (i.e., medications) into body tissues for therapeutic or diagnostic purposes. The FDA considers promotion of muscle stimulators or iontophoresis devices for any type of body shaping or contouring to be fraudulent." (Source: www.fda.gov/ora/fiars/ora_import_ia8901.html.)

BODY WRAPPING

Many salons and spas offer a cellulite/weight-loss service where the body is tightly wrapped or dressed in special garments with or without a "specialty" cream or lotion applied first. Promising to take inches off your body, these treatments may cost $65 to $500, with the range depending on the salon and if the clientele is elite enough to warrant the steep price. Scientific-sounding information makes this process seem legitimate, but in the long run all it is doing is temporarily compressing your skin. (You could probably do this yourself with plastic wrap.) The skin will then return to its original shape in a matter of time, with the duration depending on your skin's response. Impressive results often are delivered after measuring several parts of the body and adding up small, incremental changes; as a total, this ends up sounding far more impressive than it really is.

Infomercials, Internet sites, and some multilevel marketing companies sell at-home systems claiming to eliminate toxins and squeeze waterlogged fatty tissue dry. Luckily, you can't squeeze toxins out of a cell. While you may be able to squeeze water out of a cell, that same pressure would concurrently injure other cells, which isn't good for your skin. Plus, the water content would return to whatever level is natural for the body fairly soon due to homeostasis. All in all, there is no research whatsoever showing that body wrapping does anything positive, and it will not get rid of fat or cellulite (Source: Federal Trade Commission, www.ftc.gov/opa/2004/12/transdermal.htm).

SKIN PATCHES

According to the Federal Trade Commission (FTC), it "has continued its attack on bogus weight-loss claims by suing a diet patch manufacturer and a retailer that marketed the patch directly to Spanish-speaking consumers. In two separate federal court actions, the FTC charged that the patch manufacturer, Transdermal Products International Marketing Corporation, and the retailer, SG Institute of Health & Education, Inc., falsely claimed that the skin patch causes substantial weight loss. The FTC complaints in both cases also challenged false claims that the patch or its main ingredient, sea kelp, has been approved by the Food and Drug Administration (FDA). The FTC further alleged that Transdermal Products provided retailers with deceptive marketing materials that could be used to mislead consumers."

"The defendants in both cases allegedly used one or more of the seven bogus weight-loss claims that are part of the FTC's 'Red Flag' education campaign announced in December 2003. The ongoing Red Flag campaign provides guidance to assist media outlets and others in spotting false claims in weight-loss ads." According to the FTC, one of the most common false weight-loss claims is that diet patches, topical creams and gels, body wraps, and other products worn on the body or rubbed into the skin can cause substantial weight loss (Source: Federal Trade Commission, www.ftc.gov/opa/2004/12/transdermal.htm).

LIPOSUCTION

Liposuction has been used to reshape and reduce the appearance of accumulated fat layers and cellulite. However, the primary function of this procedure is to remove fat in localized areas, not cellulite. In cases where liposuction involves the removal of large quantities of stored fat, it can sometimes worsen the appearance of cellulite by creating unsupported and slackened skin, which will allow any remaining fat (and some always remains) to show through. Liposuction is an option, and for certain it will eliminate some amount of fat, but whether or not it gets rid of cellulite is not a sure thing.

CHAPTER 21
SOLUTIONS FOR WOUNDS, SCARS, OR STRETCH MARKS

THE BASICS

Follow the basic skin-care steps for your skin type or skin concern.

HOW SKIN HEALS

Whether it's a scratch, a paper cut, a scrape, cut, sore, lesion, or a really bad wound that requires stitches, one of the more amazing aspects of skin is its capacity to heal. Damaged skin regenerates and repairs itself. Only in certain circumstances, usually a result of some other illness such as diabetes, is that not true. When skin is injured, a multifaceted and complicated number of reactions take place. Many factors affect how long a wound takes to heal, and the way the wound heals affects how the skin will look, meaning what kind of scar will result. And that's not to say a scar is a bad thing—rather it's a sign that the body's repair system has kicked in so the fissure in your skin, no matter how small or big, closes up and mends.

Basically, skin goes through three fundamental and essential stages of repair. In the first stage, the scab is formed, and it's almost always accompanied by swelling, redness, and some tenderness or even pain. During the next stage, new skin tissue is formed under the scab. The final stage involves the rebuilding and reforming of the outer and inner layers of skin. Each of these stages of skin repair needs different kinds of help to aid in the healing process. What you do during the first days of a wound versus what you do after the scab has formed, or when the scab eventually comes off, is vital to the final appearance of the skin.

Stage 1, Inflammation. As soon as a cut or break in the skin has occurred, the body begins its job of preventing further injury. Signals are sent out for the blood to begin clotting and to call skin cells in to start protecting the damaged area. While the skin is working on its initial repair response, the immune system is trying to remove any foreign matter or bacteria that may have invaded the injury.

Stage 2, Regrowth. Now the body is busy producing collagen and reforming the substances that constitute the intercellular matrix. Intense collagen growth and the tightening of the surrounding tissue are the reason why we see an edge around a wound while a scab is being formed.

Stage 3, Renewal. With the inflammatory reaction calmed, and after the new skin tissue in the form of a scab and then a scar has been achieved during regrowth, it is time for the skin to focus on returning to normal. As time passes the scar becomes less noticeable and redness decreases. Then the skin texture normalizes, though it may not do so every time.

The way your body goes about this process is genetically determined. Nevertheless, outside influences can also affect the way your skin responds to being injured.

WHAT TO DO WHEN YOUR SKIN IS INJURED

Does applying aloe, vitamin E, or one of a variety of marine plants from algae to seaweed help heal wounds, prevent scars, or reduce the scarring you already have? There's no single substance or product that can address the complex issue of wound healing and scars, but there is a sensible plan you can follow to minimize scarring as much as possible. Although aloe and algae can't hurt a scar and may indeed be helpful, what is more important is the overall way you treat the wound from its first moments, when the skin is injured, to the end, when the scar has formed.

Skin's unique, but unfortunate, response to injury is scarring. But skin, almost miraculously, also regenerates quickly, essentially renewing itself in two to four weeks. Depending on your genetic makeup and the depth of the injury, scarring can range from a slightly reddish discoloration to a thick, raised red or darkened scar (described as hypertrophic or keloidal), to serious disfigurement. Even so, the way you initially take care of a wound makes all the difference in the world.

Whether it is from acne, getting cut, or an operation, when skin damage first occurs you should allow it to "breathe" as much as possible. Do not gunk up the area with creams, lotions, or vitamin E from capsules. Rubbing creams and lotions on a wound can damage fragile skin in the first stages of healing. Keep the damaged skin clean (but don't overclean it); using a gentle cleanser is the best way to do this. If you suspect there is a risk of infection, consider using an over-the-counter antibacterial such as Bacitracin.

At this stage, a lightweight gel or liquid that includes antioxidants and anti-irritants can help a great deal, but *little* is the operative word here. In the beginning, keep the injured site out of sunlight altogether, as opposed to loading up the area with sunscreen.

Heavy creams will suffocate the skin and prevent it from healing. Once the wound is healed, keep it out of sunlight as much as possible. After that, remember it's imperative to protect the area with sunscreen. Sun damages skin and doesn't promote healing. Smoking is a skin destroyer and will also prevent healthy healing of wounds.

Here's what to do when you have a wound:

1. Wounds or lesions that don't require immediate medical attention (that is, if the wound does not require stitches and is not a chronic non-healing ulcer) should not be completely or heavily covered or occluded when the damage first occurs (Source: *Archives of Dermatological Research*, November 2001, pages 491–499). After cleansing, it is best to cover the wound with a light, thin bandage. In other words, avoid heavy bandages, creams, salves, or oils, which can all impair the skin's initial healing process. Depending on where the wound or lesion is, it can be OK to wear a very lightweight bandage during the day or very lightweight moisturizers to protect the skin from getting reinjured. But if you don't have a lightweight bandage, take the coverings off at night or apply a lotion that lets air get to the wound.

2. Let a scab form and don't pick or touch it—ever! Any manipulation or removal is a serious impediment to the healing that is taking place underneath and can cause scarring that would otherwise not have taken place.

3. Do not soak the lesion in water. Too much moisture saturation prevents wound healing.

4. It is important to keep the wound clean to prevent infection. Using a gentle cleanser is essential. Topical Bacitracin is an option if you suspect a risk of infection, but use it minimally because it is very thick and occlusive and can prevent air from getting to the wound.

5. Do not irritate the skin! The skin's primary, natural reaction to a wound is inflammation, which makes blood surge to the area to aid in healing. However, inflammation must be kept to a minimum and it should not be exacerbated since that can further damage skin. Anything you do to irritate the skin more makes matters worse. That means no soaps (they're too drying), no highly fragrant products (fragrant plant extracts and synthetic fragrances are all irritating), and, as always, no alcohol, peppermint, menthol, citrus, eucalyptus, clove, camphor, or mint. If the wound in on the hand, be careful handling citrus, mint, and spices while cooking.

6. Use sun protection! Leaving a wound unprotected to sun exposure impedes the skin's healing process *and* causes further skin damage.

7. If you do want to apply something soothing to the skin, use a very lightweight moisturizing lotion or pure aloe vera gel. Aloe's benefit for wound healing is mostly anecdotal; however, because aloe allows skin to breathe and can be soothing, it is still a great option to consider in the beginning. A moisturizer with antioxidants is the best way to help the wound continue healing.

AFTER THE WOUND HAS HEALED

After the wound has healed you can use slightly more emollient products with antioxidants to keep free-radical damage to a minimum. Sunscreens in a light, moisturizing base are essential, not only to keep the skin moist but also to allow the skin to continue healing. There is some evidence that AHAs, BHA, and tretinoins (such as Retin-A, Renova, Tazorac, Avita, and generic tretinoin) can significantly reduce the appearance of scarring by exfoliating the surface skin (using AHAs) and by stimulating normal cell production (using tretinoin). Exfoliation can reduce the thick, discolored appearance of scar tissue. Tretinoins, over time, *may* help generate collagen production to possibly shore up some of what was lost from the injury.

Exfoliation, antioxidants, and sunscreens can all help minimize scarring after the skin has healed. None of them will get rid of a scar, but the possibility of greatly reducing the appearance of a scar is not to be ignored. Basically, there are no miracle skin-care ingredients or products when it comes to healing skin or reducing the appearance of scars.

Instead, practice good skin care: Don't overmanipulate the site, protect it from the sun, keep the area disinfected, keep heavy emollients off the skin, and, as much as possible, let the skin handle its own healing process.

As to nutritional issues, research shows that these definitely play a factor in healing wounds and scars. A diet high in antioxidants and omega-3 and omega-6 fatty acids can have an overall significant benefit. For a list and description of oral supplements that have been shown to help heal wounds and scars, visit the Web site www.drweil.com.

The following list describes topical factors to enhance healing wounds and scars. The most important thing, both for healing a wound and trying to improve the scar's appearance, is patience. It can take up to two years or longer depending on the depth of the lesion or wound, and it can depend on how diligent you are about caring for your skin with the following steps:

1. Once the skin has healed completely and the scab is gone, you can use nonfragrant plant oils or a lightweight moisturizer to keep the skin moist. The point here is to keep skin pliant and soft to help the skin's healing process (dry skin can fissure and tear, which can cause further skin damage). Topically applied vitamin E has not been shown to be of any special help in healing wounds or scars and may make matters worse.

2. Now that the skin is healed, it is helpful to remove the surface layers of skin where scar tissue may be forming. It is also helpful to improve skin-cell production, which may have been damaged from the wound. The damage, if any, is completely dependent on the depth of the lesion—meaning how many layers of skin were affected and how well you have left the scab alone. For gently removing the surface layers of skin, consider using an effective salicylic acid product (BHA is preferred over AHAs because BHA is composed of salicylic acid, which has anti-inflammatory properties, and reducing or preventing inflammation is essential for the healing process) as well as tretinoin (Retin-A, Renova, Tazorac, Avita) for improving cell production.

3. Once the wound or lesion is completely healed (this can take several months and up to two years), there are several options for dealing with the resulting scar. For surface discolorations and minor irregularities, microdermabrasion is an option. Acid peels (including AHA peels or trichloroacetic acid peels) as well as laser resurfacing are also significant options for reducing or eliminating scars.

4. If you have any concern about impaired healing or how the scar looks, it is important to see a dermatologist.

VITAMIN E FOR SCARS?

Let go of the long-held belief that vitamin E is a miracle ingredient for healing or scarring. If anything, the thick vitamin E in capsules or in heavy creams is occlusive and can be a problem. A report of research published in *Dermatologic Surgery* (April 1999, pages 311–315), in an article titled "The effects of topical vitamin E on the cosmetic appearance of scars" concluded that the "study shows that there is no benefit to the cosmetic outcome of scars by applying vitamin E after skin surgery and that the application of topical vitamin E may actually be detrimental to the cosmetic appearance of a scar. In 90% of the cases in this study, topical vitamin E either had no effect on, or actually worsened, the cosmetic appearance of scars.

Of the patients studied, 33% developed a contact dermatitis to the vitamin E. Therefore we conclude that use of topical vitamin E on surgical wounds should be discouraged."

Rather than worrying about one specific antioxidant, give the skin a blend of effective, non-irritating antioxidants in a gel or liquid form.

(Sources: *Journal of Drugs and Dermatology*, July 2008, pages S2–S6; and *Cancer Research*, December 2007, pages 11906–11913.)

KELOID AND HYPERTROPHIC SCARRING

Keloids are raised, thick scars that tend to extend past the original wound. Hypertrophic scars match the area of the wound and are flat, red, and somewhat swollen. Both keloids and hypertrophic scars are an area of frustration for the people who have them as well as physicians because there is no universally accepted treatment protocol. Keloid and hypertrophic scars result from abnormal and excessive collagen buildup as a wound heals. Why this happens is unclear, although it occurs more often in darker skin tones than lighter skin tones. These scars can range from presenting an unsightly problem to actually being disfiguring. Prevention is the number one solution for keloid and hypertrophic scars. Hypertrophic scars usually resolve on their own while keloids present a difficult challenge.

Once a raised scar is present, there are a several treatments to choose from. Hypertrophic scars and keloids have been shown to respond to pressure therapy, cryotherapy (where liquid nitrogen is used to freeze off the scar), cortisone injections into the scar, topical silicone dressings, pulsed-dye laser treatment, interferon, and laser resurfacing. Simple surgical excision is usually followed by recurrence unless other topical therapies are used, such as tretinoin, AHAs, and BHA (Source: *Plastic and Reconstructive Surgery*, August 2002, pages 560–571). Unfortunately, even with all these options recurrence is likely, so maintenance—including gentle skin care—is essential.

An extensive, detailed list of the various treatments available can be found at www.emedicine.com, "Keloid and Hypertrophic Scar," http://emedicine.medscape.com/article/1057599-overview.

Scar massage is not recommended because, while it can break down the material in the skin creating the raised scar, the massage can also stimulate collagen production, which caused the scar in the first place.

SILICONE SHEETS FOR KELOIDAL SCARRING

Aside from tretinoin, AHAs, BHA, and antioxidants, one way to consider treating raised scars is with a pliable sheet of silicone. Some examples of silicone sheets are ReJuveness ($39.50 to $95, depending on the size) and Syprex Scar Sheet ($20 to $40 depending on the size). It is not clear how these sheets of silicone work. They may increase the amount of water in the scar, and continuous rehydration of scars may soften the tissue, making it more elastic and pliable, thus encouraging the flattening process. (Sources: *Dermatologic Surgery*, November 2007, pages 1291–1302; and *European Journal of Dermatology*, December 1998, pages 591–595.)

There is also research that has challenged the effectiveness of these sheets. The clinical trials performed were described as either of poor quality or highly susceptible to bias, meaning they were paid for by the companies selling the sheets (Source: *Cochrane Database of Systematic Reviews*, January 2005, CD003826).

If you decide to give silicone sheets a try, there are disadvantages to think about. Users purchase one relatively inexpensive sheet of silicone that is worn over and over again. The sheet must be kept clean, which requires care and maintenance time. Most importantly, the sheet must be worn over the scar for prolonged periods of time, so you might not want to wear one on your face or other exposed parts of your body, at least not during the day. Also, the silicone sheet can stick to the skin and skin reactions such as rashes or irritation can occur.

As mentioned, you must wear the sheet for two to three months or longer for 12 to 24 hours a day to see a difference. But patience can pay off. The longer you wear it, the more likely it is that the scar will dissipate to some extent. Of course, these sheets work best over new scars, but they can make a difference with old ones, too. Even acne scarring—thick, raised scars, not pits—can be reduced if the scars have been present for less than 16 years. Do not try these if you are hoping for extraordinary results, of the kind the advertising implies. Dr. Loren Engrav, associate director and Chief of Plastic Surgery for the University of Washington burn unit at Harborview Medical Center, explains that the "silicone strips are standard treatment for helping reduce scars, and though the results may be good, they are absolutely not a miracle."

Some women buy silicone sheets to use over stretch marks, but there is no clinical evidence that this product will have any effect on them whatsoever. These sheets create a flattening process, while a raising process is what would be required for stretch marks.

STRETCH MARKS

Whether from pregnancy, weight loss, or growth spurts, the striated tracks, resembling a swatch of tire tread, that can show up on skin are frustrating to women (and lots of men, too, especially those who've lost a lot of weight). Despite cosmetics advertising to the contrary there are no solutions or preventive treatments for this problem (Sources: *Clinical Dermatology*, March–April 2006, pages 97–100). All the lotions and potions in the world, all the cocoa butter or shea butter or aloe vera you can slather on won't alter one stretch mark on any part of your body. That doesn't mean there aren't options, but research shows the results are not always what we hope they will be.

Non-ablative laser and IPL (Intense Pulsed Light) procedures and chemical peels can have benefit, but they are expensive and require multiple treatments. Moreover, the research is not exactly conclusive as to how much benefit can be derived. If your expectations are reasonable these are worth a discussion with your dermatologist. (Sources: *Dermatology Surgery*, May 2008, pages 686–691; *Aesthetic and Plastic Surgery*, May 2008, pages 523–530; and *Journal of Cosmetic Laser Therapy*, June 2007, pages 79–83.)

Topical tretinoin also can have benefit if it is applied as soon as the stretch mark is noticed. (Sources: *Experimental Dermatology*, December 2003, S35–S42; *Advances in*

Therapy, July–August 2001, pages 181–186; and *Archives of Dermatology*, May 1996, pages 519–526.)

While these studies show promise for improving the appearance of stretch marks, the word "improve" needs to be qualified. These studies were done on a small sampling of women and the improvement was evaluated as good, but the stretch marks did not disappear. What does show the most promise for reducing or even eliminating the appearance of stretch marks is laser resurfacing or chemical peels.

NEEDLING

Skin needling (also known as needle dermabrasion or percutaneous collagen induction) began in 1997 as a simple, fast, relatively inexpensive method for safely treating wrinkles. Subsequently it was found that for some types of scarring and acne scars you can have some amount of improvement (Source: *Plastic and Reconstructive Surgery*, April 2008, pages 1421–1429).

This procedure involves using very small needles (less than 0.25 millimeter) to pierce skin at or near the dermis. This controlled wounding of skin is said to stimulate collagen production, which can have a plumping effect that is supposed to improve the appearance of acne scars; the enhanced collagen production is claimed to slightly raise depressed scars. As with most medical corrective procedures, including light-emitting devices (Intense Pulsed Light therapy) and lasers, multiple treatments are required for needling before results are seen.

Needling procedures involve a topical anesthetic applied to skin beforehand so the procedure should be minimally painful, but that is not always the case depending on your own sensitivities. Side effects include redness, minor bleeding, swelling, bruising, flaking, small scabs at the injection site that have a brownish appearance, and short-term hyperpigmentation. Those side effects aren't much different from what can be expected after treatment with lasers or Intense Pulsed Light (IPL).

So is needling a good option? The research on this topic is at best sparse, so whether it is worth the investment is hard to tell at this point. What you need to be wary of, aside from the lack of published medical research proving skin needling is a viable option for improving collagen production and lessening the appearance of scars, is that the procedure can be performed by tattoo artists and aestheticians—meaning medical supervision isn't required. That puts your skin at greater risk for complications, either from using nonsterilized or nondisposable needles, or from the lack of medical backup should complications (such as a skin infection) arise. Also, there are no standards for doing this procedure, unlike the guidelines involved with the use of various chemical peels, lasers, and light-emitting devices. How would a consumer know if the person doing the needling is going too deep, inserting needles haphazardly rather than in a precise manner, or has legitimate credentials?

What makes needling more tempting than other procedures is that it is less costly than, say, Fraxel or other laser treatments or chemical peels to improve scarring. However, the lack of standards and absence of research proving its efficacy should give anyone pause. Surprisingly, some companies sell needle-rolling devices consumers can purchase to use at home. Now that's a scary thought! I've seen some of these devices and can only imagine the damage consumers could inflict if they use them improperly or too often. Once again, there's no solid proof that this is a great way to stimulate collagen production to the extent that acne or other types of scarring is significantly or even minimally improved. And at-home use could also very well lead to bacterial infections and other nasty skin issues that, you guessed it, would assuredly require medical attention.

Some people have posted before-and-after pictures on the Internet after having skin needling done (over a period of several months) and the results, I'm sad to say, aren't visually encouraging. The bottom line is that various laser devices, chemical peels, and light-emitting devices have a much better, substantiated track record of offering notable improvement for acne scars (among other skin issues). Until similar research comes to light on skin needling, it is not a practice I recommend, regardless of the facility you're considering.

MEDERMA

Mederma Skin Care for Scars ($35 for 1.76 ounces) is an overadvertised, overhyped cosmetic preparation claiming to improve the appearance of scarring. Onion extract is supposed to be the scar-changing ingredient in a formula that is as mundane and ordinary as you can get; it includes water, thickeners, onion extract, fragrance, and preservative. There is no research showing onion extract to be effective as a skin-care ingredient.

An article in the *Archives of Dermatology* (December 1998, pages 1512–1514, "Snake oil for the 21st century") from the Department of Dermatology, Harvard Medical School, stated that "With the current promulgation of skin 'products' and their promotion and even sale by dermatologists, and the use of treatments of no proven efficacy, this association between dermatology and quackery is set to continue well into the 21st century. The list of offending treatments includes silicone gel sheets and onion extract cream (Mederma) for keloids...."

Another study (Source: *Cosmetic Dermatology*, March 1999, pages 19–26) concluded that there were no discernable differences between skin treated with Mederma and skin that was treated with a placebo. Nevertheless, Mederma advertises itself as promising to get rid of scars.

More recently, a study in *Dermatologic Surgery* (February 2006, pages 193–197) concluded in a "side-by-side, randomized, double-blinded, split-scar study, the onion extract gel [Mederma] did not improve scar cosmesis or symptomatology when compared with a petrolatum-based ointment."

A customer service representative for Mederma told me that the onion extract "prevents the release of histamines which causes scarring." Even if onions could prevent the release of histamines, in reality histamines have everything to do with allergic reactions, and nothing whatsoever to do with what causes scarring. The body produces histamines in response to an allergic reaction; the body sends them in to fight the allergen that causes the redness, swelling, and itching. While histamines can cause the skin to react, that does not inhibit scar reaction. If anything, because onions release a complex mixture of sulfur-containing oils together with sulfur-free aldehydes and ammonia, all of which are more or less intensely volatile (that's what makes your eyes burn and tear when you cut into them), onion extract may be a skin irritant.

WHAT ABOUT SCARS FROM ACNE?

Severe and even mild acne can often lead to some form of scarring. A permanent scar is a defect in the skin caused by an injury to the area, such as an acne lesion. The key word here is "permanent." Most of the acne lesions that people call scars are really not scars at all, but instead post-inflammatory redness—red spots left behind after the blemish heals. What is frustrating about this redness is that it takes time for it go away—anywhere from 6 to 12 months, depending on the depth of the original lesion and how you cared for the lesion. However, there are ways to facilitate healing. Following the guidelines for treating wounds that were presented in the earlier sections of this chapter will make a huge difference in the way the skin heals.

Permanent scars develop as the skin attempts to heal itself by surrounding the acne lesion with new skin. The epidermis (outer layer of skin) grows in from the sides to the center, and underneath the sebaceous gland. When the acne finally heals, a depressed pit can remain in the skin. Scarring is unpredictable—it's impossible to know how much a particular person will scar, if at all. The best way to prevent acne scarring is through early, consistent treatment of lesions.

The best way to prevent scars is to not do anything that makes matters worse. Untreated or improperly treated acne is likely to cause the worst scarring because the problem is never mitigated and the skin has no chance to heal. Harshly attacking blemishes and creating deep scabs and sores that take a long time to heal are surefire ways to guarantee that a scar will be permanent. Using heavy or irritating facial products will also hinder the healing process. In addition, because many women don't know how to treat acne, they use ineffective topical disinfectants and exfoliants, which can also impede the skin's ability to repair itself. Unprotected sun exposure can exacerbate scarring, too. Yet, if you are good about not picking and oversqueezing blemishes from the outset, scarring can be greatly reduced. Even so, the most meticulous state-of-the-art acne skin-care routine can still result in scars. Most acne scars do fade with time, but that time can seem like an eternity when the face is yours.

Once acne and breakouts have been reduced or eliminated, the brown, pink, or purple discolorations left by acne lesions can fade a great deal in about 6 to 12 months, depending on your skin color. You can speed up that fading by continuing to use a product with AHAs, BHA, or tretinoin (which are all helpful in the treatment of acne and breakouts anyway).

Skin-lightening lotions with hydroquinone or other skin-lightening ingredients do not work on acne scarring. These lotions prevent melanin production; they do not have much effect on what gives acne scars their reddish to purple or brown color.

Once acne has healed, small areas with shallow scars or pit-type scars can be injected with dermal fillers (various substances used to lift or fill the depression), but these are not permanent fixes and require repeated treatments.

Chemical peels such as salicylic acid (beta hydroxy acid—BHA), alpha hydroxy acids (AHAs), and trichloroacetic acids (TCAs) can improve the appearance of surface scarring. (However, these peels are unwarranted for scarring if the acne is still active.) Just don't expect an AHA or BHA peel to improve the appearance of deep scarring. For larger areas of the face, laser resurfacing is absolutely the treatment of choice. (Sources: *Facial and Plastic Surgery*, November 2001, pages 253–262; and *Aesthetic Plastic Surgery*, January–February 2001, pages 46–51.)

CHAPTER 22
SOLUTIONS FOR ALLERGY-PRONE SKIN

THE BASICS
Follow the steps for your skin type or skin concern.

WHAT IS HAPPENING?

Allergic reactions occur when our skin encounters a particular ingredient or combination of ingredients, and it could be any allergen, from dust to mites and plant pollen. At that point the immune system decides whether or not it should accept, reject, or ignore the substance. If the body determines that the substance is unwanted, even when no allergic response existed before, all of a sudden it produces histamines to get rid of it.

Reactions can be subtle, such as a little itching, minor redness and swelling, or small, rashlike pimples. They can also involve a full-blown flare-up that causes intense, but temporary, discomfort and an unsightly appearance, and can even trigger a chronic condition requiring medical attention. If you have a tendency toward allergic reactions, your skin's condition can be greatly affected and you will have to pay close attention to what you use. Someone with allergy-prone skin needs to use fewer products, and the products should have shorter ingredient lists.

WHAT CAN YOU BE ALLERGIC TO?

Just about everything and anything. I would love to list ingredients that I could guarantee won't cause your skin to have an allergic reaction, but there is no single ingredient or combination of ingredients that can live up to that sweeping claim. Why not? Because everyone is biochemically different, each of us has a unique chemical makeup, and the endless paradoxical differences in the way our bodies perform is why we can react so differently when exposed to the same thing.

Because of the almost limitless combination of ingredients in all sorts of cosmetic formulations, it is truly impossible to know if, when, or how anyone's skin will react to any cosmetic. Your only recourse, and this is not the best news, is to keep experimenting until you find what works for you.

If you do get a reaction, stop using the product immediately. The next step would be to try an over-the-counter cortisone cream, which can offer almost immediate relief. If the reaction persists, you would need to consult your physician.

Finally, be patient. If you do have an allergic reaction, wait until it subsides before you venture out to try something new or different. Pare down to the absolute basics, usually just cleanser and a touch of moisturizer over very dry areas, try a bit of over-the-counter cortisone cream to reduce irritation, and stay out of the sun.

HYPOALLERGENIC?

Is there one line of cosmetics that's best for sensitive or allergy-prone skin? It would be great if there were, but it just doesn't exist. Hypoallergenic has always been a completely inane term given that no one knows what anyone is going to be allergic to. There are no agreed-upon standards or regulations that establish what ingredients are of concern, so any cosmetics company can stick the hypoallergenic claim on a label with nothing to back it up.

Allergic skin reactions are amazingly random and dissimilar. What you're sensitive to often has little to do with what someone else reacts to, and beyond that there's the intricate interaction of ingredients being combined on the face. The culprit may not be the product you think caused the problem. You may think a new moisturizer made your eyes swell, but it could be the resins from that reliable nail polish you were wearing in combination with the new moisturizer that triggered the problem.

WHAT YOU CAN DO

Aside from figuring out what you are allergic to and calming the allergic reaction, the same skin-care recommendations this book describes apply here as well. Doing what you can to reinforce the skin's barrier by giving the skin the substances it needs to repair, restore, and protect skin cells is essential to reduce the damage caused by allergic reactions. That means your skin needs the same antioxidants, skin-identical ingredients, and cell-communicating ingredients as anyone else. Just as a good diet doesn't change in terms of what's healthy, the same is true for good skin care. Of course you don't want to use some substances, even if they are healthy, if you are allergic to them. So that is part of experimenting to find the products that work best for you. What works best are those ingredients that are beneficial for skin, and you just need to find the ones that make your skin feel the best!

When it comes to dealing with allergy-prone skin you have to be a detective. Here is what you need to do when you have allergy-prone skin:

1. Primarily you need to be certain you are dealing with an allergy or sensitizing reaction to a product, and not with a skin disorder or irritation. Many skin conditions such as psoriasis, rosacea, eczema, folliculitis (an inflammation of the hair follicle), and reactions to food can account for the skin becoming irritated, swollen, red, itchy, flaky, or rashy. Irritating skin-care ingredients can cause an occurrence that looks like an allergic reaction but is not the same thing. A great resource for identifying whether what is occurring on your face is a skin disorder is the Primary Care Dermatology Atlas at www.dermatlas.org, where you can search over 10,000 images of skin problems. This gives you a way to identify whether or not your skin is similar in appearance to the images found for a particular skin disorder.

2. It would be great if you could find what product(s) or ingredient(s) are causing the problem and stop using them. Sometimes that is a simple enough procedure. If you started using a new concealer and within a few hours that area became red, itchy, and swollen, it would be clear that the concealer is the problem and you would stop using it. Unfortunately, it isn't always that easy. Even after you've stopped using the offending item or items, your skin can remain rashy, reddened, flaky, dry, swollen, and irritated for days—and for some, even months. There is no known medical reason why some skin types can't shake an allergic reaction while others improve immediately after the allergen is no longer applied.

3. For some unknown reason your skin can develop an allergic reaction over time. Further, given the number of cosmetic products women use daily, each one containing a disparate range of ingredients, it is no wonder that pinning down exactly which one caused the problem can be a challenge. To make matters even more complicated, it may not be a single product but the combination of products worn one over the other that caused the problem (maybe the concealer isn't the problem, but the mix of concealer, foundation, and moisturizer together that sparked the reaction). The key is to be patient and diligent, experimenting with the item or items you suspect and then watching how your skin responds when you discontinue using them.

4. Whether or not you've been able to identify the problem product, an over-the-counter cortisone cream can be your skin's best friend. Lanacort or Cortaid are excellent over-the-counter cortisone creams that function as anti-inflammatories. When either of these are applied to irritated, inflamed skin they can turn off the reaction that is causing the problem. It is essential to be conscientious about using these on a regular, methodical (though short-term) basis while your skin is having problems. For example, once the skin irritation shows up, keep applying the cortisone cream over the affected area for several days, even a day or two after everything seems back to normal. Remember that the skin can hold onto a sensitizing or allergic reaction for a long period of time, even after you've stopped using the offending product. And don't be afraid about the short-term use of an over-the-counter cortisone cream. It is the long-term, consistent use (for more than two or three months) of cortisone creams that can damage collagen and elastin in the skin, not short-term use.

5. While you are combating the allergic or sensitizing reaction, do not use any other skin irritants of any kind over the affected area. Fragrances, scrubs, washcloths, AHAs, Retin-A, Renova, benzoyl peroxide, skin lighteners, or other skin-care products with active or abrasive ingredients can trigger skin irritation and will only add to the problem.

6. Avoid saunas, steam, sweating (if possible), or rubbing the affected area, all of which can help re-trigger the reaction and further weaken the skin's barrier.

7. Finally, if matters don't improve after four to six weeks, or if the reaction is severe from the beginning, you should see your dermatologist for an evaluation.

8. If you suspect that you are having a serious allergic reaction (in the form of hives, extremely swollen skin and eyes, or red patches over the skin that feel warm or tingle), consult your physician to discuss varying options. Prescription-strength topical cortisone, oral cortisone, or oral antihistamines may be necessary.

CHAPTER 23
SHOULD YOU GET A FACIAL?

WHAT DOES A FACIAL DO?

That's a great question yet one that's very hard to answer because it all depends on the spa and the aesthetician. Often facials are nothing more than a series of masks and fancy machines that provide no benefit for skin other than feeling relaxing and knowing you're being pampered. Claims of getting rid of wrinkles, de-stressing, healing, cellulite removal, detoxing, and acne cures abound, yet almost without exception those services are a waste of time and money.

Many spas have very fancy-looking machines that use galvanic or some other wave energy, and claim these can drive a product's active ingredients deeper into the skin. Even if that were the case, and it isn't (there's not a shred of research showing that to be true; it has never been measured or evaluated), what's good about having those ingredients pushed farther into the skin? Antioxidants and cell-communicating ingredients, like any other worthwhile skin-care ingredients, don't work in a day. They also don't last: they are used up in a matter of hours. These ingredients have usefulness when they are applied twice a day and absorbed by skin. Depending on a single treatment would be just as problematic as eating a healthy meal only once a month.

Quality and professional capability are also factors to be wary of. Aestheticians are often poorly trained. They come out of beauty school with a cursory knowledge of hygiene, anatomy, and the same hype and misleading information rampant in the rest of the cosmetics industry. (I used to teach at a beauty school so I'm intimately aware of the limitations and what they want you to teach.) Once someone graduates from a beauty school they then seek a job at a spa or salon where they are further trained by the sales representative for the product lines being sold there. Turning your skin over to these "experts" is not a guarantee they're capable of helping your skin.

When do facials have value? It completely depends on what treatments the facialist or aesthetician does. Chemical peels, microdermabrasion, and extractions (removing stubborn blackheads and blemishes) are the procedures that offer the most long-term benefit.

While there are reasons to consider having a facial, there are no spa services that come close to duplicating the benefits of your daily skin-care regime and sunscreen. Applying a facial mask does not detox the face or change anything. It may be relaxing, but that's about it.

Let me emphasize the need to consult only a licensed aesthetician. Although "licensed" doesn't tell you anything about the capability of the aesthetician, it does mean the person has been trained in sanitation and application techniques and, more to the point, has been tested on those procedures and is certified to be able to accomplish those tasks. Of course, while that is just the beginning of what you should expect in the care of your skin, it is essential to know that your skin will be handled in as safe and hygienic a manner as possible.

WHAT SPA SERVICES MAKE SENSE?

By far the best procedures to consider from a facialist or aesthetician are microdermabrasion, AHA or BHA peels, and extractions. High-concentration alpha hydroxy acid peels and beta hydroxy acid peels can be extremely beneficial and can continue to show improvement for a period of time even after the procedure is finished. If you have an occasional or regular need to remove stubborn blackheads and deep-rooted blemishes, facials can indeed be helpful in improving the appearance of skin.

AHA peels at concentrations of 20% to 35% with a pH of 3.5, and beta hydroxy acid peels are extremely effective at providing a temporarily smooth appearance to the skin. That is within the ability of a good facialist, and the results can be very satisfying. But be extremely cautious. This is, at best, a controversial salon treatment. Many cosmetic surgeons and dermatologists (and the FDA) consider AHA peels unsafe when done by someone without medical training. That is an extremely rational concern, especially considering the wide disparity in training and licensing around the world and in the United States.

When it comes to acne, a reliable aesthetician can definitely soften the skin and safely remove blackheads and blemishes without scarring. In cases like these, there is every reason in the world to get a facial every six weeks to every other month. But please don't expect any of this to permanently stop breakouts. If anything, facialists can get carried away with applying creams and masks, and rubbing and wiping at the skin, which can stimulate the nerve endings, causing inflammation and increased oil production, and triggering breakouts and irritation.

Keep in mind that the skin-care products sold by facialists and spas are not any more effective or better formulated than those sold anywhere else. The ingredients used, the formulations, the packaging, and the performance of these spa or salon products are not unique in any way. Believing otherwise is just wasting your money and cheating your skin. If you don't really know what you are buying, or what the ingredient list is really telling you, then you are being sold on claims that don't make sense in the real world of physiology and biology.

MICRODERMABRASION

The Internet is rife with information about microdermabrasion. Some of it is backed by research, but a lot of it is sheer nonsense. Some of the research is actually meaningless, especially if it was done using a small group of women, wasn't done double- or single-blind, or if there was no histological evaluation. But this is how a process that is little more than a deep topical scrub has ended up being showcased as a solution to everything from wrinkles to acne, or being just as effective as laser resurfacing, other light devices, or chemical peels. That isn't the case, and there is no research supporting these distortions.

Microdermabrasion machines are FDA-approved Class I medical devices, which means they do not require any studies or proof that they are beneficial in any way. All it means is that the machine can be used; for example, Band-Aids are Class I medical devices. Microdermabrasion involves propelling a scrublike substance, most typically aluminum oxide crystals, onto the face at various speeds, then vacuuming off the debris using a specialized tube attached to the machine. The vacuum suction can be operated at various pressures, giving the operator the ability to control both the particle speed and suction at the skin surface. To prevent any damage to the eye area it is important that eye protection be used.

If you are interested in getting a facial, then microdermabrasion is one of the more compelling treatments to consider. It can play a role in helping skin look and feel better by removing a microscopically thin layer of surface skin. But it is not a miracle and it is pricey. A series of treatments on a regular basis is recommended, at rates that can range from $200 to $300 a session, so if you get it done once a month or every other month it adds up. And the results are not permanent; the smooth feeling most people experience afterward is short-lived, so then you have to do it again and again. You get the picture.

What results can you expect? That's a question that is hard to answer. Proponents and some research indicate a smoother appearance and feel to skin, temporary reduction in acne lesions, a general feel and look of healthier skin, and an overall improvement in dry skin. One positive side effect is that moisturizers can absorb better into skin, which can definitely improve skin texture and reduce water loss. Microdermabrasion is being evaluated for a potential role in helping topical medications absorb better. Whether microdermabrasion helps build collagen is unclear, but it does not change cell function or development.

Be aware there is no research showing that microdermabrasion gives better results than other salon treatments such as chemical peels, or medical treatments such as Thermage or IPL (Intense Pulsed Light). Most studies on the topic echo the same sentiment, which is that more research is needed to determine what benefit, aside from a glowing, smooth appearance, is gained from microdermabrasion.

Microdermabrasion should not be performed if you have any of the following problems: rosacea, surfaced capillaries, severe acne, warts, open wounds, skin rashes, psoriasis, or diabetes.

(Sources: *Journal of Cosmetic Laser Therapy*, December 2008, pages 187–192; *Natural Biotechnology*, November 2008, pages 1261–1268; *Seminars in Cutaneous Medicine and Surgery*, September 2008, pages 212–220; *Journal of Dermatologic Treatment*, August 2008, pages 1–6; and *Dermatologic Surgery*, June 2006, pages 809–814.)

LYMPH DRAINAGE

Along with the other viable and relaxing facial treatments out there, a whole host of facial masks and procedures that pass as premium skin care are just extensions of the same beauty myths that get repeated so often they have become truths in the mind of the consumer. Lymph drainage treatments are one of the many spa services that claim to rid the body of toxins, cellulite, wrinkles, and on and on. Lymph massage does have validity for those with lymphedema, a consequence of diseases such as cancer that require the removal of lymph nodes. However, the massage associated with lymphedema is not about "draining" lymph or removing toxins. Rather, it is about preventing the pooling of lymph into the extremities when the lymph system has been compromised in a given area.

The concept of draining lymph glands from the outside in to remove toxins makes as much sense as the idea of draining your hormonal system or blood system from the outside in. The lymph system carries our body's immune defenses. Lymph runs through the body like blood does, in veins and capillaries. You wouldn't want someone draining your blood or hormones (without lots of proof that it was safe and worthwhile), and the same goes for the lymph.

DETOXING THE SHAM OF DETOXING

Myths, much like anything else you hear or read about often enough, tend to become facts in the mind of many consumers. Once that happens they are eager to seek out the benefits of what amounts to little more than snake oil. The notion of purging toxins from the body and skin is one of these myths, on par with the perceived need to drink lots of water (and often too much water) to keep skin hydrated. Neither is based on fact.

And this isn't a conspiracy of the medical world, as many Web sites argue. (Actually, you could just as easily argue that the myth of detoxing is a conspiracy by those who take your money for bogus treatments and procedures.) But the medical world has nothing to gain from keeping someone from a treatment or medication that works. In fact the medical world discourages people from smoking and overeating, and encourages exercise and other beneficial behavior in the most direct campaigning possible, with solid research and studies on why you should follow their advice. If detoxing made sense, they would definitely have something to say, so it's no surprise the medical field hasn't jumped on the "let's purge toxins" bandwagon. If purging toxins from your body could help, then physicians would be at the forefront of getting the information out to you as soon as it was shown to be true. Doctors would make money from those treatments just as any other alternative service provider would. But truth doesn't always sell products. Oftentimes you'll get more people's attention, and dollars by promoting fiction-based fear instead.

When it comes to fiction, snake-oil salespeople are supreme at quick fixes and euphoria. I love the drink more water example, because if your water intake is greater than what your body needs all you do is go to the bathroom more. Nothing in your body changes. And it absolutely doesn't change the status of "toxins" in your body or how dry your skin is. Kids who don't drink enough water don't have dry skin because of it. Dry skin, for most adults, is the result of sun damage, genetics, health issues, certain medications, and their environment, not water intake. Believe me, I wish alleviating dry skin was as easy as increasing water intake!

In terms of skin and the purging of toxins, we move into the absurd. At least with routine (not excessive) water intake it does help to stay hydrated and not be thirsty. When it comes to purging toxins from the skin there isn't a particle of evidence it is even possible, let alone helpful. Yet somehow efforts to suck toxins out of your pores or between skin cells have become a basic part of many women's attempts to achieve flawless skin. As a result of this flawed belief, detoxifying the skin, a concept supported by the cosmetics industry or earnest spa attendants and aestheticians, as well as the vitamin/herbal supplement world, has become a sizable business.

WHAT TOXINS ARE BEING DETOXED?

Exactly what is a toxin? If you consult the dictionary it defines a toxin as any poison. So what poison is lurking in your skin needing removal? Again, there is no answer from anyone in any corner of the alternative cosmetics or herbal worlds. What you may hear are more general, vague terms such as bacteria, airborne pollutant particulates from cars and city life, bad fats (this is a big lie in cellulite treatments), or faulty lymph systems that build up who knows what. Even fast food and secondhand smoke require purging in this part of the cosmetics industry. Listening to all of this is enough to make some people want to live in a sterilized, airtight bubble for the sake of whole-body purity, but there's no need to take such a drastic step.

What isn't ever explained is exactly what is being eliminated when so-called toxins are being purged. No one has measured how much (of whatever stuff it may be) is supposedly being removed during the process of cleansing. The reason no one is doing such testing is because many consumers don't need facts to make decisions about their skin. And so we end up with a big myth that is good for business but not for you.

Without ever doing even basic testing, the people selling these detoxifying skin-care products or treatments leave it up to the consumer's imagination, and they are adept at creating imaginary, unspecified toxins that are causing wrinkles, open pores, oily skin—you name the skin-care complaint—and then suggesting that purging the skin is supposed to help. That expensive spa treatment that wraps your body in herbs, salts, fragrant oils, clay, or minerals might feel good and for a short time make your skin feel smooth, but in reality no skin condition has changed: your wrinkles haven't gone away, your cellulite is still there, your pores haven't changed, yet your pocketbook is lighter. Now that's what I call purging.

Many of these products claiming to detox the system, at least as far as the cosmetics industry and spa world are concerned, are fairly benign and do little, if any, harm. Overheating the body with saunas, Jacuzzis, and facial steaming can cause more problems than they help by damaging the skin's ability to hold moisture, causing capillaries to surface, and increasing oil production. Putting fragranced salts into your bath can irritate the vaginal skin lining. Not good news but not terrible. Mostly it is just a waste of money, and following myths is not the best recipe for good skin care.

SNAKE OIL AT ITS BEST

What has me concerned is some research I saw on really dangerous snake-oil type treatments, as reported on a blog/podcast site at http://skeptoid.com, which had several posts written by Brian Dunning, a computer scientist who debunks pseudoscience reports as a hobby (I confirmed that the content is accurate and all quoted material below is from the author's blog.)

Mucoid plaque is supposedly a toxin naturopaths and herbal charlatans say everyone has growing inside their bowels; in fact it is created by the pill sold to purge the plaque. In other words, the supposed cure is causing the problem, making people assume the malady is real.

What you get to cure mucoid plaque is a "bowel cleansing pill, said to be herbal, which causes your intestines to produce long, rubbery, hideous looking snakes of bowel movements, which they call mucoid plaque. There are lots of pictures of these on the Internet, and sites that sell these pills are a great place to find them. Look at www.DrNatura.com, www.BlessedHerbs.com, and www.AriseAndShine.com, just for a start.

"Imagine how terrifying it would be to actually see one of those come out of your body. If you did, it would sure seem to confirm everything these web sites have warned about toxins building up in your intestines. But there's more to it. As it turns out, any professional con artist would be thoroughly impressed to learn the secrets of mucoid plaque (and, incidentally, the term mucoid plaque was invented by these sellers; there is no such actual medical condition). These pills consist mainly of bentonite, an absorbent, expanding clay similar to what composes many types of kitty litter. Combined with psyllium, used in the production of mucilage polymer, bentonite forms a rubbery cast of your intestines when taken internally, mixed of course with whatever else your body is excreting. Surprise, a giant rubbery snake of toxins in your toilet.

"It's important to note that the only recorded instances of these 'mucoid plaque' snakes in all of medical history come from the toilets of the victims of these cleansing pills. No gastroenterologist has ever encountered one in tens of millions of endoscopies, and no pathologist has ever found one during an autopsy. They do not exist until you take such a pill to form them. The pill creates the very condition that it claims to cure. And the results are so graphic and impressive that no victim would ever think to argue with the claim."

Another detoxing gimmick I came across is about some electrical foot-bath products on the market. "The idea is that you stick your feet in the bath of salt water, usually with some herbal or homeopathic additive, plug it in and switch it on, and soak your feet. After a while the water turns a sickly brown, and this is claimed to be the toxins that have been drawn out of your body through your feet. One tester found that his water turned brown even when he did not put his feet in. The reason is that electrodes in the water corrode via electrolysis, putting enough oxidized iron into the water to turn it brown. When reporter Ben Goldacre published these results in the *Guardian Unlimited* online news, some of the marketers of these products actually changed their messaging to admit this was happening – but again, staying one step ahead – now claim that their product is not about detoxification, it's about balancing the body's energy fields: Another meaningless, untestable claim.

"But detoxifying through the feet didn't end there. A newcomer to the detoxification market is Kinoki foot pads, available at BuyKinoki.com and many drugstores. These are adhesive gauze patches that you stick to the sole of your foot at night, and they claim to 'draw toxins' from your body. They also claim that all Japanese people have perfect health, and the reason is that they use Kinoki foot pads to detoxify their bodies, a secret they've been jealously guarding from medical science for hundreds of years. A foolish claim like this is demonstrably false on every level, and should raise a huge red flag to any critical reader. Nowhere in any of their marketing materials do they say what these alleged toxins are, or what mechanism might cause them to move from your body into the adhesive pad.

"Kinoki foot pads contain unpublished amounts of vinegar, tourmaline, chitin, and other unspecified ingredients. Tourmaline is a semi-precious gemstone that's inert and not biologically reactive, so it has no plausible function. Chitin is a type of polymer used in gauze bandages and medical sutures, so naturally it's part of any gauze product. They probably mention it because some alternative practitioners believe that chitin is a 'fat attractor', a pseudoscientific claim which has never been supported by any evidence or plausible hypothesis. I guess they hope that we will infer by extension that chitin also attracts 'toxins' out of the body. Basically the Kinoki foot pads are gauze bandages with vinegar. Vinegar has many folk-wisdom uses when applied topically, such as treating acne, sunburn, warts, dandruff, and as a folk antibiotic. But one should use caution: Vinegar can cause chemical burns on infants, and the American Dietetic Association has tracked cases of home vinegar applications to the foot causing deep skin ulcers after only two hours.

"Since the Kinoki foot pads are self-adhesive, peeling them away removes the outermost layer of dead skin cells. And since they are moist, they loosen additional dead cells when left on for a while. So it's a given that the pads will look brown when peeled from your foot, exactly like any adhesive tape would; though this effect is much less dramatic than depicted on the TV commercials, depending on how dirty your feet are. And, as they predict, this color will diminish over subsequent applications, as fewer and fewer of your dead, dirty skin cells remain. There is no magic detoxification needed to explain this effect."

What remains indisputably true is that the country of Japan is not selling these toxin-purging foot pads like hotcakes, everyone is not using them, and the Japanese have health problems like any population.

Trying to eliminate wrinkles and other skin woes with false hopes that essentially involve throwing your money down the toilet on products that can't help doesn't really make sense. When there are brilliant things you really can do for your skin, wasting money isn't the way to go. Purging yourself of the myths the industry loves instigating and perpetuating, and learning what you really should do instead are the best ways to take care of your skin.

DERMATOLOGISTS IN THE SPA BUSINESS

Nowadays many dermatologists' offices have become spa centers offering many of the same services a salon or spa would, such as light chemical peels, microdermabrasion, and even facials (applying masks to the skin), waxing, and manicures. Going to a doctor's office for these kinds of spa procedures can be pricey because you end up paying a premium for getting it done there even when the procedure is performed by an aesthetician, nurse practitioner, assistant, or often just a receptionist the doctor has trained.

When dermatologists enter the spa business it's controversial. Some doctors see it as a natural evolution of what dermatologists already do, that is, taking care of skin. In defending the potential breach of ethics, physicians often assert that they take spa procedures and make them more "medical," or make these treatments safer and more effective. There is no research showing that to be true, but doctors too can be vulnerable to exaggeration, fluff, and bogus declarations of efficacy.

What medical spas can provide that salons and nonmedical spas can't are prescriptions like Renova or Retin-A, liposuction, removing surfaced veins or capillaries, and injection of dermal fillers and Botox. While those additions are nice, there is no regulation or industry standard for medical spas, so the name on the door does not guarantee you any official standard. The general guideline is to make sure the spa is indeed run by a dermatologist or plastic surgeon and not by an internist or dentist (yes, dentists have gone into the medical spa business).

Adding to the questionable facade of medical ethics, some physicians sell skin-care products claiming they are cosmeceuticals and somehow special and different from products sold by the rest of the industry. Sadly, there is no truth to this; it is false advertising at its best. When you hear the word "cosmeceutical," you're supposed to think the product is a blend of cosmetic ingredients and pharmaceutical-grade ingredients and, therefore, it must be better for your skin. The fact is, "cosmeceutical" is just a trumped-up word that has no legal or recognized meaning as to what ingredients it contains versus the content of any "non-cosmeceutical" cosmetic.

A quick comparison of ingredient lists reveals that there is nothing any more unique or pharmaceutical about cosmeceuticals than any other cosmetic in the cosmetics industry. There are no ingredients used in products formulated by physicians that can't be used by any other cosmetics company, and there are lots of cosmeceutical lines that aren't as well formulated as other product lines without the medical marketing strategy.

Bottom line: The FDA does not consider the term "cosmeceutical" to be a valid product class, so the term isn't regulated. There are no unique formulary standards or special ingredients for these products. Cosmeceutical is merely a marketing term, and nothing more. Anyone can use that term to represent their brand's identity (Source: www.fda.gov).

According to the American Academy of Dermatology (www.aad.org), "the answer to whether or not cosmeceuticals really work lies in the ingredients and how they interact with the biological mechanisms that occur in aging skin." But of course that's true for any cosmetic. Even doctors can be seduced by their own hype into using a coined, misleading term so they can sell skin-care products and market them as different.

CHAPTER 24
HAIR REMOVAL

WAY TOO MUCH HAIR

Having too much hair on the parts of the body where you don't want it is technically called hirsutism. Hirsutism is a disorder in women where excessive growth of thick, coarse hairs occurs in areas of the body that are easily activated by androgens (male hormones), such as the chin, jaw, forearms, or moustache area. This excess hair growth is often, but not always, associated with measurably elevated androgen levels.

Androgens are male hormones that are natural in women, where they are balanced along with the female hormone estrogen as part of the body's hormonal equilibrium. Both androgens and estrogens are produced in women by the ovary and adrenal glands, and peripherally from skin and fat cells (so that the more fat cells you have, as in being overweight, the more risk you have for excess hair growth).

The most common cause of hirsutism is polycystic ovarian syndrome. Other causes are late-onset congenital adrenal hyperplasia, Cushing's syndrome, and the HAIR-AN syndrome. Pituitary, ovarian, and adrenal tumors can be factors that are important, but they are rarely causes of hirsutism.

If you are struggling with excessive or abnormal hair growth, ranging from moderate to severe, or you experience a sudden onset of excessive hair growth, it can be helpful, if not essential, to have a medical evaluation to determine the cause and options for treatment. Identification of the underlying causes usually doesn't alter the management of the condition, but it can identify women at risk for infertility, diabetes, cardiovascular disease, and endometrial cancer. (Source: *Dermatologic Therapy*, September–October 2008, pages 376–391.)

HAIR-BRAINED IDEAS?

From the onset of adolescence, the desire to get rid of unwanted body hair can become an almost daily obsession. Whether it is shaving legs or underarms, struggling with dark hair above the lip or on the chin, or concern about dense hair growth on the arms, finding a way to effectively and efficiently deal with this problem is a recurring issue.

If a beauty need exists, lots of cosmetics companies are more than willing to manufacture products with sham claims, insisting they are the solution you've been looking for. However, most of these end up sounding far more effective than the way they actually perform. Infomercials and ads in fashion magazines seem to have the answer for the hair you're longing to get rid of, but alas, these products either can't live up to their claims or they are just standard depilatories or waxing options that offer little to no improvement over what has been around for years.

Believe me when I say I would love to find an easy way to achieve a smooth bikini line or a hairless upper lip without trouble or bother, but hair removal just isn't that simple. The following are some of the more popular options, each described with its own pros and cons (and everything in this category has pros and cons). Depending on your budget, available time, and the area you want to make hair-free, you can explore these options and choose what works best for you.

DEPILATORIES

Depilatories literally melt and dissolve hair with strong ingredients like calcium hydroxide and sodium or calcium thioglycolate. There are many reasons why this group of products is not great for everyone. The most compelling one is that they pose the risk of causing serious irritation or (in the extreme case) possible burns to the skin and eyes. It is essential to test the depilatory on your arm first as a precaution against allergic reactions or skin sensitivities. Hair and skin are similar in composition, so chemicals that destroy the hair can also destroy the skin.

Depilatories, much like shaving, remove only the hair on the surface, which means the hair comes back in just a few days. To get the best results from your depilatory, first apply warm to hot (but not too hot) compresses, which help soften the hair and pores (where the hair is growing), allowing the depilatory to be absorbed better. Then apply an extremely thick, generous layer of the depilatory completely over the entire length and base of the hair shaft area and let it stay on for the full recommended time, but no longer than between 4 and 15 minutes, depending on how fine or coarse the hair is. Because depilatories dissolve the hair, applying pressure can help remove more of the shaft. Instead of simply washing the depilatory away, use a washcloth and wipe the cream off, using a firm back-and-forth motion.

Depilatories should never be used for the eyebrows or other areas around the eyes, or on inflamed or broken skin.

WAXING

Waxing is an excellent and inexpensive way to deal with most hair removal situations on the body or face. Waxing leaves the area smoother than shaving does because it pulls the hair out below the top layer of skin, which makes it grow back slower and less uniformly. You can do waxing at home by yourself, and beauty supply stores sell all the equipment you need, from the wax to spatulas, strips of cotton, and anti-inflammatory lotions. There are even hair-remover kits with strips of wax or waxlike ingredients that you just peel open, place on the skin, and then rip off. No heating or mixing. This is by far the most convenient and easiest way to peel off hair from large areas such as the legs, bikini line, and arms. For smaller areas such as the upper lip, a wax that is melted in the microwave (instead of on the stove) and applied with a small spatula offers the most control.

In hot waxing, a thin layer of heated wax is applied to the skin in the direction of the hair growth. The hair becomes embedded in the wax as it cools and hardens. The wax is then pulled off quickly in the opposite direction of the hair growth, taking the uprooted hair with it. Cold waxes work similarly. Strips precoated with wax or a cool, sugar-based substance are pressed onto the skin in the direction of the hair growth and pulled off in the opposite direction.

Before you consider doing this yourself, visit an aesthetician with experience in this method of hair removal. It's tricky to get the technique right, and getting it wrong can mean a sticky mess on your body, in your kitchen, and around your bathroom. It also smarts a bit when the hair is ripped off. You can't wax again until the hair grows out to a noticeable length.

Sugaring

What makes this kind of hair removal different is that it literally uses sugar instead of wax. With its thick, caramel-like consistency, it works identically to regular waxing, only instead of spreading a wax substance over the skin you're spreading caramel. Is sugaring better than waxing, as many companies claim? As far as your hair is concerned, the effect is identical. You spread the sugar substance over the hair you want removed (there needs to be some hair length or there won't be anything for it to grab). Then you rip it off and the hair comes off, same as waxing.

However, there are two main positives to sugaring over waxing. First, sugaring's mess washes away while wax has to be peeled or scratched off (and that isn't easy). Plus sugaring doesn't usually require heating while waxing often does, and adding heat is far more damaging to skin! Easy cleanup and a relatively easier application (no risk of burn) are the incredible benefits of sugaring.

Claims for waxing and sugaring usually state that they are more effective than other at-home methods because when the hair is extracted it includes the roots, so regrowth is softer, finer, and slower. That isn't true. Hormones and genetics determine hair growth and hair thickness, not the hair-removal method. What does happen when you "tweeze" hair is that, because it has been removed closer to the root, the new hair takes longer to grow back to the top of the skin, in contrast to shaving, where the hair is removed only from the surface, so the hair pops back out faster. Also, because each hair follicle has a different rate of growth, there will be less of it as it grows back than what was present when you first waxed or sugared, making the hair seem softer.

There are also claims that sugaring prevents ingrown hairs. Ingrown hairs are unrelated to the way hair is removed. Ingrown hairs occur when a hair that has been removed below the skin's surface has trouble finding its way back to the surface as it regrows. That applies to hair removal in general, regardless of whether you shave, tweeze, sugar, or wax.

Tweezing or Threading

Tweezing is not only a painful option, but also an extremely time-consuming one. It is OK for occasional stray hairs or very small areas (think eyebrows), but it is not the best for large areas or areas with dense hair growth. Tweezing works virtually the same way as waxing—by pulling the hair out from the root—which means the effects last far longer than shaving. Some women worry that tweezing will increase the growth or make the texture of the hair heavier, but it won't. If plucking (or waxing and shaving) altered hair growth, we would all have bushy eyebrows! Actually, pulling out hair can eventually shut down the hair follicle by causing repeated shock and injury, though this takes a very, very long time. For the most part, any texture change is a result of the initial re-growth phase, when the hair reemerges from the pore.

Threading is a Middle Eastern technique that plucks hair from the root by using a twisted piece of thread. It is a fascinating process to watch. The person doing the treatment holds the thread in her mouth and hands and plucks away the hair faster than you can imagine, leaving the area smoother then you could do on your own with a tweezer. However, threading has no benefit over and above tweezing in terms of regrowth. All threading does is yank out a hair, the same thing that tweezing does.

BLEACHING

Bleaching is a great, inexpensive option if the issue is not the density of the hair but its darkness. This method is particularly effective for the upper lip or other parts of the face, neck, and arms. There are many options for facial bleach products at the drugstore or on the Internet. One of the best Internet sources for a range of inexpensive options is www.folica.com. Please be aware that this site also sells an array of products that exaggerate their claims or simply mislead as to what they can really do for skin.

ELECTROLYSIS

Electrolysis is the only permanent form of hair removal, at least so far, but it requires repeated treatments that can take up to a year and it can be pricey, especially when you take into consideration the time commitment. The biggest hurdle is finding an extremely skilled technician to achieve satisfactory results. Before you see someone, check out the clients who have had permanent success with this tricky, but effective, method of hair removal.

There are two types of devices that use electric current to remove hair: the needle epilator and the tweezer epilator. (Tweezer epilators are discussed in the next section.) Needle epilators introduce a very fine wire under the skin and into the hair follicle. An electric current travels down the wire and destroys the hair root at the bottom of the follicle. The loosened hair is then removed with regular tweezers. Every hair is treated individually. Needle epilators are used in electrolysis because this technique destroys the hair follicle. Thus, this is considered a permanent hair-removal method. The hair root may persist, however, if the needle misses the mark or if insufficient electricity is delivered to destroy it. However, the intrinsic stimulus for hair growth can never be permanently removed. For instance, you can't control hormonal changes that may cause new growth (Source: FDA *Consumer* magazine, September 1996).

The major risks of using electrolysis include electrical shock, which can occur if the needle is not properly insulated; infection from a nonsterile needle; and scarring resulting from improper technique. In addition, there are no uniform licensing standards regulating the practice of electrolysis. Only 31 states require electrologists to be licensed, and among those the license requirements vary from as few as 120 hours to 1,100 hours of study, which means that to set up shop many electrologists only need a machine and very little else.

The American Electrology Association and the Society of Clinical and Medical Electrologists have certification programs based on a written exam. A list of licensed and certified electrologists is available from the International Guild of Professional Electrologists, 202 Boulevard Street, Suite B, High Point, NC 27262; (800) 830–3247 or on the Web at www.igpe.org/.

HOME ELECTROLYSIS

Technically, these devices work the same way as those that the professionals use (they also carry the same health risks). However, the risks for the home-use machines are not very great because the voltage and current output are not very high, and that means they aren't as effective. I know we've all seen those little machines you can buy via mail order (for about $100) that claim to remove hair painlessly and permanently. They've been advertised for years and years. I remember them from when I was a kid. The chances of operating these successfully yourself are at best slim. You probably would end up just tweezing instead of zapping the hair because getting the device to work right is extremely tricky and incredibly time-consuming. Given the time it takes for a hair to grow back, it could take months before you knew if it was really working (Source: FDA *Consumer* magazine, September 1996). There is no research indicating these machines do anything but tweeze the hair. The low voltage makes these machines extremely low risk, but they are also ineffective. What a waste.

SHAVING

Shaving is fine, but we all know the problems associated with it. Shaving is the method most of us go back to for our legs and bikini line, but the hair grows back way too fast and the stubble or redness it can cause on the thigh and crotch is obnoxious. There are ways around the redness, such as shaving with a good topical lotion like a hair conditioner or body wash and applying a nonfragranced moisturizer afterward. Also, one of the best options for preventing red bumps is applying aspirin topically to the skin. Aspirin has potent anti-inflammatory properties even when applied to the surface of skin. Simply dissolve one or two aspirins in about a quarter cup of water and then use a cotton ball to apply the solution to the area you just shaved! This works on any part of the body you shave. You will be impressed by the results.

On the legs, using a mild scrub of cornmeal mixed with Cetaphil Gentle Skin Cleanser can help keep flaky skin at a minimum, which means you can get a closer shave. Skin should never be shaved while dry; wet hair is soft, pliable, and easier to cut. Contrary to what many believe, shaving does not change the texture, color, or rate of hair growth. Hair density is genetically and hormonally determined; it has nothing to do with what you do topically to the skin (unless you traumatically damage the hair follicle via injury or burns).

LASER HAIR REMOVAL

Since the advent of the first FDA-approved laser hair-removal system in 1995, its popularity has made laser hair-removal a financial cornerstone for many dermatologists and plastic surgeons. The original laser hair-removal machine was The Soft Light Hair Removal System developed by Thermolase Corporation. Since then the growing popularity of and demand for this treatment from eager consumers reading ads and articles in fashion magazines has prompted many laser manufacturers to seek FDA clearance for their laser hair-removal machines. The market is growing so quickly that the FDA cannot maintain an up-to-date list of all laser manufacturers whose devices have been cleared for hair removal, as this list continues to change. However, to learn if a specific manufacturer has received FDA clearance, you can check the FDA Web site at www.fda.gov/cdrh/databases.html. You will need to know the manufacturer or device name of the laser. You can also call FDA's Center for Devices and Radiological Health, Consumer Staff, at 1-888-INFO-FDA or (301) 827-3990, or fax your request to (301) 443–9535 (Source: FDA Center for Devices and Radiological Health, *Laser Facts*, May 2001, online at www.fda.gov/cdrh/consumer/laserfacts.html).

One of the significant FDA regulations regarding all companies that promote approved laser hair-removal systems is that "manufacturers may not claim that laser hair removal is either painless or permanent…. The specific claim granted is 'intended to effect stable, long-term, or permanent reduction'…. Permanent hair reduction is defined as the long-term, stable reduction in the number of hairs regrowing after a treatment regime, which may include several sessions. The number of hairs regrowing must be stable over time—greater than the duration of the complete growth cycle of hair follicles, which varies from four to twelve months according to body location. Permanent hair reduction does not necessarily imply the elimination of all hairs in the treatment area." That is a very convoluted way of saying that laser hair removal is not permanent and that there are no studies showing it to be so even after several treatments. However, the consumer is usually not told what the FDA's regulation verbiage is.

When laser hair-removal arrived on the scene, many exaggerated, largely unsubstantiated claims about its efficacy, risks, side effects, and long-term effects were asserted (Source: *Journal of Cutaneous Laser Therapy*, March 2000, pages 49–50). Far more research has taken place since then and there's much more data (both clearer and more precise) regarding statistical analysis of performance and adverse outcomes. Several studies have looked at various other laser systems, including some showing more promise for darker skin tones (Source: *Annals of Plastic Surgery*, October 2001, pages 404–411).

The risks in laser hair removal can include skin discoloration (either darkening or lightening of skin), swelling, inflammation, and infected hair follicles. Laser hair removal is particularly problematic for those with tans or darker skin colors (Source: *Cosmetic Dermatology*, November 2001, pages 45–50). Because of the potential for complications and the plethora of hair-removal machines available, it is essential to have this procedure performed by a physician who is familiar with the research and who can make the correct choice about which procedure is best for you.

AT-HOME LASERS? MAYBE!

Lots of cosmetics companies have advertised their products as being able to replace and reproduce the effects of medical procedures such as Botox, dermal injections, and lasers. There have always been skin-care products making absurd claims that were absolutely not possible or even remotely true. No skin-care product can remotely work like a medical corrective procedure. But now there are companies selling small hand-held machines claiming they can replace what laser hair removal treatments physicians are licensed to do. But do they work? The answer is yes and maybe.

Yes, they do have ability to reduce hair growth and when combined with shaving and tweezing during intervals net fairly impressive results. But do they work as well as the lasers used in doctors' offices? Maybe, but it's hard to be certain. Because so much of the research about laser hair removal is sponsored by the companies who sell the machines the studies are questionable. Plus, if you go to a physician's office and ask about lasers for hair removal they will always have a strong bias about the machines they own or rent. I have yet to see an exception to that axiom.

Of the research that does exist, it seems of all the things you can buy to test against the claim are these hand-held, at-home lasers for hair removal. Some of them are almost identical to those used by physicians. For example, TRIA is an 810 nanometer diode laser with research showing it can reduce hair growth. The claims go beyond the pale, but you should see some percentage of hair reduction, just not as much as they claim.

One claim about these machines to ignore is the part where they brag about their FDA status of being a Class I medical device, which is often used by companies wanting to make their machines sound more impressive than they are. To keep it in perspective, according to the FDA, Class I devices are subject to the least regulatory control. They present minimal potential for harm to the user and that's about all that classification represents. Examples of Class I devices include elastic bandages, examination gloves, and hand-held surgical instruments such as scalpels or dental scrapers. Class I devices are exempt from any notification of efficacy.

Using the term laser is clever, too, because even the flashlight pointers used to project a red light during slide presentations are referred to as lasers. As a term, lasers do not have to be related to the medical world.

My recommendation? Go ahead and give these at-home laser devices a try. The results from home-use devices are decent (some would argue impressive) but still inferior to office-based lasers and light devices.

(Sources: *Seminars in Cutaneous Medicine and Surgery*, December 2008, pages 292–300; and *Lasers in Surgery and Medicine*, July 2007, pages 476-493.)

VANIQA

Manufactured by Bristol-Meyers Squibb, Vaniqa ($37.50 for 1.05 ounces) is FDA-approved as a prescription-only topical cream for reducing and inhibiting the growth of unwanted facial hair (it has not been studied for its effect on hair on other parts of the body). On the surface, Vaniqa might sound like a depilatory (those nonprescription, drugstore products that topically dissolve hair away), but Vaniqa's effect on hair and skin is unrelated to the way a depilatory works.

The active drug in Vaniqa is eflornithine hydrochloride, which has been used as an oral medication for certain cancers and to treat African Sleeping Sickness. Many disconcerting side effects are associated with this drug when it is taken orally, ranging from anemia to diarrhea, vomiting, and hair loss. The notion that topical application of eflornithine hydrochloride could also affect hair loss probably stems from its hair-loss side effect when taken orally. However, the product information insert for the medication states that, when applied topically, eflornithine hydrochloride, "is not known to be metabolized and is primarily excreted unchanged in the urine with no adverse systemic side effects."

The information insert for Vaniqa explains that eflornithine hydrochloride affects the skin because it "interferes with an enzyme found in the hair follicle of the skin needed for hair growth. This results in slower hair growth…. [However] Vaniqa does not permanently remove hair or 'cure' unwanted facial hair…. Your treatment program should include continuation of any hair removal technique you are currently using…. [Further] Improvement in the condition occurs gradually. Don't be discouraged if you see no immediate improvement. Improvement may be seen as early as 4 to 8 weeks of treatment … [and] may take longer in some individuals. If no improvement is seen after 6 months of use, discontinue use. Clinical studies show that in about 8 weeks after stopping treatment with Vaniqa, the hair will return to the same condition as before beginning treatment."

There are warnings that accompany this cream and there is still research to be done. Note that the insert warns, "You should not use Vaniqa if you are less than 12 years of age…." Plus, there are animal studies that showed definite fetal problems. That means pregnant women should not use this drug, and lactating women probably should not either, though there is no research about that risk. Also, "Vaniqa may cause temporary redness, stinging, burning, tingling or rash on areas of the skin where it is applied. Folliculitis (hair bumps) may also occur," as well as acne.

So, should you consider Vaniqa? Well, that depends on how you look at the statistics, because clearly for some women it can work very well to reduce the amount of facial hair while others will be disappointed. It seems to work even better in conjunction with laser hair removal. At the very least, it is certainly an option when experimenting with serious hair-growth problems. (Sources: *European Journal of Dermatology*, January–February 2008, pages 65–70; and *Journal of the American Academy of Dermatology*, July 2007, pages 54–59.)

HAIR-REMOVAL WARNING!

All treatments for hair removal are contraindicated after any facial peel or laser procedure. It can take six to eight weeks for the skin to completely heal after a peel. Any trauma to the skin during the recovery period can cause discoloration or even scarring.

Hair removal is also extremely problematic if you are using AHAs, BHA, topical retinoids, azelaic acid, or taking Accutane. These treatments can make skin more susceptible to tears, wounds, and irritation, and attempting hair-removal at the same time can prove to be uncomfortable as well as damaging.

CHAPTER 25
GROWING HAIR

HAIR GROWTH SCAMS

Regrowing hair that has been lost is a tantalizing hope for both men and women. As a result, hair-loss scams are one of the more pervasive and prevalent marketing deceptions found on the fringes of the cosmetics industry. Few major cosmetics companies dally in this arena; instead it is populated by small, fly-by-night companies. These companies say just about anything to get you to buy their products. You can barely avoid the snake-oil sales pitches aired on TV and radio infomercials, on Internet sites, and in print ads. Almost without exception what you are told are lies, deceptions, and twisted interpretations of actual scientific information.

In reality, once hair begins to fall out, for any of a variety of reasons, it is very difficult to grow it back. There are only two products with substantiated, published research showing they can reduce hair loss and regrow hair. But even those two drugs (Propecia and minoxidil) have limited results. When a company asserts that its product stops hair loss, prevents thinning hair, or regrows what you've lost, it simply can't be true. Even when they showcase their research, those studies aren't published, and the results are simply too good to be true.

What you don't know about your hair will waste your money and it won't give you the head of hair you want. Either way, you're left with less, not more of what you want.

HOW DOES HAIR GROW?

Depending on the individual, approximately 5 million hair follicles cover the surface of the body at any given time. Of that total, about 100,000 to 150,000 strands are growing on the head. Surprisingly, blondes usually have more hair on their heads than those with red or darker hair colors. All those millions of hair follicles are developed and in place before a person is born. Biologically, it is impossible to grow more hair after birth—all the hair you are ever going to have is already there when you arrive in this world (Source: "Hair Loss and Hair Restoration," www.aad.org/public/publications/pamphlets/common_hairloss.html).

Inside the hair follicle, deep below the skin, hair is going through a life cycle all its own. At any given time, each hair on your body is in one of three phases—growing, resting (or dormant), or shedding. The first phase is the anagen (growth) phase. At this point, the hair is very busy developing in the hair follicle, the pocket-like structure that houses the bulb-shaped root of the hair. At the very base of this root is an intricate network of capillaries and nerves that feed the developing hair. During the growth stage, each individual hair is formed by rapidly dividing cells that push forward and up through the follicle. As they multiply and expand, the cells reach the surface, where they die and harden into what we know (and see) as hair. The growth stage can last anywhere from two to six years. During this phase, hair grows an average of about half an inch per month, or six inches per year (but that is only an average and it varies drastically from very active hair growth to very slow growth for different people).

Over the entire growth phase, the hair can reach a length of approximately three feet, about the middle of the back for most women, before it stops growing and proceeds to the catagen (resting) phase. Naturally, there are variations in length potential, and women with tresses six feet long have been reported, but there are also women who can't grow hair much past their shoulders. The reason for these variations is that the length of hair is genetically predetermined, which explains why some women feel they can never get their hair to grow past a certain point, while other women can't seem to get to a hairdresser often enough to keep up with the grow-out.

The catagen phase also includes a transition (intermediate) phase. After about three to six years of growth, the hair cells stop reproducing and the growth process is over. For about two to six weeks, the hair just lies around taking it easy while the root slowly moves up to the skin's surface.

Entering its last phase of life, the hair is ready to literally jump ship and shed. The telogen (final) phase is short-lived. At this point the hair root has moved almost to the surface (near the opening of the oil gland), where it is completely separated from the base of the follicle. In a matter of weeks the anagen (growth) stage will begin again at the base of the hair follicle. Hair cells again start dividing and multiplying, generating a new shaft. When the new hair sprouts to the surface, it simply pushes the old hair out of its way. So all that hair collecting on your brush, in the bottom of your drain, or on your clothing—about 25 to 100 hairs a day—is usually hair that has passed from the growth phase through the transition plateau and into the final period of shedding.

At any given time, approximately 88% of scalp hair is in the anagen phase, 1% in the catagen phase, and 11% in the telogen phase. Thankfully, hair is predominantly in the growing phase (at least if male pattern baldness or some other form of hair loss has not started to occur), which explains why we end up having more hair than less, despite the strands we lose daily.

Although everyone's hair goes through the same life cycle, not all hair is the same; hair has very distinct inherited differences. African hair grows mostly in an alternating curved/flat sequence that imparts a coiled, corkscrew-like shape to the hair, a form that produces weak spots at every turn. Asian, Native American, and Hispanic hair is straight to slightly wavy, coarse, thick, and almost always black. European and Hindu hair textures vary greatly, from straight to curly, thick to thin, and fine to coarse, and they also have a wide range of colors. Generally, what distinguishes African hair from European or Asian hair is its tight, spiral growth pattern.

(Sources: www.aad.org; *Hair Loss: Principles of Diagnosis and Management Alopecia*, by Jerry Shapiro, Taylor & Francis Group, December 2001; *Disorders of Hair Growth: Diagnosis and Treatment*, McGraw-Hill, Inc., 1994; *Dermatology Clinics*, October 1996, pages

573–583; *The Molecular and Structural Biology of Hair*, Annals of the New York Academy of Science, 1991.)

WHY DOES HAIR STOP GROWING?

Alopecia is the technical name for hair loss, but that's just the beginning of the story. There are so many complicated and multifaceted factors that affect hair growth the subject is too vast and complex for this book to tackle in detail.

For example, reasons for hair loss can include scarring alopecia (also referred to as pseudopelade, a condition where for no known reason the hair follicle is destroyed, resulting in permanent hair loss); nonscarring alopecia (also referred to as alopecia areata, which results in hair loss that can grow back); androgenetic alopecia (more commonly known as male pattern baldness); scleroderma (a chronic connective-tissue disease believed to be an autoimmune rheumatic disease); some tick bites; lichen planopilaris (an inflammatory disease of unknown origin that usually affects the skin but can also affect hair and can result in permanent hair loss); psoriasis; lupus (an autoimmune disorder causing chronic inflammation, especially of the skin, but that can also affect hair growth); seborrheic dermatitis; trichotillomania (an impulse-control disorder that causes people to pull out their own hair); traction alopecia (resulting from inadvertent pulling on hair from styling hair too tightly); physical injury (particularly burns that destroy hair follicles); hemochromatosis (an inherited disorder that causes the body to absorb and store too much iron, damaging the organs in the body); surgery; cancer; rapid weight loss; thyroid abnormalities; and high blood pressure are all contributing factors.

There is also a long list of medications that can cause hair loss, and there are no cosmetic products that can reverse their effect, though hair growth is almost always restored once the drug is not being taken. These include the cholesterol-lowering drugs clofibrate (Atromis-S) and gemfibrozil (Lopid); the Parkinson's medication levodopa (Dopar, Larodopa); the ulcer drugs cimetidine (Tagamet), ranitidine (Zantac), and famotidine (Pepcid); the anticoagulants coumarin and heparin; drugs for gout treatment, including allopurinol (Loporin, Zyloprim); anti-arthritics penicillamine, auranofin (Ridaura), indomethacin (Indocin), naproxen (Naprosyn), sulindac (Clinoril), and methotrexate (Folex); drugs derived from vitamin-A isotretinoin (Accutane) and etretinate (Tegison); anticonvulsants for treating epilepsy like trimethadione (Tridione); beta-blocker drugs for high blood pressure such as atenolol (Tenormin), metoprolol (Lopressor), nadolol (Corgard), propranolol (Inderal), and timolol (Blocadren); and the anti-thyroid medications carbimazole, iodine, thiocyanate, and thiouracil.

But by far, the most typical cause of hair loss is something called male pattern baldness caused by certain androgens (male hormones) destroying the hair follicle. Yes, despite the name, more then 21 million women are affected by male pattern baldness.

Before you even begin to think about what products to use for hair growth, you must know the source of your hair loss. Each of these causes requires medical evaluation and a determination of treatment. Hair loss is not merely an aesthetic issue, it can also be a health issue.

(Sources: *European Journal of Dermatology*, May–June 2007, pages 220–222; *Facial and Plastic Surgery*, November 2008, pages 414–427; *Cosmetic Dermatology*, December 2003, pages 48–51; *Journal of the American Academy of Dermatology*, October 2003, pages 667–671, and April 2000, pages 549–566; "Anagen Effluvium," August 14, 2000, www.emedicine.com; American Academy of Dermatology, www.aad.org; and American Hair Loss Council, www.ahlc.org.)

MALE PATTERN BALDNESS

Although there are many forms of alopecia, the most prevalent by far is androgenetic alopecia, better known as male pattern baldness. About 95% of all cases of hair loss are the result of male pattern baldness, but this number also includes women, who can have a version of hair loss referred to as female androgenetic alopecia or female pattern baldness. Approximately 25% of men begin balding by age 30; two-thirds begin balding by age 60. For women, androgenetic alopecia was found in 3% of women ages 20 to 29 years, 16 to 17% of women ages 30 to 49, 23 to 25% of women ages 50 to 69, 28% of women ages 70 to 79, and 32% of women ages 80 to 89. In some research, statistics indicate that 40% of women are affected by androgenetic alopecia. As you can tell by these numbers, female pattern baldness increases dramatically just before and after menopause.

For men, male pattern baldness develops in a horseshoe pattern, with the hair receding from the forehead back toward the neck. Male pattern baldness can also take place from the center of the scalp out toward the sides. For women, the location is more diffuse, with hair loss taking place all over the scalp (Sources: *Male Pattern Baldness*, American Medical Association Medical Library, www.medem.com; *Hair Loss & Restoration in Women*, International Society of Hair Restoration Surgery, www.ishrs.org; and *Dermatologic Surgery*, January 2001, pages 53–54).

The key element you need to be aware of to understand whether the products being sold to improve or restore hair growth will work is how hormones affect hair growth. This is because, for both male pattern baldness and female pattern baldness, hormones are the primary cause of hair loss. First, let's start with some basic information about the hair growing on your head.

Hair growth basically has a lot to do with hormonal activity, and is especially related to the male sex hormone group called androgens. (Androgens are male hormones such as testosterone and dihydrotestosterone.) Many different types of hormones influence hair growth, but androgens are believed to have the largest impact on the process. Testosterone and dihydrotestosterone (DHT, a hormonal by-product of testosterone) are produced in large quantities by the testes in men, and in smaller quantities by the ovaries in women. These hormones are responsible for the development of secondary male sex characteristics for both genders. They are also responsible for increasing the size of hair follicles early in life, and, ironically, for decreasing and shrinking the hair follicles later in life.

Technically, what is in part believed to be taking place in the hair follicle is that over time testosterone is changed to dihydrotestosterone (DHT) by the enzyme 5-alpha reductase

(5AR). When DHT becomes concentrated in the hair follicle it eventually slows, and ultimately stops, hair growth. It is also believed that the effect of DHT is compounded or enhanced by an individual's genetic hair-follicle traits.

(Sources: *Journal of the American Academy of Dermatology*, October 2008, pages 547–566, and May 2004, pages 777–779; *British Journal of Dermatology*, April 2004, pages 750–752; *Journal of Investigative Dermatology*, December 2003, pages 1561–1564; *American Journal of Clinical Dermatology*, 2003, volume 4, issue 6, pages 371–378; *Androgenetic Alopecia*, October 2, 2003; www.emedicine.com; and *Journal of Alternative and Complementary Medicine*, April 2002, pages 143–152.)

For women, it appears that their increased levels of estrogen (the primary female sex hormone) act against the effects of male androgens on hair growth. This explains why, when estrogen levels decrease as women approach menopause, androgen-related balding can begin to appear. There is some research indicating that topical application of estrogen can induce hair growth in women (Source: *Journal of Investigative Dermatology*, January 2004, pages 7–13).

BLOOD FLOW AND HAIR LOSS

While research concerning hair loss has focused primarily on the involvement of hormones, there is a good deal of discussion about another concept, especially on Web sites selling products claiming to regrow hair. According to these sources, the status of the hair involves the issue of blood supply to the hair follicle. Some hair-care companies want you to believe that reduced or impeded blood flow is the primary factor affecting hair growth. Improve the blood flow, they say, and you should be able to improve hair growth. As logical as that sounds, it doesn't work that way in reality.

Although an adequate oxygenated blood supply is necessary for any and all of the tissues of the body to function properly, not all disorders of the body (including hair loss) are related to decreased blood flow. Consider this: When hair follicles are transplanted from the back of the head to the front they do not become thin and they do not fall out. There seems to be plenty of blood flow in the same bald areas where the newly transplanted hair thrives. If the areas that became bald were damaged as a result of poor blood flow, then the transplanted hair follicles should suffer the same fate—yet they don't. If anything, the new hair becomes beautifully thick and healthy. Plus when your scalp suffers a wound, it bleeds, and profusely; if that weren't the case then perhaps there would be a more solid argument about blood flow and hair loss (Source: *British Journal of Dermatology*, February 2004, pages 186–194). Needless to say, this is one example of a hair-loss solution that sounds plausible, but the facts paint a different picture.

CAN THEY REALLY STOP HAIR LOSS?

I'm sure you've seen the ads: Grow Hair in 12 Weeks! Stop Hair Loss Today! Stop Baldness Without Costly Drugs, Chemicals, or Surgery! Turn Fallout into Grow-out with Only One Hour of Your Time a Week! Wouldn't that be nice? Then all you'd have to do is send in your three easy payments of $29.95 and receive a combination of vitamins, a special shampoo or conditioner, several scalp masks, a battery-operated scalp massager, and who knows what else, and you, too, would look like the before-and-after pictures in the advertisements. Bald spot one day, waves of bushy hair a few weeks later. If any of this were possible, why would anyone be bald? There wouldn't be a naked scalp in the house!

Some popular ingredients such as emu oil, zinc, superoxide dismutase, and green tea have some minor studies showing they have some ability to generate hair growth, but the research is not enough to warrant much attention. Nonetheless, these ingredients are promoted and glorified to the point of absurdity by companies selling products that contain them. The information enthusiastically states that there is abundant definitive research proving efficacy, when in reality the research is at best questionable, not done double-blind, and there are no additional, follow-up studies to verify the results of earlier studies. One study alone cannot by anyone's definition generate conclusive evidence. That means the evidence is more like guessing than anything, and that's something you shouldn't bank on with your hair follicles.

Regrettably, almost all of the concoctions being sold for hair growth are nothing more than snake-oil treatments, here today and gone tomorrow. You would be better off throwing your money out the window; at least then you wouldn't be funding the unscrupulous businesses that lure other hopeful but soon-to-be-deceived consumers into wasting their money.

MINOXIDIL

Minoxidil is still the only over-the-counter, topical pharmaceutical whose claims regarding hair regrowth have been approved by the FDA. Minoxidil, at one time available only under the trade name Rogaine, is now available under different names from several different companies and can increase hair growth by a statistically significant percentage in both men and women. Extensive research and statistics suggest that this fairly inexpensive treatment works incredibly well for some people and is even more effective for women with male pattern hair loss then men (and most women struggling with hair loss have androgen dependent hair loss which is referred to as male pattern baldness). (Sources: *Clinical Interventions in Aging*, February 2007, pages 189–199; and *Journal of the American Academy of Dermatology*, April 2004, pages 541–553.)

Using minoxidil (the active ingredient in Rogaine) at the available strengths is extremely safe (Source: *Journal of Cutaneous Medicine and Surgery*, July–August 2003, pages 322–329). Two strengths are available, 2% and 5% concentrations, and for women it seems that the 5% strength works better than the 2%. A study reported in the *Journal of the American Academy of Dermatology* (April 2004, pages 541–553) looked at 381 women who used either the 5% or 2% minoxidil solution for hair loss. Both the 5% and 2% solutions were superior to using nothing, which means both helped hair grow back, but the group that used 5% minoxidil demonstrated better hair growth than the 2% minoxidil group.

Despite this success, there is concern for women that both the 2% and 5% strengths can cause hair growth where you don't want it, namely on the face and other parts of the body, but that is easily adjusted by stopping usage. A study published in the *Journal of the European Academy of Dermatology and Venereology* (May 2003, pages 271–275) found that in a review of 1,333 women who were using either 2% or 5% minoxidil, 4% experienced unwanted hair growth, and that there was a higher incidence of unwanted hair growth in the group using the 5% strength. The study also pointed out, however, that a large percentage of the women in a part of this study (27%) reported that they experienced facial hair growth before they began using minoxidil, so it's possible that the women who reported the unwanted hair growth before applying minoxidil had stronger potential for that growth when using minoxidil. It is important to note that the unwanted hair growth is not permanent and reverses itself once you stop treatment.

The question is: Would you fall into the 4% group who experienced hair growth in annoying places, and is that worth the risk to you? If you already have a problem with too much hair growth in unwanted places, perhaps minoxidil isn't right for you. I should mention that personally I use the 5% strength. I had been using the 2% strength and didn't see the improvement I was hoping for. I changed to the 5% strength and the receding areas at my hairline grew back in just under four months. I also found that I was allergic to Rogaine (it made me itch and flake terribly), so I changed to the generic version of minoxidil and it worked just fine with no problem in the several months I've been using it. And it's definitely less expensive.

No one is certain yet just how topical minoxidil works, though work it does, although once you stop using it any hair that grew as a result of the drug will fall out. The most common side effects with this medication are itching and skin (scalp) irritation at the application site.

PROPECIA

Propecia (technical name finasteride) is an oral medication that was approved by the FDA in 1998 to treat men with male pattern baldness. It works by inhibiting the 5 alpha-reductase enzyme, the enzyme that converts testosterone into DHT, the hormone that causes male pattern baldness. The FDA's Dermatologic and Ophthalmic Drugs Advisory Committee agreed in discussions that Propecia is efficacious in treating male pattern baldness. Three studies involved 1,879 men, ages 18 to 41, who had mild to moderate but not complete hair loss. These studies, which lasted 24 months, demonstrated that treatment with Propecia prevented further hair thinning, and significantly increased hair growth in the majority of men (86%). However, 46% of the men using the placebo also saw improvement.

But don't get too excited—there are negatives to taking this drug. Propecia can cause birth defects for pregnant women and may decrease men's libido. However, as several doctors pointed out to me, the research showed the libido decrease was minor and that it was not significantly different from that of the placebo group. What the study warnings didn't point out was that in some people finasteride raised the levels of testosterone and increased the libido! For some that's a great side effect, and you may get some of your hairline back at the same time. (Sources: *European Journal of Dermatology*, January–February 2002, pages 38–49; *Archives of Dermatology*, August 1999, page 990; and *Journal of the American Academy of Dermatology*, June 1999, pages 930–937.)

There is also research showing that a combination of applying minoxidil topically while taking the oral medication Propecia has the most impressive and long-lasting results (Sources: *Dermatologic Surgery*, November 2003, pages 1130–1134; and *Journal of Dermatology*, August 2002, pages 489–498).

I should point out that one study, published in *Dermatologic Surgery* (May 2004, pages 761–763) and conducted at the University of California Los Angeles, showed significantly fewer desirable results than every other study published about finasteride (Propecia). A total of 1,261 patients were monitored every three months with telephone calls after finasteride was initially prescribed. After 12 months, a detailed questionnaire was sent to all patients. The study noted that 32% (414 men) continued to take finasteride daily for one to three years, that 24% (297 men) discontinued the drug between 3 and 15 months because of poor results, and that the remaining 44% (549 men) dropped out of the study for unknown reasons. Of the 414 men who continued to take the medication, less than half returned their detailed questionnaires; a small percentage of this group felt that they grew hair and the others noted poor results.

SAW PALMETTO

Saw palmetto is a popular herbal supplement sometimes recommended for hair growth. However, there are absolutely no reliable studies that have investigated saw palmetto in relation to hair growth. A few of the studies you see on the Internet were done by the companies selling saw palmetto supplement or were done on a small number of people. There is a study in the *Journal of Alternative and Complementary Medicine* (August 2002, pages 143-152) that was done on 10 people and the results were lackluster. There is no reliable information you can construe from that kind of research.

There are abundant studies for saw palmetto in relation to its ability to improve benign prostatic hyperplasia (BPH). Saw palmetto got its reputation for hair growth inadvertently due to the relationship between BPH and male pattern baldness, both of which are affected by the production of DHT. If saw palmetto could affect DHT, it was only a short stretch to assume that it might be effective in treating male pattern baldness, too. But theory isn't always good medicine. There is also research suggesting that saw palmetto does not affect DHT and that it exerts some other action that may be the reason for the improvement in BPH symptoms.

Having said all this, for $10 you can get saw palmetto as a supplement and see if it works for you after discussing this option with your physician.

(Sources: *Cutis*, February 2004, pages 107–114; www.naturaldatabase.com; *American Family Physician*, March 2003, pages 1281–1283; *Urological Research*, June 2000, pages 201–209; *Cochrane Database of Systematic Reviews*, 2002, volume 3; *Journal of the American Medical Association*, November 1998, pages 1604–1609; and www.hairlosstalk.com.)

TRETINOIN

Tretinoin (trade name Retin-A or Renova) is a topical cream or gel that may influence improvement in cell development, making it beneficial for many skin-care problems ranging from acne to wrinkles. Surprisingly, no one is actually sure why tretinoin can do that, but there are lots of studies indicating that it does. Some dermatologists have begun formulating their own treatments for male pattern balding by mixing tretinoin with minoxidil for topical application. It is thought that tretinoin can increase the absorption of minoxidil into the scalp. However, subsequent research has disproven tretinoin to have any effect at all either by itself or in combination with minoxidil (Source: *American Journal of Clinical Dermatology*, 2007, pages 285–290)

AZELAIC ACID

Azelaic acid is typically prescribed for rosacea and some acne conditions. Recently, the potential for using azelaic acid to treat androgenetic alopecia has been discussed. According to Kevin J. McElwee, an immunologist/dermatologist involved in research on hair loss and regrowth, "Studies carried out in France in the late 80's were to assess the effects of zinc sulfate and azelaic acid on the human skin. The result of these studies demonstrated that at high concentrations, zinc could completely inhibit the activity of 5-alpha reductase. Azelaic acid was also shown to be a potent inhibitor of 5-alpha reductase. Inhibition was detectable at concentrations as low as 0.2mmol/l and was complete at 3mmol/l. When zinc, vitamin B6, and azelaic acid were added together at very low concentrations, which had been ineffective alone, 90% inhibition of 5-alpha reductase was achieved" (Source: *British Journal of Dermatology*, November 1988, pages 627–632). However, there is no other research showing azelaic acid to be useful for hair regrowth. Even the Web sites that claim there are numerous studies list no other sources.

TAGAMET

Tagamet (active ingredient cimetidine) is an oral medication commonly used for acid indigestion and to treat stomach ulcers and other digestive discomforts. However, Tagamet has been shown to have an anti-androgenic effect, meaning it blocks the binding of DHT, and that can in turn reduce hair loss (Source: *International Journal of Dermatology*, March 1987, pages 128–130). However, for women, there is research showing that cimetidine can also induce hair loss (Sources: *The Journal of Clinical Endocrinology & Metabolism*, January 2000, pages 89–94; and *Therapie*, March–April 1995, pages 145–150).

KETOCONAZOLE

Ketoconazole is a topical and oral antifungal medication. It is used topically to reduce the presence of fungus that might be triggering dandruff, and orally to reduce systemic fungal infections. It has been observed that oral doses of ketoconazole can lower serum testosterone and thereby reduce the presence of DHT (Sources: *Journal of Dermatological*

Science, January 2007, pages 66-68; and *Hormone and Metabolic Research*, August 1992, pages 367–370). However, there are serious side effects to taking ketoconazole orally, including dizziness, nausea, and headaches. Due to the associated problems with taking ketoconazole orally, there are those who think that applying it topically, in the form of the anti-dandruff shampoo Nizoral, can produce the same testosterone-lowering effect as the oral dosage. However, there is no research of any kind demonstrating this to be the case.

HORMONE BLOCKERS

Hormone blockers (such as spironolactone, cyproterone acetate, and flutamide) are oral drugs that specifically reduce the production of testosterone by the adrenal glands and can thereby prevent DHT from having an effect on the hair follicle. But these are serious drugs and are not a consideration for men due to their feminizing effects, but can be considered an option for women, especially when combined with minoxidil. Studies indicate a good success rate especially when combined with the topical use of minoxidil. (Sources: *British Journal of Dermatology*, March 2005, pages 466-473; and *The Journal of Clinical Endocrinology & Metabolism*, January 2000, pages 89–94.)

BIRTH-CONTROL PILLS

Birth-control pills definitely affect hormones, and there are many conflicting opinions about their effect on hair loss or hair regrowth. Regrettably, there are few scientific studies on female pattern baldness, and even fewer when it comes to the effect of birth-control pills on this condition. The small amount of research that does exist shows that some birth-control pills have more testosterone-like activity, which can possibly promote hair loss by increasing the likelihood of testosterone being converted to DHT. That would cause a number of hair follicles to lapse into the telogen phase (shedding) and then not begin the anagen phase (growth) again. Further, the presence of testosterone can increase secondary male sex characteristics such as facial hair growth. It can also increase the likelihood of acne, because acne is frequently caused by androgen activity involving testosterone and DHT, the same hormones that trigger hair loss.

Many birth-control pills also contain minimal amounts of testosterone, or have anti-androgenic properties (meaning they inhibit testosterone). These formulas can therefore reduce hair loss and may actually help hair growth on the head, while also reducing the risk of acne. When birth-control pills contain estrogen, they can help reduce hair loss because estrogen makes hair stay on the head longer.

Because there are so many other complicated and significant health issues related to taking birth-control pills, hair loss and hair growth should not be the primary reason for taking them. It is essential for you to discuss all the pros and cons of these drugs at length with your physician.

(Sources: *Contraception*, May 2008, pages 337–343; *Current Drug Safety*, August 2006, pages 301–305; *Obstetrics and Gynecology*, May 2003, pages 995–1007; *Drugs*, 2003, volume 63, issue 5, pages 463–492; and *American Journal of Clinical Dermatology*, 2002, volume 3, issue 8, pages 571–578.)

MELATONIN

Melatonin is an herbal supplement. One study, published in the *British Journal of Dermatology* (February 2004, pages 341–345), stated that because melatonin has been reported to have a beneficial effect on hair growth in animals, it was of interest to evaluate the effect of melatonin on hair growth in women with male pattern baldness. The double-blind, randomized, placebo-controlled study was conducted in 40 women suffering from diffuse alopecia or androgenetic alopecia. Either a 0.1% melatonin solution or a placebo was applied on the scalp once daily for six months. The results showed melatonin led to a significantly increased growth rate in comparison to the placebo group. However, this is the only study that indicates melatonin has this effect.

HAIR TRANSPLANTS

Mention hair transplants to someone and it will immediately conjure up images of obvious, unsightly plugs of hair dotting someone's scalp like bad patches of grass on a lawn. Hair transplants from a decade ago did use strips of hair, grafts of scalp, and the results appeared like rows of planted hairs growing from a black plug on the scalp. Or you imagine little plugs dotted over the head appearing like sprouts of chives growing over the head. Fortunately, those days are over, and new techniques in hair transplants create a completely natural look. Today's techniques implant only one to four hairs, with no detectable base in sight. This state-of-the-art procedure is called the follicular-unit grafting technique, a process that relies on microscopic dissection at the back of the head to produce the hair grafts. It is an expensive, complicated procedure, but the results are remarkable and the hair does grow with minimal to no risk of further hair loss or thinning.

(Sources: *Facial and Plastic Surgery Clinics of North America*, August 2008, pages 289-297; *Journal of Plastic and Reconstructive Aesthetic Surgery*, November 2006, pages 1162-1169; *Archives of Facial Plastic Surgery*, September–October 2003, pages 439–444; *Plastic and Reconstructive Surgery*, January 2003, pages 414–424; *Dermatologic Surgery*, September 2002, pages 783–794; International Society of Hair Restoration Surgery, www.ishrs.org; and Hair Transplant Medical, www.hairtransplantmedical.com.)

Before you decide to consult a physician for a hair-transplant procedure of any kind, keep in mind that any licensed physician in the United States and Canada can perform hair surgery. That means a doctor who was previously a gynecologist, without taking one course, could hang out a shingle tomorrow declaring him- or herself a hair-transplant specialist. It is that easy, and it happens all the time. This lack of licensing or coursework requirements means that it's easy for the consumer to end up with disappointing and inferior results, such as visible scarring, patching, fuzzy hair, or even more hair loss. Before you book an appointment, find out if the doctor you are considering is in good standing with the International Society for Hair Restoration Surgery (ISHRS); contact them through their Web site at www.ishrs.org, or contact the American Academy of Facial Plastic and Reconstructive Surgery at (800) 332–3223 or www.plasticsurgery.org.

BALD BUSTING—SCAMS OR SOLUTIONS?

The number of hair-growth products on the market is literally hair-raising! Sadly, however, very few actually grow hair, although the companies that sell them are taking in a lot of your money. Several products and product lines make claims about hair growth, including Avacor, BioFolic, Fabao 101, Folliguard, Folligen, Hair Factor PX-2000, Hairgenesis, Hair Prime, Helsinki Formula, Nioxin, Nisim, Nutrifolica, Proxiphen, Pro-Genesis, Regenix, Revivogen, Shen Min, and I'm sure dozens—perhaps hundreds—more.

"[First,] most alopecias are not a gradual progressive hair loss. Most, including androgenetic alopecia, develop in spurts and then stop. There may even be some improvement for a short time before the hair loss begins again. Someone using a hair growth product might falsely attribute this slowdown or temporary reversal to the use of the [product they purchased].

"Second, people who want to believe will believe. When real drug companies test products for hair regrowth they run at least two methods of analysis side by side. One method is entirely empirical evidence. They mark an area on the volunteer's head and count the hair density in the area before and after treatment to see if there is improvement. The other analysis method they run is more subjective. They give a questionnaire to the volunteer and ask how the volunteer tester perceives the drug is working. Most human trials of drugs for alopecia are classic double-blind studies involving a group that receives the drug and another control group that receives an innocuous placebo compound. No one knows whether they are using the drug or placebo. Frequently what is found is that volunteers on the drug or placebo indicate they believe they have regrowth of hair, but when comparing their positive comments to the hair count/density data it is revealed there is no actual improvement and there may even be a deterioration. Call it optimism or an overactive imagination, it is an important factor for professional scam artists" [because they can tell you a product works when it only appears to work due to a placebo effect]." (I have added my comments in square brackets.) (Source: www.keratin.com.)

GROWING EYELASHES—A BEHIND-THE-SCENES EXPOSÉ

Eyelash growth-enhancing products are starting to be sold by a small but growing number of cosmetics companies. In one form or another, products like these have been around for some time without much success. The success ratio changed when Jan Marini launched her Age Intervention Eyelash product, which contained an ingredient the company merely referred to as "eyelash growth factor." There is no such thing as eyelash growth factor, so that made-up marketing term was meaningless.

But who cared what they called it, because after a few weeks this product worked, and I mean really worked. My lashes actually became amazingly, almost preposterously long and darker, and putting mascara on made it almost look like I was wearing false eyelashes. Every woman using it in my office was also experiencing the same thing. A cosmetic product that really works (and it worked fast) doesn't happen every day or even a few times per year.

It turned out that the mysterious eyelash growth factor was something the FDA did care about because the ingredient causing the lashes to suddenly grow was the glaucoma drug bimatoprost. Marini was using this prescription-only drug without following regulations.

As a result of FDA pressure, Marini slightly renamed the product Age Intervention Eyelash Conditioner and listed the lash-growing ingredient on the label with its ridiculously long chemical name of 7-(3, 5-dihydroxy-2-(3-hydroxy-4-(3-(triflormethyl) phenoxy)-1-butenyl) cyclopentyl), N-ethyl,) 1R-(alpha(Z), 2beta (1E,3R), 3alpha, 5alpha)). No wonder she wanted to leave that off the label!

This nearly indecipherable ingredient is similar to a class of ingredients known as prostaglandin analogues. These drugs, including latanoprost, bimatoprost (the drug present in Marini's original formula), and travoprost, are used in eye drops to treat eye health problems such as glaucoma or ocular hypertension. One of the common side-effects of using these prescription-only glaucoma eye drops is that eyelashes grow, darken, and become thicker. Adapting this to a cosmetic made sense, so Marini stuck it in a tube, and added a thin brush to help with application. You simply brushed it along the lashline once a day, in much the same way you would apply liquid eyeliner. It was flying off the shelves in no time, and quickly became a celebrity favorite.

The "active" ingredient listed above is, according to Marini, a customized analogue her lab had created and therefore was not a drug. Therefore, she was not in any trouble with the FDA for using a prescription drug in a cosmetic product. At least that's what Marini and her staff were telling the public. Behind the scenes, the company was embroiled in a battle with Allergan, a pharmaceutical company that holds a patent for using bimatoprost in their own lash-enhancing product. Allergan was also spending lots of money getting it approved through the proper channels for a new drug application with the FDA. Its new drug status? Growing longer, darker, thicker eyelashes, of course! On the other hand, Marini was attempting to get around Allergan's patent and the FDA at the same time. It didn't work.

Patent infringement and FDA regulations aren't something to sneeze at. In 2007 the FDA seized over 12,600 tubes of Age Intervention Eyelash (the original formula) and sales were stopped. The FDA accused Marini of using a drug (bimatoprost) and misbranding it, which she was. So what was the danger? If a woman uses Age Intervention Eyelash containing a form of this glaucoma medication and they are already using glaucoma eye drops to treat the disease she could be at increased risk for optic nerve damage and eye inflammation, both of which can have serious consequences, including blindness.

Given that most of the public didn't know what was going on and that both the original product and its successor had already gained a strong following, Marini made the decision to reformulate again and renamed her product Marini Lash. This version does not contain bimatoprost or anything else even remotely similar. Instead, it now contains peptides that Marini claims works better than the previous version. Yet there is no research anywhere proving any peptide can grow longer, thicker, or darker eyelashes so it is NOT a lash-enhancing product I can recommend.

What happens now with Allergan's patent and FDA approval? As this book goes to press Allergan is hoping to enjoy unprecedented success with the launch of their eyelash-growing product, which they've named Latisse. Latisse's active ingredient is 0.03% bimatoprost, and it will come in a brush-on formula to be applied to the lash line, just like Marini's original lash product.

A major difference between Marini's former Age Intervention Lash products (as well as those from other brands selling the same thing, and more on that in a moment) is that because Latisse is classified as a drug, it is available by prescription only. Not only will this require a trip to or consultation with your physician, but the cost is considerable: $120 for a one-month supply. Marini's former lash product wasn't cheap either at $160 per tube, but at least it lasted several months with once-per-day use.

There is every reason to believe that Latisse will have a noticeable impact on the length, color, and thickness of your eyelashes. However, there are still side effects to consider such as a stinging sensation on skin where Latisse is applied, potential skin discoloration, and a permanent change in pigmentation of the iris (the colored part of the eye). Incidences of such side effects are low, but, as with any drug, you need to discuss the pros and cons with your prescribing physician or pharmacist. By the way, these same side effects were potentially present with the Marini product, she just didn't tell anyone. If anything, she went on and on about how safe her product was.

One question I've pondered since Allergan and Marini were at odds with each other is why the FDA (and Allergan, for that matter) only went after Marini for using a glaucoma drug off-label. Several other companies are selling products with the same drug or with another type of prostaglandin analogue. They include Peter Thomas Roth Lashes to Die For, MD Lash Factor, Revitalash, Lilash, and Neulash. As of this writing, all of these products are available, all are expensive, and none have been seized by the FDA or called into question by Allergan. In any event, it continues to bother me. Why should Marini take all the financial loss while other companies continue to enjoy success selling lash-enhancement products that work because, surprise, they contain prostaglandin analogues? If the FDA and Allergan wanted to make an example of Marini, the mission was accomplished. But to be fair, they should've endeavored to make an example of any company selling this type of product.

(Sources: *Clinical and Experimental Ophthalmology*, November 2006, pages 755–764; www.nlm.nih.gov/medlineplus/druginfo/medmaster/a602027.html; http://dermatology. cdlib.org/93/commentary/alopecia/wolf.html; www.medscape.com/viewarticle/443657; *Drugs of Today*, January 2003, pages 61–74; www.elixirnews.com/newsView.php?id=1149; www.reuters.com/article/pressRelease/idUS122104+18-July-2008+BW20080718; and www.truthinaging.com.)

CHAPTER 26
MEDICAL COSMETIC CORRECTIVE PROCEDURES

SKIN CARE ALONE WON'T DO IT

It's an undeniable fact: all the expensive or inexpensive skin-care products in the world, even those that are brilliantly formulated, won't prevent your skin from "aging" or wrinkling. Hormone loss, genetics, the simple act of growing older, gravity, muscle movement, sun damage, bone loss, and fat loss, all inevitably take their toll on skin. No matter how cautious you've been about sun exposure and how regularly you've used sunscreen, the realities are that sun damage begins when we are young, even the best sunscreens can't provide complete protection, and damaging UVA rays come through windows. We can slow the process but these factors add up to what we see on the face as "aging."

Had you taken all the money you wasted on expensive anti-wrinkle and anti-aging products and started saving from the time you were in grade school you would have the money in the bank to pay for medical procedures that can in the long run truly make you look younger, if that's your goal. It's not that state-of-the-art skin care doesn't play a part—because it does help—but it can only do so much. And it can't replace the arsenal of rejuvenating procedures a cosmetic surgeon or dermatologist can offer.

The desire to look younger is pervasive, and the accessibility of options that can make a huge difference by erasing years from your face makes the chance to achieve it beyond enticing for many men and women. When these procedures are done well the results are often outstanding. But when they are overdone or the treatment is performed by an unskilled physician, things often go from bad to worse.

Many celebrities provide perfect examples of how bad you can look when cosmetic corrective procedures go awry (or too much is done at once). Lots of celebrities have had their looks altered by cosmetic surgery or have had Botox, dermal injections, or laser resurfacing. But often you can tell at a glance whose physician overdid it because the celebrity's face is so tight she or he looks constantly surprised or incessantly half-smiling, or distorted in away that appears preternaturally odd. And there are way too many celebrities to list that fit this description. Perhaps in no other arena is one thing clearer: Celebrities are not the best informed about beauty. Those examples aside, the good news is that you don't need to avoid the benefits of what is available; you just need to avoid the same mistakes.

In short, you need to know the pros and cons about all cosmetic corrective procedures, including plastic surgery. What you don't know can hurt, and that doesn't mean just your appearance but also your health and your pocketbook. To help you think about this, I'd like to give an overview of what is available, how to plan what you want to achieve, and what you can afford, along with a discussion of the risks and/or benefits of different procedures and how the different services work.

ONE PROCEDURE IS NOT ENOUGH

As if taking care of your skin isn't complicated enough, and even though I hate to say it, there isn't a single overall medical corrective procedure that by itself will result in helping your entire face look younger. A realistic, multifaceted approach is the only option that can make achieving a complete picture of youth possible (assuming that is what you are aiming for). I know that can get expensive, and many of the procedures (especially dermal injections, Botox, laser and light treatments) are not permanent and need to be redone to maintain benefits. Granting all that, each procedure, regardless of what it is, can only impact a part of the face or a particular condition. The lesson is, don't expect to find one procedure that will take care of all your concerns.

For example, an eye tuck (blepharoplasty) can make the skin around the eyes look younger and reveal an eyelid that has long been hidden, but it won't change sagging at the chin, wrinkles, or crepey skin anywhere else on the face. Botox can smooth out a lined forehead and crow's feet (I do not recommend getting Botox anywhere else, but I'll get to that discussion later in this chapter), but that won't change the under-eye area, sagging, or wrinkles and crepey skin on the rest of the face. Dermal injections can work wonders for the lines between the eyebrows, laugh lines (the deep folds that run from the nose to the corner of the mouth), and receding lips, but there a lot of other areas that won't improve. Even a face-lift won't change the texture of skin, brown discolorations, wrinkles on the forehead (unless a brow lift was included in the procedure), sagging areas around the eyes (unless an eye tuck is included), or overall skin texture.

Deciding what to do requires balancing what you can afford with what you want to achieve. One laser or IPL machine treatment, or a single surgery, Botox injection, or dermal injection is unlikely to get you what you want. Any physician who is selling you a treatment or surgery as being a panacea for looking younger is not giving you the whole picture.

EVERYONE'S FACE IS DIFFERENT

Not everyone has the same face—that's a given!—and every difference in structure and genetics can affect how the skin ages. Some women have a thinner, narrower face, which causes more sagging skin especially at the jawline. Others have less fat content in the face, meaning there is less cushioning underneath the surface to prop up and support the layers of skin. You can have more sun damage than someone else, resulting in deeper wrinkles, skin discolorations, and surfaced capillaries being visible. Eyelids that genetically droop more than someone else's, or a puffy lower eye area (caused by fat and muscle movement) will be different person to person. All these elements and more, to one degree or another, are what identify an older looking face.

Over and above a physician's advice and talent, the array of procedures is large, and they also differ based on what you want to achieve, what you are comfortable with, what is in your budget, and what your short- and long-term goals are. There's no one-size-fits-all menu, but in fact it does take choosing from a menu if this is the route you want to take.

Unfortunately, doctors performing cosmetic corrective procedures can be salespeople too, and often they bend or manipulate your needs to fit the services they offer and not necessarily those that would work best for you. It is the rare physician who says "I can't do that, but this other doctor could really help you." It is essential to get a variety of opinions about what is possible for your face.

WHEN TO HAVE A PROCEDURE

When should you do it? When should you start having Botox? Dermal fillers? A face-lift? IPL or laser resurfacing? Perhaps you've discussed this with your friends, especially when chatting about the people you know who have had procedures, or when you're considering one. You know, those conversations where you pull your skin back from your jaw to your ear saying, Doesn't that look better?

Inevitably someone in the group says you don't need to do that, you look great. I always wonder what that means. Are you supposed to wait to have a procedure until one of your friends finally says to you: Your skin is hanging down around your neck and your wrinkles look like pleats in a drape; you look terrible! Go see a plastic surgeon now!

Of course not, because no one needs to get Botox or a face-lift, it's a personal decision, a personal prerogative, based on what you want. Medical cosmetic corrective procedures are about wanting to look younger and choosing realistically how you want to accomplish that goal. Period. The choice is yours.

STRATEGIC PLANNING

Timing is all about what you feel is right for you, weighed against what your goals are. Some procedures are better done sooner than later because they prevent further damage, rebuild the skin, and repair some amount of damage. Planning is everything. Knowledge and careful strategy is the smart way to approach this entire topic.

The options for changing your body and face are almost limitless, and the results can be stunning. Traditional surgical procedures that cut off leathery, thick, lined, and sagging skin long abused by the sun can subtract years from a person's appearance. Laser resurfacing can create smooth skin and remove skin discolorations. Dermal fillers can plump up wrinkles and acne scarring. Botox can erase forehead wrinkles almost immediately. IPL treatments can reduce skin discolorations and zap surface capillaries.

Having procedures done at a younger age, before you "need it" can mean having healthier-looking skin for years as opposed to making an abrupt change when you finally decide you can't take it anymore and begin searching out a physician.

Some physicians claim that if you do things as they crop up there's less trauma, better healing, and, because younger people generally have more elasticity and fat in their skin, the results should last longer and look more natural. Less-invasive and relatively minor procedures can extend the time before major surgery is eventually needed, and there is something to be said for having the face you want now as opposed to later. I think that is a reasonable approach.

We are in a new era where the possibility of looking younger is more accessible than ever before. Some people are pleased to know their face doesn't have to look as old as they really are and that they can have a choice about what to do about it. As long as the results are impressive (and they can be), people will want to stay young-looking via procedures that have as little risk as possible. That's not bad or good; it is just a legitimate option for creating the look you want. Plus, it beats wasting money on creams and lotions that do nothing for the wrinkles. As one plastic surgeon I spoke with noted, "Women have been buying wrinkle creams by the truckload, and yet they still get wrinkles and I'm still in business because none of those cosmetic products work to dramatically stop or change wrinkling."

LOOKING YOUNGER: A GAME PLAN

I rarely share my personal experiences as a way to educate or relate information about skin care or any issue related to beauty because I always prefer facts and research to anecdotes. However, in this section I would like to share my thinking and course of action about my face in regard to medical cosmetic corrective procedures. I do so because my process and decision making may possibly provide insights for you about what options you might want to consider. Again, everyone is different, yet many of our concerns about an older-looking face are similar and the long list of options is the same for everyone. The selection process is where the choices come into play.

For me, I felt my forehead wrinkles, the folds between my brows, the folds that run from the nose to my mouth (the nasal labial folds), the lines around my mouth, and the wrinkles under my eyes were the most bothersome. I was 49 years old when I thought it was time to start considering medical cosmetic corrective procedures.

To start, I felt Botox was my best option. My reasoning was that it was fast, relatively inexpensive, had no real downtime, minimal to no risk, required only one treatment to see results (as opposed to lasers or IPL treatments that need multiple treatments before you realize a noticeable benefit), and my wrinkles were supposed to be gone in 48 hours to a week. Botox lived up to my expectations and I have continued getting Botox injections every six to seven months.

A year later I decided that the lines from my nose to the corners of my mouth were becoming more noticeable and it was getting trickier to keep my makeup from sliding into those lines. I decided to have a dermal filler injected. I considered many options (there are over 30 fillers doctors can use) and opted for Artecoll, a synthetic filler that is considered semi-permanent; it can last anywhere from two to seven years.

There are risks with Artecoll, and there is disagreement between doctors about those risks. Mostly the concern is that because Artecoll is semi-permanent, various factors come into play. All dermal fillers pose a risk of moving into areas you don't want them to go, or there can be overcorrection (think of celebrities with overblown lips), and there's the possibility of granulomas (small, hard bumps under the skin). With a semi-permanent filler, these problems would not go away. Understanding that risk, I decided to have this procedure anyway. Artecoll had a historical safety profile that showed only a small percentage of unwanted results, it's results were relatively long-term (over five years for me), and the idea of having to go back every six months to a year for more injections did not suit me in the least. I'm high maintenance, but I lead a busy life, and given what I wanted to accomplish the less time I needed to be in a doctor's office the better.

Artecoll worked beautifully for me. My lip line (which was starting to recede), the laugh lines, and the lines between my brows were injected and the results did last for five years. I did have some complications with slightly tender lumps along my lips that I could feel but that weren't visible. They did stay and have been slightly bothersome, but for me that has been a minor complication in comparison to going through the pain of injections every six months or once a year (dermal injections are painful and you can look swollen for several days!). I actually could have waited another two to three years before having more Artecoll but decided to have a touch-up after five years. (Permanent fillers do last a long time, but the face continues to age, requiring more if you desire to keep the same appearance.) The results have been impressive.

Treatments to smooth the surface of skin, build collagen, and reduce the appearance of surfaced capillaries fall in the realm of treatment with lasers and IPLs (intense pulsed light), and all those issues were among my concerns and things I wanted to fix or reduce. I chose to do a combination of both. IPLs work best for skin discolorations and surfaced capillaries, while lasers smooth the surface of skin and build collagen. (IPLs do build collagen but far less dramatically.)

I began with IPLs, and after five treatments I did see a reduction in brown discolorations and surfaced capillaries. After 18 months they started to show up again (despite the fact that I don't tan and I'm diligent about wearing sunscreen with titanium dioxide and zinc oxide). That's disappointing, but I am going to do another series.

I decided ablative lasers were not an option for me even though they have the most dramatic results. They impressively smooth and tighten skin and build collagen, but they also have over a 4% risk of causing damage or color loss. However, I did try a new form of laser that reduces the risks associated with traditional laser resurfacing, called fractional resurfacing. This type of laser pixilates, or breaks up, the laser emission to greatly reduce any risk yet still garners similar results. It wasn't a pleasant treatment, it does require four to six treatments a year and then maintenance treatments, and there was downtime, but the results were noticeable, especially around my eyes, after two treatments. Of course, now I have to schedule time for this procedure, but the results are worth it.

At one point I did have liposuction to remove the fat from under my chin to prevent my neck from looking like a turkey wattle. It worked very well but that procedure was a bit of a gamble because I chose not to have surgery to tighten the jaw and neck area, which had been recommended. I was taking the chance that my neck would have enough elasticity so the skin would bounce back and not just hang (minus the fat). It was a good gamble because my skin did bounce back.

I have tried Thermage but was unimpressed with that. I have also considered a face-lift, but right now the noninvasive procedures I've had seem to have postponed that decision for awhile.

So for me, a combination of dermal injections, Botox, IPL, fractional resurfacing, and liposuction of my chin has made quite a difference and I'm happy with my choices. I know things could have gone wrong along the way, but I went into all of these having done my research and weighing the pros and cons and assessing my risk potential along the way. As you make decisions about your face and possible options for rejuvenation your thought process needs to follow the same pattern. What you absolutely never want to do is believe the marketing claims that make any particular procedure sound like a risk-free miracle. No such procedure exists.

How to Choose Your Doctor

Before I get to the details about the various corrective medical procedures that are available, I want to address the most important consumer challenge of all: Who should do your procedure, regardless of what you decide to have done. Given the growing number of doctors with cosmetic or plastic surgery practices and dermatologists who are performing cosmetic corrective procedures (and the advertisements are about as prevalent and some of them as insufferable as those for car dealerships), it is very difficult to know where to go and how to get started.

Most women use one of four methods to select a physician: articles in fashion magazines; finding out where celebrities went (everybody loves knowing where the stars are going for anything and everything, regardless of how they look); getting a referral from a friend or a friend of a friend; and, last but not least, checking out the doctors who advertise their services.

Though I wouldn't call these the worst plans of action, they should just be the beginning of the process. The most important thing to know is whether your physician is board certified. That doesn't guarantee you might not encounter complications or have less than optimal results, but at least you have a better chance of avoiding problems. Doctors of any background can perform cosmetic corrective procedures; you want one who has been specifically trained to work in that field. The Internet makes it easier than ever before to find out the qualifications of the physician you want to see. Here are the steps to follow.

If you are considering plastic or cosmetic surgery, at the very least be sure that your doctor is certified by the American Board of Plastic Surgery (www.abps.org). If you want to see a dermatologist in the United States, be sure they are certified by the American Board of Dermatology (www.abderm.org). To verify that your doctor is legitimately board certified, go to the American Board of Medical Specialties at www.abms.org. Certification lets you know the physician has had the training required to earn the title of specialist.

Each country will have its own resources for board-certified physicians, surgeons, and dermatologists who work in these areas of expertise. What gets confusing is that there are lots of boards that claim to be able to accredit physicians, but not all of them are legit. Don't be fooled by other similar, professional-sounding boards.

When it comes to surgery, you will also want to find out if your doctor has hospital privileges. Even if the procedure will not be performed at the hospital (and 53% of cosmetic surgeries are not), some feel it is important to know that your doctor is qualified and has the necessary training to be accepted. The American Society of Aesthetic Plastic Surgery states that "it is important to find out if the doctor has operating privileges in an accredited hospital for the same procedure you would like to have performed. Before granting operating privileges, hospital review committees evaluate a surgeon's training and competency for specific procedures. If the doctor does not have hospital privileges to perform your procedure, look for another surgeon." (Source: www.surgery.org)

Of course, there are great dermatologists and plastic surgeons who are not board certified, but the odds of getting someone who is inexperienced are greatly reduced when you take the time to find out if that person is board certified. To be certified by the ABPS, a physician must have at least five to six years of approved surgical training, including a two- to three-year residency in plastic surgery. He or she must also have been in practice for at least two years and pass comprehensive written and oral exams in plastic surgery.

THERE ARE RISKS

When you consider that over 13 million medical cosmetic corrective procedures, ranging from face-lifts to collagen injections, were performed in the United States in 2008, and a vastly larger number around the world, it's clear that lots of people are attempting to look younger or to improve some aspect of their skin. This popularity, plus the money-making prospect for doctors—as well as new procedures with limited track records—all mean you have to be careful about your decision-making process.

Shockingly, many physicians downplay any risks. If anything, many physicians offer a hard sell more than a trustworthy medical perspective. A quick review of several cosmetic surgery Internet sites or cosmetic dermatology–related sites reveals a scarcity of detailed information about what can go wrong during or after a procedure. Yet each and every medical cosmetic corrective procedure has risks. Yes, the risks are few and far between, but on average about 1% to 4% of people having these procedures have had problems or negative outcomes. An even larger number of people, ranging from 10% to 50% depending on the treatment, are disappointed in the results. These statistics are a bit elusive because these numbers are dependent on whose data you use, what procedures you are including, and what definition of adverse event, complication, or dissatisfaction is being included. Regardless, it is wise for you to decide if you want to chance being one of those who may fall into any of these statistics.

Being proactive about any cosmetic procedure is incredibly important, but let me reiterate that it is even more vital with cosmetic surgery. After all, this surgery is usually elective and completely up to you; there is (or ought to be) nothing life-or-death about these procedures. Furthermore, cosmetic surgery is a very lucrative business—most surgeons get paid up front before you go under the knife or laser. So, before you hand over your hard-earned money, your very appearance, and your well-being, you have to be knowledgeable about every detail.

WHAT TO ASK

Once you've dealt with the issue of board certification, it's time to ask lots of questions and then look for answers that make you feel comfortable and make the most sense to you in light of the research you have done. Not all physicians will come up with the same game plan for your face. Each one has techniques he or she prefers, sometimes regardless of whether these actually represent the best or most current technology. That's not necessarily bad. Some use the latest technology not because it is better or has proven more effective but in response to pressure from their elite clients, who expect or demand what's new regardless of the risks.

Many doctors love to use computer imaging to "close the sale" on the cosmetic procedure they are recommending. A picture of your face or body is taken and scanned into a computer program, allowing the surgeon to then demonstrate how you would look if you were pulled a little here, tucked a little there, and lifted a little all over. As impressive as this is, it is only a computer image and not real life. It is a great tool for getting an idea of what you can expect, but it isn't an exact blueprint, and real-life results are never the same. Don't let this imaging be the deciding factor in your final decision.

One of the most important questions you can ask when interviewing a doctor is how often per month they perform the specific procedure or procedures you are considering. It is best, but not essential, to get a doctor who specializes, as opposed to a doctor who tries to do it all. If you want to go for Botox, it is probably better to find a physician who has done thousands of Botox injections than someone who only does a few every week.

When it comes to cosmetic surgery, it is imperative to ask how many surgeries the doctor performs in a day. If the doctor schedules more than three procedures a day, most likely another doctor or nurse will do the prep work and/or the finishing work. That may not mean poor results, but it does mean the doctor is not giving you his or her full attention.

Make sure the doctor you are consulting or want to work with will be the only doctor working on your face or body, and that he or she will never leave the operating room during your procedure. You would be shocked how often the doctor allows his assistant to do the surgery and how seldom the doctor may be present for the entire operation.

It is also valid to ask if the doctor charges for redos and touch-ups. Though it isn't something doctors like to admit, going back in for fine-tuning or to correct mistakes is common, and you don't want to be charged to have the doctor repair what you don't like.

Be insistent about understanding every nuance of the postoperative procedure. Many complications can occur when the patient doesn't realize her part in the healing process. For example, scar tissue can cause problems for a breast implant. One of the ways to minimize that risk is to keep your breasts tightly bound and your arms firmly at your side, with little to no movement and no lifting for four to seven days.

PRETREATMENT

Are there steps you can take to get the most out of your procedure? Absolutely, but they aren't any different from what you should already be doing to keep your skin vital, nourished, healthy, repaired, and stable. However, these daily essentials become even more important if you're going to undergo a cosmetic corrective procedure. Don't smoke, stay out of the sun, use a sunscreen daily, use gentle cleansers (irritation and dryness hurt the skin's ability to heal), consider using a retinoid such as Renova or Tazorac, exfoliate (to remove any unhealthy build-up of dead skin cells), and use a product (such as a gel, liquid, or cream) loaded with antioxidants and skin-identical ingredients. All of these will help your skin be at its best and help support the results you are going after.

Some women have been told that before they have a chemical peel, laser resurfacing, or any cosmetic corrective procedure they need to purchase and use special products, especially the expensive ones sold by their dermatologist or plastic surgeon, starting two to four weeks ahead of the treatment. First, of all the skin-care products sold by dermatologists or plastic surgeons, none are in any way preferred to other well-formulated skin-care products that are usually readily available elsewhere for a lot less money. If a doctor tells you otherwise they are not telling the truth. Second, reputable doctors can sell their own products, but ethically they should recommend products other than their own and that cost less. Plenty of products being sold by physicians are not only overpriced but also poorly formulated. Don't let your doctor dupe you with this deceptive scam that claims products being sold in doctors' offices are somehow better, because they absolutely are not.

Theoretically, pretreatment seems to make sense, but there is no research showing a specialized skin-care routine is necessary. As an article published in *Cosmetic Dermatology* (March 2000, "Pre-Treatment of Skin for Laser Resurfacing: Is It Necessary?") states: "Retinoic acid derivatives [tretinoin such as Retin-A or Renova] have been studied most thoroughly and have been shown to accelerate wound healing. On the other hand, the preoperative use of AHAs, hydroquinone, and ascorbic acid [vitamin C] has proven to be of no apparent clinical benefit. Since these compounds appear to affect only superficial epidermal melanocytes [skin cells] (which are vaporized upon ... laser irradiation)... they have no effect on the lower layers of skin." That means you can save your money by avoiding expensive pretreatment products being sold by the physician.

In terms of topical tretinoin cream, daily use does help repair some amount of sun damage and does offer an advantage in wound healing, but that is very different from the cosmetic products many doctors are selling these days (Source: *Journal of Cellular Physiology*, May 2008, pages 506–516).

Although cosmetic skin-care products are not helpful for use as a pretreatment, what does make sense, at least in terms of helping your skin handle the procedures better, is the ongoing use of well-formulated products every day. They will go a long way toward helping you keep the results you achieved and also will ensure that your skin is as healthy as it can be all the time.

POSSIBILITIES FROM A TO Z

None of these procedures come with a guarantee of happiness—they are just a way to buy the kind of body and face you want. (If that designer outfit didn't make you happy, don't expect new breasts or a face-lift to provide peace of mind!) Every plastic surgeon I've spoken with has told me that among their patients those most pleased with the results of their surgery were the ones who had the most realistic expectations. What are unrealistic expectations? Expecting to end up looking like a supermodel, or believing you will now find the perfect relationship. Plastic surgery should be about your self-esteem associated with societal standards of beauty—nothing more and nothing less.

Important details: Keep in mind that everyone scars differently, and that scarring often has little to do with the skill of the surgeon. You could be left with lines wherever an incision was made. In general, the paler your skin, the more prone you may be to red, welt-like scarring, and the darker your skin, the more prone you may be to thick, dark, keloidal scarring.

There are serious risks with all cosmetic corrective procedures, and recovering from the more serious surgeries, such as face-lifts, tummy tucks, and breast implants, can be a daunting, frightening experience. For example, eye tucks can damage the tear ducts or permanently destroy eyelashes, face-lifts can leave painful scars and pockets of dimpled flesh, laser or chemical peels can render skin tone uneven and cause discolorations, dermal injections can cause lumps and the material can migrate to areas where it wasn't intended to go, and breast implants can leak or become encapsulated and painful.

All cosmetic surgery procedures have limitations as to how long the change will last, depending on skin type, age, the surgeon's technique, and postoperative care (including using sunscreen). Do not expect any cosmetic surgery to be permanent, especially laser peels, dermal filler injections, chemical peels, and Botox (discussed later in this chapter).

Note: As indicated below, prices for these procedures vary widely. The region of the country you live in, the popularity of the surgeon, the specific techniques used (the more invasive or complex, the more expensive), the combination of techniques, and discounts given for doing more than one procedure can all greatly affect price.

FROM THE NECK UP

BOTOX (BOTULINUM TOXIN A) *($300 TO $1,000)*

Botox is the number one noninvasive cosmetic corrective procedure around the world. When injected into specific muscles Botox (botulinum toxin A) prevents muscle movement by partially and almost completely paralyzing them. Botulinum toxin inhibits the release of the chemical acetylcholine, which stimulates nerve endings attached to the muscle, thereby inhibiting muscle movement. The resulting inability to use those face muscles causes the wrinkles in that area to completely disappear.

Most typically Botox is used to eliminate the wrinkles of the forehead and reduce the wrinkles around the outside corner of the eye (the crow's feet area). It has also been used for other parts of the face but those techniques are somewhat controversial and the naturalness of the appearance it imparts is less clear.

By now Botox is not new. It has been used by ophthalmologists since 1973 to treat patients suffering from disabling eye ticks, as well as to treat crossed eyes. It is also used by other medical specialists to treat spasmodic neck muscles, spasmodic laryngeal muscles, multiple sclerosis, cerebral palsy, some post-stroke states, spinal cord injuries, nerve palsies, Parkinson's disease, facial spasms, and, most recently, migraine headaches. However, the research on the effectiveness of Botox for headaches or other analgesic benefit is inconclusive.

(Sources: *Head and Face Medicine*, August 2007, page 32; *Cochrane Database Systematic Review*, July 18, 2007, CD000319; and *Journal of Neurology*, February 2004, pages S119–S130.)

This history of extensive use (and the corresponding research) has shown that Botox has a great success rate, with minimal risk of detrimental side effects, but that doesn't mean they don't exist. An inexperienced physician, for example, may cause the most complications, since if they inject the wrong areas you may experience temporary facial or eye drooping, long-lasting bruising, or jaw and neck weakness. These problems almost always last only for the duration of the Botox, and so go away in three to six months, but there are rare cases where the problem has persisted.

Moreover, different formulations of botulinum toxin type A are not identical and may behave differently in clinical practice. The reportedly lower incidence of adverse effects with one formulation (from Allergan, Ltd.) relative to another (from Ipsen, Ltd.) may be due to differences in the degree of migration of the neurotoxin-protein complex from its injection site (Source: Journal of Cosmetic Dermatology, March 2008, pages 50–54).

(Sources: *Skin Therapy Letter*, July–August 2008, pages 1–4; *Clinical Dermatology*, March–April 2008, pages 182–191; *Journal of Cosmetic Laser Therapy*, September 2007, S23–S31; and *Facial and Plastic Surgery Clinics of North America*, February 2007, pages 41–49.)

MYOBLOC (BOTULINUM TOXIN B) *($300 TO $1,000)*

Myobloc (botulinum toxin type B) was approved by the FDA in December 2000 "for the symptomatic treatment of patients with cervical dystonia (CD) to reduce the severity of abnormal head position and neck pain associated with CD." Cervical dystonia is a neurological movement disorder in which a person's neck and shoulder muscles are subject to contractions that force the head and neck into abnormal and sometimes painful positions, making it difficult for some people to function normally in their daily activities.

For those receiving Myobloc treatments for CD, the side effects may include dry mouth, dysphagia, dyspepsia, and injection site pain. These adverse effects are generally mild to moderate, transient, self-resolving, and more common only with higher doses. The side effects are also related to the location of the injection site and the muscles involved and not the drug itself. Myobloc was formerly known as BotB and is marketed outside the United States as Neurobloc.

Few trials have compared the efficacy of Botox with Myobloc. Overall, the evidence suggests that although both are safe and effective, Myobloc has a more rapid onset but a shorter duration of action, and may be associated with slightly more discomfort at the time of injection. Myobloc is mostly useful for people who receive minimal or no results with Botox, although this is a rare problem.

(Sources: *Journal of Cosmetic and Laser Therapy*, September 2007, pages 186–192; and *Dermatologic Surgery*, May 2003, pages 519–522.)

CHEEKBONE (MALAR) AUGMENTATION *($2,000 TO $3,500)*

Improving the shape of the face is usually considered separately from the issue of facial rejuvenation, although it can serve both purposes. For many women, having a more sculpted face is an aesthetic goal, and, therefore, cheekbone augmentation is among the more common procedures in facial plastic surgery practices. Cheekbones are reshaped and built up by placing an implant (made of plastic or some other inorganic material) over them to build up their structure. But beyond wanting to have higher cheekbones, this procedure can be helpful for an aging face. This is because with aging the volume of the cheekbone's fat pad and bone structure diminishes, one of the reasons an older face can become gaunt. Cheek implants can correct this appearance.

Cheek implants are considered a safe, relatively simple technique with generally good results, although like any surgery it can have its problems both in terms of adverse events and results that are disappointing or upsetting.

The inorganic implant is usually inserted via an incision within the mouth, but it may be done through a lower eyelid or brow incision. Perhaps the biggest mistake made during this procedure is overcompensation. When cheekbones are so enlarged they look like they belong on someone else, the effect is fake-looking (think Disney's cartoon character Cruella de Vil).

Alternatively, the buccal fat pads under the cheekbone, which are located above the jawline near the corners of the mouth, just below the cheekbone, can be removed in individuals with an excessively round face if they want a more angular appearance. This procedure imparts a more contoured look, sometimes referred to as the "waif look," à la Kate Moss. However, plastic surgeons warn that, in many individuals, removal of the buccal fat pads can lead to a more drawn, hollow-cheeked look as the naturally occurring aging progresses continues, making the face look older, not younger.

(Sources: *Plastic and Reconstructive Surgery*, February 2008, pages 620–628; and *Facial and Plastic Surgery Clinics of North America*, February 2008, pages 11–32.)

CHEMICAL PEELS *($500 TO 2,700)*

Peel solutions may contain alpha hydroxy acids (glycolic or lactic acid), beta hydroxy acid (salicylic acid), tricholoracetic acid (TCA), or phenol as the peeling agent. Each of these is categorized by the percentage of its concentration and the resulting depth of the peel that takes place on the skin. Fine lines and wrinkles, skin discolorations, reduction in the appearance of skin discolorations and scars, along with overall improvement in skin texture and subtle rebuilding of the skin's collagen are all possible outcomes of chemical peels.

There are definite drawbacks to consider, but what these may be is largely dependent on the depth of peel. The risk of complication is directly related to the amount of benefit desired. Superficial peels (almost always either glycolic acid or lactic acid) have little to no associated risks, but also produce less dramatic results. Low-concentration glycolic acid and salicylic acid peels can have rare side effects, and prolonged redness, swelling, and increased skin sensitivity do occur.

When more significant results are desired, the complications increase proportionately. Skin discoloration can occur in medium and deeper peels (called hypo- or hyperpigmentation) where the skin becomes either darker or lighter in certain areas. Many more complications and scars are recorded from TCA peeling than from phenol, perhaps because of the care with which phenol peels must be performed, and the implied safety of TCA (Source: *eMedicine Journal*, February 14, 2002, volume 3, number 2).

Chemical peels are performed by the application of the specific solution that peels away the skin's top layers, either on the entire face or on specific areas. Often, several shallow to medium-depth peels can achieve results similar to one deep-peel treatment, with less post-procedure risk and a shorter recovery time.

Alpha hydroxy acids (AHA) use glycolic acid as the chemical ingredient. Various concentrations can be applied, but most commonly 30% to 70% concentrations are used. Lower-concentration peels can be used by an aesthetician and are a popular spa procedure. Again, the lower the concentration of AHA, the less impressive the results will be.

Low-concentration AHA peels are effective in improving skin texture; they cause some collagen and elastin rebuilding, somewhat reduce the appearance of acne scarring, and reduce the appearance of skin discolorations. The effects are all temporary and subsequent treatments, spaced anywhere between six weeks and two months apart, are required (Source: *American Journal of Clinical Dermatology*, March–April 2000, pages 81–88).

AHA peels are not medical procedures and as a result are not regulated by the FDA. A physician usually performs higher-concentration peels, but this is not always the case. In lower-concentration peels, often performed by aestheticians, repeated treatments are necessary to achieve and maintain the results seen immediately after the peel is performed.

Beta hydroxy acid (BHA) or salicylic acid peels are not as popular as AHA peels, yet they are equally as effective and have specific advantages for some skin types. A solution of salicylic acid can work in a way that is similar to a glycolic acid peel, but irritation is much reduced. Salicylic acid is a compound closely related to aspirin (acetylsalicylic acid), and it retains its aspirin-like anti-inflammatory properties. A deep BHA peel can be superior for many skin types because the irritation and inflammation are kept to a minimum due to the analgesic action of the BHA compound. Salicylic acid is also lipid soluble, which means it is a good peeling agent for blemish-prone skin with blackheads. The most common concentrations used today are 20% to 30% (Source: *Dermatologic Surgery*, March 1998, pages 325–328).

Trichloroacetic acid (TCA) peels in concentrations of 10% to 35% have been used for many years and are considered effective and safe (Source: *Dermatologic Clinics*, July 2001, pages 413–425). TCA can be used for peeling the face, neck, hands, and other exposed areas of the body. It has less bleaching effect than phenol (see the next paragraph) and is excellent for "spot" peeling of specific areas. It can be used for medium or light peeling, depending on the concentration and method of application. TCA peels are best for fine lines but are minimally effective on deeper wrinkling (Source: *eMedicine Journal*, December 5, 2001, volume 2, number 12). However, at higher concentrations, such as 50% and above, TCA has a tendency to scar and is less manageable than other agents used for superficial peels.

Phenol is sometimes, though rarely, used for full-face peeling when sun damage or wrinkling is severe. It can also be used to treat limited areas of the face, such as deep wrinkles around the mouth, but it may permanently bleach the skin, leaving a line of demarcation between the treated and untreated areas that must be covered with makeup. "Although phenol produces the most remarkable resolution of actinic damage and wrinkling among the various [chemical peels] … it also possesses some of the more significant [serious side effects]. Many have abandoned phenol in favor of other agents or laser resurfacing…. Hypopigmentation may occur in all skin types, noticeably lightening patients with darker skin and making lighter-skinned patients appear waxy or pale. A clear line of demarcation may be present between treated and untreated skin" (Source: *eMedicine Journal*, July 20, 2001, volume 2, number 7). Given the positive results that can be achieved with other resurfacing procedures and the extreme risks associated with phenol, this method is actively discouraged and rarely used.

Buffered phenol offers yet another option for severely sun-damaged skin. One such formula uses olive oil, among other ingredients, to diminish the strength of the phenol solution. Another, slightly milder formula uses glycerin. A buffered phenol peel may be more comfortable for patients, and the skin heals faster than with a standard phenol peel, but it is still a risky procedure that can depigment the skin (Source: *Facial Plastic Surgery Clinics of North America*, August 2001, pages 351–376).

CHIN AUGMENTATION (MENTOPLASTY)
CHIN REDUCTION *($1,700 TO $5,000)*

Chin augmentation can strengthen the appearance of a receding chin by increasing its projection. (Look at pictures of Michael Jackson when he was young, then look at a recent picture; it's hard to ignore his mega-chin implant.) The procedure does not affect the patient's bite or jaw, and can be done using one of two techniques. One approach is to make an incision inside the mouth, move the chin bone, and then wire it into position; the other requires the insertion of an implant through an incision inside the mouth, between the lower lip and the gum, or through an external incision underneath the chin. Hydroxyapatite granules, a bone substitute made from coral, can also be used to enhance facial contours, such as forming a more prominent chin or cheekbones. The substance also has reconstructive uses in craniofacial surgery.

From another perspective, even if the shape of the chin may not be an issue, with aging excess skin can start pouching along the jawline, creating the appearance of a double chin or a turkey neck. Having liposuction to remove the excess fat and then a chin tuck to shore up the sagging skin is one way to address this issue. You and your surgeon can also decide if reshaping a too-narrow chin should be part of the effort.

(Source: *Facial Plastic Surgery Clinics of North America*, February 2008, pages 79–85.)

COLLAGEN INJECTIONS *($325 TO $1,400)*

See Dermal Fillers in this chapter.

Cosmetic Tattooing *($750 to $1,500)*

Cosmetic tattooing, or micropigmentation, can be used to create permanent eyeliner, eyebrow color, or lip color. It can also be used for permanent blush or eyeshadow, though this is uncommon. Other uses include re-creating the coloration of the areola around the nipple following breast reconstruction; restoring the color of dark or light skin where natural pigmentation has been lost through such factors as vitiligo (a whitening of the skin from an autoimmune response), cancer, burns, or other scarring; and eliminating some types of birthmarks or previous tattoos.

While cosmetic tattooing can be useful there are significant risks both aesthetically and medically. Because makeup fashions change and the face ages, tattooed eyebrows or lip lines may look nice and even when you're in your thirties or forties, but as you near 50 and your face starts to droop the tattoo will go with it. Additionally, your style preferences can change. A brown or bright red lip color imprinted on your mouth may look good today, but in five or ten years it can look strange and out of date. Many cosmetic surgeons and dermatologists I've interviewed have commented that removing tattooed-on lip liner, eyebrows, and blush has become a lucrative business due to the large number of botched applications.

Dermabrasion *($1,000 to $2,500)*

Dermabrasion is a procedure in which a high-speed wheel, similar to a rotary sander using fine-grained sandpaper, is used to abrade the skin. As a method of resurfacing, dermabrasion can be an effective way to treat deep acne scars and deep facial wrinkling. Its strong point is that the procedure can be done without the heat damage that lasers or acid burns of chemical peels can cause. However, some expected side effects, both transient and long-term, are considered normal and do occur. Transient effects can include spot bleeding for several days after surgery, swelling, breakouts, and hyperpigmentation. Hypopigmentation, the permanent loss of skin color, occurs in 20% to 30% of patients. Possible scarring can also occur but that is true for any of the deeper chemical peels and ablative laser resurfacing (Source: *eMedicine Journal*, October 17, 2001, volume 2, number 10).

Despite these daunting considerations, dermabrasion may still be recommended for deep acne scarring, provided there is a firm understanding about the risk of depigmentation.

Dermal Fillers *($500 to $3,000)*

No matter what it's called—tissue augmentation, injectable fillers, soft-tissue fillers, implants, or dermal filler injections—one of the more popular ways to improve the appearance of wrinkles or acne scars is to fill them in with a variety of substances. These fillers work just the way they sound: by literally being injected or implanted into a wrinkle or a scar so that the material (either synthetic or natural) then fills in the depression (temporarily or semi-permanently), creating a smoother impression. Almost all fillers can also work to plump up lips or alter the shape of the face, but their primary use is to fill in wrinkles and acne scars.

Filling in wrinkles or scars using any form of tissue augmentation can be done in combination with other cosmetic procedures. These can range from Botox injections to laser,

IPL, or chemical peel resurfacing (as well as face-lifts) to achieve optimal results in obtaining the smoothest looking skin you can get.

If you're considering injectable fillers of any kind, the following information will help give you a realistic guideline for comparisons, risks, and expectations. It is vital to understand that, as with any cosmetic corrective procedure, there's no single best option. Quite the contrary—there are many excellent alternatives available, and the final decision should be determined by your doctor's skill, your budget, how much risk you're willing to take, and what kind of realistic results you're looking for.

Some of the typical risks of all dermal fillers are a possible reaction to the needle or device used to place the material in the skin, pain, bruising, inflammation, discoloration, and swelling. These often resolve within a few days to a few weeks. On rare occasions discoloration can last for up to year if a blood vessel was affected. Other adverse reactions can be allergic reactions, granulomas (palpable bumps under the skin), red discoloration from injections that are too superficial and can be felt on top of the skin, overcorrection, migration of the substance, persistent lumpiness, and infection.

The price of dermal fillers depends on many factors but primarily it is about the cost of the filler itself and the amount used. If you only chose to inject and plump up the folds from the nose to the mouth, it will cost less money than also treating the marionette lines that go from the corners of the mouth down to the chin and the frown lines between the eyes.

(Sources: *Journal of Plastic Reconstructive and Aesthetic Surgery*, January 2009, pages 11–18; *British Journal of Dermatology*, November 2008, pages 1036–1050; *Dermatologic Surgery*, June 2008, pages S92–S99; and *Journal of Cosmetic and Laser Therapy*, December 2005, pages 171–176.)

NON-PERMANENT VERSUS PERMANENT FILLERS

The number of available filling agents has increased dramatically, improving the range of options available to select from. Getting some information about the different characteristics, capabilities, risks, and limitations of the varying options can help an informed consumer understand what results they can expect and how much risk they face in terms of potential complications.

Fillers are classified as temporary/nonpermanent, semi-permanent, or permanent. Temporary fillers stay in the tissue for less than a year, semi-permanent fillers for up to one or two years, and permanent fillers are substances that remain in the tissue more than two years (so technically, they're not really permanent). Beyond their permanent versus nonpermanent status, fillers are also classified by their source: human, animal, or synthetic.

Nonpermanent and semi-permanent fillers have the disadvantage of spontaneously disappearing so they have to be redone every six months to two years to maintain the effect. Ironically, the advantage of nonpermanent and semi-permanent fillers is that if any problems do arise they dissolve in a relatively short period of time. Permanent fillers obviously have the advantage of not requiring additional treatments for many years if at all, but if there are complications with these the problem(s) may not resolve on their own and could even require surgical removal if rare, serious problems occur. In terms of risk, rare, long-lasting side effects have been reported even with temporary fillers.

(Sources: *Journal of Plastic, Reconstructive and Aesthetic Surgery*, January 2009, pages 11–18; and *Journal of Oral Implantology*, April 2007, pages 191–204.)

ANIMAL-DERIVED COLLAGEN FILLERS

Brand names: Zyderm 1, Zyderm 2, Zyplast, Fibrel

Major risks: Allergic reactions and necrotic (non-living) areas of skin can occur. These can have a hard feel, and may look lumpy or uneven under the skin. Primarily, the risk of an adverse effect is 3% and that's considered a significant amount.

Stability: Benefits can last three to six months.

Collagen is found in all living tissue, and in the skin its basic function is to provide support and structure. The FDA approved injectable collagen in 1981. For most of the 1980s and 1990s, collagen injections were one of the primary methods used to fill in wrinkles. Zyderm and Zyplast are derived from cow collagen; Fibrel is derived from pig collagen. Injectable animal collagens are used less frequently in Europe than in the United States due to the risk of their association with bovine spongiform encephalopathy (BSE, or Mad Cow Disease). Collagen injections derived from animal sources are now used less frequently than other dermal fillers in the United States, but that is largely due to a substantial risk of allergic reaction (according to the FDA, "about 3 percent of the population is allergic to collagen") and the short duration of the results.

Because of the potential for allergic reaction (particularly for cow collagen), it is essential to have a pretest at least four to six weeks prior to treatment. A small amount of the collagen is injected into the arm or thigh and the area is monitored closely for any signs of inflammation, swelling, irritation, rashes, or itching. Once it has been determined that you are not allergic to the material it can be injected into the wrinkle underneath the skin. Repeated injections may be necessary until optimal results are achieved.

HUMAN-DERIVED COLLAGEN OR DONOR FILLERS

Brand names: Dermalogen, Autologen, Isolagen, AlloDerm, Micronized AlloDerm (trade name Cymetra)

Major risks: Minimal to no risk of allergic reaction, but the area injected can have a hard feel under skin and the skin may look lumpy or uneven.

Stability: Benefits can last three to nine months and possibly longer, though there is no research establishing the exact length of time. Requires several injections over a period of time to obtain results and significant initial overcorrection is required.

Dermalogen is derived from human cadaver collagen, Autologen is derived from your own skin's collagen, and Isolagen is made of cells that are actually cloned from your own skin. The primary benefit of human-derived collagen injections is that there is almost no chance of having or developing an allergic reaction.

Autologen can be harvested during cosmetic surgery procedures such as tummy tucks, face-lifts, and breast augmentation or reduction. The skin removed from those procedures is sent to a laboratory where it is processed to become injectable collagen filler. Depending on the results you are trying to achieve you may receive a series of injections over a period of a year. Some doctors claim that Autologen achieves permanent results, but that has not been proven, and for many women is definitely not the case. Plus it can take several series of injections over a few weeks to see results.

Isolagen, as futuristic as it sounds, is made of cells cloned from your own skin. It's done by simply removing a small piece of skin (about the size of a dime) from your neck or behind your ear. The skin is sent to a lab that, in about four to six weeks, can grow your own injectable collagen from it. Generally, three to four injections are delivered over a two-month period. Each subsequent injection produces increased improvement. After the last injection, continued improvement may still be seen because, unlike all other injectable procedures, Isolagen uses live cells and that stimulates further smoothing out of wrinkles for a period of time.

The process of creating Dermalogen is similar to that for creating both Isolagen and Autologen. Dermalogen, however, is derived from skin tissue removed at the time of death, much as other organs are removed from human donors. All three—Autologen, Isolagen, and Dermalogen—are thought to last longer than animal-derived collagen, but that is yet to be proven. A primary benefit of Dermalogen over Isolagen and Autologen is that it doesn't require any skin removal (at least not from you); and there's no waiting time for preparation.

AlloDerm, technically called acellular cadaveric dermis, refers to the use of donor tissue obtained from dead bodies. Much as donor organs are removed from cadavers at the time of death, skin tissue can also be surgically removed and then processed to be used as filler material for wrinkles or to improve facial contours. The donated human tissue undergoes a complex treatment process, and then is finally freeze-dried in a way that preserves the integrity of the dermal matrix. When it is ready to be used it is rehydrated and surgically inserted under the skin where recountouring is desired. Once implanted, AlloDerm merges with your own skin and stimulates your body to produce its own collagen until it essentially becomes a part of your skin. Although Alloderm is not widely used as a filler for wrinkles, it has been successfully used in thousands of skin-graft operations and is considered exceptionally safe, stable, and reliable for creating natural-looking results. There is little research showing its benefit for wrinkles. (Source: *Archives of Facial and Plastic Surgery*, October–December 2002, pages 252–257.)

Overall, these fillers have taken a back seat to many other options that are less expensive, last longer, and are far less complicated for the physician to prepare. (Sources: *Facial and Plastic Surgery*, February 2004, pages 21–29; and *Journal of Burns and Wounds*, March 2005, page 4.)

BIOENGINEERED HUMAN COLLAGEN FILLERS

Brand names: CosmoDerm I, CosmoDerm II, CosmoPlast

Major risks: Minimal to no risk of allergic reaction, but the area injected can have a hard feel under skin and may look lumpy or uneven.

Stability: Benefits can last three to nine months and possibly longer, though there is no research establishing exact length of time.

Because of the risk of allergy with bovine-derived collagen fillers, several companies were motivated to develop human-derived collagen dermal fillers. Since these agents do not contain any bovine collagen, no allergy testing is required prior to treatment and treatment can begin immediately. Furthermore, no cross-reactions have been documented in patients with a history of allergy to the bovine collagen fillers, so any patient with a documented allergy to bovine collagen may be treated with bioengineered human collagen.

Dermal fibroblasts are harvested from bioengineered human skin and placed into a three-dimensional mesh. These fibroblasts synthesize collagen and extracellular matrix proteins, which are then used as a dermal filling agent. In March 2003, the FDA approved three bioengineered human collagen dermal fillers, CosmoDerm I, CosmoDerm II, and CosmoPlast. These human-based dermal fillers probably have the least patient downtime of any dermal filler available (Source: *Plastic and Reconstructive Surgery*, November 2007, pages 17S-26S).

FAT TRANSFER FILLERS

Technical names: Autologous Fat Transplantation, Fat Injections, Microlipo-injection, Fat Grafting

Major risks: There are risks associated with liposuction procedures. From the injection itself there can be some local swelling, redness, and bruising. Scar-tissue buildup is possible, and it is possible to temporarily lose sensation in the treatment area due to nerve damage or swelling. Long-term or permanent loss of sensitivity is possible. There is also the risk of an asymmetrical appearance.

Stability: Your body will absorb about 65% of the fat within the first six months. The remaining 35% can remain in place for longer, but exactly how much longer varies greatly from person to person. For some reason some people's bodies just can't hold on to the injected fat, even when it's their own.

Getting rid of your own fat from areas you don't want excess and then injecting it into your wrinkles to eliminate them does sound like the best of all worlds, but fat injections are a more complicated process than other injectables and they don't last as long. So even though the concept of redistributing fat from an area where you don't want it (like the thighs and buttocks) to areas where it may be of better use (like wrinkles) is very appealing, the benefit of fat transplantation is limited by the body's dramatic reabsorption of fat grafts.

The first step is to remove fat from your own body, and it is usually taken from the abdomen or buttocks. It is important that the fat being used has a soft texture so it can more easily adapt and be contoured to the shape of the face. Once the fat is extracted it is processed to make it usable, so it can be injected precisely beneath the wrinkle to fill in and reshape the area. This injection process is repeated until the desired enhancement is attained.

Another added benefit of fat injections is that when physicians extract fat from a liposuction procedure, breast augmentation, tummy tuck, or some other reduction surgery, they can store the fat in a freezer to be used in future fat-injection procedures.

Because of the amount of absorption that takes place within the first few months of treatment, many physicians overfill the treated area to help improve the long-term results. This overfilling can create a strange appearance by making the face look swollen and puffy. The puffiness does diminish over a period of weeks, but be aware that this is a potential problem for the short term.

(Source: *Archives of Facial Plastic Surgery*, May–June 2008, pages 187-193; and *Plastic and Reconstructive Surgery*, May 2006, pages 1836-1844).

HYALURONIC ACID DERIVED FILLERS

Brand names: Restylane, Hylaform, Perlane, Juvederm, Rofilan Hylan gel, and Captique

Major risk: Hypersensitivity can occur in 1 out of every 2,000 treated patients. There have also been cases of persistent inflammation and noninfected abscesses, which may persist for up to a year, or until the injected material is fully absorbed.

Stability: Benefits can last 3 to 6 months and occasionally for one year, and may sometimes last for up to 18 months.

Restylane, Hylaform, Perlane, Juvederm, Captique, and Rofilan are all different forms of hyaluronic acid (either derived from bacteria or rooster combs) that has been formed so that it can be injected into wrinkles to fill them out. Restylane is probably the most popular filler worldwide, and has practically become a household name when the subject of cosmetic corrective procedures is brought up.

Each of the hyaluronic acid fillers has specific benefits for different parts of the face, but Restylane is the most used and is generally preferred over the others. Aside from their natural origin and rare occurrence of complications, results from these fillers are short-lived, meaning that when complications do occur they resolve in a short period of time.

Hylaform, Perlane, Rofilan, and Restylane have many similarities. The primary difference is in their consistency: Hylaform, Perlane, and Rofilan are viscoelastic gels, which means that they are more viscous and pliable than Restylane. This makes them better for treatment of deeper lines than for superficial wrinkles, where they can feel thick and be visible under the skin. Restylane, on the other hand, is better for treatment of superficial wrinkles.

(Sources: *Journal of Cosmetic Dermatology*, December 2008, pages 251–258; *Dermatologic Surgery*, June 2008, pages S92–S99; *Plastic and Reconstructive Surgery*, November 2007, pages 41S–54S; *Dermatologic Therapy*, May–June 2006, pages 141–150; and *Dermatologic Clinics*, April 2005, pages 343–363.)

FASCIAN FILLERS

Technical name: Irradiated Human Cadaveric Preserved Fascia Lata

Brand name: Fascian

Major risks: Depending on the amount of material and the size of the needle used, the injected site can become swollen or bruised. The area may also feel thick or lumpy, though typically this softens in time. Allergic reactions are rare.

Stability: Benefits can last 6 to 12 months.

Fascian, much like Alloderm (described above), is obtained from donor tissue from dead bodies. In this case the donated material is fascia, the substance covering your muscles (and some organs) in large, thick, white sheets, keeping them compact and supported yet limber. Fascia's unique property is that it is a firm yet pliable type of human tissue, qualities that make it adaptable for use in improving the appearance of skin. The main drawback of this procedure is its expense when compared with the length of time results remain, which is not much longer than other injectables.

(Sources: *Plastic and Reconstructive Surgery*, November 2007, pages 8S–16S; and *Facial and Plastic Surgery*, May 2004, pages 149–152.)

SYNTHETIC GRAFTS/IMPLANTS

Brand names: Gore S.A.M., Softform

Major risks: These grafts and implants require surgery. There can be unpleasant firmness and a risk of the implant breaking through the skin. Thinner strands of Gore S.A.M. (Subcutaneous Augmentation Material) and Softform may reduce the risk of over-firmness. Synthetic implants are not recommended for lip enhancement due to the potential for an uneven or hard, unnatural appearance of lips. Your body can reject the implant. Scarring can occur.

Stability: Benefits can be permanent.

Gore S.A.M. and Softform are technically not injectable fillers but rather synthetic grafts of material surgically placed under the skin to plump up wrinkles. For those of us who live in the Northwest, Gore-Tex is a well-known, durable, synthetic fabric that works well in all weather conditions. It is essentially a form of Teflon. Gore-Tex has remarkable flexibility, and in the form of Gore S.A.M.—created by the same company that developed Gore-Tex, W. L. Gore and Associates—it can be used for cosmetic corrective procedures. The actual implant material is called expanded polytetrafluoroethylene (ePTFE). Implanting threadlike strips of Gore S.A.M. under the skin around the lips or along the nasal labial folds (the lines that run from the nose to the mouth) can improve the appearance of the face.

Gore S.A.M. is porous, and therefore allows the body's own tissue to attach itself to the material, creating a very durable, stable implant. However, Gore S.A.M has limited uses. For example, those with thin skin would find that the implant can easily be felt or even seen under the surface. It also should not be used on the lips because of the risk of stiffness, making the mouth look unnatural.

The Softform implant is made from the same material as Gore S.A.M. The major difference between Softform and Gore S.A.M. is that Softform threads are hollow, as opposed to Gore S.A.M., which is porous. Softform's hollow structure allows your own tissue to grow through the cylinder to help make it more stable and durable. (Source: *Journal of Oral Implantology*, August 2007, pages 191–204.)

ARTECOLL

Brand names: Artecoll (in Canada), Artefill (in the United States), Dermalive/Dermatech

Major risk: Artecoll has the same potential for allergic reactions as collagen injections because of the bovine vehicle substance. Dermalive/Dermatech has minimal risk of allergic reaction because it is suspended in hyaluronic acid, a non-sensitizing vehicle.

Stability: Benefits range from five to seven years but are most likely permanent, though this is still under investigation.

Artecoll and Dermalive are combination injectables; they are made up of a synthetic substance called polymethylmethacrylate (PMMA) and collagen (similar to Zyderm and Zyplast, described above) for Artecoll, and hyaluronic acid for Dermalive. The FDA has only recently (2006) accepted Artefill as a filler.

Artecoll has been around for the past 50 years as a bone substitute and it is approved in Canada and Europe as an injectable filler for wrinkles; it's referred to as Dermalive in Europe. Results of a debate in the dermatologic community about the adverse events for both have yet to settle out; some research says it is no greater risk than other injectables, while other research has shown different outcomes. What needs to be considered, as is true with any permanent filler, is that when a problem such as lumping or migration does take place it doesn't go away, as would be the case for a nonpermanent filler.

Artecoll is injected in the same manner as collagen, and has the same initial results; Dermalive avoids this risk. With Artecoll, however, after the collagen is absorbed or broken down by the body, the synthetic material PMMA remains, stimulating the formation of new collagen and connective tissue in the area surrounding the PMMA, and this is true for Dermalive as well. One or two injections are enough to obtain good results. The results are thought to be permanent, but are definitely long lasting, with some research showing effectiveness for at least five to seven years, with ongoing improvement as the new collagen matrix is being formed.

(Sources: *Clinics in Plastic Surgery*, October 2006, pages 551–565; *Plastic and Reconstructive Surgery*, September 2006, pages S64 and S76; *Expert Review of Medical Devices*, May 2006, pages 281–289; and *Dermatologic Surgery*, June 2003, pages 573–587.)

SILICONE INJECTIONS

Brand name: Silikon

Major risks: Allergic reactions can occur. It can have a hard feel under skin, and may look lumpy or uneven under the skin.

Stability: Because migration and lumping can occur several years after having the injections, its stability is questionable.

Liquid injectable silicone is a permanent soft-tissue filler that is injected into wrinkles to produce fibrous tissue and a gradual increase in volume. Use of large quantities of impure silicone has led to a number of serious complications, including migration of the product, deep tissue infection, cellulitis, and even death. Use of small amounts of pure liquid silicone, via the microdroplet technique, is thought to have a low complication rate (less than 1%). However, lumps can occur weeks to years after treatment.

(Sources: *Plastic and Reconstructive Surgery*, December 2007, pages 2034–2040; and *Journal of Plastic, Reconstructive, and Aesthetic Surgery*, January 2007, pages 11–18.)

SCULPTRA/NEWFILL

Brand name: Sculptra (called Newfill in Europe)

Major risks: Similar to all dermal injections, but it is unlikely to cause an allergic reaction so no skin test is required prior to treatment.

Stability: Benefits can last between one to three years.

Sculptra is the trade name for the dermal filler poly-L-lactic acid. It differs from all other agents in several aspects. Poly-L-lactic acid is a synthetic but also is a biodegradable, biocompatible, immunologically inert peptide polymer that is believed to stimulate fibroblasts to produce more collagen, thus increasing facial volume. In the United States, poly-L-lactic acid is only FDA approved for the treatment of HIV-associated fat loss, which makes the face look gaunt and haggard. It is also routinely used off-label for the correction of skin folds such as the lines that run from the nose to the mouth. It is approved in Europe for filling wrinkles. Sculptra's main limitation is that two to three treatments are needed to achieve results and they need to be done four to six weeks apart.

Use of Sculptra on the hands has increased; unfortunately, however, the incidence of nodules in this location may be as high as 10% and the nodules are often visible, unsightly, and difficult to treat.

(Sources: *Journal of the American Academy of Dermatology*, December 2008, pages 923–933; and *Journal of Cosmetic and Laser Therapy*, March 2008, pages 43–46.)

RADIESSE

Brand name: Radiesse (previously called Radiance)

Major risks: No risk of allergic reaction. Otherwise, it has the same risk of any dermal injection, though it can have a hard feel under skin, and may look lumpy or uneven under the skin.

Stability: Can last up to 18 months

Radiesse was FDA approved in December 2006 for the correction of facial wrinkles and folds and for the correction of HIV-associated facial atrophy. This dermal filler is composed of 30% calcium hydroxylapatite, which is a natural substance, and 70% of a carrier gel. Calcium hydroxylapatite has safely been used in the body for many applications, including dental surgery where bone replacement is needed, and it can be used in facial implants. When injected in soft tissue, away from bone, it stimulates fibroblasts to build what is reportedly a non-scar-tissue collagen type, thus creating volume in the treatment area.

Calcium hydroxylapatite may induce the production of new collagen, although further research is needed. No skin test is required prior to treatment, and the product is stored at room temperature.

(Sources: *Clinical Interventions in Aging*, 2008, volume 3, issue 1, pages 161–174; *Journal of Drugs in Dermatology*, September 2008, pages 841–845; and *Dermatologic Surgery*, June 2008, pages S53–S55.)

EAR SURGERY (OTOPLASTY) *($2,000 TO $3,000)*

If you've worn heavy earrings for most of your life, your earlobes may be swinging down closer to your shoulders than you ever thought possible. A simple, 30-minute earlobe reduction can be performed in a plastic surgeon's office or at the same time as a face-lift. Aesthetically speaking, or at least to be sure your earlobes don't wobble, the earlobe should not be more than 25% of the total length of the ear. If it exceeds this, an L-shaped wedge can be cut away, and the earlobe edges can be brought together and sutured.

The earlobes can also protrude from the head. This protrusion can be part of the entire ear sticking out or be caused by an oversized ear shape that looks out of proportion to the shape of the head. Earlobe surgery can achieve an appearance that makes the ear more in balance with the face. One way to accomplish this is to position the ears closer to the head by reshaping the cartilage (supporting tissue). Otoplasty can be performed on children as early as age five or six.

(Source: *Facial Plastic Surgery Clinics of North America*, May 2006, pages 89–102.)

EYELID SURGERY (BLEPHAROPLASTY) *($2,500 TO $5,000)*

Eyelid surgery is one of the more popular cosmetic surgeries because it is relatively simple, it requires minimal postoperative recovery, and the results can be stunning. This operation involves cutting away the fat that causes bags beneath the eyes and removing wrinkled, drooping layers of skin on the eyelids.

Blepharoplasty is often performed along with a face-lift or with other facial rejuvenation procedures, especially forehead lifts. Incisions follow the natural contour lines in both upper and lower lids, and the thin surgical scars are usually barely visible and blend into the eyelids' natural lines and folds, although that can depend on how your skin scars.

A talented surgeon can avoid some of the typical mistakes, such as creating a scar that sits above the fold of the upper eyelid, overpulling the skin, or removing too much of the fat pad areas, which would create a sunken, drawn appearance. Risks of dry eye and damaged tear ducts are also a concern. (Sources: *Plastic and Reconstructive Surgery*, January 2009, pages 353–359; and *Survey of Ophthalmology*, September–October 2008, pages 426–442.)

Transconjunctival blepharoplasty, a variation of eyelid surgery, is performed by making an incision inside the lower eyelid. It avoids any scarring on the lower lid and may reduce the possibility of the eyelid pulling down, a postoperative complication in some patients. It is a useful technique when fat only, and not skin or muscle, needs to be removed from the eyelid area.

It is important to note that the upper eyelid may improve, negating the need for surgery there, if a forehead lift can produce a more positive effect. This also reduces risk to the eye area or obvious scarring. This option should absolutely be discussed with your surgeon.

FACE-LIFT (RHYTIDECTOMY) *($5,000 TO $10,000)*

"Although there are a multitude of techniques currently used for performing face lifts, there is no general agreement as to which, if any, of these techniques is most effective. There may never be a definitive answer to this issue because of the highly subjective nature of aesthetics, variability among surgeons, differences in patient anatomy, and specific patient desires" (Source: *Plastic and Reconstructive Surgery*, 1998, volume 102, pages 878–881). That statement is even truer today. The scientific literature is filled with studies of the different techniques used to surgically cut away and recreate a younger looking face.

The art of the face-lift is extremely complicated and the choices read like a menu with too many entrées, because it can include eye tucks, a forehead lift, chin tuck, and on and on. All of these, when combined, can dramatically reduce sagging skin on the face, neck, eye, and jaw. As impressive as this cosmetic procedure can be in creating a youthful, taut visage, it can also create an overly pulled, masklike appearance, with the face drawn up in a stretched, permanent smile. This is one cosmetic procedure where you want to see the doctor's work on someone else up-close and personal.

During this complicated, elaborate procedure, incisions are made in the hairline both in front of and behind the ears (the exact design of the incisions may differ from patient to patient, and surgeons' personal techniques can vary widely). For younger patients, more-limited incisions may be appropriate. When necessary, fatty deposits beneath the skin are removed or repositioned, and sagging muscles are tightened. The slack in the skin itself is then taken up and the excess cut away. Scars can usually be concealed, but when things go wrong thick, obvious, scars may be seen, or the hairline behind the ear or along the forehead may be altered in such a way that it creates an unnatural, strained appearance.

Most face-lifts also involve repositioning the muscles and fat pads of the cheek that have slipped forward, causing deep lines near the mouth (laugh lines), as well as dealing with the sagging of the muscle along the chin. Face-lifts that only tighten the skin without repositioning the muscles and fat pads can cause the face to look gaunt and unnatural. Face-lifts also have limitations as to the areas of the face they can affect. Other areas require a forehead lift, chin tuck, or endoscopic repositioning of those muscles and fat pads. Likewise, wrinkles by the eyes and mouth are not affected by a face-lift alone and require additional procedures (such as laser resurfacing) that are often done at the same time the face-lift is performed. Here is a partial menu of face-lift options a doctor can select from:

CLASSIC OR TRADITIONAL FACE-LIFT

This is what most of us think of when we think of a face-lift. Sagging, wrinkled skin is cut away and the remaining skin is repositioned to create a smoother and tighter visage. Cutting the skin is only one part of this procedure; to create the most natural finished appearance, the muscles and fat pads under the skin need to be repositioned so the realigned skin is formed over a structurally youthful base.

SMAS-LIFT (SUPERFICIAL MUSCULOAPONEUROTIC SYSTEM)

The SMAS face-lift is a term that has become familiar to those looking into plastic surgery. SMAS refers to the superficial musculoaponeurotic system. The skin on the face is composed of the superficial layers of skin, both the top and lower layer as well as the underlying layer of fat. Beneath the skin, fat, and muscle is a gliding membrane composed partly of connective tissue and partly of muscle. This gliding tissue is the SMAS, which is responsible for our ability to have facial expressions. Realigning this structure is considered a valid option for re-creating a youthful appearance for the face. However, when you cut under the muscle layer you can negatively affect nerve endings, and that is the major risk of this procedure. However, if you pulled only the top layer of skin and the fat layer, the muscle layer (which also sags and causes an aged appearance to the face) would not be corrected. Many surgeons feel that addressing the SMAS layer of skin, along with other procedures, is necessary to avoid giving a flat or unnatural appearance to the face. (Sources: *Facial and Plastic Surgery*, March 2000, pages 215–229; and *Plastic and Reconstructive Surgery*, 2000, volume 105, pages 290–301.)

SUBPERIOSTEAL LIFT

Periosteal refers to the thick membrane that covers the surface of bones. The subperiosteal lift is a technique used for the mid- and upper-face area, an area that is not helped by the typical face-lift (cutting and pasting skin around the ear area) or by endoscopic face-lifts (which reposition fat tissue and muscles without cutting and pasting). This is an aggressive technique that removes all the tissue and muscles attached to the bone and reshapes them into a more youthful position over the face. The benefit of the subperiosteal approach to the midface is the ability to lift the center of the face, improving the appearance of the nasal labial folds, smoothing the cheek area, and tightening the eye area. (Sources: *Journal of Plastic, Reconstructive and Aesthetic Surgery*, December 2007, pages 1287–1295; and *Plastic and Reconstructive Surgery*, September 1999, pages 842–851.) However, anytime work is done deeper under the skin the risk of impairment to nerve endings increases.

NECK LIFT

A woman's neck area is often the place that can look the most aged. Traditional face-lifts do not address this area. Sagging of the neck results when the platysma muscle loosens and becomes elongated. Typically, when an SMAS-Lift is performed the platysma muscle is reshaped and repositioned at the same time. Excess skin and fat can also be cut away at this time. (Sources: *Plastic and Reconstructive Surgery*, May 2006, pages 2008-2010, and November 1999, volume 104, pages 1093–1100.)

S-LIFT OR MINI-LIFT

This technique may be helpful for minor jowls or sagging skin. One source describes its objective this way: "To develop a safe and effective method to lift the jowl either as a single procedure or combined with other rejuvenation methods, S-shaped incisions are marked and then cut from the area just in front of the tragus [the front part of the ear]" (Source: *Dermatologic Surgery*, January 2001, pages 18–22). Once the small S-shaped flap of skin is cut and lifted away from the face the skin is rejoined, tightened, and repositioned along with the underlying muscles and fat tissues. If necessary, excess fat can be removed from this area at the same time.

Temporal Lift

The temporal face-lift refers to the area along the sides and top of the forehead. This technique is also referred to as a brow-lift. It is meant to smooth out the lines of the forehead and some of the eye area by repositioning the forehead skin along the hairline. At the time of the cutting and pasting for this area, the muscles of the forehead would also be repositioned (Source: *Facial Plastic Surgery*, February 2001, pages 57–66). This technique is described in more detail below.

Deep-Plane Lift

A deep-plane face-lift simply refers to how deep under the skin the surgeon works to perform any given face-lift procedure. Although it is similar to the SMAS-Lift, the deep-plane face-lift goes even deeper. It involves lifting and repositioning the various layers of the face—skin, fat tissue, muscles, and other structures—as a single unit rather than separating and lifting them individually. Because of its complexity, this procedure is not widely performed. However, while it is technically demanding the results are considered more satisfactory than those of a traditional or more superficial face-lift (Sources: *Current Opinion in Otolaryngology & Head and Neck Surgery*, August 2007, pages 244–252; and *Ophthalmology*, March 2000, pages 490–495).

Fat Implants

See Dermal Fillers, above.

Forehead Lift *($2,500 to $7,000)*

Endoscopic Face-Lift or Brow Lift

An endoscope is a small surgical instrument that can be inserted under the skin through small incisions, allowing a surgeon to perform a cosmetic corrective procedure via microsurgery. The endoscope itself is a miniature camera with a light fitted on one end of a long tube. When inserted under the skin the camera transmits magnified images to a television monitor.

During the procedure the surgeon watches the screen as the endoscope functions as the doctor's under-skin eye. Simultaneously, the surgeon inserts and uses other small surgical instruments, including scalpels, scissors, or forceps to actually perform the operation. These are used to remove excess fatty tissue and to reshape facial muscles and tissue that have become loose over time. In this way, many of the key factors contributing to sagging or drooping in the face are resolved.

Endoscopic face-lifts are an optimal way to minimally impact the skin and yet achieve impressive results for some types of wrinkles and sagging, and can have results similar to a traditional face-lift but without cutting and pasting sections of skin.

It turns out that a good deal of the skin's tendency to sag over time is a result of the face's muscles and fat pads shifting down and in toward the center of the face. This is what happens with the deepest furrowed lines on the face, particularly on the forehead and with the nasal labial folds from the nose to the mouth.

Let's say your jawline is beginning to sag. Using the somewhat simple surgical procedure called endoplasty, the surgeon makes a mere quarter-inch-long cut underneath the chin and at each edge of the jaw, and then, via microsurgery (the surgeon watches what is being done via a television screen), sutures the platysma muscle, which extends from jawline to jawline under the chin, back where it belongs.

For reasons similar to those causing skin to sag, the deep frown lines and vertical creases in the mid-forehead result from a literal slippage of the forehead muscles downward and inward, as well as just simple frowning and movement of the forehead. The same endoscopic technique used to anchor the platysma muscle can be used on the forehead muscles, and an additional separating of the muscles between the eyebrows can reduce the fold lines there. This operation can be done via three tiny incisions inside the hairline, allowing the surgeon to anchor the slipped muscles back in place and to cut away a small section of the muscles between the eyebrows.

There is a great deal of research showing that endoscopic face-lifts can achieve impressive results. However, because it is a very difficult surgery and requires a physician be skilled in microsurgery, it is not a popular method, although it has minimal to none of the risks associated with traditional surgical procedures.

(Sources: *Archives of Facial and Plastic Surgery*, January 2009, pages 34–39; *Facial and Plastic Surgery*, February 2007, pages 27–42; *Plastic and Reconstructive Surgery*, January 2002, pages 329–340; *Facial Plastic Surgery Clinics North America*, August 2001, pages 439–451; and *Aesthetic Plastic Surgery*, January 2001, pages 35–39.)

FOREHEAD LIFT (BROW LIFT—TRANSBLEPHAROPLASTY BROW LIFT)

The forehead lift is designed to correct or improve wrinkling, as well as the sagging of the eyebrow area that often occurs as part of the aging process. The procedure may also help to smooth horizontal expression lines in the forehead, smooth vertical frown lines between the eyebrows, and reduce the sagging appearance of the eyelids. Behind the hairline, incisions are placed above the ear and over the top of the head, although in some cases incisions may be made in front of the hairline. Forehead lifts are often (and usually should be) accompanied by repositioning the muscles of the forehead, which are partly responsible for the furrowed lines of the brow. The major downside of this procedure is that the hairline may be pulled farther back than desired.

Often referred to as a coronal forehead lift, this procedure involves an incision across the top of the head, running from ear to ear. Through this incision excess skin from the scalp is cut away as the muscles of the forehead are realigned and the fat pads repositioned. It is the most established cosmetic surgery technique available. Results can be impressive, with no visible scarring to be seen from any angle, though the major disadvantage is that your hairline can be raised by at least a half inch to an inch depending on the amount of correction needed.

(Source: *Archives of Facial and Plastic Surgery*, January–February 2009, pages 13–17).

SUBCUTANEOUS BROW AND FOREHEAD LIFT

Most forehead and brow lifts are usually done via an incision made at the top of the head, thus placing the scar where it won't be seen. However, this can raise the forehead and hairline, and for someone with an already large forehead this can be an undesirable outcome.

Endoscopic forehead lifts address this concern with almost no visible scarring or change to the forehead and hairline position but the procedure itself is a highly technical, difficult operation requiring a great deal of skill on the part of the surgeon. Subcutaneous forehead lifts neither change the hairline or forehead positioning and for a doctor who knows what he or she is doing, can be done quickly and resulting in immediate improvement, a slight headache and almost no recovery time. This technique is the least commonly performed of all brow lifts because of the small amount of skin involved but it is definitely an option for you to consider. All of the same techniques used in a coronal forehead lift (repositioning of the muscles and fat pads, cutting away the excess) are used, but in the subcutaneous forehead lift the scar is placed across the top of the forehead, basically following the hairline. Obviously, the major disadvantage with this technique is that you may have a noticeable scar at the hairline. Whether this scar is any more desirable than having your forehead raised is a discussion to have with your physician. There is research indicating that the scar in this procedure heals reasonably well. (Source: *Dermatologic Surgery*, October 2008, pages 1350–1361.)

PHOTOREJUVENATION
LASERS, INTENSE PULSED LIGHT, & OTHER ENERGY PRODUCING DEVICES
($1,200 TO $7,500)

Issues involving cosmetic corrective surgical procedures are complicated as it is, but when the topic turns to light or energy devices to reduce wrinkles, skin discolorations, surfaced capillaries, or acne scarring, what you find is a clutter of equipment that's almost impossible for the consumer to wade through on their own or even with the help of their physician (even many physicians can't sort through the mess). Not only are there dozens and dozens of machines with different energy outputs, wavelengths, purposes, and results, but the politics behind the laser/light/energy devices are also fraught with paid endorsements, paid research, and questionable studies.

An article in the *Archives of Facial Plastic Surgery* (January–March 2002, pages 6–7, "Laser Madness in Facial Plastic Surgery") summed up the problem beautifully: "In facial plastic surgery, many articles written by physicians promoting … facial resurfacing lasers appear in both peer-reviewed and non–peer-reviewed journals. These articles can read more like advertisements than science, overestimating the advantages of laser surgery, while underestimating the disadvantages and complications. Furthermore, the public's fascination with high-tech procedures related to cosmetic surgery has further exacerbated the unchecked outbreak of laser madness. Currently, it is unclear who is benefiting from laser madness in medicine. Is it the patient, the physician, or the laser company?"

Despite the challenges, at some point you will most likely want to consider treatment with one of these devices because, depending on your concern, these machines produce great results that are not possible, either with any other form of cosmetic surgery or with cosmetic corrective procedures (such as dermal injections or Botox).

Where you can get lost in this tangle of technology is the fact that one machine never does it all, no matter what you are told. For example, devices that treat brown skin discolorations and surfaced capillaries don't build much if any collagen or remodel skin.

Your physician can get lost because physicians are easily sold on a machine that ends up in a relatively short period of time not being as good as another machine. In other words doctors often invest in a device that subsequent research shows isn't all that exciting. Some physicians are also limited by the size of their practice and can only afford one machine when multiple machines are needed to provide the range of options patients require. Financially, the doctor can become stuck between a rock and a hard place and you are left in the middle being encouraged to use a machine that might not offer the best results for your concerns.

WHAT PHOTOREJUVENATION DOES

Lasers, as well as light-emitting, ultrasound, and radio energy generating machines, produce frequency waves in a wide variety of forms and intensities that are aimed at different parts of the skin and the structures of skin. Which device is selected and what its output will be in order to treat a particular problem are determined by the physician or technician. Some wavelengths target blood and therefore reduce the appearance of surfaced veins and capillaries, while others affect melanin in order to reduce or eliminate brown skin discolorations; still others stimulate collagen production, reduce wrinkling, and improve the appearance of scars.

Just to be clear, all photorejuvenating machines hurt, some more than others, but none of them are pleasant. Ironically, the more it hurts, the better the results.

Of the many machines a doctor can use, which include intense pulsed light (IPL) or radiofrequency (Thermage), by far the most well-known are lasers. Laser is an acronym for Light Amplification by Stimulated Emission of Radiation. Lasers work by generating a concentrated and penetrating stream of pulsed bright light that can be controlled and strategically directed over the skin.

Two types of lasers are used in photorejuvenation, **ablative** and **nonablative**. An ablative laser literally vaporizes and removes deep wrinkling and scars from the surface of skin and penetrates deeper into skin tissue, reorganizing and stimulating production of collagen and elastin fibers in the process.

Ablative laser resurfacing uses extreme heat to remodel the collagen in skin and it is very effective for that purpose, offering dramatic results. However, ablative lasers absolutely do cause damage to skin, healing takes awhile, and the procedure runs a far higher risk of complications. Strangely enough, the positive impact ablative lasers have on skin is a direct result of the damage they cause. Ablative lasers include the CO2 Pulse laser, the Er:YAG laser, and the Q-Switched Ruby laser.

To address the issues associated with ablative laser resurfacing, a new generation of lasers was developed that pixilated or created fractional light output of the pulsed light, reducing the damage and risk. These machines cause severe redness, similar to a severe sunburn, and require subsequent treatments, but have fairly impressive results (Source: *Lasers in Surgery and Medicine*, September 2008, pages 454–460). One of these types of machines is called the Fraxel.

Nonablative laser treatments use a level of energy that does not damage skin. They pose minimal risk but also have less-impressive results and require multiple treatments and yearly maintenance. Lots of nonablative lasers are being used today, but some of the more popular ones include the N-lite laser, Nd:YAG laser, Flashlamp laser, the Pulsed-Light laser, and the CoolTouch laser.

THE EQUIPMENT

The following is a summary covering a range of machines and the skin conditions they address. Selecting which one to use depends mostly on the physician you see, what machines they may own or lease, and their skill with those particular machines.

CO2 Pulse Laser (trade names Feather Touch or Ultra Pulse): This is one of the oldest types of ablative machines around. Although it can create more lasting and noticeable results than any other laser, it is also associated with the most risk and potential skin damage. The skin can take one to two weeks to heal and can be red for one to two months afterward. Risks of scarring, skin discoloration, and uneven texture must be weighed against the intended outcome, although these side effects are rare when the doctor is experienced with this kind of procedure. (Sources: *Dermatologic Surgery*, April 2004, pages 483–487; *International Journal of Dermatology*, June 2003, pages 480–487; and *Lasers in Surgery and Medicine*, May 2003, pages 405–412.)

Erbium:YAG Laser: This ablative laser is far less invasive than the CO2 Pulse laser and is considered effective for minor or superficial wrinkling. However, if the intensity of the machine is increased, deeper wrinkling can also be treated. Another option is the **Variable Pulse YAG Laser**, which alternates frequency with pulses that heat the skin and cause ablation that resurfaces the skin almost as effectively as the CO2 laser but with fewer side effects. (Sources: *Dermatologic Surgery*, August 2004, pages 1073–1076; *Archives of Dermatology*, October 2003, pages 1295–1299; and *Archives of Facial Plastic Surgery*, October–December 2002, pages 262–266.)

A combination of CO2 and Er:YAG laser treatments is now gaining popularity. In this treatment, the Er:YAG laser is first used to remove the epidermis, followed by use of the CO2 laser to achieve contraction of the underlying collagen. This produces the collagen-tightening benefits of CO2 therapy but with minimal damage to surrounding tissues. (Sources: Department of Otolaryngology/Head and Neck Surgery at Columbia University and New York Presbyterian Hospital, www.entcolumbia.org/laserskinresurf.htm; and *Dermatologic Surgery*, February 2000, pages 102–104.)

Long-Pulsed YAG Laser (trade names CoolTouch and Lyra): This nonablative laser is often used for treating wrinkles and reducing the appearance of acne scars. As is true with any nonablative laser resurfacing, it takes several treatments to achieve very subtle results.

The CoolTouch has a built-in cooling device that protects the top layer of skin but it can still feel like a rubber band snapping against the face as it is used. Types of the Long-Pulsed YAG Laser can be used for hair removal and removing surfaced capillaries. (Sources: *Lasers in Medicine and Science*, April 2004, pages 219–222; *Seminars in Cutaneous Medicine and Surgery*, December 2002, pages 288–300; and Laser Abstracts from the 14th Annual Congress of the American College of Phlebology).

Q-Switched Ruby Laser: This laser is minimally ablative and is primarily used to selectively remove skin pigment, as in freckling, sun-damage spots, and actinic keratosis, without damaging the surrounding tissue. It is also useful for removing birthmarks. It usually takes several treatments to see the desired results. One of the popular uses for the Q-Switched Ruby laser is cosmetic tattoo removal. Many physicians have noted that eliminating impulsive tattoo designs, as well as the poor work done by inexperienced or poorly trained aestheticians who tattoo lip liner, eyeliner, and eyebrows on women, now constitutes a large portion of their laser work (Sources: *Dermatologic Surgery*, November 2008, pages 1465-1468; and *American Journal of Clinical Dermatology*, February 2001, pages 21–25).

Pulsed Dye Laser, Short- and Long-Pulsed: This nonablative laser gives impressive results in removing surfaced capillaries on the face, port wine marks, hypertrophic scarring (thick or raised scars), and hemangiomas (red dots on the surface of skin). It doesn't cause skin damage but it almost always causes temporary bruising. Several treatments may be required (Source: *Dermatologic Surgery*, January 2004, pages 37–40).

Long-Pulsed Alexandrite Laser (trade names GentleLASE and Cool Pulse): This nonablative laser is another option for hair removal, and for removing surfaced capillaries and leg veins. This machine can quickly cover large areas of skin. (Sources: *Lasers in Surgery and Medicine*, May 2002, pages 359–362; and *Dermatologic Surgery*, July 2001, pages 622–626.)

Fractional Laser Resurfacing: This method is intended to offer the best of both the nonablative and ablative systems, that is, significant improvement with low risk and minimal downtime. "Fractional" refers to the way the laser light is emitted to small areas of skin at any one time, pinpointing tiny sections smaller than a human hair and wounding the underlying collagen, which stimulates more production. An effective treatment regime is three to five sessions spaced two weeks to a month or longer apart. (Sources: www.mdlive. net/xfractional.htm; *Photodermatology, Photoimmunology, and Photo-medicine*, August 2005, pages 204–209; *Archives of Facial Plastic Surgery*, November–December 2004, pages 398–409; *Journal of Cosmetic and Laser Therapy*, May 2004, pages 11–15; and *Lasers in Surgery and Medicine*, May 2004, pages 426–438.)

Intense Pulsed Light (IPL): This is a "light" modality that uses high-intensity pulses of light that do not involve lasers; it is considered to be exclusively nonablative. Though the IPL's beam of light is similar to lasers in many ways, its range is limited when it comes to the depth of resurfacing it can produce. This technique is not meant for those with extensive sun damage and skin discolorations, but it can reduce surfaced capillaries or veins, port wine marks, hemangiomas, and brown spots, as well as tighten the skin to some degree. The number of side effects is minor, but it can take several treatments (typically four to six) to see the desired results. There are a range of IPL machines, including PhotoDerm VL, PhotoDerm PL, PhotoDerm HR, EpiLight, and Quantum. (Sources: *Plastic and Reconstructive Surgery*, May 2004, pages 1789–1795; *Lasers in Surgery and Medicine*, February 2003, pages 78–87; and www.emedicine.com, "Non-ablative Resurfacing," June 30, 2003.)

PhotoDerm VL (for vascular lesions): Light pulses are directed at spider and varicose veins as well as vascular birthmarks. The tissue targeted is the red pigment (hemoglobin) in the blood, which is heated by the light pulses that destroy it without affecting the skin or other tissue.

PhotoDerm PL (for pigmented lesions): Light pulses are directed at "age spots," freckles, flat pigmented birthmarks, and other types of discolorations. The tissue targeted is the melanin in the skin's surface. The melanin is heated by the light, and the resulting damage or destruction removes the skin discolorations.

PhotoDerm HR and EpiLight (hair removal): Light pulses are directed at the hair follicle, causing the hair to fall out and preventing further growth, although this method is not permanent.

Radio frequency (RF) resurfacing involves neither a laser nor IPL. Rather, it is a form of electromagnetic energy very similar to microwaves. It is considered a nonablative resurfacing treatment. The RF treatment passes radio frequency electricity through the skin to heat up tissue. This is supposed to make the tissue contract and, as happens following any injury to skin, it then begins making collagen. The most popular RF machine is known as Thermage. Another device, called the Aurora, uses IPL and RF together for a unified procedure, supposedly to give patients the best of both modalities. (Source: *Journal of Cosmetic Dermatology*, January 2002, page 142.)

You may have heard claims that RF treatments are painless and have no adverse effects or complications, yet the research, though extremely limited, demonstrates otherwise. First, RF is considered by some as one of the most painful nonablative procedures, requiring localized anesthesia because it intensely heats up the skin (Source: *Cosmetic Dermatology*, December 2003, pages 28–34).

A study published in *Lasers in Surgery and Medicine* (November 2003, pages 232–242) reported that "fifty percent (41/82) of subjects reported being satisfied or very satisfied." Keep in mind that means 50% of the subjects were less than satisfied or were unhappy with their results. Further, second-degree burns did occur and "Three patients had small areas of residual scarring at 6 months." Scabbing and edema (skin swelling) occurs in some patients and though it does resolve, it can take six months to do so. Technically, the improvement measured in this study saw an average lift of 0.5 mm. Half of one-millimeter is 0.019 of an inch. That may not be exciting for what can be a costly procedure.

LIP AUGMENTATION OR REDUCTION *($2,500 TO $4,000)*

While thin lips may not seem like a cosmetic issue, for some women looking for perfection fuller lips are considered more attractive. Moreover, as you get older the lip area begins to recede, becoming thinner and narrower, or may fold in on itself, with obvious lines extending outward around the perimeter.

Aside from dermal fillers (described above), one of the more interesting methods for augmenting the lips is to surgically advance the lip forward via incisions placed inside the mouth. Fat implants or collagen injections (see the Dermal Fillers section above) may then be positioned under the lining of the lip to add additional plumpness. Neither collagen nor fat is permanent, however, and the procedure must be repeated periodically to maintain results.

A lip lift is a technique that surgically lifts the corners of an aging mouth to eliminate the pronounced droop and unhappy facial expressions that often develop with advancing age. Cutting away small diamonds of skin just above the corners of the mouth raises the border of the lips into a slight smile.

If thin lips have an unfashionable aspect, it isn't hard to imagine that overly full lips can also be viewed as too much of a good thing. In lip reduction, a small section along the top lining of the lip is surgically removed to narrow the lips to the desired proportion. The small scars on the outside of the lips are often barely noticeable, though it all depends on how you scar.

MICRODERMABRASION *($300 TO $1,000)*

See Chapter Twenty Three, *Should You Get a Facial?*, for details on microdermabrasion.

NOSE RESHAPING (RHINOPLASTY) *($4,000 TO $6,000)*

Rhinoplasty is usually performed to alter the size and shape of the bridge and tip of the nose. Reshaping is generally done through incisions inside the nose, but sometimes an incision across the central portion of the nose between the nostrils is also made. Narrowing the base of the nose or reducing the size of the nostrils involves removing small wedges of skin at the base of the nostrils. The nose is reduced, or sometimes built up, by adjusting its supporting structures, a process that involves either removing or adding bone and cartilage. The skin and soft tissues are then redraped over this newly created structure.

An open rhinoplasty technique can sometimes benefit patients who need more complex correction or who are undergoing a secondary rhinoplasty procedure. A small incision is made outside the nose across the columella (the tissue that divides the two nostrils). This enables the plastic surgeon to turn the outer tissue of the nose back, providing a view of the structures inside. Additional incisions, like those used in the traditional closed approach, are made inside the nose as well. The scar from the incision on the outside of the nose eventually becomes barely visible.

As one of the most commonly performed cosmetic surgeries, rhinoplasty has a strong success rate but given the various ways the procedure can be done (and each has its pros and cons) it is imperative to find a surgeon familiar with them so you can discuss which method will work best for you (Source: *Facial Plastic Surgery*, August 2006, pages 198–203).

FROM THE NECK DOWN

ABDOMINOPLASTY (TUMMY TUCK) *($4,000 TO $8,000)*

Sometimes, after multiple pregnancies or major weight loss, a person's abdominal muscles weaken and the skin in that area becomes flaccid and hangs below the pubic bone. Abdominoplasty can tighten the abdominal muscles and, in some instances, banish stretch marks (because they are cut away, never to be seen again). In both men and women, the procedure removes excess skin and fat. Generally, an incision is made across the pubic area just above the bikini line and around the navel. The skin is lifted up and away from the sides of the body and up to just under the breasts, then pulled down and reshaped firmly along the body. Liposuction may be used to remove excess fat along the back area just in front of where the skin is lifted away from the body. Often the stomach muscles, which may have separated and pulled apart, are stitched back together, re-creating the natural girdle you had when you were younger. The excess skin is then cut away, and what remains is stitched back together around the navel and at the original incision above the pubic bone.

The complication rate for this type of surgery is significant. Primary problems include wound infection, the wound splitting open, blood-filled swelling, blood clots, and intestinal obstruction. It is a serious operation with potentially excellent results, but it is not a procedure to venture into lightly without taking all the risks into consideration. (Sources: *Annals of Plastic Surgery*, January 2009, pages 5–6; and *Plastic and Reconstructive Surgery*, 2001, volume 107, pages 1869–1873.)

ARM LIFT (BRACHIOPLASTY) *($3,000 TO $6,000)*

All the weight-lifting in the world won't build up enough muscle to pick up the excess skin that can hang and flap under the arm, particularly if you have lost a great deal of weight or have a tendency to gain weight in that area. Excess fat in the upper arms can sometimes be reduced through liposuction alone, but loose, drooping skin may need to be excised. To that end, an arm lift is an impressive way to shore up that area, making the skin smooth and taut again. Incisions are hard to hide for this operation, because they can run lengthwise from the armpit to just above the elbow. The risks for this operation are the same as for the tummy tuck procedure.

BREAST IMPLANTS, BREAST AUGMENTATION (AUGMENTATION MAMMOPLASTY) *($4,500 TO $8,500)*

In 2008, about 350,000 women in the United States had breast augmentation, 57,000 had breast reconstruction, 106,000 underwent breast reduction, and 14,000 had their implants removed. Those are interesting numbers. Since the advent of breast implants in 1962 it is estimated that over 2 million women have had breast augmentation (Source: American Society of Plastic Surgeons, www.plasticsurgery.org).

Breast augmentation is typically performed to enlarge small breasts, underdeveloped breasts, or breasts that have decreased in size after a woman has had children or lost weight. It is accomplished by surgically inserting an implant behind each breast. The implant is soft and pliable, and it resembles a plastic bag filled with water. An incision is made either under the breast, around the areola (the colored skin surrounding the nipple), or in the armpit. A pocket is created for the implant either behind the breast tissue or behind the muscle between the breast and the chest wall.

Textured-surface breast implants are made with the same silicone material used for the shell of other types of breast implants, but a special manufacturing process creates a textured surface. Some studies have suggested that this surface texture may help reduce the incidence of capsular contracture—tightening of the scar tissue that forms naturally around the implant—which can make the breast feel heavy and hard.

The controversy surrounding implants over the past several years has to do with health risks associated with the contents of silicone gel–filled implants leaking into the body and causing autoimmune disorders. Large-scale epidemiological studies conducted independently by leading research institutions have provided some reassuring data. One large-scale study of this kind conducted by the Mayo Clinic and published in the June 16, 1994, issue of the *New England Journal of Medicine* found no connection between silicone breast implants and connective tissue diseases such as rheumatoid arthritis and lupus. Similar conclusions were reached in an extensive study reviewed in the November 2001 issue of *Arthritis and Rheumatism* (pages 2477–2484).

A press release from the National Cancer Institute (http://newscenter.cancer.gov/pressreleases/siliconebreast.html) on Monday, October 2, 2000, stated that "In one of the largest studies on the long-term health effects of silicone breast implants, researchers from the National Cancer Institute (NCI) in Bethesda, Md., found no association between breast implants and the subsequent risk of breast cancer…. Of the implant patients in the study, 49.7 percent received silicone gel implants, 34.1 percent double lumen implants, 12.2 percent saline-filled implants, 0.1 percent other types of implants, and 3.8 percent unspecified types of implants…. The participants had cosmetic surgery during a time (between 1962 and 1988) when a great number of changes were taking place in the manufacturing of breast implants such as the shell thickness, the type of shell coating, and the gel composition. However, the researchers found there was no altered breast cancer risk associated with any of the types of implants."

Due to the controversy regarding implants, in 1994 a new version was launched for clinical trials. Called the TrilucentTM implant, it was filled with a soybean oil derivative that developers hoped would allow for better results and less risk. Despite the natural sound of the soybean material, this implant has since been withdrawn from the market and it has been recommended that all women who received the Trilucent implant have it removed. It turns out that the breakdown of the soybean oil filler resulted in substances that had a toxic effect on the body. (Sources: FDA Center for Devices and Radiological Health, www.fda.gov/cdrh/breastimplants/indexbip.html; and *British Journal of Plastic Surgery*, December 2001, pages 684–686.)

There are a wide variety of options when it comes to implants. These now include round or anatomical pre-filled saltwater implants, adjustable implants (that are filled with salt water at the time they are placed in the body), and double-lumen or "stacked" implants (this implant has two layers, an inner sac filled with silicone gel and an outer sac filled with salt water). Each has its own set of positives and negatives, so the choice depends on what you and your surgeon prefer.

A review published in the *Aesthetic Surgery Journal* (July 2000, pages 281–290) concluded that "the round and anatomical saline implants have similar teardrop shapes and essentially the same proportions relative to height and volume when the patient is in an upright position, but that round implants behave more like a natural breast when the patient is lying down. When both the upright and the recumbent implant shape is considered, the round implant is the more [natural in appearance]."

Another review in the same issue of the *Aesthetic Surgery Journal* (pages 332–334) stated that "Adjustable breast implants allow women to adjust their breast size up or down within a certain time period following breast augmentation surgery. They also give surgeons the ability to improve breast shape and symmetry, and may be useful in treating capsular contracture (breast firmness), the most common problem associated with breast implants. The technique involves overfilling the implant to stretch the breast tissues, then removing some of the saline solution to obtain the final result." Stacked implants were also discussed in this issue (pages 296–300): "The stacked implant has two compartments, each able to be filled to a different volume, so that greater fullness can be achieved at the base of the breast with a gradual slope in the breast's upper portion." This can also be helpful when breast reconstruction is done, allowing the operated breast to be filled to match the other side more precisely.

Although having large, full breasts can be a tempting possibility, be sure your physician is sensitive to your body type and will veto your preconceived notion of what a desirable body looks like if it is not appropriate for your size and shape. It is best to have breasts that look like they are a part of you, not two huge lumps pointing straight out and up from your chest.

Be sure the physician you see is familiar with the differences between saline, silicone gel, and textured-surface implants. Also, your physician should be aware of the need for strict postoperative treatment and should explain it to you at length. For example, it is essential that there be no movement of the hands or arms above the waist for several days after surgery. Also, the breasts must be bound for from several days to three weeks after surgery. All this ensures healing and minimizes the chances of the implant becoming encapsulated.

There are significant risks with breast augmentation surgery, and they can include any and all of the following.

Capsular contracture, the most common problem associated with breast implants, occurs when the body rejects the implant or when scar tissue builds up and pushes against the implant, causing a hardening of the area. The result of this encapsulation around the implant can produce hard breast tissue. It is not a health concern, but depending on the extent of the encapsulation it can be extremely painful and can also make mammography screening more difficult. The likelihood of capsular contracture is fairly high, occurring in more than 54% of breast implants.

Deflation, rupture, and leakage are highly probable. It is very important to understand that breast implants are not lifetime devices and cannot be expected to last forever. Some implants deflate or rupture in the first few months after being implanted and some deflate after several years; others are intact ten or more years after the surgery, though the incidence of rupture is less likely with saltwater-filled implants than with silicone gel–filled implants.

Other physical complications can include pain, infection, swelling, and changes in the physical sensation of the breast and nipple.

Cosmetically undesirable side effects can include wrinkling or puckering of the skin around the implant, asymmetry, implant shifting, thickened or noticeable scarring, and an obvious movement of the sac's content. Also, the breast tissue can shrink around the implant.

Again, perhaps the most serious associated problem is that breast implants can interfere with mammography.

BREAST LIFT (MASTOPEXY) ($3,000 TO $5,000)

Frequently, a woman elects this surgery after losing a considerable amount of weight or when she has lost volume and tone in her breasts after having children. The plastic surgeon relocates the nipple and areola (the pink skin surrounding the nipple) to a higher position, repositions the breast tissue to a higher level, removes excess skin from the lower portion of the breast, and then reshapes the remaining breast skin. Scars occur around the areola, and extend vertically down the breast and horizontally along the crease underneath the breast. Variations on this technique, in some cases, may result in less noticeable scarring.

BREAST REDUCTION
(REDUCTION MAMMOPLASTY)
($4,000 TO $8,000)

Perhaps no other form of elective cosmetic surgery is more life-changing than a breast reduction procedure. A woman with massive breasts struggles with the extra bulk, which is extremely uncomfortable and awkward and curtails physical activity. Additionally, because of the substantial extra mass, detection of breast cancer is compromised and the skin tissue under the breast area can be incessantly lacerated and infected by rubbing, irritation, and perspiration. With the development of successful reduction mammoplasty procedures, there is no reason for any woman to struggle with this kind of physical distortion.

Unlike most other types of cosmetic surgery, breast reduction is normally classified as a reconstructive procedure rather than a cosmetic one because oversized breasts greatly interfere with normal daily activity and physical activity, not to mention related health issues such as infection and problems with breast cancer screening. Depending on your insurance company's policy regarding breast reduction, the entire procedure may be paid for in full by your health insurance provider. Generally, the determination is made according to how much tissue (by weight) is removed. A certain minimum gram weight must be met to prove to the insurance company that the procedure is corrective and not just aesthetic. However, regardless of the insurance company's position, there is an important aesthetic component to the operation because the plastic surgeon can improve the shape of the breasts and the nipple area, and enhance a woman's physical profile.

Breast reduction involves removing excess breast tissue and skin, repositioning the nipple and areola, and reshaping the remaining breast tissue. Some of the risks are fairly serious, including noticeable scarring, loss of sensation, and the inability to breastfeed, along with other surgery-related complications. But for women with heavy, pendulous breasts, a breast reduction can be a godsend. (Sources: *Aesthetic Surgery Journal*, March–April 2008, pages 171–179.)

BREAST RECONSTRUCTION
(TRAM FLAP OR PROCEDURE)
($8,000 TO $10,000)

Usually as a result of breast cancer, a woman may have one or both breasts removed. Other traumas to the body can also take place that result in a loss of breast tissue. In these instances, rebuilding one or both breasts can return the body to its original condition or even to a perceived enhanced appearance. This surgery involves a fairly complicated procedure that uses the muscles of the abdomen. The abdomen has two large, parallel muscles, called rectus abdominus. When only one breast is reconstructed, relinquishing one of these muscles poses no risk of impairment to a woman's health or physical activity. However, when both breasts need to be reconstructed, using both muscles can cause abdominal weakness, so that some movements (such as sitting up from lying down) are harder to do.

During breast reconstruction, the abdominal muscle is used to move the skin and fat from the abdomen to the chest for the construction of a new breast. This flap is referred to as the TRAM flap, or the Transverse Rectus Abdominus Muscle flap. The skin, fat tissue, and the muscle are cut away intact from the abdomen while remaining attached to the body. Because the TRAM remains attached to the body, blood vessels remain unbroken, allowing the tissue to remain vital and functioning. The TRAM is then repositioned underneath the skin and adjusted and shaped via an opening where the original breast used to be. It is an amazing operation, and many of the same risks associated with abdominoplasty (a tummy tuck, describer earlier in this chapter) can occur. However, once complications are resolved, a woman has the benefit of a more natural looking body shape and a tummy tuck at the same time.

BUTTOCK LIFT *($4,500 TO $7,000)*

Excess fat and loose skin in the buttock area can be reduced by performing a buttock lift in combination with liposuction (see the "Liposuction" section below). Incisions required for skin removal can often be hidden in the fold beneath the buttocks. Though the results are impressive, the scarring can be quite noticeable, meaning you'll look great in pants but in the buff your backside might look like a road map.

CALF AUGMENTATION *($3,000 TO $5,000)*

Increased fullness of the calf can be achieved by using hard silicone implants, which are inserted from behind the knee and moved into position underneath the calf muscle.

LIPOSUCTION *($1,000 TO $2,000)*

Liposuction (also referred to as lipoplasty) allows a doctor to remove localized collections of fatty tissue from the legs, buttocks, abdomen, back, arms, face, and neck by using a vacuum device that literally cuts up and then sucks up fat tissue. Depending on the area treated, the procedure leaves only minute scars, often as short as one-half inch in length or less.

The use of refined equipment allows removal from delicate areas such as calves and ankles. Liposuction does remove fat, but it cannot eliminate dimpling (cellulite) or correct skin laxity, which are the result of the skin's structure and are not caused by the presence of the fat itself. In fact, the result of the procedure can actually cause an increase in the appearance of cellulite or sagging skin because the fat is no longer there to support the skin. A talented physician should know that and always leave some amount of fat in place.

For some patients whose skin has lost much of its elasticity, a plastic surgeon may also recommend a skin-tightening procedure such as a thigh lift, buttock lift, or arm lift, all of which leave more extensive scars.

Most women consider liposuction a method of weight loss, but that makes it a very high-risk, expensive way to "diet." Plus, in terms of total fat removed, the typical amount is less than ten pounds and it is easily gained back.

Suction-assisted liposuction, where a long, needlelike tube is inserted into the skin and the fat is literally suctioned out of skin under anesthesia, remains the traditional method for body sculpting. However, newer technologies may increase efficiency, decrease surgeon fatigue (yes, doctors get tired during procedures, which increases mistakes), and minimize complications. Power-, ultrasound-, and laser-assisted devices are being used in cases where large volumes of fat tissue are being removed in areas with dense fibrous tissues as an adjunct to traditional liposuction. (Tumescent anesthesia is a method of eliminating pain during a liposuction procedure by injecting lidocaine and epinephrine into the area, causing it to become tumescent, which means swollen and firm. This makes the area easier to work on and there is no need for additional, riskier anesthesia.)

Power-assisted liposuction devices and traditional liposuction ones differ in that the tube-like tip of the power-assisted version vibrates. This vibrating vacuum moves at an ultra-high speed that generates a frequency powerful enough to emulsify fat cells, making them easier to suck up and remove from the body. This also causes less trauma and bruising to the surrounding tissues and makes the procedure easier for the physician.

Ultrasonic liposuction uses high-pulse sound waves to liquefy excess fat, which is then removed. The procedure has both advocates and detractors; some complain that the equipment is cumbersome, and others consider it time-consuming to use.

Laser-assisted liposuction was introduced in 2007, and the machine called the SmartLipo is the first laser to be approved by the FDA to be used for liposuction. As the laser wand is inserted into the skin, piercing the fat tissue, the laser pulses liquefy the fat. Just like power-assisted and ultrasound-assisted liposuction, laser-assisted liposuction still requires the use of tumescent anesthesia and a standard liposuction vacuum to suck up and remove the now-liquefied fat.

Interestingly enough, despite the creation of these new devices, research has shown that the effects of ultrasound-, power-, and laser-assisted liposuction basically differ from traditional liposuction in only two ways: the improved initial healing process, and greater ease of use for the physician (something of value for the patient if the doctor finds the procedure less tiring to perform).

(Sources: *Seminars in Cutaneous Medicine and Surgery*, March 2008, pages 72–82; *Plastic and Reconstructive Surgery*, 2006, volume 118, pages 1032–1045; *Annals of Plastic Surgery*, March 2001, pages 287–292; *Aesthetic and Plastic Surgery*, November 1999, pages 379–385; and www.fda.gov/cdrh/pdf6/K062321.pdf.)

Overall, liposuction is considered a low-risk cosmetic procedure. An article in *Plastic and Reconstructive Surgery* (November 2001, pages 1753–1763) reviewed 631 liposuction cases over 12 years and found "Results showed the majority of patients to be women, aged 17 to 74 years old. Of the preoperative weights, 98.7 percent were within 50 pounds of ideal chart weight.... Cosmetic results were good, with a 2- to 6-inch drop from preoperative measurements, depending on the area treated. Ten percent of patients experienced minor skin contour irregularities, with most of these patients not requiring any additional surgical procedures. One year after surgery, 80 percent of patients maintained stable postoperative weights. No serious complications were experienced in this series. The majority of the complications consisted of minor skin injuries and burns, allergic reactions to garments, and postoperative [swelling]. The more serious complications included four patients who developed mild pulmonary edema and one patient who developed pneumonia postoperatively. These patients were treated appropriately and went on to have [successful] recoveries. The results show that large-volume liposuction can be a safe and effective procedure when patients are carefully selected and when anesthetic and surgical techniques are properly performed. Meticulous fluid balance calculations are necessary to avoid volume abnormalities, and experience is mandatory when performing the largest aspirations. Cosmetic benefits are excellent, and overall complication rates are low."

It is important to keep in mind that scraping fat out of your body is an intense medical procedure. Liposuction can be painful, and the pain can last for several weeks. Adhering to postoperative guidelines is essential for success. Touch-up work may be necessary because even the best techniques can remove fat unevenly, resulting in unwanted bulges and contours. Moreover, if you gain weight, depending on how your body distributes fat, it can all be added exactly where the liposuction was performed. Now that is some fat to chew on!

SCLEROTHERAPY ($250 TO $1,000)

The most typical and successful treatment for getting rid of surfaced red and blue veins on the legs is sclerotherapy, a procedure that involves injecting a solution into the veins of the leg or thigh that destroys the vessel's lining. The solution causes the walls of the veins to collapse, destroying the source of the problem. (Source: *Aesthetic Surgery Journal*, September–October 2008, pages 573–583.)

One solution used for sclerotherapy is polidocanol (aethoxysclerol), which was originally developed as a local anesthetic. Polidocanol turned out to be undesirable as an anesthetic because it shut down veins wherever it was injected, but it was perfect for sclerotherapy. It is relatively painless. It is also one of the few drugs you can inject into the skin that doesn't leak into the other veins, so it affects only the vein it is injected into. That means there is little to no risk associated with this treatment. Your doctor will want to choose the best option for your condition, but make sure he or she is familiar and skilled with all available options. For more serious, larger varicose veins, a more potent choice is sotradecol. It is similar to polidocanol, but sotradecol can cause sores (ulcers) if it leaks.

Deciding whether to choose laser removal of surfaced veins or sclerotherapy may not be a simple matter. The method the physician prefers is usually what makes the difference and not the methodology as such. Both lasers and sclerotherapy have a place in treating small leg veins. A study in *Lasers in Surgery and Medicine* (2002, volume 30, issue 2, pages 154–159) compared "a long pulsed Nd:YAG laser with contact cooling to sclerotherapy for treating small diameter leg veins by evaluating objective and subjective clinical effects.... Patient surveys show 35% preferred laser and 45% chose sclerotherapy." Other research has shown sclerotherapy has the edge (Source: *Dermatologic Surgery*, August 2002, pages 694–697).

Aside from the type of treatment, it is important to determine the underlying cause of a problem to prevent recurrences. A surfaced vein is distended and visible because it is connected to a high-pressure system that has gone wrong. You can visualize what happens with these surfaced veins as being similar to the experience of driving along and all of a sudden finding heavy traffic backed up several miles from the actual problem.

When veins work normally, they collect blood from tissues and pump it around the body in an even flow, without hitches, stops, or abrupt starts. When things go wrong, the blood can actually go in the wrong direction or all of sudden get blocked. This occurs because the valves in the vein no longer function properly or the blood volume in the vein increases (often because of trauma); often both conditions occur together and are interrelated.

This misdirected blood flow can build up pressure, creating painful swelling and protrusions. A vein that becomes permanently dilated is called a varicose vein. Theoretically, any vein can develop varicosity, but certain veins, such as those in the legs, are more likely to. This can be due to an injury, to pregnancy hormones (which make the valves in the veins soft and floppy, causing damage), to being overweight, or just to bad veins. And the problem can spread from one bad vein to others (sort of like a bad traffic jam spreading to nearby roads).

REMOVING VARICOSE VEINS *($500 TO $2,000)*

Varicose veins are twisted, dilated veins and are most commonly located on the calves and thighs. Risk factors for getting varicose veins include chronic coughing, constipation, family history of venous disease, being female, obesity, older age, pregnancy, and prolonged standing. The exact pathophysiology is not clear, but most experts agree it involves a genetic predisposition, improperly working veins, and increased blood pressure in the veins of the legs.

Varicose veins are not only an aesthetic issue. They can also create a sensation of heaviness in the leg, along with itching, burning, and discomfort. Potential complications include infection, leg wounds that don't heal, and blood clots. Avoiding long periods of standing or straining, elevating the legs, wearing support hose for external compression to help evenly distribute blood flow, and wearing loose clothing on other parts of the body to prevent pushing blood flow into the legs can all help. Medical options include external laser treatment, sclerotherapy, endovenous laser ablation (EVLA) treatments, and surgically removing the veins from the leg. The choice of therapy is often affected by cost, available medical resources, and physician training. (Source: *American Family Physician*, December 2008, pages 1289–1294.)

Among the treatments, EVLA is considered by far the most reliable; it offers the best long-term results, is less invasive, and is the least painful of all the options for varicose veins. Outcomes from EVLA appear to be equal to or better than stripping, with better quality-of-life scores in the postoperative period, but in addition EVLA has been shown to improve and strengthen the veins, preventing further occurrences (Source: *Journal of Vascular Surgery*, July 2008, pages 173–178).

EVLA works by destroying the varicose vein through the introduction of heat. A thin tube is inserted into the vein and a tiny laser pulse is emitted; a variety of wavelengths can be used, such as 810, 940, 980, 1064, and 1320 nanometers. When the laser is triggered, it generates targeted, intense heat to the specific vein, destroying it; the tissue is then reabsorbed by the body (Source: Emedicine, November 7, 2008, http://emedicine.medscape.com/article/1085735-overview).

THIGH LIFT *($5,000 TO $7,500)*

Losing a lot of weight or suffering a lot of sun damage can cause the thigh area to sag, making cellulite look worse and excess weight appear more noticeable. Liposuction alone won't lift up the skin that hangs down and causes pouching and folds. Thigh lifts can be performed, along with liposuction, to tighten sagging muscles and remove excess skin in the thigh area. However, because a thigh lift leaves noticeable scars in the inner or outer thigh area, it is not a frequently performed procedure.

For more detailed information on the subject of plastic surgery and cosmetic corrective procedures these two books are excellent sources: *Straight Talk about Cosmetic Surgery*, Yale University Press Health & Wellness, Author Dr. Arthur W. Perry and *Your Best Face Without Surgery*, Author Dr. Brandith Irwin.

CHAPTER 27
BODY AND NAIL CARE

> *Skin is skin, head to toe—so why waste money on*
> *specialty products that aren't specially formulated?*

FROM THE NECK DOWN

Neck creams, throat creams, breast creams, thigh creams, and creams for the elbows, knees, and heels abound throughout the cosmetics industry. While the cosmetics industry loves to sell products for every corner of your face and body, the basic fact is that, with very few exceptions, what applies to the face applies to the body. That means almost every aspect of skin care designed to work from the neck up will work (to one degree or another) fine from the neck down. Dry skin; cracked, callused heels; acne on the back and chest; and skin discolorations all require the same skin-care formulations as the face. The names on the products may differ to fit a company's marketing campaign, and lots of body-care products are less elegantly formulated than those for the face, but when it comes to the health and appearance of your skin it's always about content and results.

Of course there are differences. If you shave your legs or underarms there are techniques for that, manicures and pedicures are unique, and vaginal care has special nuances as well. But those differences are anatomical—they aren't about skin care.

Dry or cracked skin on heels, elbows, or knees can require more emollient, even greasy or heavy formulations than the face, but the basics about exfoliation, antioxidants, cell-communicating ingredients, and skin-identical ingredients still apply.

Interestingly enough, when it comes to body care women often neglect their skin from the neck down. Many women tell me they would never tan their face because they want to prevent sun damage and the inevitable wrinkling and discoloration it can cause, yet they happily brown and bake the rest of their body. Sometimes there is a disconnect between head and body—or perhaps there is a misconception that the legs, arms, and chest are tougher or aren't subject to the same ruination caused by sun damage. Nothing could be further from the truth.

Unprotected skin anywhere on the body develops the same thickened, brown-spotted, lined, and rough texture as skin on the face does, and is subject to the same skin cancers. There are women who fly into a tizzy at the appearance of one facial blemish, but who ignore breakouts on their chest and legs, never thinking of applying the blemish-fighting basics to any other part of the body. This is also misguided. Skin is skin, head to toe—so why accept artificial boundaries between parts of the body?

The number of products dedicated to bathing and body care is growing, but they tend to be all about pampering, fragrance, and indulging ourselves rather than addressing concerns about blemishes, wrinkles, sun damage, exfoliation, and reducing irritation. A veritable deluge of overly fragranced moisturizers, cleansers, bath salts, scrubs, bubble baths, hand creams, and massage oils, in every aromatic combination imaginable, promises to soften, scent, stimulate, smooth, and soothe your body, yet more often than not those products have nothing to do with really helping your skin.

You can't find a square inch of the body that has been neglected by the cosmetics industry. Large cosmetics companies, small cosmetics companies, prestigious lines, simple lines, and even businesses for whom body care is just a sideline, all want us to soak, scrub, and moisturize everything from dry skin to stress and emotional woes out of our lives with bath oils, bath salts, loofahs, body masks, fragrant moisturizers, and perfumes. And we love buying the stuff. Bath and body-care products and fragrances account for more than 33% of all cosmetics sold! Yet more often than not these products are poorly formulated, don't contain sunscreen, are overly fragranced (which causes irritation), or contain other skin irritants, and in general they just don't measure up to the quality of products we put on our face.

SPA TREATMENTS

One interesting wrinkle (no pun intended) in this story is the number of body-care lines that include the word "spa" as part of their name. Marketing finesse gives spa lines an authoritative aura and healthful image when it comes to skin care, particularly from the neck down. This misperception can waste money and also cause skin problems.

Spa products are not the result of any particular enlightenment, nor are they specially formulated in any way. In fact, spa products sold at cosmetics counters and specialty spas are notoriously similar to the ones sold in drugstores. I think most women would be shocked to discover that the "spa" formulations for various body washes, bath salts, body moisturizers, and bath oils are really almost identical to the drugstore formulations. Moreover, spa lines, like most body-care products, are highly fragranced, and fragrance is no better for skin on the body than it is for facial skin.

Far be it from me to deny anyone the pleasure that can be derived from pampering, soothing body care. Taking care of the body should include relaxing in deliciously warm water or being gently massaged. But skin-care problems can occur all over the body, and they require more than sweetly scented bath salts and oils, which are often enough the very same things responsible for red, flaky, irritated skin. Despite the allure of spa treatments and their high price tags, the products used rarely, if ever, seriously address the issues of sun damage, blemishes, skin sensitivity, antioxidants, anti-irritants, or skin disorders such as rosacea or psoriasis.

Doing all they can to appear more natural and superior to other product lines, spa lines tend to add an eccentric marketing flare. How can you convince a consumer that your products are really different? You throw in exotic ingredients from some remote part of the world and claim it is the new miracle for your skin. These novel ingredients always come from a part of the world like the remote deserts of Africa or the Amazon rainforest, since of course they would never come from someone's backyard in Dallas or Miami. If it sounds out of the ordinary and mysterious, women are eager to believe it must have glamorous benefits for skin. That is never the case. Whatever foreign plant extract is being heralded as the answer for your skin today will be replaced in a few months by another rare and heretofore unknown plant extract, maybe from China, that will unleash its youth-bestowing benefit for you. So however you look at it, you are being played for a sucker and wasting your money.

For example, in marketing their facial services and skin-care products, one line boasted that their products contained truffles that were handpicked and mixed into their treatments. While handpicked truffles (is there another kind?) might be great for a salad or steak, the skin can't tell the difference. What does matter is whether or not truffles can have a positive effect on skin. It turns out that there is a small amount of research showing black and white truffles to be effective for inhibiting melanin production and for some antibacterial properties. (Sources: *Federation of European Microbiological Societies (FEMS) Microbiology Letters*, April 2000, pages 213–319; and *Pigment Cell Research*, February–April 1997, pages 46–53.) However, there are many different products that contain other effective skin-lightening or antibacterial ingredients with less spin, less expense, and with vastly more researched efficacy.

Caviar is often touted as an especially extravagant ingredient in some products. Exclusivity aside, what is caviar's benefit for skin? It turns out that caviar does contain essential fatty acids similar to the ones found in skin. But lots of living substances, from fish to animals and plants, are replete with identical or better fatty acids (like phospholipids and triglycerides). Caviar is not a superior or even desirable source for these skin-care ingredients. Plus, only a tiny amount—and I mean it's barely detectable—of caviar is included in products like this, rendering it almost impossible to exert any effect on skin whatsoever.

A cornerstone for almost any spa service is the ever-popular mud mask. Some kind of mud from some exotic part of the world is showcased to get the consumer's attention, because how could mud from your backyard be worth $50 to $100 a treatment? How appealing would mud from Idaho be in comparison to mud from Ishia or Austria? "Parafango" mud gets a lot of attention in spa treatments, but "parafango" is merely Italian for "protecting mud"—it isn't a kind of special earth from some distant, far-off land.

But could there be parts of the world where the dirt is better for your skin than it is from somewhere else? I have looked for the evidence, and to tell you that there is no research showing mud that is beneficial for skin is an understatement. Further, having a mask applied once a month at a spa is similar to dieting once a month; it ends up being of little help in keeping your body healthy day in and day out. It may feel good to be wrapped or to soak in mud, but the benefit is purely emotional and unrelated to any real effect on your skin.

THE JOY OF BATHING

While there is no joy or beauty in wasting money on useless body products, the pleasure of a wonderful luxurious bath offers many emotional benefits that should not be ignored. There is no denying the amazing amount of relaxation you can derive from a quiet interlude in a serene, carefully prepared bath. By adding a few aesthetic touches to your bathroom and locking the door you can create a tranquil refuge right in your own home. And none of these products have to be expensive or contain irritants. In fact, the less-expensive ones (like pure almond, olive, or sunflower oil, Epsom salts, or nonfragranced body moisturizers) all work beautifully.

Where the body is concerned, fragrance can be a serious skin irritant. If you use fragranced oils and salts in the bath, the perfume component can be especially sensitizing for the vaginal area as well as other parts of the body. But you can still gain the comforting, tranquil benefit of fragrance by lighting scented candles or spraying the room with a special scent. Keeping the fragrance out of the tub and off your skin is the ideal way to have your cake and eat it too, figuratively speaking.

But back to indulgence. Simply feeling beautiful and tranquil is the main goal of a leisurely bath. Steamy water, drizzled with nonfragranced plant oils and foaming bubbles, accompanied by scented candles flickering in the mirror (that way you don't need to put fragrance in the bathwater, and your olfactory sense can still participate), and at least a half hour of spare time is all it takes.

Later, when you're done soaking, after gently exfoliating your skin, shaving unwanted hair from your legs and underarms, and applying an unscented moisturizer, your body will feel silky in a way it doesn't after your usual morning ritual of shower and moisturizer.

Without trying to burst anyone's bubble, and because my job is to tell you what I know to be true from current research, I must mention that, as blissful as all this can be, the only benefits are psychological. Regularly soaking for long periods, especially in hot water—and that includes Jacuzzis—is actually not the best for the long-term health of the skin. Oversaturating the skin with water can break down its immune and healing responses and even actually make it drier. (Source: *Contact Dermatitis*, December 1999, pages 311–314.)

The best approach is to bathe infrequently—or, if you bathe regularly, to soak for no more than five to ten minutes. Occasionally it is fine to soak for longer periods, but make that the exception instead of the rule. Whether it's for five or ten minutes, or the infrequent twenty- to thirty-minute soak, the repose and quiet serenity of a bath can give you the time to feel the texture changes in your skin and to calm stressed-out, responsibility-weary nerves.

What is the best way to go about this indulgent ritual? It is definitely easier and far less expensive if you use something other than the products lined up at the cosmetics counters and specialty salons, that's for sure.

Here is one scenario for how to enjoy a relaxing bath.

- Start running the bath using water that's only slightly hotter than normal, but only slightly; water that is too hot can be hard on the skin and may cause problems over the long haul. It shouldn't hurt to get in the tub.
- Turn on relaxing music.
- If you have normal to dry skin, drizzle in some almond, olive, or sunflower oil, or mineral oil (but use only a teaspoon or two or you'll feel like you're soaking in an oil spill). If you have oily, blemish-prone skin from the neck down, oils of any kind are not the best idea.

- You can use bubble bath, but dish detergent from your kitchen can work just as well. Both bubble bath and dish detergent can be drying, but the teeny amount used for either to produce copious suds in a bath negates any negative effect on skin.
- If you are keen to add bath salts to your bath experience consider adding Epsom salts instead. They are far more soothing and helpful for the body than fragranced bath salts. These are a great and incredibly inexpensive addition to any bath.
- Rather than pouring fragrance into the bath, which can be irritating for the skin, you can light a scented candle or two and place them in strategic locations so the light can flicker on the water and in the mirror. You can also buy tiny oil lamps that help radiate fragrance throughout the room.
- If you plan to give yourself a manicure or pedicure after your bath, take the time now to file your nails into the shape you want. Filing nails when they are wet can damage them and cause splitting. If you plan to cut your nails, wait until after you are done soaking, when they are softer and less likely to be damaged.
- Turn down the lights or turn them off altogether and bathe by candlelight.
- Enter the bath slowly, even gracefully; the experience is everything, try seeing if you can do this without disturbing the water or bubbles.
- Prop a towel or bath pillow behind your head, and stretch out.
- While you're soaking, take the time to gently, and I mean gently, buff a washcloth over your body. (Be careful with loofahs—they can be hard on most skin types and if they are not cleaned regularly or replaced can be a source of bacteria.)
- Use a body cleanser or body wash, alone or with a gentle washcloth. Soap can be too drying on skin.
- If you want to shave your legs, do not scrub your legs. Shaving will provide enough exfoliation. Save shaving your legs till the end when the water is going down the drain and not sitting in the tub with you. Use unscented shave cream or your hair conditioner for the smoothest results. (Shaving the legs is much easier and causes far less irritation and fewer bumps if the legs have been soaked for a period of time. Also, sitting in water filled with used shaving cream is hardly luxurious.)
- You may want to shower off as your final step. If you don't like the feeling of bath oils left on your feet, underarms, or genitals, this is the time to wash those areas again to remove the oil or bath salts from your skin.
- When you're done, exit as slowly as you entered. This is still part of the ritual, so keep the candles lit.
- Dry your skin with a fresh towel, dabbing your skin lightly. There is no benefit to further scrubbing or buffing skin with a towel, especially not if you've used a wash-cloth or loofah in the bath.
- If you haven't used a body exfoliant in the bath, you can use your towel to give your legs and arms a good but gentle rubdown. But take it easy; hard rubbing can irritate the skin.
- If you haven't shaved, you can apply an AHA or BHA moisturizer over your legs and arms, especially on your knees, elbows, and heels. The exfoliation prevents dead skin

cells from building up, which can cause rough texture and dry flaky skin and also allows the moisturizer you apply to absorb and be more effective. Exfoliation with an AHA or BHA provides the same benefit for the body as it does for the face.

- Next apply a moisturizer. (Do not apply moisturizer to areas of the body that tend to break out.) A richer, emollient balm or pure shea or cocoa butter can be used on heels, knees, and elbows.
- If you bathe in the morning it is essential to apply an effective sunscreen over those parts of the body that will be exposed to daylight.
- Finally, if this has been an evening ritual, slip on something very soft, like cotton leggings and a cotton top, or a silky robe, and enter the world slowly, refreshed and renewed. Don't forget to blow out the candles.
- If you have extra time, this is the perfect opportunity to give yourself a pedicure and manicure.

BODY WASHES

Body cleansers, body washes, and body shampoos are just what they sound like—they use the detergent cleansing agents typically found in hair shampoos to clean the body—and they are excellent for all skin types. They tend to be less drying than bar soaps and bar cleansers, they leave no residues from the bar on the skin, and the chance of irritation or dryness is greatly reduced. (A moisturizing body wash can leave a slight film on the skin if it contains oils, but that's how these body cleansers moisturize the skin after you get out of the bath or shower.) Bar soaps and bar cleansers can be problematic for the body, just as they are for the face. Body washes are just as effective as soaps are, without any of the problems soaps can stir up, such as clogging pores or drying out the skin.

Please do not be fooled by the claims high-end cosmetics companies make about the body cleansers they sell. There is absolutely nothing that differentiates an expensive body wash from an inexpensive body wash. It is pathetic how brazenly identical the ingredients are between the pricey versions and the less pricey ones. Spending your money on these products is a waste regardless of your financial wherewithal and wasting money is never pretty.

Many body washes designed for dry skin claim all kinds of moisturizing properties. What they contain is simply some kind of oil. Vitamins, proteins, amino acids, and other fancy water-binding agents may be in there, too, making you think you're getting something special, but while these ingredients can be good moisturizing agents in a cream or lotion you leave on the skin, in a body wash they are just rinsed down the drain.

Oils tend to stick around a bit longer and are not easily washed away, so they do provide some emollient benefit for dry skin. Some people don't feel quite as clean after using a moisturizing body wash. They prefer the gentle cleaning effect of a regular body wash, followed by a moisturizer applied after getting out of the shower, but the choice is yours.

Here's a list of great body washes to consider: Aveeno Daily Moisturizing Body Wash ($6.79 for 12 ounces); Aveeno Skin Relief Body Wash Fragrance-Free ($6.79 for 12 ounces); Burt's Bees Naturally Moisturizing Milk & Shea Butter Body Wash ($8 for 12 ounces);

Caress Exotics Oil Infusion Japanese Cream Oil Body Wash ($5.99 for 15 ounces); Doctor Bobby Body Wash ($15 for 8 ounces); Dove Beauty Body Wash Sensitive Skin ($8.79 for 24 ounces); Eucerin Calming Body Wash Daily Shower Oil ($7.49 for 8.4 ounces); Ivory Simplement Body Wash Fresh Snow ($5.59 for 24 ounces); Jason Natural Cosmetics Fragrance-Free Satin Shower Body Wash ($10.99 for 16 ounces); Johnson's Softwash Body Wash Extra Care ($5.99 for 20.3 ounces); Nature's Gate Hemp Velvet Body Wash ($7.49 for 18 ounces); Neutrogena Rainbath Deep Moisture Body Wash Butter Cream ($8.49 for 6.7 ounces); Olay Quench Body Wash ($8.79 for 23.6 ounces); Olay Ultra Moisture Body Wash ($8.79 for 23.6 ounces); Paula's Choice All Over Hair & Body Shampoo ($12.95 for 16 ounces); Softsoap Skin Essentials Nutraoil Moisturizing Body Wash ($5.99 for 18 ounces); and St. Ives Collagen Elastin Moisturizing Body Wash ($4.89 for 18 ounces).

BODY SCRUBS

Exfoliating skin from the neck down provides the same benefits as it does from the neck up: It helps the skin absorb moisturizer better, unclogs pores, and allows healthier skin cells to surface. There are lots of ways to help get dead skin cells off the body. You can use anything from a gentle washcloth to a well-formulated AHA or BHA product. Topical scrubs are also an option, but are no better than a washcloth. Even though the skin on the body can handle mechanical scrubbing a bit better than the skin on the face can, you still need to be gentle with this kind of physical scouring (except on the heels—callused heels can take a bit more rough treatment to get the built-up layers of thickened dead skin cells off).

Loofahs have one major drawback you need to be aware of. Because they hang around in the shower and are often not cleaned or rotated with a new one, they are an ideal breeding ground for bacteria such as staphylococcus. Overscrubbing or scrubbing over blemishes and cuts with an old loofah that has not been properly cleaned is unwise. Washcloths are easy to throw in the laundry and tend to be less rough and less irritating on the skin and that is always a benefit.

Unequivocally and without exception, no amount of scrubbing or beating at the skin will change or eliminate one dimple on your thighs. The only benefits from exfoliation are those discussed earlier in this book and above, and that's really it. You might feel your thighs look better after you have scrubbed them and applied various lotions and gels, but all these products and massaging actions do is temporarily swell the skin on the thighs, making them look momentarily smoother.

ANTIBACTERIAL CLEANSERS

It's hard to imagine that the popularity of antibacterial cleansers is a cause for concern, but for a variety of reasons it is. Antibacterial cleansers are usually effective against many types of bacteria on the skin but they end up causing problems for just that very reason. The widespread use of antibacterial agents has created strains of resistant organisms that will compromise the wider usefulness of triclosan, the most typical antibacterial agent in these products (Source: *American Journal of Infection Control*, October 2001, pages 281–283).

The national Centers for Disease Control and Prevention (Source: CDC, www.cdc.gov) states that hand-washing in warm water with plain soap for at least ten seconds is sufficient in most cases (even for healthcare workers) to eliminate germs.

There are now more than 700 antibacterial products available to the consumer. According to the CDC, "The public is being bombarded with ads for cleansers, soaps, toothbrushes, dishwashing detergents, and hand lotions, all containing antibacterial agents. Likewise, we hear about 'superbugs' and deadly viruses. Germs have become the buzzword for a danger people want to eliminate from their surroundings. In response to these messages, people are buying antibacterial products because they think these products offer health protection for them and their families…. Besides resistance, the antibacterial craze has another potential consequence.

"Reports are mounting about a possible association between infections in early childhood and decreased incidence of allergies. In expanding this 'hygiene hypothesis,' some researchers have found a correlation between *too much* hygiene and *increased* allergy. This hypothesis stems from studies that revealed an increased frequency of allergies, cases of asthma, and eczema in persons who have been raised in an environment overly protective against microorganisms. In one rural community, children who grew up on farms had fewer allergies than did their counterparts who did not live on farms. Graham Rook, University College, London, has likened the immune system to the brain. You have to exercise it, that is, expose it to the right antigenic information so that it matures correctly. Excessive hygiene, therefore, may interfere with the normal maturation of the immune system by eliminating the stimulation by commensal microflora [normal and safe bacteria that live on the skin]."

Even if the hypothesis that antibacterial products help create strains of resistant bacteria doesn't prove out and the theories about "exercising our immune system" fail to be true, antibacterial products may not be the help many think they are. Antibacterial products are marketed under the notion that they will lower the risk of disease. However, flus and most colds are viral infections, not bacterial ones, so antibacterial cleansers are useless as a protection against them.

BATH OILS

Bath oils are primarily just that: oils derived from all sorts of sources, including sunflower, almond, coconut, and jojoba—and from a virtual plethora of plants and flowers. Some bath oils contain volatile (fragrant) oils that can potentially cause allergic reactions. Other bath oils are formulated with slip agents (ingredients that help the oils move over the skin) as well as with mineral oil (mineral oil can be more soothing for the skin than plant oils because it poses minimal to no risk of irritation). Some even contain water-binding agents, which are hardly necessary since the skin will be water-laden whether they are present or not, and because their effect is washed down the drain.

If there is any distinction between oils, it has more to do with how greasy they feel and how much irritation they can cause than with any healing benefits they may have. Plain mineral oil can be an excellent bath oil because it is fragrance-free, gentle and emollient, and unlikely to cause irritation or breakouts. Safflower, sesame, almond, avocado, and even olive oil can add the slip and emollience needed by dry skin because they stay on the skin and are not rinsed down the drain before you step out of the bath or shower.

BATH SALTS

Bath salts can be beneficial for many skin types. Salts and minerals, regardless of their source, can soften water and, depending on the specific salts used, reduce inflammation and swelling. Epsom salts are probably the best-known type; they work quite well and are wonderfully inexpensive. Most of the salts added to bath products are just fine, although ingredients such as borax, sodium sesquicarbonate, sodium carbonate, and phosphate can cause irritation and probably should be avoided. Table salt and sea salt can also be a problem, because if they don't get rinsed off well they can pull water from the skin and cause dryness and irritation.

Many cosmetics lines, particularly spa lines, brag about how their products contain minerals from all kinds of sources: mineral springs in France, volcanic waters in Italy, Dead Sea salts from Israel, and on and on. The question is whether minerals and salts from exotic sources have any special effect on skin. In the long run, unless you have a skin disorder such as psoriasis or seborrhea, those salts and minerals have no positive effect. Epsom salts are preferred both for their skin-softening and anti-inflammatory properties, and because they pose a minimal risk to sensitive skin.

AROMATHERAPY?

Fragrance is one of the most important aspects of body care, at least to many consumers. Ironically, it is one of the least important for the health of the skin. For some people, fragrance can be as much a problem from the neck down as for the neck up. Although the body is generally less susceptible to sensitizing reactions than the face, this can vary from person to person; there can also be a problem even if you don't feel a reaction.

Popularity has given aromatherapy a prominence in the world of body care, and it can be difficult to avoid. Despite the risk to the skin, most body and bath products are highly fragranced, and things are getting worse, not better. While women are becoming more and more aware that fragranced skin-care products can cause problems for the face, they are nevertheless likely to purchase bath and body-care products because of their scent.

Can a particular scent or blend of scents provide special benefits for your skin or your emotions? When it comes to skin, fragrant oils are not helpful for any part of the face or body because they can cause irritation, skin sensitivities, rashes, inflammation, and allergic reactions. Fragrance is especially problematic for the genital area (Source: *American Journal of Contact Dermatitis*, December 2001, pages 225–228).

However, as far as your emotions are concerned, only you can know for sure. Lots of women indeed feel less stressed out after indulging their senses with interesting fragrant blends, but they are also taking time out from their busy day while doing it. Does the fragrance cause the effect or the time out? That's hard to say. What is easy to say is that scent has nothing to offer the skin and everything to offer the nose.

Most people are greatly affected by pleasing aromas, and almost everyone feels invigorated or supremely relaxed after a good long soak. Because fragrance can play such a significant role in this experience, there is no reason not to partake. However, I would encourage you to find other ways to please your olfactory sense than putting fragrant products in the bathwater or all over your skin. Scented candles, plain candles drizzled with fragrant oils, and oil lamps or diffusers (you can purchase the latter at most health food stores or specialty body-care shops) are a great way to fill the air with sublime scents and leave your skin unaffected. That is better for your nose and great for your skin.

PERFUME AND ITS MYSTERIES

Women the world over use perfume and have been doing so for eons. When it comes to buying perfume or cosmetics, one of the first things a consumer does is smell the product. Why? Because a pleasing scent can make a woman feel confident, sensual, and happy. With all that, who cares if it helps the skin?

Buying perfume is an entirely sensory experience. Minute drops applied to the "warm" spots on the body—behind the ears, along the cleavage, inside the thigh, and on the pulse points on the wrist, neck, inside elbow, and behind the knee—can provide all the radiating scent you need to attract someone's attention. Perfume is almost exclusively about love and sex, and not necessarily in that order.

Unless you've been visiting another planet for the last 30 years, you won't be surprised when I say that sex is used as a sales tool for almost every product from shoes to deodorant (if advertisers could figure a way to make the Pillsbury Doughboy into a sex symbol, they would do it to sell more biscuits). Perfume ads almost always feature young, sultry, long-legged, breathless women; half-clothed, hard-bodied men; or both, in couples who can barely keep their hands, lips, or low-lidded eyes off each other.

Most of us throw logic out the window when confronted with the hope of increased desirability, and that's what sells perfume, because there is nothing utilitarian, professional, or rational about it. In short, perfume is a difficult subject for a consumer reporter because it defies logic, and that's as it should be. But let me throw in just a little information to help you in making your selection. Other than allergic reactions, there are no risks when it comes to wearing perfume. How much you like a scent and how it affects the people around you, specifically the people who get close to you, are all that count.

Speaking of the people around you, it is a complete mystery to me why some women or men or teenagers (the explosive growth of the Axe products comes to mind) feel a need to saturate themselves with a conspicuous amount of fragrance. The air around men and women who have generously anointed themselves with their favorite perfume or eau de toilette or aftershave can be so thick and pungent that their presence is announced by an overpowering hit of fragrance. This is definitely one of those beauty steps that can be overdone and lose its original purpose, which in this case is to exude a subtle scent for those you want to be close to.

Perfume should not be so pungent an emission that it overwhelms strangers in an elevator or business associates around a conference table. In addition, an overpowering scent can trigger allergic reactions in others. I suspect many women put on extra fragrance in the morning to make it last longer. Yet it is simple enough to touch up fragrance as the day goes by, just as you would makeup. Most women who overdo their perfume would never apply 20 layers of makeup to make sure it stayed on all day!

While we're on the subject, the endurance of a fragrance has nothing to do with natural ingredients versus synthetic ones or with how many products you apply. If anything, synthetic ingredients create more stable products by taking the unreliability of plant extracts and oils out of the equation. Yet there is no way to know which ingredients are used in any perfume or eau de toilette because this is the sole area where the cosmetics industry doesn't have to reveal formulas. Consequently, fragrance recipes truly are secrets (Source: www.fda.gov).

Several master perfumers have told me that most fragrances are created from a vast combination of fragrance components that are both natural and synthetic. The art of creating a nuanced, resplendent bouquet involves bringing together varying aromas in a cohesive, unified scent that pleases the olfactory sense. That secrecy and complexity is why fragrance knock-offs and inexpensive imitations just don't work. Some perfumers have blended hundreds of flower oils, plant extracts, and synthetic scents to create one perfume. How can a formula that complex be duplicated unless you know the exact recipe? It can't. And that's why a cheap version of the perfume you like won't make your nose as happy.

Without ingredient lists to turn to, there are only two ways to determine how long a fragrance will last on your body: product type and testing. In terms of product type, you can count on cologne (which is about 1% to 3% fragrance) and eau de cologne (about 3% to 5% fragrance) lasting two to three hours; eau de toilette (about 5% to 7% fragrance) lasting two to four hours; eau de parfum (about 12% to 18% fragrance) lasting four to six hours; and perfume (about 15% to 30% fragrance) six to eight hours or more. Consider purchasing perfume (which is oil-based) instead of cologne or eau de toilette (which are water- and alcohol-based) if longevity is an issue for you. Perfume is more expensive, but it does have a better potential for lasting the whole day because the oil and the fragrance concentration cling better to skin, so it tends not to wear off as easily as alcohol- and water-based fragrances.

Testing is the next step. Body chemistry can greatly affect any fragrance a person applies. How long any fragrance, regardless of type, will last or how well it will retain its scent during the day is anyone's guess. A fragrance can smell different at the beginning of the day than it does by the end. Trying on a fragrance (only one at a time) is the best way to determine how well it endures and which one you prefer. Do not choose a fragrance based on the way it smells in the bottle or on a card because that is not usually representative of what it will be like on your skin.

Should you buy body products that all have the same fragrance as your perfume? In a word, no. As you already know by now, I would rather you not apply scented skin-care products of any kind all over the body. It is best if your fragrance comes from a perfume or cologne applied to the inside part of your elbow, knee, neck, and cleavage. That's plenty.

You do not need an additional bath product, dusting powder, body cream, perfume, or cologne to make a fragrance stick around longer; that's fragrance overkill.

One more point of interest: The most expensive part of any fragrance is the bottle (about 40% of the cost). Then comes the advertising (another 30% of the cost) and the celebrity endorsement or designer insignia (another 10% to 15% of the cost). That leaves about 15% to 20% actual fragrance cost. Now that stinks!

SMOOTHEST LEGS IN THE WORLD

Shaving is one of the primary ways women remove hair from their legs. Before I get into the discussion about how best to tackle this often-daily event, you might want to read Chapter Twenty-Four, *Hair Removal*, which presents the various options for this repetitive task.

Most women barely get out the door on time with their teeth brushed, their kids off to school, and their makeup on evenly before they commute to the office, so shaving is a luxury that gets put on the bottom of the to-do list. But when the long, cold days of winter are a memory and the shorts and no-nylons time of year begins, there is no more hiding. Women, bring out your razors!

Several lines of cosmetic products are dedicated to the art of shaving. A brochure for one of these lines says a perfect shave requires an understanding of the fundamental principles of wet shaving and the use of five easy products (their products, of course). But you can easily do the five steps and not use their products (which were way overpriced for what they contained, especially considering the few bells and whistles would just be rinsed down the drain). Shaving involves a few basics: getting the legs wet, applying shaving cream or gel, shaving, and rinsing. You only need two shaving products, the razor and a non-fragranced shaving cream or gel, followed by a moisturizer, a sunscreen for daytime if your legs are going to see daylight, and a well-formulated moisturizer for night if your skin is dry.

There is no real trick to shaving. We all know how to do it, but not everyone knows how to get the best results and the softest legs. The following tips are the basics of a great, smooth shave:

- It is essential for your legs to be wet for at least two or three minutes before starting. Few things are as irritating or chafing as shaving dry or slightly damp legs.
- Find a razor that works well for your skin. Given the pressure you use while shaving, the texture of your skin, and the density of hair growth, this takes some experimentation. No single type of razor works well for everyone, but the three- and four-bladed razors are gentler by far and produce better results than throwaway or single-use razors. After that, the main thing is to change the blade frequently—dull razors make for poor shaving results.
- When it comes to shaving creams, for both men and women, those that contain emollients (usually those identified as being good for sensitive, dry skin) work perfectly on the legs! There is absolutely no reason to buy shaving gels or creams in pretty pink containers when in truth they are virtually identical to those in more masculine or unadorned packages.

- Avoid shaving products that contain irritants. Used over newly shaved skin, irritating ingredients can cause red bumps and ingrown hairs. When I find myself without shaving cream in the shower, I use hair conditioner or body wash instead, which is far easier on the legs than bar soap or bar cleanser.
- For best results, shave against the growth of hair, and be careful.
- After you are done, do not use a loofah or washcloth; shaving is enough exfoliation for your legs. Any extra abrasion can cause too much irritation and create problems.
- At night, apply a moisturizer, and during the day, if your legs are going to be exposed to sun, apply a moisturizer with sunscreen (SPF 15 or greater) that contains the UVA-protecting ingredients avobenzone, titanium dioxide, zinc oxide, Tinosorb, or Mexoryl SX.
- Do not use an AHA or BHA lotion over newly shaved skin; they can be unnecessarily irritating at this time.

PREVENTING RED BUMPS AFTER SHAVING

As many women know, in addition to the occasional nicks and cuts incurred during shaving, it isn't unusual to also have an aftermath of uncomfortable and unattractive razor bumps (red, inflamed blemishes), particularly along the bikini line. Hair follicles are attached to oil glands, and both are attached to nerve endings. Shaving can easily irritate the skin, the hair follicle, and the oil gland, causing a rashlike breakout of annoying bumps. Ingrown hairs can also present a dilemma. Ingrown hairs are curly, wiry hairs that turn, curl, and dig into the adjacent skin as they grow out, or hairs that grow back in the wrong direction, causing a bump that can become infected.

As widespread a beauty problem as this can be, for women and men alike, the lack of products addressing the issue is surprising. One of the more effective products for this problem are those formulated with aspirin in a glycerin base without alcohol. Aspirin, or acetyl salicylic acid, is a potent anti-inflammatory when taken orally yet has the same properties when applied topically. Unfortunately, it is hard to find products of this kind that are formulated without alcohol (alcohol would only add to the redness and irritation, making matters worse, not better). So why not consider formulating this yourself? You can easily mix together two aspirin tablets, a tablespoon of water, and a teaspoon of glycerin (you can buy this at the pharmacy) in a small cup or bottle. Once the aspirin is dissolved you can use it like a toner over the areas you've just shaved. This works for the face (for men), bikini line, legs, and underarms. You can apply your moisturizer after the aspirin solution is absorbed into the skin. If that sounds like too much effort, consider the aspirin-based Skin Relief Treatment I created for my Paula's Choice line. It has a toner-like consistency and works beautifully to soothe redness and razor bumps.

If you find the bumps do not respond well to the aspirin, try occasionally using an over-the-counter cortisone cream to reduce the redness and irritation. However, if the bumps get infected you will need to disinfect them with an over-the-counter antibiotic like Neosporin, Polysporin, or Bacitracin. All three are excellent for quick relief from small topical infections.

WHAT ARE ALL THOSE BUMPS ON MY ARMS AND LEGS?

Some people have a troublesome inherited skin problem called keratosis pilaris. This is the technical name for a condition in which hundreds of hard, clogged pores cover a person's shoulders, upper arms, buttocks, and upper thighs. It can seem to be a persistent case of acne, but these lesions rarely become inflamed and rarely become a pimple—though they will become inflamed if you pick at them. On darker skin the plugs can look like a sea of blackheads. What to do?

Gentle cleansing, exfoliating, and disinfecting can cause a huge reduction in the number of bumps. First, wash the skin gently with body wash (avoid soap, which can not only be too harsh but also may leave behind a film that can clog pores). If you like, you can use a clean washcloth gently over the bumpy areas. Do not overscrub. You can't rip these bumps off, and inflaming the area will only make matters worse.

After bathing, dry the area gently. When the skin is dried, apply a BHA lotion, gel, or toner over the problem area. BHA (salicylic acid) is the perfect option because it is lipid soluble. Lipid soluble means it can exfoliate inside the pore where the plug exists, improving the shape of the pore to allow a normal flow of oil. That makes it the best choice for reducing and potentially even eliminating the problem. If the bumps you have tend to become pimples or are infected after the BHA, apply a topical disinfectant of either 2.5% or 5% benzoyl peroxide. Do not apply moisturizer to these areas unless they are dry. During the day it is best to keep the area covered by clothing to avoid the use of sunscreen, which can make the problem worse. However, if the skin is going to be exposed to sun then it is essential to apply a well-formulated sunscreen. It will take some experimenting until you find the sunscreen that works for you. (Source: *Cutis*, September 2008, pages 177–180.) If you are unable to use or do not get noticeable results from a BHA product, an AHA lotion or gel with glycolic acid is also worth considering.

BLEMISHES, WRINKLES, SKIN DISCOLORATIONS, DRY SKIN, SUN PROTECTION, AND MORE

All of the same treatments explained in earlier chapters for any skin concern for the face apply to every other part of your body. Please refer to those sections for answers to your skin-care needs from the neck down as well. Even the application process from the neck down doesn't differ from the face, so you can follow the same course of action for both. During the day, after cleansing, apply an AHA or BHA lotion, cream, or gel over skin and then Retin-A or Renova over the sun-damaged areas. You should then apply a sunscreen over areas of the body that will be exposed to daylight. At night, if necessary, you can apply an additional moisturizer over particularly dry areas.

SERIOUSLY DRY HANDS

Struggling with dry hands can be painful. There is no question that being diligent about keeping them protected when doing housework or gardening, and unfailingly applying moisturizer whenever the opportunity arises can make all the difference in the world. Yet even those following this due diligence can still suffer from bone-dry, cracked, parched hands. Clearly, it is essential to protect your hands from dish detergent, laundry detergent, excessive washing (medical professionals have a rough time with this one), and irritating ingredients, and also when doing potentially irritating manual work. Wearing gloves to prevent contact with these types of products and ingredients is of the utmost importance. However, a significant number of women may find they are allergic to latex gloves. About 10% of the population has negative reactions, ranging from mild to severe, if they come in contact with latex. If this turns out to be a problem, ask your physician or pharmacist where you can find nonlatex gloves.

The faster you get an emollient moisturizer on your hands after washing, and the longer you can keep it on, the better. It helps to keep small tubes or bottles of emollient moisturizer all over the house, including near the kitchen sink, in the bathroom, at the bedside, and in the garage. Keep more in your car, purse, briefcase, and desk drawer. That way it is never out of reach for a quick application. The best moisturizers for daytime are moisturizing sunscreens whose active ingredient is either avobenzone (butyl methoxydibenzylmethane), titanium dioxide, zinc oxide, Tinosorb or ecamsule. However, titanium dioxide and zinc oxide provide an occlusive barrier that can act as a protective layer to retain moisture in the skin while keeping the sun's rays off the skin. (Bear in mind that brown "sun spots" on the back of hands and arms are a direct result of relentless, daily, unprotected sun exposure.)

Moisturizers such as Palmer's Cocoa Butter Formula, Eucerin Dry Skin Therapy Plus Intensive Repair Cream or Lotion, Curel Extreme Care Body Lotion, Jergens Advanced Therapy Lotion, and countless others are all excellent for use at night. The best approach is to apply moisturizer every chance you get. It is also incredibly helpful to purchase an over-the-counter cortisone cream such as Lanacort or Cortaid to help treat cracks and fissures that may occur, but cortisone creams are only to be used intermittently, not on a regular basis.

BODY ITCHES

Assuming you are following the skin care information I've provided so far but you still find that every time you shower your entire body begins to itch and the problem lasts for either a brief span of time or longer, you may have an allergy to the bath or hair-care products you are using. It will take experimentation to find out exactly what the culprit ingredient is, but the best strategy is to switch to products that have no fragrance whatsoever. However, you may also want to check out the possibility that the laundry detergent or fabric softener you use for your clothes or linens may be the real offender. Fabric softener sheets pose an interesting chemical problem. These sheets are heat-activated in the dryer. When you shower and towel dry, a little of the fabric softener residue comes off on your skin. Then, the next time you take a hot shower, the residue is heat activated on your skin, causing the itching. The itching stops after about twenty or thirty minutes, as your body cools down again. Laundry detergent can also be a problem. Using laundry detergents that have less potential for causing skin irritation, such as Cheer Free, All Free & Clear, Arm &

Hammer Free, or Tide Free, can make a huge difference. Sleeping on pillowcases and sheets that have detergent or fabric softener residue can be a serious problem when you have dry, sensitive, or acne-prone skin.

Hot water and showering can also cause problems for sensitive skin and can stimulate itching. I have advocated the use of tepid water for some time, particularly for the face, and it can make a difference for the body from the neck down if itching and rashes are an issue.

Another source of body itches can be the extremely irritating and drying salts that get deposited on the skin when you sweat. Instead of washing with bar cleansers or soaps, consider using a fragrance-free body wash. You will also want to avoid scrubs, loofahs, washcloths, bubble baths, and bath salts, all of which can trigger itchy skin.

Tight clothing such as jeans, nylons, tights, and leggings can also stimulate itching. The only way to prevent that is to loosen things up or do without. Nylons may be hard to give up, but for those with itchy thighs, wearing pants and cotton socks may be the only way to solve the problem.

HARD AS NAILS

While some women have naturally great nails, others search endlessly for anything that will help make their nails strong, thick (but not too thick), and long (sometimes too long). Sadly, you can't fool Mother Nature. What is genetically predetermined cannot be permanently transformed. If you are lucky enough to have strong, fast-growing, perfectly shaped nails with smooth, even cuticles, only trauma and damage to the nail bed will change the health and appearance of your nails. If you have naturally brittle, soft nails and thick cuticles, there is also no way to alter what you've inherited. There is a lot you can do to make your nails look and feel better (there's plenty you can do to make matters worse, too), but changing the way your nails naturally grow is as impossible as changing the way your hair grows.

I know there are dozens of nail products made by everyone from Revlon and Sally Hansen to Barielle, Orly, and Cutex, plus new ones being introduced monthly, all claiming they can repair the irreparable. Don't any of them work? If they did, we'd all have long, beautiful nails. Yet millions of women have struggled with weak, brittle, soft nails, trying an endless assortment of strengthening, lengthening, and fortifying nail products, only to give up in frustration. It is almost impossible for a woman who wants to improve the appearance of her short, fragile nails not to wonder about all of the products that claim to feed the nails, engorge them with vitamins, or build them up from the outside in. I would love to say those claims are legitimate and tell you which ones perform the best, but all the claims are bogus; changing the way a nail grows can't be done by putting something on it topically. Also, there's no research showing that vitamin supplements such as biotin or eating gelatin can change the way the nails grow, either.

Physiologically speaking, the nail is simply a protective covering composed of dead cells filled with a thick protein called keratin, quite similar in essence to the hair. Although the part of the nail you can see is dead, the matrix (the part of the nail under the skin) is very much alive. The white crescent area of the nail is called the lunula and is part of the matrix. The nail grows out from the matrix, and as the growth of new cells builds up and dies it is pushed forward and out toward the surface. The cuticle is the protective layer of skin between the outside environment and the matrix. Keeping the cuticle intact is perhaps the single most important element in preserving the health of the nail.

Despite the nail's basic attributes, several long-standing myths about getting the talons of your dreams make the coffee-klatch rounds every now and then. Perhaps you've heard some of these nail delusions before, such as that tapping your nails on a hard surface will help nails grow and make them stronger. That isn't true in the least. You can't strengthen the nail by exercising it, assuming the nail needs the same training as a muscle. If anything, tapping will do just the opposite of what you want. Repetitive pressure or strain on the nail will lead to breakage and splitting. Another inane nail fiction is the notion that eating gelatin makes nails healthier. Gelatin probably got its reputation as a nail builder because of its relationship to protein. Like your nails and your hair, gelatin contains protein, but no form of food can go directly to the nail or hair to help it grow. There are no studies or data demonstrating that eating gelatin will improve the condition of anything. Eating a balanced, low-fat, nutritious diet (meaning lots of fresh fruits, vegetables, and whole grains) is certainly an important factor in overall good health, but feeding the nail directly just isn't feasible.

FLUORIDE

Several nail-care products want you to believe that "What's good for your teeth is great for your nails," so you can "Harness the power of fluoride with strengtheners, base and top coats, and cuticle care." If only that were possible! It would be a dream come true to have a product that could make nails as strong as teeth, or even relatively as strong. Alas, unless you were born with naturally strong nails, fluoride isn't going to help your nails the way it helps teeth.

First, teeth are unrelated to nails. Teeth are made of a bony substance composed of various mineral compounds, mostly calcium phosphate. Nails have no mineral content but rather are composed of hardened keratin, basically the same substance that comprises skin and hair. Further, fluoride doesn't "strengthen" teeth, but rather, according to the American Dental Association, has varying influences that work with saliva and the growth of developing teeth to prevent decay. One function of fluoride is to reduce the constant reaction taking place between the tooth's surface, saliva, and bacteria in the mouth. When we eat sugar or starchy foods the number of bacteria in the mouth increases, which raises the acidity of our saliva, which in turn slowly, over time, demineralizes the surface of the tooth. As the acidity subsides, the tooth's surface becomes remineralized. Fluoride reduces the presence of bacteria in the mouth, which reduces the acidity of the saliva and in turn reduces or eliminates tooth decay. None of that, to put it mildly, has anything to do with nail growth or nail problems.

One more point: Given that almost all of us drink and wash with fluoridated water, our nails are consistently exposed to fluoride. If fluoride were important for healthy nails—which it isn't— the amount we get in our drinking water would be more than enough.

The nail-care industry has tried to build up many ingredients in the effort to convince us that we can grow stronger nails. For years protein was a big one that showed up in nail-care products, though protein can't feed the skin or nail from the outside in. Diligently applying most nail-care products does help, but it is the protective coating they provide that does the trick, not these impressive-sounding-yet-do-nothing special ingredients.

CALCIUM

Perhaps the last piece of nail improbability is the belief that applying calcium to your nails will make them strong. Calcium, along with lots of other minerals and vitamins, shows up in many nail-care products owing to the assumption that you can feed the nail from the outside in. You can't feed the nail directly, though even if you could, calcium and other minerals are unlikely ingredients for this purpose. Calcium and minerals may help build strong bones (bones are primarily calcium), but that is unrelated to the content of nails. The notion of having nails as strong as bone does make calcium sound appealing. However, even by itself calcium can't build bone; the body needs other vitamins and minerals to use the calcium. Moreover, there is virtually no calcium in nails; they're made of keratin and that's about it.

CUTICLE CARE

Although trying to affect the matrix and change the inherent growth of the nail with nail-care products is a waste of time and money, there are many things you can do to improve your nails. Without question, the most important element to pay attention to is the skin around the nail, namely the cuticle. The best way to keep your nails healthy, whole, and as free from problems as possible is to push your cuticles back as little as you can. The less you manipulate and cut your cuticle the better off your nails will be. Aside from inherited problems and physical trauma (getting smashed by a hammer or door can permanently alter the physical attributes of the nail), damage from overpushing or overtrimming the cuticle is the number one cause of nail problems. I know this may seem shocking and contrary to much of what you've heard, but excessively pushing back the cuticle and cutting it off is a huge no-no. Removing too much cuticle can damage the nail.

Overtrimming the cuticle can destroy the integrity of the matrix, which is the source of healthy nail growth. There is no way around this one. The cuticle is the body's form of protection for the area between the exposed dead part of the nail and the living matrix where the nail grows from. Anything that damages this seal puts the nail at risk.

If you cut too much cuticle away it can result in weak, brittle, ridged, dented, peeling, or unevenly growing nails (where one part of the same nail grows at a different rate), and once these problems occur they won't go away until the nail grows out, which can take anywhere from three months to a year. Orange sticks and metal cuticle tools, even when padded with cotton on the tip as most manicurists do, can cause damage to the nail if they are not used carefully.

Almost every dermatologist I interviewed agreed that cuticle damage negatively affects nail growth. You can test this for yourself. Stop manipulating, pushing, or overtrimming your cuticles. For the next six months, simply take care of your nail shape (I'll explain more about that later in this section) and only minimally trim hangnails or excess skin around the nail. Do not overmanipulate the cuticle in any manner whatsoever. Within a relatively short period of time you are likely to see a radical change in the growth of the nail. I know this is a hard one to get used to but it will pay off in the long run.

Another thing you can do for the cuticle is to moisturize it as often as possible, and during the day be sure you use a moisturizing sunscreen with avobenzone, Tinosorb, ecamsule (Mexoryl SX), titanium dioxide, and/or zinc oxide. It doesn't have to be a special nail or hand moisturizer with sunscreen—as long as the SPF is 15 or greater and the active ingredients are the ones I've been mentioning, it will do just fine. If the cuticle becomes dry and flaky (or sun damaged), the protective barrier for the matrix will break down, which can absolutely and quickly hurt nail growth. Yet in some ways it is almost impossible to keep the cuticle moist and healthy. Think about how often you wash your hands and use them every day for everything from office work to housework to sports. Also, the hands are incessantly exposed to the sun and it is difficult to keep them constantly protected with sunscreen. Yet doing so is essential. In short, don't overdo trimming cuticles, keep nails protected from the sun, and use a moisturizer to prevent dryness.

MANICURES AND PEDICURES

While leaving the cuticle alone is the best thing you can do for the growth of the nail, leaving the length of the nail alone is also a wise part of nail care. The part of the nail that extends past the quick is long dead and vulnerable to damage. Overfiling can tear at the nail's structure, and that can never be replaced. Once filing tears or starts lifting the fibrous nail material, it can begin a cycle that is hard to stop. Nails are softened by water, and soft nails are more susceptible to damage and tears. Shape the nails only when they are completely dry. It is also essential to avoid metal or extremely coarse nail files. Use the gentlest file with extremely gentle pressure to achieve the shape you want. You'll use up more nail files faster than you did before, but stronger nails will be the result of the extra expense and trouble. You've probably heard the one about filing in one direction only. That is completely unnecessary. Regardless of the direction you file, if you don't do it gently you will damage the nail.

When you do take the time to indulge in a full manicure or pedicure, it is essential to keep it simple.

The following is a great system for creating the perfect manicure or pedicure:

- First, remove any previously applied nail polish. It doesn't matter whether you use a nail-polish remover that contains acetone or not. It also doesn't matter whether the nail-polish remover contains moisturizing ingredients. If a nail-polish remover can remove nail polish it is going to be harsh stuff, but that is the price of nicely painted nails. Use as little nail-polish remover as necessary to remove the polish. Never soak the nail in nail-polish remover! Nail-polish remover is extremely drying and damaging to the entire nail, especially the cuticle. Keeping contact with nail-polish remover to a minimum is crucial for the well-being of the nail and cuticle.

- Gently file the nails into the shape you want, using the least-abrasive emery board you can find. Avoid shaping your nails into long talons or severe shapes (too square or pointy).

- Softening the cuticle around the nail is necessary only if you plan to remove just a tiny bit of excess cuticle. Soak the nails in plain warm water for no more than three minutes. Oversoaking hurts the nail and the cuticle. Avoid soapy or detergent-filled water, which only dries the skin and damages the cuticle. If the hands or feet are dirty, wash them first and that's it. Minimal contact with cleansers is best for any part of your body, including the nails!

- Trim the cuticle and avoid pushing it back as much as possible, being exceedingly careful not to pull, lift, tear, rip, force, or cut into the cuticle in any way.

- Trim the nails carefully, using sharp manicure scissors or nail clippers. Nails are definitely easier to trim after bathing or soaking. Fingernails should be given a slightly rounded edge to protect the nail growth; toenails should be trimmed straight across, slightly above the quick. Avoid cutting nails too short because doing so increases the chance of developing ingrown nails, which can be particularly uncomfortable for toenails.

- Moisturize the cuticle with an emollient moisturizer. Almost any moisturizer for dry skin will do. It is not necessary to purchase special cuticle creams, but some companies make brush-on, oil-based cuticle moisturizers that are quick and convenient to use.

- Before you polish your nails it is essential to remove the moisturizer from them. Moisturizing ingredients prevent nail polish from adhering to the nail. Use nail-polish remover just over the nail's surface to take off any moisturizer. Avoid getting nail-polish remover on the cuticle; that's the area you want to keep the moisturizer on.

- Polish your nails in layers, allowing them to dry between coats. A minimum of three coats is standard. If you have weak or brittle nails, place one or two coats of ridge-filling nail polish on the nail as the base coat. This is the best way to shore up the nail. Two coats of a colored nail polish are next, followed by a top coat to add shine and luster.

- Allow plenty of time for the polish to dry. Quick-dry polishes and some quick-dry top coats of polish often contain alcohol, which can cause the polish to peel and chip more easily, so you want to avoid those. Using a quick-dry oil or spray after you're done polishing is a great way to ward off smudges, but these won't prevent nicks or dents in the polish, so be careful.

- Do not dry your nails with a blow dryer or any other heat source. Heat causes the polish to expand and lift away from the nail.

- Touching up polish every other day with a layer of top coat can help make a manicure last longer. Carry a bottle of top coat in your purse, and when you have a moment or break in your day, quickly do a once-over. A single layer dries quickly and makes all the difference in keeping up appearances.

NAIL POLISH THAT LASTS

After spending way too much money on nail-care products and nail polishes, many women complain that for this kind of money their nails should be ten times stronger and the polish should last ten times longer. A nice thought, but that isn't the case. The price of a nail polish has no connection with how long it will last. Nail polishes are produced by only a handful of manufacturers, so there are no secrets, and the formulations vary only slightly because only a handful of ingredients will stay on the nail.

Lots of women complain that if they want their nails to look good it takes practically a full-time effort, and they can't live life like a normal person. I've gone around walking like a surgeon to be sure my nails don't come in contact with any surface anywhere. Though it doesn't take money to improve the appearance of your nails, it does take diligence and care. Those two things can't be avoided. Unfortunately, some polishes do tend to chip more than others (but this is determined by formulation, not cost). I wish I could offer some insight into which formulations work best, but no matter how many surveys I do or how many cosmetics chemists I interview, I have found no consensus as to which products last better. More often than not, polish longevity has to do with the process of applying the layers in the right order, including the base coat (preferably a ridge-filler-type product), color, and top coat; applying layers that are thick enough but not too thick; allowing plenty of time for drying; and then treating your nails carefully (wearing gloves, avoiding water, having minimal contact with soaps or cleansers, and not using the nails as tools).

Polishes are often given names like SuperWeave Base Coat, Color Lock No-Chip Sealer, Strong Wear Nail Strengthener Polish, Extra Life Top Coat, Nail Building Base Coat, Color Shield, Fortifier Hydrating Base, or Nail Protector. They are all great names that promise wonderful things they can't even begin to deliver. Nails are dead, and all the protein, amino acids, and other familiar and exotic conditioning agents in the world won't help them live.

I wish I could find a line of nail polishes that last, but it doesn't exist. So many factors affect how well your nail polish holds up. For example, do you wear gloves when you clean? What kind of daily work do you do with your hands? Are your nails oil- and cream-free before you start polishing? I also get frustrated trying to separate one nail product from another because they have so much in common. The resins, lacquers, and basic products are all essentially the same. Most women experience about the same amount of wear from product to product, and it's about one to three days. All nail polishes begin to chip on the third to fourth day after application, regardless of the claim on the label (but you already knew that, didn't you?). Reapplying your top coat daily and avoiding fast-drying nail polishes will increase the chances of having your polish last. Finding the discipline to do that isn't easy, but it is the cheapest and most reliable way to make a manicure stick around until the end of the week.

By the way, it is completely unnecessary and actually a bad idea to store nail polish in the refrigerator. Condensation and cold negatively affect nail polish, making it too thick to use reliably.

FAKE NAILS—REAL PROBLEMS

The long and short of artificial nails is that there are risks associated with having them applied. I won't get into the aesthetic issues here, though it is a mystery to me why women can consider this a valid expenditure of their hard-earned money or believe that anyone thinks these are real—that's another story altogether. What is of more concern is the number of women every year who see a physician because of nail-related disorders that are directly related to the application of artificial nails. The most typical problems are horizontal nail grooves that develop close to the cuticle. This abnormality, according to an article by Dr. Zoe Draelos in the January 1998 issue of *Cosmetic Dermatology*, is seen in chemotherapy patients and women who wear artificial nails. When it's unrelated to chemotherapy, this nail damage is probably a result of the drill used by the manicurist to buff out the acrylic nail, or to rough up the real nail to allow better adhesion of the fake nail. It is far less damaging to use an emery board to file the nail, but salons are using the drill procedure to speed up an otherwise time-consuming process.

The thinning of the nail plate is another problem that occurs, especially when the acrylic nails are finally removed. To address this, it is quite typical for the manicurist to recommend oils, vitamins, or other treatments ranging from calcium to oxygen infusions, none of which will improve the appearance of the nail. The weakened, fragile part of the nail is long dead, and there is nothing that can be done to change the damage that took place when the artificial nail was applied and then repeatedly damaged with each reapplication. The only option is time, enough of it to grow out the damage, assuming that you are not doing anything else to your nails to cause more damage to the nail or cuticle.

Inflammation of the nail area is almost always a direct result of the chemicals used to apply artificial nails, but it can also be an allergic reaction to the acrylic material. However, if the inflammation persists or swells, it is essential to use a topical disinfectant such as Bacitracin. If the swelling continues or becomes more painful, it is imperative to see a physician who can treat the possible infection.

Another typical and more painful problem is something called onycholysis, which is the separation or loosening of a fingernail or toenail from its nail bed. What makes acrylic nails often more amazing than your own nails is, according to Dr. Draelos, "that the adhesion between the artificial nail and the natural plate is stronger than the adhesion between the natural nail plate and the nail bed." If you twist your nail, it is far easier to have your own nail become detached from your skin than it is for the artificial nail to pop off your natural nail. This means you need to avoid misuse (and not think the artificial nail can withstand any amount of pressure). It is imperative to pay attention to any loosening of your own nail and to be careful how you use the artificial nail. Because the artificial nail may be stronger than your own, it can put your real nail at risk.

One other possible problem for fake-nail wearers is infection. If you see a yellow or green discoloration, you can attempt to treat it yourself with Bacitracin. But if this doesn't produce any improvement then it is essential you contact your physician.

NAIL STRENGTHENERS

If only nail-strengthening products really existed! What I wouldn't give for that, and I've tried them all. As it turns out, many of the products that claim to strengthen nails contain extremely drying ingredients such as formaldehyde or toluene, which do toughen the nail temporarily, but also make it more brittle. Formaldehyde goes by other names on ingredient lists, so watch out for names like toluene, toluene sulfonamide, and toluene sulfonic acid. Toluene and toluene-like ingredients are illegal in the state of California because of the serious health risks they pose, including cancer and respiratory problems.

Some formaldehyde-free nail strengtheners just coat the nail, like the ridge-filling products. So-called strengthening creams contain thick, waxy ingredients, like lanolin, that smooth over the nail and are hard to wash off. If you are good about reapplying these several times a day (sans polish, of course, because they can't penetrate polish), you might just see a change in your nails, because they help protect the cuticle and prevent the nail from drying out, but it takes discipline. Keep in mind that you can't wear polish over any kind of moisturizing product because polish won't adhere to a moist, lubricated surface. You can apply these products over polish; but then they won't help the nail, although they can moisturize the cuticle.

NAIL DO'S AND DON'TS

Surprisingly, there are more don'ts than do's when it comes to taking care of your nails. Most dermatologists will tell you that what you don't do to your nails is by far more important than what you do to them when healthy, strong nails are what you want. This list summarizes some of the things I've mentioned above, but the information bears repeating, given the amount of deceptive nail information and the number of nail products being sold and advertised all over the cosmetics world:

- Do coat the outside of the nails with nail polish or ridge fillers, which can help protect the nail and prevent breaking and splitting, at least while the manicure lasts.
- Do moisturize the cuticle area to prevent cracking and peeling, which can hurt the matrix.
- Do wear gloves to protect nails and cuticles from housework, gardening, and doing dishes.
- Do be cautious when doing office work. Nails and cuticles can take a beating from filing, opening letters (use a letter opener), typing (use the flat of your finger pads on the keyboard instead of the tips of your nails), and handling papers.
- Do apply a hand cream frequently, especially after you're done washing your hands, and pay attention to the cuticle area.
- Do wear a sunscreen during the day on the hands and cuticles to prevent sun damage, which can hurt the nail, and reapply it every time you wash your hands.
- Do meticulously clean all nail implements and change nail files often. Bacteria and other microbes can get transferred by the nail tools you use, causing infection or harm to the matrix.

- Do disinfect any tears or cuts to the cuticle, and treat ingrown nails as soon as possible. Nail infections are not only unsightly, but they can also cause long-lasting damage to the nail. Any drugstore antibacterial ointment, such as Polysporin, Neosporin, or Bacitracin, will do.
- Don't use nail products that contain formaldehyde or toluene. They pose health risks for the nail and for your entire body as well.
- Don't use fingernails as tools to pry things open.
- Don't use your fingers as letter openers. That destroys the cuticles, which destroys the nail matrix and affects nail growth and strength.
- Don't soak nails for long periods, and never use any kind of soap or detergent when soaking. Nails and cuticles that become engorged with water weaken, and the longer soap or detergent is in contact with skin and nails (despite the advertisements for Palmolive dish detergent) the greater the potential for damaging the nail and cuticle structure.
- Don't overuse any kind of nail-polish remover. Use a minimal amount on the nail and avoid getting too much on the cuticle and skin.
- Don't push the cuticle back too far. Trim only the part of the cuticle that has started to lift away from the nail.
- Don't allow any manicurist to touch your hands with utensils that have not been properly sterilized. The importance of this step cannot be stressed enough. Risking your health and well-being for a manicure is just not worth it, and that is a definite possibility with bacteria-laden nail instruments!
- Don't pull or tear at hangnails. Always gently cut them away, leaving the cuticle intact and as untampered-with as possible.
- Don't ignore nail or cuticle inflammation. Disinfect the skin as soon as you can with an antibacterial or antifungal agent. Any change to the nail's appearance (see the next section) needs to be checked out by a dermatologist.

WHEN THE NAIL GETS SICK

There are times when nail care requires a dermatologist. Fingernails and toenails are extremely vulnerable to infection and damage. If you have been diligent about leaving your cuticles alone and avoiding all the don'ts and performing most of the do's in the list above and you are still having nail problems, make an appointment with your dermatologist. Nails that are brittle, discolored, dull, abnormally thick, distorted, crumbling, loose, or subject to unusual debris under the nail are a medical problem, not a cosmetic one.

It is quite normal for the skin to host a variety of microorganisms, including bacteria and fungi. Some are useful to the body, but others can multiply rapidly, leading to infections. Specifically, fungal infections are caused by microscopic plants (fungi) that thrive on the dead tissue of the nails and outer skin layers, particularly the cuticle.

Fungal nail infections are most often seen in adults, can be difficult to treat, and often recur. Toenails are affected more often than fingernails. People who frequent public swimming pools, gyms, or shower rooms; people who perspire a great deal; and people who wear tight, occlusive shoes are most likely to develop toenail infections because the fungi flourish in warm, moist areas. Prolonged exposure to moistness on the skin, minor nail injuries, and damage to the cuticle area can also increase susceptibility to fungal infection. Please be aware that fungal and bacterial infections are extremely contagious and can be spread through direct contact with another person who has the problem, and even through contact with contaminated towels, shower and pool surfaces, and nail implements such as cuticle clippers, nail clippers, orange sticks, and cuticle pushers.

Nail infections can be cleared with the persistent use of a prescription antifungal or antibacterial cream or lotion. Because nails grow slowly, treatment must be continued for 3 to 6 months for fingernails and 6 to 12 months for toenails (the time it takes to grow a new nail). There are oral medications for these problems, but they are best discussed with your doctor.

In terms of preventing problems for the feet, it is essential to keep them clean and dry. Change shoes and socks frequently. Dry the feet and hands thoroughly after bathing. Powders such as baby powder with corn starch or talcum may help keep the feet dry. Of course, avoiding any damage to toenails and fingernails is of utmost importance.

To minimize the risk of damage to the nails, keep them smooth and properly trimmed. Trim the fingernails weekly. The toenails grow more slowly and may be trimmed as needed, about once a month. Nail-polish remover of any kind can weaken and dry the nails. Nail polish may coat and protect the nails slightly, but if you choose to use it remember that all polishes are basically identical, despite advertising claims to the contrary. Nail strengtheners can discolor or break the nails and damage the nail, too. Artificial nails may produce allergic reactions under the nail and can create a perfect environment for bacterial or fungal growth.

INGROWN NAILS

Ingrown nails are another inelegant but typical nail problem. Often they are the result of cutting the nail too deeply or filing the nail too much, setting the scene for abnormal growth. Pain, swelling, infection, and discharge can result when the nail edge then grows into the surrounding skin. Many women love to wear shoes that crunch their toes into unnatural positions, and this, too, can interfere with nail growth and impair a normal healing process.

How can you prevent ingrown nails? Give your toenails plenty of room. That means wearing shoe styles that do not force the foot into an unnatural shape. Also, when you trim your fingernails and toenails, it is essential to avoid radically changing the natural shape of the nail by overfiling or by cutting the nail below the tip of the finger or toe. Also, do not cut or push the cuticles; damage there can significantly affect the nail's growth.

If an ingrown nail does become infected, thoroughly clean the area and try to minimally trim away the portion of the nail that is digging into the skin. Overcutting can simply re-create the problem, so be cautious. Disinfect the area with an over-the-counter antibacterial ointment like Polysporin, Neosporin, or Bacitracin. If the problem does not improve, it may require medical care.

CORNS, CALLUSES, AND BUNIONS

Taking a closer look at our feet can be depressing. Statistically, eight out of every ten adults have calluses, bunions, and corns to deal with. Blisters are a common occurrence as the latest shoe fashions are broken in. Athletically inclined adults (or adults with athletically inclined family members) run a high risk of struggling with athlete's foot. Depending on how careful you are with pedicures, you can also be subject to painful ingrown nails that can become infected and swollen! There are ways to prevent these problems from occurring and there are solutions to most of these foot infirmities, but some are going to be hard to adopt and adapt to your lifestyle. Try to stick with it though, because soft, smooth feet, without squished toes and lumps and bumps, are definitely the way to go!

There is nothing glamorous about corns and calluses but they are abundant and occur more often than just about any other foot malady. Corns are thickened lumps formed on the outer layer of skin and occur over bony areas, such as toe joints, especially on the tops or sides of toes. Corns are most recognizable by a small, tender, and painful raised bump that has a noticeably hard-textured center. Corns can be tender and painful, depending on how large they are and how much pressure shoes put on them.

Calluses are larger, and almost always are a painless thickening of skin caused by repeated pressure or irritation on the heels or balls of the feet. Calluses can become painful when they become so dry and cracked that the area becomes sore and tender to the touch.

In essence, corns and calluses are the body's way of protecting the feet from injury. For women, the most typical source of injury is from the shoes they wear. The pressure exerted on the foot, especially the toes, when it is forced into high heels or narrow shoe widths is nothing less than torture for the toes, heels, and arches of the feet. Your feet respond to this burden by growing skin cells at a faster rate to form a protective covering as a way to cushion the bones of the foot. It's this overgrowth of skin cells that forms calluses and corns.

Our feet would almost be picture perfect if women wore better shoes. High heels, narrow toe boxes, tight fits, and strange shapes (that don't match the proportions of the foot) are all disasters waiting to happen. If stopping the growth of calluses and corns isn't enough of an incentive, it also turns out that wearing high heels can cause back, hip, knee, and ankle pain brought about by a change in one's gait due to severe discomfort; it can also cause degenerative changes in the joint (Source: *Lancet*, May 1998, pages 1399–1401).

A study reported in *Health News* (June 1998, page 5) established that regular walking in high heels may also cause arthritic knees and hips, conditions that affect twice as many women as men. High heels prevent the ankles from functioning as they should, causing added strain to the hips and knees. For those of you who are saying "I don't have severe discomfort wearing heels; heels are just part of my life and I'm used to them," you are only fooling yourselves. Consider Chinese women at the turn of the century who had their feet bound. For some of them, the inevitable, daily pain was just part of their life, too.

As you may have guessed, it is really useless to try and treat corns and calluses until you remove the source of the problem. Once you do that, you can use good old-fashioned corn and callus pads to reduce pressure on irritated areas in your new, comfortable, well-fitting shoes. Many women try to peel or rub the thickened area with a pumice stone, but irritation and pressure will only make things look slightly better temporarily, and probably only exacerbate the problem in the long run. It is also a big no-no to try and slice away the offending areas with a razor or to use scissors or clippers to cut them off. That's a sure way to cause injury or infection. A better fix is to exfoliate with a high-concentration beta hydroxy acid product designed for warts. First soak your feet in warm water and then apply a 5% or 10% salicylic acid cream (which may need to be specially compounded by your pharmacist). In general, if you see any signs of infection developing around a corn or callus, such as redness, swelling, pain, heat, or tenderness, see your doctor immediately.

Bunions are another story altogether, except that wearing ill-fitting shoes can also be (and often are) the cause. The technical name for a bunion is "hallux valgus." If you have a lump or bump on the inside edge of your foot around the big toe, especially one that's red, swollen, or hurting, you probably have a bunion. Another telltale sign is the direction your big toe points. If your big toe is angling inward and the joint is jutting outward, you're probably looking at a bunion.

There's no way around this one—you've got to change your shoes or you will never get rid of the bunion. The toes of any shoes you wear should be round or square, not pointy. And think flat! Heels are just asking for trouble. If you're experiencing pain, it is best to see your doctor, but you can try icing the area or taking aspirin or ibuprofen to reduce the inflammation. Really severe bunions, however, may require surgery.

NO MORE DRY, CALLUSED HEELS

Dry, cracking heels (xeorosis) is a condition where the skin on the feet becomes thick and then starts fissuring and almost splitting open. Calluses and corns all occur for the same reasons: skin becomes thick over time and with age in reaction to pressure. A callus generally refers to a larger area of thickened skin (more common on the heels but can occur under the ball of the foot and toes), whereas a corn is a thicker, more focal area (more common on the toes). A corn can occur under and be surrounded by a callus.

For most people this is nothing more than an unattractive and uncomfortable cosmetic problem. But if this has been a long-term problem, and you really have tried everything, then other health problems need to be considered first before you jump into other skin-care options. For example, dry, cracking heels or wounds on the feet that don't heal can often be signals of vascular problems or the presence of diabetes. It is essential to rule out any of those possibilities before following my suggestions.

Personally, I am obsessive about my heels. I dislike the look of crusted-over, cracked, dry heels. Unfortunately, just getting regular pedicures is not enough to keep these at bay. It takes daily care, just as it does for the face. I can guarantee that if you follow these steps exactly and on a regular basis (as long as there are no other underlying health problems) your heels will be beautiful all year long. Here is what you can do:

1. In the bath or shower keep a pedifile or foot-file and a callus preparation used by manicurists called Callus Eliminator. Both of these can be found at any beauty supply store.

376 THE ORIGINAL BEAUTY BIBLE

2. Three to four times a week apply some of the Callus Eliminator to the pedifile and gentle scrub over your calluses.

3. Three times a week, after you get out of the shower before you put on your socks or nylons or before you get into bed apply a cream or lotion containing 2% salicylic acid (BHA—beta hydroxy acid).

4. On the days or nights when you don't apply a BHA product apply an emollient, thick moisturizer such as pure shea butter or cocoa butter that you can buy at most drugstores or health food stores.

5. Avoid any foot products that contain irritants such as peppermint or lemon, or abrasive scrubs that would only hurt the skin.

You'll need to follow this treatment regimen for several nights in order to attain notable improvement. Once the skin improves, ongoing use of a non-irritating moisturizer in this area is recommended, as well as occasional use of a BHA exfoliant. You will love how your feet feel and look!

ATHLETE'S FOOT

The fungus among us, or at least among our feet, are nasty critters that cause the problem called athlete's foot (technically known as *Tinea pedis*). The damp, dark area between toes is just heaven for these fungi, which are what cause those spots to tear, ooze, itch, burn, and just feel downright uncomfortable. The most common way to catch athlete's foot is by walking barefoot in public showers and locker rooms. Even if you're good about wearing sandals or flip-flops in gyms and spas, if someone in your family isn't, it is almost a slam-dunk certainty that they will pass athlete's foot on to other family members when they come home and walk around barefoot in the bathroom.

Nevertheless, there is a cure—it just takes persistence and reapplication (and reapplication and reapplication) of an antifungal medication even several weeks after the cracks and tears between the toes disappear. Over-the-counter products containing tolnaftate, such as Aftate or Tinactin, or products containing miconazole nitrate, such as Micatin, are sure-fire successes when used as directed and applied frequently. The other issue is moisture. Athlete's foot fungi can't survive without that, so you must find creative ways to keep your feet as dry as the desert. You can try Zeasorb-AF (found at most drugstores), an absorbent foot powder that can keep your feet bone dry. It also helps to wear cotton socks (nylons are out) to be sure moisture doesn't get trapped and enhance the environment the fungi crave. Whenever possible, removes shoes and socks and go barefoot so feet are exposed to air, which keeps excess moisture away. Whichever route you take, eliminating a case of athlete's foot requires persistence and patience.

For more information about feet or to find a podiatrist in your area, contact the American Podiatric Medical Association at (800) FOOTCARE (366-8227) or visit their Web site at www.apma.org.

CHAPTER 28
PROBLEMS? SOLUTIONS!

WHEN SHOULD I THROW OUT A PRODUCT?

Problem: I've heard a lot of different information regarding when I should throw away a cosmetic. Is there a time limit when products should be thrown away?

Solution: There isn't an easy answer to this question because there are no regulations or agreed-upon guidelines on the expiration times for skin-care or makeup products, and the FDA has no rules on the issue whatsoever. Cosmetics companies generally test their products for stability, but some do one-year assays while others do three-year assays. Clouding the stability testing issue even more is that the cosmetics companies typically look only at temperature variables (freezing or overheating, for instance). The testing doesn't take into account how consumers use the products. Cosmetics that have been improperly stored—for example, exposed to sunlight, left open, or become contaminated (any product packaged in a jar has almost a 100% risk of being contaminated)—may deteriorate substantially before a year is up. On the other hand, products stored under ideal conditions may be acceptable long after the suggested "use by" dates. An additional stability issue, which is not related to stability testing, is that there is no way to tell how long a product has been sitting on a shelf before you buy it.

So what should you do? In general, it's best to toss out cosmetics that you place near the eye (mascara, for example) after four to six months, and to dispose of face products (moisturizers, foundations) after one to two years. The toss time for eye-area cosmetics is more limited than for other products because of repeated microbial exposure during use by the consumer, which poses the risk of eye infections. Some industry experts even recommend replacing mascara after only three months from the date of purchase. Another thing: If mascara becomes dry, discard it. Don't add water or, even worse, saliva to moisten it, because that will introduce bacteria into the product. And if you have an eye infection, consult a physician immediately, stop using all eye-area cosmetics, and discard those you were using when the infection occurred.

Among other cosmetics that are likely to have an unusually short shelf-life are certain "all-natural" products that contain plant-derived substances conducive to microbial growth. It's also important, for both consumers and manufacturers, to consider the increased risk of contamination in some "natural" products that contain nontraditional preservatives or no preservatives at all.

Sharing makeup also increases the risk of contamination, and the testers commonly found at department-store cosmetics counters are even more likely to become contaminated than the same products in your home. If you must test a cosmetic before purchasing it, apply it with a new, unused applicator, such as a fresh cotton swab. But remember, these are merely suggestions; they are not based on any established research or guidelines (Source: FDA *Office of Cosmetics Facts Sheet*, March 9, 2000, "Shelf Life-Expiration Date").

DARK CIRCLES

Problem: I have dark circles that seem to get worse as the day goes by! What can I do to make my concealer last?

Solution: Dark circles can be caused by several factors, and each needs to be dealt with in a different way. Dark circles can be caused by sun damage, veins and capillaries that show through skin, irritation, the natural dark pigment that can occur in this area, and by dry skin that just makes the area look dull and tired. Dark circles can also be the result of natural shadows that fall within the eye area due to the fact that the eye is set back and the brow bone can cast a shadow, making that area appear darker.

Be sure you are using a lightweight moisturizer (gel or silicone-based moisturizers are best) under the eye area; too much moisturizer or too heavy a moisturizer can make your concealer slide off. And always use a sunscreen over this area during the day, or wear sunglasses, to prevent the sun from stimulating melanin (dark pigmentation) production.

Matte-style (rather than creamy or greasy) concealers are best to cover natural shadows or natural dark pigmentation, and concealers such as Clinique All About Eyes Concealer, Elizabeth Arden Flawless Finish Concealer, or Maybelline New York Instant Age Rewind Double Face Perfector work particularly well. The color of the concealer must be light enough to cover the dark circles, but not so light that it gives the appearance of a white mask around the eyes. Avoid using greasy pencils along the lower lashes, and stay away from mascara that smears; these can both slide during the day, making the under-eye area even darker. Use only a powder to line the lower lashes, and then the thinnest line possible, or wear no lower liner at all. City pollution can get to your eyes by day's end, too, so you may want to consider using an air filter in your home or office (talk to the building or office managers to see if they are willing to accommodate this request).

If you have allergies that get worse as the day goes on, you may want to consider taking an antihistamine. Although uncommon, food allergies may also be to blame, but this would need to be confirmed by an allergist.

If all else fails, you may want to consider laser treatments for lightening (and in some cases eliminating) dark circles. Traditional skin-lightening products used for sun or hormone-induced skin discoloration do not have any effect on dark circles. For more information on lasers, refer to Chapter Twenty Six, *Medical Cosmetic Corrective Procedures*.

LASHES FALLING OUT

Problem: My lashes are falling out! Is there anything I can do to stop this from happening?

Solution: It is natural for lashes to shed and then regrow, but if you are noticing bald spots along your lash line, you may need to change some habits that might be making the condition worse. For example, don't wipe off eye makeup (or any makeup, for that matter) because wiping and pulling at the eyes can pull out lashes. Don't rub your eyes, even if they itch, especially when you are wearing mascara. Also, do not overuse mascara. I know it's tempting to have long, dramatically thick lashes, but the weight of the mascara (and what it takes to remove it later) can be too much for delicate lashes. Waterproof mascaras are the most difficult to remove and often take many lashes with them, so you might want to consider changing mascaras. It is unlikely that you are allergic to your mascara, but on the remote possibility that it may be the cause of the fallout, switch brands and see how that works.

By the way, you aren't using an eyelash curler are you? Over time, that consistent tugging can certainly pull out lashes. Another possibility is that noncosmetic allergies could be playing a part in your eyelash dilemma. Your only recourse, if that turns out to be the cause, is to use antihistamines, or to eliminate from your environment the allergens causing the problem. For example, if you are allergic to the down in your pillows, use pillows with a synthetic fill. Hay fever can also cause the eye area to swell severely, damaging eyelashes, a problem that could be alleviated by using over-the-counter or prescription antihistamines.

Medically speaking, doctors refer to the loss of eyelashes as *madarosis*. According to ophthalmologist Dr. William Trattler, "While it may seem like mainly a cosmetic problem, the condition can be an indicator of something more serious, such as eye trauma, eyelid infections and even cancer of the eyelid. In addition, metabolic conditions such as hypothyroidism and pituitary insufficiency can cause madarosis." (Source: http://ivillagehealth.com)

It is also possible that the eyelash loss can be attributed to the presence of a mite called *Demodex folliculorum*. When it is active in small hair follicles and eyelash hair follicles it can consume epithelial cells, causing the hair follicle to become swollen, inflamed, and plugged. All of this can cause the eyelashes to fall out. Fortunately, this problem is easily treated once correctly diagnosed, so consider seeing your dermatologist for an evaluation. (Source: *eMedicine Journal*, May 11, 2001, volume 2, number 5.)

If your loss of eyelash hair is chronic, you should see an eyelid specialist (called an oculoplastic surgeon) and have him carefully examine your eyelid to determine the cause of the madarosis.

Latisse, a prescription product from Allergan, has been proven to make eyelashes grow longer, thicker, and darker. It does this by means of a drug known as bimatoprost, which was originally used for glaucoma. Use of this drug by glaucoma patients made it clear that one if its unexpected side effects was longer, thicker eyelashes Topical application of a low dose of this drug (Latisse is applied once daily like a liquid eyeliner) has demonstrated impressive efficacy and safety, and was granted FDA approval in early 2009. Latisse isn't cheap (as this book goes to print, a 30-day supply costs $120) but you should see impressive results after 8 to 12 weeks of using it. Ongoing use is required to maintain results. Of course, don't ask your doctor for Latisse until you have been examined and other potential causes of eyelash loss have been ruled out or treated.

SELF-TANNER MISHAPS

Problem: I tried an expensive new self-tanner from the spa line Decleor. It just smelled so much better than the one I was using from Coppertone, and the packaging was so much prettier. Now my palms are striped, one leg is darker than the other, and my knees and elbows look mottled!

Solution: Believe it or not, the expensive self-tanner is not at fault for your chameleon-like dilemma; rather, it is most likely due to uneven application. First, almost all self-tanners, regardless of price, use the same ingredient, dihydroxyacetone, to create the color change in your skin. The scent that attracted you to the Decleor product (some women tell me the Clarins, Origins, and Lancome self-tanners smell great, too) helps mask the naturally sweet smell of this ingredient. However, the fragrance is temporary and fades in a brief period of time. The color, on the other hand, affects the skin cells, and it takes time to get your skin back to its normal color because the cell itself changes color. Sloughing can remove altered skin cells, but at this point you can't quickly slough off all the layers of skin that have been affected. That takes time. Well-formulated AHA or BHA products can make mistakes fade faster and sometimes even remove them entirely. For less prominent problems, you can try baking soda mixed with Cetaphil Cleanser, sea-salt scrubs, or even a washcloth massaged over the problem areas twice a day. Still, in most cases when complete fading of botched areas is hoped for, time is the only real cure.

Once your skin is back to normal, you can try again. Remember that when it comes to self-tanners, application is everything! Be patient. Apply the self-tanner only over a clean, dry, exfoliated body, giving special attention to the knees, elbows, and heels. Do not apply self-tanner in a steamy, hot room where perspiration or condensation may make it run. Do one area of your body at a time. Watch what you are doing, and apply the self-tanner thoroughly and evenly. If you miss an area, you are going to look noticeably streaked or blotchy. Wash the palms of your hands as soon as you are done applying the self-tanner (or wear gloves during application and use a makeup sponge to apply self-tanner to the top of your hands), and then stand still until it is completely absorbed, with no after-feel. Some women think that using a fast-darkening self-tanner is best because it changes the skin's color immediately and you can more easily see your mistakes and correct them. Others prefer a self-tanner that changes color slowly, so you can build a tan slowly and evenly. The choice is yours.

Small Lips

Problem: I have small lips. Any lipstick color I put on seems to make this more noticeable. What should I do?

Solution: The best way to deal with small lips is to not overline them to make them look larger. That technique of creating a new lip line works great in photographs, but in real life it looks like you missed your mouth. Also, to maintain the look, you have to diligently touch up your lipstick and use your pencil the moment any of the color wears off. What works best is lining just to the outside or edge of your true lip-line with a lip liner that matches your natural lip color as closely as possible. Do not wear dark lipstick, because dark colors applied to any surface make it look smaller. A true red or any vivid color will make your lips look bigger. Of course you can always consider a cosmetic corrective procedure such as collagen injections or other dermal fillers that enlarge lips, either temporarily (about 3 months to a year) or semipermanently (18 months to 3 years), or permanently (5 years or longer).

FLAKING EYESHADOW

Problem: Whenever I apply eyeshadow, I always find eyeshadow sprinkles on my cheeks and under-eye area. What am I doing wrong?

Solution: Sprinkles are almost inevitable, but knocking the excess powder off the brush before you apply your eye makeup will help a lot. Some eyeshadows are more powdery than others and cause more sprinkles. Eyeshadows made by M.A.C., Physicians Formula, Shu Uemura, Bobbi Brown, Jane, Estee Lauder, and Dior are more reliable in this respect. Another technique that some makeup artists use is to apply foundation and concealer to the eye area first; then the eyeshadow, liner, and mascara; after that, apply foundation to the rest of the face, touching up the concealer if "drippies" have made a mess of things. Although I find that approach time-consuming, it does help eliminate any trace of stray eyeshadow. Another trick is to apply a bit of loose powder under the eye area. Any excess eyeshadow should fall on this area, and you can brush the mix off when you're done, leaving a smooth, sheer, powdered finish.

BLEEDING LIPSTICK

Problem: I like a sheer lipstick look, but every one I've tried (and I've tried them all) just feathers into the lines around my mouth and looks like a mess! I've tried several of the lip paints, but they look so hard and dry unless you keep applying the glossy top coat, and pencils are useless. I'm too young to have this problem. Is there something out there I've missed?

Solution: No, you haven't missed anything! Sheer lipsticks—which are just glosses in a stick form, and this goes for both the expensive and inexpensive ones—are slippery by nature and don't stay put. Pencils are helpful, but they can't block a creamy, glossy lipstick all day. If you have any lines around your mouth, and that's not necessarily related to age, sheer, creamy lipsticks and lip glosses in general will follow those pathways. Your only option is to give up the notion of a completely sheer look. Try a semi-matte lipstick such as Clinique Long Last Soft Matte Lipstick, Laura Geller Creme Couture Soft Touch Matte Lipstick, or for a more creamy feel with staying power, Max Factor Vivid Impact Lipcolor.

Once you apply it, blot with a tissue until it looks more or less sheer. I know it won't have the sheen you're looking for, but it also won't travel into the lines around your mouth. Don't try to put a gloss over it; that will only encourage the lipstick to bleed. Matte lipstick isn't a shield that's impervious to the effect of the gloss. Gloss creates movement no matter what it goes over.

BLOODSHOT EYES

Problem: I have red, bloodshot eyes that just look awful. It seems to have nothing to do with sleep and I don't drink alcohol, so what am I doing wrong, or, better yet, what should I be doing right?

Solution: Many things can cause the blood vessels in the eye to swell and look more obvious. Lack of sleep and alcohol consumption are only two possibilities; there are lots more. For example, contact lenses, exposure to smoke, rubbing the eyes, allergies, dry air (from heat or air-conditioning), makeup particles getting in the eye and causing irritation, bad pollution days, staring at a project or computer monitor all day without giving your eyes a break, and overusing redness-relieving eyedrops can all make the tiny blood vessels in the eye look like roadmaps.

A humidifier in your home or office can help, and so can remembering to blink regularly during the day, especially when working at the computer. Not wearing contact lenses all day, using antihistamines for allergies, keeping your hands away from your eyes, and zealously keeping makeup out of your eyes are all exceptionally helpful. To reduce dryness, the "natural" tear products and eyewashes found at the drugstore are a great option (but use only disposable eyecups; repeatedly using the same eyecup can cause or aggravate problems such as eye infections or irritation). Avoid "gets the red out" eyedrops such as Visine, which if used repeatedly can actually aggravate the problem by causing a rebound effect, making the blood vessels swell even more (Sources: Visine product warning label; *Ophthalmology*, November 1991, pages 1364–1367). You would want to use Visine-type products only occasionally, not as a regular routine.

PUFFY EYES

Problem: I have puffy eyes every morning that sometimes don't go away until midday. They look awful and I've tried lots of eye products that don't change a thing.

Solution: There are no cosmetics or miracle eye moisturizers that can alter puffy eyes, but lots of things, including water retention, can cause the skin around the eye area to swell. Lack of sleep is probably not as big a factor for puffy eyes as it is for bloodshot eyes. If anything, sitting up instead of lying down would prevent fluids from collecting in the tissues around the eye. Of course, no one should sit up day and night! Sleeping with your head slightly elevated, and making sure you give your neck the support it needs, can help prevent fluid retention. Alcohol consumption and a diet high in salt also can cause water retention and increase the puffiness around the eyes.

Another factor to consider is contact lenses, which can cause irritation and swelling of the eye, so be sure you are wearing the most comfortable type available for your vision correction. As with bloodshot eyes, exposure to smoke, rubbing the eyes, allergies, dry air (from heat or air-conditioning), makeup particles getting in the eyes, allergic reactions to skin-care or makeup products, bad pollution days, leaving makeup on overnight (which can cause inflammation), and using irritating skin-care products around the eyes can all make the eye area swollen.

Be sure to take your makeup off meticulously at night, don't rub your eyes during the day, and take an antihistamine if you have allergies. If you are allergic or sensitive to certain skin-care or makeup products, avoid them.

Preventing dryness around the eyes can also help reduce irritation and swelling that can cause a puffy appearance. If that's your problem, a lightweight, fragrance-free moisturizer will help a lot. Be certain the moisturizer does not contain any irritating ingredients that could make matters worse, such as witch hazel, volatile plant oils, and sensitizing plant extracts like lemon oil or forms of mint (including menthol). If you have time in the morning, place cool compresses on the eyes (low temperatures can make the skin contract); if you don't have time for that, leave your moisturizer in the refrigerator so it's cool when you apply it in the morning.

If none of these things help alleviate the problem, it may be that your eye area is just naturally puffy. Most typically this results from overly large fat pads around the eye (everyone has fat pads around the eye) creating a puffy-looking bulge. If that's the case, the only way to get rid of the problem is with cosmetic surgery, which in most cases is incredibly effective at eliminating the puffiness.

CHAPPED LIPS

Problem: What should I do about my eternally chapped lips? No matter what I use, the chapping never goes away.

Solution: Whether they are responding to cold weather, an arid climate, or are just naturally dry, chapped lips are a pain. Cracking, flaking, and chapping are not only uncomfortable but also unsightly, and lipstick only seems to make the situation worse. You can solve those dry-lips blues with consistency and patience. Chapped lips are not going to disappear in a day, and missing even one day of treatment can drive lips back to dryness.

Lips are more vulnerable to the environment than any other part of the face. This means that keeping your lips moist and sealed against the weather is essential. There are lots of emollient lip products that do just that, and the more emollient they are, the better. Ingredients like lanolin, oils of any kind (including castor oil, lanolin oil, safflower oil, almond oil, and vegetable oil), and shea and cocoa butter are all excellent, especially if they are listed at the beginning of the ingredient list. However, many lip products are little more than waxy coatings that make lips feel thickly protected when they are applied (ChapStick is a great example), but they don't really moisturize or provide adequate protection from the weather or from the dry heat and air-conditioning you find indoors.

Lots of lip products also claim to be medicated. "Medicated," however, is at best a dubious term, and it has no regulated meaning when it comes to lip balms. These "medicated" products usually contain camphor, menthol, peppermint oil, and eucalyptus, but these are not medicines for dry lips! They mostly irritate and can actually make lips burn, which is neither disinfecting nor helpful for lips that are already dry and chapped. Products like classic Blistex, which includes 0.5% phenol, are the exception, because they truly are medicated; phenol kills anything that gets in its way. However, phenol is strong stuff and can actually trigger serious irritation and dryness all by itself. It is not something I would recommend for anything but extremely limited use.

You may have heard a rumor that lips can adapt to or become addicted to lip balm. It isn't possible. But if the lip balm you are using contains irritating ingredients (and lots of them do), your lips will stay dried up. When a lip product contains irritating, drying ingredients, there is no way the other, more emollient ingredients can help. Likewise, if you are using a lip product that is just waxy, with no emollients or water-binding agents, it can only plaster down the dry skin; it doesn't reduce the dryness.

At night you can apply almost any lip balm that contains some of the emollients I mentioned above, but no irritants. For daytime care, it is best to use an SPF 15 lip balm that contains either avobenzone, Tinosorb, ecamsule (Mexoryl SX), titanium dioxide, or zinc oxide. However, if you wear an opaque lipstick, it may not be essential to have that kind of SPF protection. Research has shown that women who apply lipstick more than once a day are at a much lower risk of getting lip cancer than women who apply lipstick only once a day (Source: *Cancer Causes and Control*, July 1996, pages 458–463). Theoretically, opaque lipsticks have enough sun-blocking protection to enable them to screen out the sun's cancer–causing rays. Still, you may as well play it safe and use a lip balm or lipstick with sunscreen daily, especially if you are outside for long periods of time in the sun or if you live in a sunny climate. Chanel, Clinique, Neutrogena, and Paula's Choice each offer very good lipsticks with broad-spectrum sunscreen.

DRY SKIN AROUND THE LIPS

Problem: For some time now I have had a strange red, dry irritation, just along the skin around my mouth. Moisturizers don't seem to help and I don't know what else to do!

Solutions: One of the first things you can do is determine whether you've developed an allergic reaction to fluoride toothpaste. Fluoride can cause irritation around the mouth. Try a fluoride-free toothpaste for a while and see what happens. If that seems to be the solution, check with your dentist to see how this will affect your dental health.

The dryness and irritation around your mouth could also be caused by a significant other who happens to have a rough beard. There isn't much you can do about that, but occasionally using a little cortisone cream around the area can help minimize the irritation from almost any source. Another possibility is frequent, unconscious licking of the lips. Saliva can be an irritant for the lips, causing flaking and dryness. Lip balm won't be able to keep up with this bad habit.

If the area around the mouth is dry and irritated, that can also affect the lips. What's important here is to treat the root of the problem, which in this situation may require using an emollient moisturizer around the edge of the mouth as well as a lip exfoliant and lip balm for the lip area.

PERIORAL DERMATITIS—RED BUMPS AROUND THE MOUTH

Problem: I can't seem to get rid of these red, swollen, sometimes crusty bumps around my lips and at the sides of my nose. Nothing seems to help, including over-the-counter acne products and cortisone creams. What can I do?

Solutions: What you describe sounds like an almost classic case of perioral dermatitis. According to the American Academy of Dermatology (www.aad.org) "Perioral dermatitis [POD] is a common skin problem that mostly affects young women [20 to 45 years of age]. Occasionally men or children are affected. Perioral refers to the area around the mouth, and dermatitis indicates redness of the skin. In addition to redness, there are usually small red bumps or even pus-filled bumps and mild peeling. Sometimes the bumps are the most obvious feature, and the disease can look a lot like acne. The areas most affected are within the borders of the lines from the nose to the sides of the lips, and the chin…. Sometimes there is mild itching and/or burning."

POD is actually quite common and, according to most dermatologists, is increasing in incidence (Source: *Australasian Journal of Dermatology*, February 2000, pages 34–38). While little is known about what causes this disorder, there are theories that overuse or chronic use of topical cortisone creams, fluoridated toothpaste, or heavy or occlusive skin-care ointments and creams may be responsible. Exposure to sunlight, heat, and wind can also make matters worse (Source: http://emedicine.medscape.com/article/1071128-overview).

You can experiment by stopping the use of any of the potentially problematic products mentioned above. It would be a great idea to stop using topical cortisone creams, but be advised that this step can initially make matters worse before any improvement takes place. That can feel self-defeating, but be patient, at least for a few weeks, to see if the condition finally improves.

It would also be helpful to find out if fluoridated toothpaste is the source of the problem. You can try brushing with fluoride-free toothpaste such as Tom's of Maine Natural Fluoride-Free Toothpaste or Squiggle Enamel Saver Toothpaste and see if that makes a significant difference. If fluoride-free toothpaste turns out to be the solution, check with your dentist to see how this will affect your dental health.

If these experiments lead you to suspect POD is indeed the cause of the bumps around your mouth and nose, it is best to see a dermatologist because there are no cosmetics or over-the-counter medications that can treat the condition. A dermatologist can prescribe topical metronidazole (MetroGel, MetroLotion, or MetroCream), alone or in combination with either oral tetracycline or erythromycin. Even though topical cortisone creams may be the cause of POD, you may be prescribed a low-potency cortisone cream to reduce the inflammation and to help you wean off the stronger topical cortisone cream you may have been using (Sources: *Seminars in Cutaneous Medical Surgery*, September 1999, pages 206–209). For more information on POD, visit www.aad.org/public/publications/pamphlets/common_perioral.html.

EXPENSIVE VERSUS INEXPENSIVE

Problem: I'm not one to fall for a company's enthusiasm for its products, but surely some companies can have secret or special ingredients and formulas, or use more expensive, superior ingredients. A friend mentioned that her chocolate chip cookies contain flour, sugar, shortening, eggs, vanilla, chocolate chips, and nuts, but they still don't taste like Mrs. Fields'. I have used your inexpensive recommendations and they have worked great, but I am so tempted to buy the more expensive stuff!

Solution: I understand the concept your friend is suggesting when it comes to her cookies. However, some people may prefer Mrs. Fields cookies while others would prefer your friend's. If this company does have a secret ingredient, that may taste great to you but not to someone else. With a cosmetic the situation is a little different, because here you are asking, Is it really any better for skin? And, What is the product's impact on the skin; as well as What is its overall benefit (or detriment) to your body?

When it comes to shopping for skin-care products, there are unquestionably great formulas out there that work better for different skin types and different needs, in all price ranges, but most of that is about the texture of the product, not the beneficial ingredients. Think of it like your diet. Dark green leafy vegetables, deeply colored fruits, fish rich in omega 3 and omega 6 fatty acids, flax seed and olive oil, and herbal seasonings such as curry, turmeric, and curcumin all offer the body numerous health benefits. How you eat them, whether in a salad, barbecued, grilled, sautéed, raw, or mixed in some kind of ethnic culinary delight is up to you, because the preparation (as long as it's healthy) doesn't significantly change the benefit (some types of high-heat cooking can destroy nutrients). What counts are the ingredients; not the cuisine.

The same is true for skin care. Whether you prefer a gel, cream, lotion, liquid, serum, or balm, those qualities are separate from the value of the bioactive ingredients the product should contain. The healthy ingredients for skin should all be in there, and the texture is simply the way you prefer to feel them delivered to your skin.

It is a complete fallacy that expensive products are better than inexpensive products, not to mention there isn't a shred of research supporting this concept. Our own empirical evidence also tells us this is true because we've all bought expensive products we didn't like.

After interviewing dozens of cosmetics chemists and cosmetic ingredient manufacturers, I have yet to find any that agree with the notion that secret ingredients provide superior benefits for the skin. There also aren't any secret ingredients, because all ingredients have to be listed on the label or the company will be in violation of almost every cosmetics regulatory board in the world.

There are ingredients that can make a difference, but almost without exception they are accessible to every cosmetics manufacturer. I rate hundreds of expensive and inexpensive products on a range of excellent to poor, so I've come to know that judging by price alone can hurt your skin and waste your money.

USING DIFFERENT PRODUCTS FROM DIFFERENT LINES

Problem: I've been following your advice and am using products from several different lines. My skin is doing great, but all the cosmetics salespeople say it is a mistake to mix brands. They say products are designed to work together, and that is what helps the skin best.

Solution: Stop listening to the cosmetics salespeople; they are wrong. If every line had SPF 15 sunscreens with the requisite UVA protection, gentle cleansers with nonirritating ingredients, foundations that aren't peach-colored, and on and on, I would agree that you don't need to mix and can be brand-loyal. But I have found good and bad products in every line (and I've reviewed hundreds of cosmetics lines and thousands of products). Many lines don't have adequate sunscreens, have products that contain irritating ingredients, or offer rose, peach, and ashen foundation colors, though they may have superior mascara and blushes. Staying with the same line for all your skin-care or makeup needs almost always ensures that you end up with some bad products! Mixing and matching is the only way to go. You don't wear clothes from one designer, buy furniture from one manufacturer, take medicine from one pharmaceutical company, or eat food from just one company. The only way to develop a successful skin-care or makeup routine is to select what works best for your skin type and needs, not what one line happens to be selling (or telling you).

FEELING BEAUTIFUL DURING THE TRAUMA OF CANCER

Problem: I have a dear friend who has just been diagnosed with breast cancer. I want to be a supportive and I know how important feeling beautiful is for her. Any suggestions from you would be truly appreciated.

Solution: I've spoken with many women who have lived through the ordeal of radiation and chemotherapy, and they all agreed that paying attention to how they looked helped their emotional well-being a lot during the trauma of diagnosis and treatment. Having gone through this life-threatening event with my older sister, I had a reason to look further into these issues, and now I have the opportunity to share some solutions and possibilities with you and your friend. Given the number of women who have breast cancer or other cancers, surely most of us know someone who can benefit from this information. One thing my sister found immensely helpful was talking openly about her cancer experience without embarrassment or reservation. Perhaps your friend or someone else in your life would appreciate that kind of support and openness.

Body care: Because chemotherapy and radiation make the skin ultra-sensitive and even sunburned, as a general rule it is best not to use any types of adhesives, tints, bleaches, waxes, harsh or irritating chemicals, or to take hot baths or showers. Even deodorants and shaving can be problems. Saunas, Jacuzzis, loofahs, strong soaps, and washcloths can also exacerbate irritation. Anything you can do to reduce the hypersensitivity will go a long way to making the skin feel soothed and less irritated.

Instead of bar soap, which can be extremely drying and harsh on sensitive skin, try a gentle liquid body cleanser (it's almost hard to find anything other than a gentle body cleanser). The least-expensive ones are formulated the same as the most-expensive ones.

Keep the skin moist with lightweight gels that don't trap heat, such as pure aloe vera (found at most health food stores). If the skin becomes dry, use a nonfragranced, nonirritating moisturizer (the fewer plants it contains, the better) such as those from CeraVe, Cetaphil, or Eucerin. Take tepid or slightly warm showers and baths, and try to enjoy cool baths whenever possible, adding a little bit of light oil, such as safflower or sunflower oil, to the water. Avoid heavy oils such as vitamin E. Despite the fact that vitamin E has a reputation for healing the skin and can help the skin after the radiation and chemotherapy are over (as can other antioxidants), in the midst of treatment keep in mind that vitamin E is a potential allergen, and that its occlusive attributes can trap heat in the skin when it needs to dissipate heat instead.

Many women worry that even washing the skin may increase irritation. It turns out that gentle washing is better for skin than just leaving it alone. According to an article in

Radiotherapy & Oncology (March 2001, pages 333–339), "Washing the irradiated skin during the course of radiotherapy for breast cancer is not associated with increased skin toxicity [or irritation] and should not be discouraged."

To keep her skin feeling soft and light, one of the first things my sister and I did before she went in for her radiation was to buy silk underwear, including T-shirts, underpants, teddies, and pajamas. She had to give up wearing a bra because the irritation from the straps and the tightness around the breast was just too uncomfortable. The silk was not only soothing, it also helped her feel more feminine and attractive.

Hair care: Some women feel compelled to shave their head in anticipation of losing their hair. That can be the worst possible solution for dealing with the inevitable. Shaving your head may look exotic, but unless you plan to shave every day, it can itch like crazy when it starts to grow back between treatments. It's best to cut your hair very short and consider wearing designer baseball caps or wigs. Scarves always make it look like something is wrong, while baseball caps and wigs are quite normal nowadays.

By the way, the American Cancer Society can provide you with a free wig; call (800) 227-2345. The wigs have been donated and are clean, but use them as a springboard for finding one that is perfect for you. You can buy a wig at a specialty salon or wig shop, but the trick is to find a good one and go to someone who knows how to style it. Wigs almost always need to be cut and styled to match your face. If you live in or near a large metropolitan area, your absolute best option is to find out who styles wigs for the women in the Orthodox Jewish community. For religious reasons, many Orthodox Jewish women cover their own hair with a wig. The shatel-macher (wig maker) is a mainstay of the Orthodox community and knows better than anyone how to make a wig look natural and attractive. Just call the Orthodox synagogue in your area and ask for the number of the woman who styles wigs for the community. The larger the metropolitan area, the more choices there will be.

One woman told me that after she purchased her first quality wig (around $100 to $500), she was a changed woman. "Not only did it fit great, but it looked so real that no one could believe it was a wig. I still wear it now and then, and get the biggest kick out of telling people it's a wig."

When your hair starts growing back, you may find that it grows back in thicker and straighter or curlier than it was. As tempting as it will be to dye your hair or perm it, be patient. Wait for the hair to go through a few normal cycles of growth before using chemicals on it. The skin and hair may still be sensitive or altered by the radiation and chemotherapy, and could react in a way that can cause problems.

Skin care: All of my recommendations for gentle skin care are doubly true during radiation and chemotherapy. And it is even more imperative than usual to avoid the sun, because the skin can become photosensitive. Sunscreen is essential, and the less the body and face are exposed to the sun, the better. That means wearing hats; light, tightly woven cotton pants; and light, long-sleeved blouses whenever possible. Because the skin can become dry, it is important to follow my recommendations for dry-skin care, which include using a gentle cleanser, a skin-softening toner, an emollient moisturizer, and plant oils such as evening primrose, jojoba, olive, or sunflower oil over dry patches.

Eyebrows and eyelashes: Accompanying the loss of hair on your head is the probable loss of eyebrows and eyelashes. Avoid the natural tendency to pencil in new brows, which look fake and dated. Instead, try powder shadows to draw on a soft arch of a brow. If you have any eyebrow hair left, consider using the colored brow gels from Bobbi Brown, Origins, or Paula's Choice; these can add definition and shape to the eye area. Another option is to use a water-proof mascara or a waterproof eye pencil that matches your brow color. Although waterproof mascara and waterproof eye pencils can look slightly more artificial, they are worth trying because chemotherapy or other drugs can bring on menopause or menopausal symptoms, and the accompanying hot flashes, followed by profuse sweating, will wash the others away. This one takes some experimenting, so be patient until you find what works for you.

If you do lose your eyelashes, it's best to not use any mascara, even if you have a few lashes left, because gaps in your application will be quite noticeable and mascara can shorten the life of the lashes you still have. Instead, consider lining the eyes with a dark brown shade of powder that you draw on more as shading than as a line. Lining with a pencil or liquid liner and no mascara can look odd, but shading the eye with a dark powder can look smoky and defining without making the lack of lashes more obvious.

Remember that brows and lashes grow back quickly, so that part is the most temporary!

Makeup: When it comes to concealer, foundation, blush, lipstick, and the rest, do whatever you are used to doing. Not only will it make you feel good, it will also normalize much of the process.

One woman wrote me a wonderful e-mail about this issue: "I cannot stress enough the concept that *look good and feel better* really works. I thought I was doing OK and I was, until I found out what it felt like to go out in public with hair and makeup (eyebrows) that looked real. I never lost my sense of humor or my positive outlook; but when I got a great wig and wore makeup (and eyebrows), I felt fantastic."

One of the most powerful things you can do for yourself is to pay attention to your physical appearance and experiment to find what works. Don't try to pretend that feeling and looking beautiful doesn't matter during this time or that it is a waste of your energy. It may provide some of your most pleasant and uplifting moments until you are on the other side of your treatment.

FOUNDATION SETTLING INTO PORES AND LINES

Problem: What causes foundation to settle into the pores and leave tiny little spots, or settle into laugh lines? I do not know whether my moisturizer is too heavy or not heavy enough, whether the foundation is too heavy or too light, or whether I have not waited long enough for the moisturizer to be absorbed.

Solution: Most foundations contain ingredients that allow some amount of movement. If they didn't, they wouldn't blend easily and would feel dry and matte on the skin, making wrinkles look worse. But that also means that those foundations can easily slip into pores, making the skin look mottled. Moisturizing when you don't need it creates even more slip-page. Unless you have dry skin, there is no reason to wear a moisturizer under foundation.

Most foundations for normal to dry skin have enough emollient ingredients to make an extra moisturizer unnecessary. Too much moisturizer (not too little) or too much foundation can absolutely cause slippage into lines and pores. Once you've blended on a foundation, apply a light dusting of powder to set your makeup. Also, try blending on your foundation with a sponge or a foundation brush, not with your fingers. A flat sponge can pick up excess foundation from the skin and blend it on in an even layer. Most important, if you have normal to dry skin, you may want to consider changing to a satin matte or matte finish foundation to avoid slippage. If you have oily skin then you may want to consider an ultra-matte foundation, which won't move throughout the day. I list several top foundation options on my Web site, www.Beautypedia.com.

EYELASH DYES

Problem: A friend of mine gets her eyelashes and eyebrows dyed at the hair salon. The effect is really rather impressive and I'm tempted to try this myself. Her blonde lashes look dark and long, even without mascara. What do you think?

Solution: Unfortunately, my solution isn't much of a solution, because all I can do is strongly say, "Don't!" The only safe solution for making lashes and brows more visible is to use mascara on the eyelashes, and to shade your eyebrows either with an eyeshadow that matches your hair color, an eyebrow pencil, or a brow mascara like Bobbi Brown's Natural Brow Shaper. But first let me give you a little history on why my answer to your question is such an emphatic "no." Back in 1933, a congressional controversy was brewing over the need for new and stronger food, cosmetic, and drug laws. At the time, the FDA had no authority to move against a cosmetic product called Lash Lure that was causing allergic reactions in many women. Two women, in fact, suffered severe reactions to the product; one woman became blind and the other woman died. When the new Food, Drug, and Cosmetic Act was passed in 1938, Lash Lure was the first product seized under its authority. A lot of time has passed since then, but although hair dyes (and that includes lash dyes) have changed a great deal, they are still formulated with peroxide and ammonia or ammonia-like ingredients. If a hair dye doesn't contain those ingredients, it can't affect hair color.

No one should ever dye her eyelashes or eyebrows. An allergic reaction to the dye formulation could prompt swelling, inflammation, and susceptibility to infection in the eye area. These reactions can severely harm the eye and even cause blindness. The FDA absolutely prohibits the use of hair dyes for eyebrow and eyelash tinting or dyeing, even in beauty salons and other licensed, seemingly professional establishments. The FDA has also continually warned the public about the use of coal-tar dyes on the eyebrows and eyelashes, stating that such use could cause permanent injury to the eyes, including blindness. (Using eyelash and eyebrow dyes or hair dyes for the eyes or brows should not be confused with using mascaras, eyeshadows, eyebrow pencils, and eyeliners, which contain ingredients that have been approved by the FDA for use in the eye area.)

Be aware that there are no natural or synthetic color additives (or coloring agents) approved by the FDA for dyeing or tinting eyelashes and eyebrows—either in beauty salons or for use at home. In fact, the law requires all hair-dye products to include instructions for performing patch tests before use, to identify possible allergic reactions, and to carry warnings about the dangers of applying these products to eyebrows and eyelashes. The health hazards of permanent eyelash and eyebrow dyes have been known for more than 70 years. These dyes have repeatedly been cited in scientific literature as capable of causing serious reactions when placed in direct contact with the eye.

Seasonal Changes

Problem: During the winter I use an emollient moisturizer you recommend and it works great, but during the summer it seems a bit much. Should I change what I do with the seasons?

Solution: Summer weather can absolutely require a change in skin-care products, particularly moisturizers. Instead of the richer or more emollient moisturizers you were wearing during winter to combat the dry heat indoors and the dry cold outdoors, consider using lighter moisturizers that come in gel or gel/lotion consistencies. Keep in mind that the major concept here is to cut back on the amount of moisturizer you use. Moisturizer is for dry skin, so if you don't have dry skin, you really don't need moisturizer (but there are other ways to give skin essential ingredients, such as serums).

Please ignore the fact that many moisturizing products are labeled "oil-free." This is a meaningless term. What makes these products good for those with minimally dry skin is that they contain fewer thickening agents and emollients. Also ignore words and phrases such as "oil-control," "lift," and "firming." None of these products can control oil, lift the skin anywhere, or firm it in a noticeable way.

Whiter Teeth

Problem: I would so love to have a perfect white smile. I hate the color of my teeth. I want them to look like the way models' and celebrities' teeth look. What should I do?

Solution: There are many reasons why someone may have yellow or stained teeth. Mostly it's genetic: Some people just have teeth with a yellowish or off-white appearance. But if silver fillings have grayed the surrounding tooth enamel, changing those for the new, tooth-colored material dentists are using can make a world of difference. Foods like coffee, tea, red wine, and berries can also cause stains. You can cut back on the foods causing the problem, but who wants to give up their coffee in the morning, much less fresh berries and red wine (like a beautiful pinot noir or cabernet sauvignon at the end of the day)! Smoking is perhaps the worst offender because not only does it discolor the teeth, it also kills healthy gum tissue, causing serious health risks for your mouth. Serious staining and discoloration, natural or otherwise, cannot be corrected with toothpaste no matter what the claim on the label says. But the teeth whitening, lightening, and bleaching products, from your dentist or at the drugstore, in the form of strips, liquids, or gels can work miracles.

The whole subject of improving the color of your teeth gets complicated because the terminology has been regulated, but the regulation is too confusing to be of help to consumers.

According to the FDA, the term "bleaching" is permitted for use on products that can "whiten" or "lighten" teeth over and above their natural color. Plus bleaching products must contain "bleach" (not the kind for your laundry), but the kind that "bleaches" teeth, making the color lighter, with the typical ingredients being hydrogen peroxide or carbamide peroxide.

Now here is where it gets really confusing, because the term "whitening," can only be used on products that clean teeth, meaning toothpaste. So any product that cleans the surface of a tooth can be labeled a whitener. However, because the term whitener sounds so much better than bleaching (which we think of in terms of Clorox and the washing machine, not our teeth), "bleaching" products call themselves whiteners or whitening to sound more appealing to the consumer. Yet the term whitening is only about cleaning your teeth, not changing the color.

One more bit of confusion to clear up. As mentioned, the two ingredients used in bleaching products are almost always either carbamide peroxide or hydrogen peroxide. Hydrogen peroxide is the stronger of the two. In order for carbamide peroxide to be effective it has to break down into hydrogen peroxide. That means a 10% solution of carbamide peroxide (CP) is about one-third the strength of the same percentage of hydrogen peroxide (HP). As a general rule, keep these numbers in mind: 3% HP equals 10% CP; 6% HP equals 20% CP; and 9% HP equals 30% CP.

Before you jump in to make any choice for teeth whitening, be aware there is a risk of mild to painful gum sensitivity. Mild to moderate isn't bad, but when it's painful, believe me, it isn't pleasant. However, one way to resolve that problem is to brush your teeth with a toothpaste containing potassium nitrate. Research shows that this desensitizing, teeth-friendly ingredient can make a huge difference in reducing some of the side effects.

Dentists would like you to believe that they are the only solution for teeth whitening but that isn't the case. Most teeth whiteners ("bleaches") work incredibly well, so you can either choose by cost or just start with whatever is most readily available, which would be at the drugstore. All teeth whiteners use the same type of ingredients, either carbamide peroxide or hydrogen peroxide, but with different strengths to lighten teeth. The higher the percentage of the active ingredient, and the type of ingredient, determines how fast you see improvement, which is usually within 1 to 14 days depending on the product you buy and how diligently you follow the application instructions.

If you choose the in-office dentist procedure it would cost on average about $500 per visit. Dentists can also give you take-home kits that you can only buy from them (though there are Web sites that sell the exact same product to consumers as well, such as www.aplussmile.com). The cost for the dentist-sold kits ranges from $100 to $300 (expect to pay about half that from most Web sites selling the same products). At the drugstore the "bleaching" kits cost between $20 and $100, and they often go on sale.

Teeth-whitening kits at the drugstore or from various Web sites come in many different forms, from strips, to paint-on types, to gels that are used with a mouth guard. Choosing which one is all about your own personal preference because they all pretty much work as claimed when they contain the same active ingredients; just follow the ratio of effectiveness I explained above.

No matter what the claim on the label may say, there are pros and cons to each type of application. Strips can slip off the teeth, creating uneven results. Some people don't like dental trays. Paint-on products require more time to evenly cover each tooth surface. Strips are also limited because they can only cover the front teeth, which means only those teeth will be affected, leaving the others as they were.

Another problem is that bleaching kits of any kind cannot change the color of dental crowns, bonding material, porcelain veneers, fillings, or any other material in your mouth other than your teeth. You can imagine how strange an appearance you can end up with if each of your teeth were a significantly different color from the other. None of these treatments is very effective if your teeth are grayed rather than yellowed, or if they are completely yellowed. Teeth-bleaching systems work best for partially yellow or food-stained teeth.

Keep in mind that bleaching products have a short shelf-life. This is because the active ingredient is a form of peroxide and it is an exceptionally unstable ingredient. It can happen that by the time you find, buy, and start using your whitening strips the peroxide may have become inactive.

Other than bleaching, if the yellow or dull color of your teeth is from tartar buildup, get your teeth cleaned, and have them cleaned regularly. If you can, avoid foods that can grab onto teeth and make them look darker, such as chocolate, dark-colored berries, red wine, and coffee. Milk can also bond onto front teeth and cause a yellow tartar buildup. Clearly, it would be best to brush immediately after eating these foods, but if that isn't possible, rinse your mouth well with water and then chew sugarless gum. Many dentists recommend using the Sonicare automatic toothbrush to prevent tartar or plaque buildup. You definitely cannot manually brush your teeth as well as the Sonicare can, so it is a worthwhile option to check out.

Word of warning: There is no FDA approved laser for use in teeth whitening. There are studies that have looked into using lasers or other light sources to activate the hydrogen peroxide or carbamide peroxide, but results so far show they have caused problems as well as successes.

(Sources: *Operative Dentistry*, July–August 2008, pages 379–385; *Journal of Dentistry*, February 2008, pages 117–124; *Dental Materials*, May 2007, pages 586–596; *Cochrane Database Systematic Reviews*, October 18, 2006, CD006202; *Journal of Contemporary Dental Practices*, February 2004; pages 1–17; *Compendium of Continuing Education in Dentistry*, June 2003, pages 461–464; *Journal of Clinical Dentistry*, 2002, volume 13, pages 91–94; and *Journal of Esthetic and Restorative Dentistry*, 2001, volume 13, number 6, pages 357–369.)

SKIN TAGS

Problem: I have developed small, brownish pieces of skin that are dotted all over my neck. This is so unattractive and seems to be getting worse. What are these things and what can I do about them?

Solution: The good news is the growths that you see are almost certainly benign and nothing more than an unattractive pouching of the skin called skin tags, but or course your skin should be examined by your dermatologist or physician to be sure.

Technically called an acrochordonor, a skin tag is a small, benign, growth of skin connected to the body by a tiny or even imperceptible branchlike protrusion of tissue. Skin tags look like tiny bits of brown or flesh-colored tissue hanging loosely off of the skin. Typically they occur in sites where clothing rubs against the skin or where there is skin-to-skin friction, such as the underarms, neck, under the breasts, chest, back, chin, and sometimes the groin and eyelids.

Skin tags almost never develop when we are young; for some reason they occur as we get older, and there may even be a genetic component, though no one knows for sure. Occasionally a skin tag can become gnarled in such a way that the blood supply to the protrusion is cut off and the tag can turn red or black.

Getting rid of skin tags is probably one of the easiest cosmetic corrective procedures a physician can perform. All a doctor has to do is cut it off. Almost without exception the skin heals without any trace or remnant of the tag, there's no scarring, and the tag won't grow back. Of course you can still grow other skin tags but the one that was removed is gone forever.

Some physicians suggest removing the tag yourself by tying off the small stem that attaches the protrusion to the skin. This can be done by simply taking a piece of thread or dental floss and tightly tying off the tag; in a few days it simply falls off. However, if the skin tags are around the eyes it is essential to have them removed by an ophthalmologist.

SEBACEOUS HYPERPLASIA

Problem: I recently went to the dermatologist and she told me the little whitish-yellowish bumps on various parts of my face are a disorder called sebaceous hyperplasia. She explained to me that the only way to permanently get rid of these bumps was to come in for laser treatments (probably three sessions) with the Smooth Beam laser. I just had my first treatment and my face looks awful to me. What can you tell me about sebaceous hyperplasia? No one seems to have an answer as to what causes it in certain people. Second, what do you know about the Smooth Beam laser treatment? Do you know what a person should expect in his/her results after a treatment?

Solution: Sebaceous hyperplasia is an extremely common, exceedingly stubborn, though completely benign condition of the oil gland. "Sebaceous" refers to the oil gland, and "hyperplasia" describes an abnormal but benign increase in cells (in this case sebaceous cells) that causes the oil gland to increase in size.

Sebaceous hyperplasia typically occurs in people 40 years of age or older and the effect looks exactly like what you described—white to yellowish soft bumps. You can have more than one, and they occur in areas where we have oil glands, mainly the nose, cheeks, and forehead. If you look close enough or with a magnifying mirror you can see a small depressed area in the center that looks like an open or clogged pore.

Oil glands in general are extremely sensitive to the status of hormone production, and although the number of oil glands you have never changes their activity and size does. As hormone levels change with age, cell production in the oil gland can become distorted and the result is these strange-looking facial blemishes. What is most frustrating is that no matter what you seem to do these types of blemishes never go away. Trying to squeeze them may release some sebum, but that rarely changes anything and usually just makes matters look worse.

Cosmetics companies have no solution for sebaceous hyperplasia. The bumps are not pimples or blackheads and therefore don't respond to benzoyl peroxide or topical exfoliants. Unless the lesion is removed and the oil gland excised or destroyed, the condition won't go away.

There are several medical treatments that can achieve this goal, including lasers, but your doctor could also have suggested far less-expensive options as well. Cryotherapy (liquid nitrogen—where the lesion is burned off), cauterization or electrodesiccation (these are other forms of burning off the lesion with heat), and topical chemical treatments (application of a deep peel such as trichloroacetic acid) all have research showing they work. Lasers, including the Smooth Beam, which is a nonablative, pulsed-dye laser, have research showing treatment can be effective, but there are risks, as there are with any medical option.

It should also be pointed out that retinoids, particularly tretinoin (as in Renova or Retin-A) can also help prevent the problem from happening in the first place, along with preventing recurrences from showing up. That would be an important maintenance consideration regardless of the treatment you decide to try.

(Sources: *Clinical Dermatology*, January–February 2006, pages 16–25; *Journal of the American Academy of Dermatology*, July 2000, pages 49–53; *Journal of Investigative Dermatology*, February 2000, pages 349–53; and *Dermatology*, January 1998, pages 21–31.)

CHAPTER 29
MAKING SENSE OF MAKEUP

MAKEUP: A PHILOSOPHICAL APPROACH

Several years ago a documentary produced by the British Broadcasting Corporation went into entertaining detail and analysis of this salient point. *The Human Face* was written and directed by comedy legend John Cleese and featured some rather candid comments from dermatologist Dr. Vail Reese on how we perceive skin flaws while watching films, and the way we make character assumptions based on things like facial asymmetry or scarring.

According to Reese, the clear-skinned, smooth-faced individual is almost always the hero, while anyone with a skin defect is relegated to the role of bad guy. In most societies skin becomes a reflection not just of health and beauty, but also of moral content and integrity, not to mention sex appeal. While we know rationally that appearance has no relevance to a person's being ethical, studies have shown that people interacting with others who have clear, flawless skin feel more comfortable and relaxed than they do with those who have facial scarring or some other skin imperfection. When skin was marred in some way, spectators were more hesitant, more wary, or even fearful of the people who did not have good skin.

In terms of cosmetic adornment, Reese commented that women who use makeup to minimize skin imperfections and enhance their eyes and lips, thus giving the impression of flawless skin, create more positive human interaction (Source: www.skinema.com).

History Professor Arthur Marwick of Open University, Milton Keynes, England, maintains that there are many types of beauty and that with modern travel and the mass media we have become increasingly flexible. There is Chinese beauty, African beauty, Latin beauty, Nordic beauty, and more, yet only a tiny minority within each type is truly beautiful. Beauty is what the overwhelming majority, on sight, recognize as beautiful. Beauty is in the eye of all beholders but most people doing the beholding have a similar notion of how beauty is defined, regardless of cultural influences.

The Human Face goes on to reveal how studies from all over the world found that certain similar qualities about women are considered most attractive. It seems that people everywhere rate smooth skin, big eyes, and plump lips as signifying beauty. Interestingly, women and men of all sexual persuasions also rate the same faces as beautiful.

Women's desire for self-appointed personal enhancement is as strong as ever, and although the reasons we use makeup have evolved, looking beautiful continues to involve using makeup, and it has for eons.

SHOULD YOU JUDGE A BOOK BY ITS COVER?

Whether or not you should or shouldn't judge a book by its cover, in truth most of us do, at least upon initial contact. When we meet a stranger, consciously or unconsciously our reaction is as much a result of societal standards as a genetic, instinctive reaction is. If someone is pretty, the initial and even subsequent interactions are going to be better.

You can believe beauty is more than skin deep and that physical beauty has little meaning compared with the importance of an individual's positive contribution to the world we live in. Yet it only takes a quick scan of Hollywood's A-list actors and actresses or models in advertisements and fashion magazines to notice that what we pay attention to and revere is all about looks. We project or infer meaning into someone's appearance. People's good looks have a way of letting us assume almost without hesitation that these are good, smart people. When they are a spokesperson for a cosmetics company (or any other consumer good from motor oil to toothpaste) we assume they have our best interests at heart or know what they are talking about, as opposed to the fact that they are being paid handsomely for their endorsement whether they like, care, or even know about what they are hawking.

It would be foolish to ignore the fact that personal appearance has enormous consequences in life. I don't know if Brad Pitt, Jennifer Aniston, Daniel Craig, or Julia Roberts are good people, but they are simply stunning to look at. Looking beautiful has power in most societies. Ignoring the significance of that impact may be virtuous, but it can also be unrealistic and get in our way.

WHY WEAR MAKEUP?

Wearing makeup is a personal decision and is hardly a mandate or the only way for women to look attractive. Nonetheless, applying makeup can be about looking and feeling more beautiful—and it can be exciting and fun. When done right, it can also express a great deal of personal power and élan. Whatever your choice, if you do want to wear makeup, applying it deftly can make the difference between looking attractive instead of strange, out of place, or sloppy.

Throughout this chapter, I try to guide you through the maze of options and help you create a beautiful makeup look for yourself that feels comfortable and fits like a glove. Although fashion statements can be taken to extremes—from following the whims of everything the fashion magazines portray or that your favorite celebrity decides to do, to holding on to looks that are long gone—ignoring fashion is a mistake. Finding your own balance between fashion, comfort, and personal style is the most logical and beautiful choice.

DRESSING YOUR FACE—WHAT'S IN FASHION?

When fashion is the topic, there are enough opinions and viewpoints to fill thousands and thousands of pages in hundreds of women's magazines every single month, 12 months a year. With such a storm of possible options screaming at us from the pages of *Vogue*, *Glamour*, *In Style*, and all the rest, choosing a direction may seem impossible. One model may wear a minimal sweep of tan blush on her cheeks, a hint of lipstick, taupe eyeshadow used both on the lid and crease, and a thin coating of mascara. Another model may have on an elaborate blend of contour shading; blush on top of that; an array of eyeshadow colors; dramatic, thick liner across the upper lashes and another thick sweep of liner along the lower lashes; and lots of mascara. The variations are endless.

To make things even more confusing, each month there are new announcements about what is fashionable and what isn't. One month red lipstick is hot, the next month it's sheer plum, and the next pink, and then you read that blue eyeshadow is coming back and you have to avoid wearing anything more than a hint of blush. Following these dictates can be maddening, not to mention expensive and more often than not inappropriate for you.

So where do you fit in? There are no hard and fast rules, though I know that's what we all want to hear—a clear path of exactly what to use to make us look picture perfect. In the long run, and among an nearly endless array of choices, the final decision is yours. Once you get these basics down—how to choose and apply concealer, foundation, powder, contour (if you want), blush, eyeshadow (one is plenty, but you can choose more), eyeliner (optional), eyebrow color (if needed or desired), mascara, lip liner (optional), and lipstick—wearing as little or as much color or using as many of these steps as you feel comfortable with is completely up to you. That's not to say I won't be throwing in my opinions of what I think works and looks best. If you use lip liner that smears, eyeshadows that streak and flake, mascara that clumps, blush that goes on choppy, eyeliner that smudges, or concealer that creases into the lines around your eyes and mouth, you and your makeup will not look beautiful in the least—and the goal is to look and feel more beautiful.

DOES MAKEUP CHANGE WITH AGE?

Whether or not you choose a new approach to your makeup based on your age is entirely dependent on what you're doing at the moment and how that makes you feel, but it is not essential or necessary. Just because more and more candles are finding a way onto your birthday cake, you don't have to hightail it to the nearest cosmetics counter for a makeover.

If you have reached a point where you truly feel comfortable and confident in your own skin, what you adorn it with should reflect this. For most women at any age, this may mean a sheer foundation that matches their skin exactly, a neutral-toned, creaseless concealer that does not play up wrinkles, a light dusting of sheer, non-shiny powder, soft matte eyeshadows in a variety of neutral hues, lightly defined and shaped brows, a great mascara that makes the most of your eyelashes, a softly blended blush color that adds vibrancy and color to your cheeks, and a lipstick color that seems "just right" no matter what other makeup you use. Sticking with well-chosen, adeptly applied and blended makeup in flattering shades gives a timeless look that can make ordinary features stunning.

However, if you breezed through your teens and twenties choosing makeup on a whim or enjoyed using bold, shiny eyeshadows, obvious blush, overly greasy or glossy lipsticks, heavy or mismatched foundation and too-thick concealer, and a kaleidoscopic array of eyeshadows and liners that were "out" as soon as you discovered they were "in," then you really should consider making adjustments to your routine. The same holds true if you feel as if you've been a slave to the latest makeup fads or styles, be they a retro Marilyn Monroe look with liquid-lined bedroom eyes and pouty red lips, or the Crayola crayon–colored eyeshadows and obvious false eyelashes seen in countless ads.

I'm all for self-expression—and when you're younger the limits of this are justifiably something to test—but as an adult, if your goal is to be taken seriously and be respected, why not think twice before heading to the office or grocery store wearing taxicab-yellow eyeshadow, clumpy mascara, and blue-tinged lipstick?

WHERE TO BEGIN

Three of the most difficult aspects of makeup are choosing the right colors, discerning the differences between products, and learning the correct application techniques. Though these major issues need to be addressed, they are still only part of the picture. Wondering where to put your blush or how to blend your foundation before you know what type of foundation or what color of blush you should wear is putting the cart before the horse. Before you even choose specific makeup colors, discriminate between products, or deal with application, it is important to have a clear idea of the makeup look and style you want to create. Just as you choose what clothes to wear that are appropriate for where you are going—you wouldn't put on a jogging suit to go to a formal dinner or wear a long gown for a grocery run—the same guidelines are true for makeup selection.

Color, style, and fashion are all essential elements in clothing, and they are also essential to putting together a great makeup look. Too often women shop for or apply makeup with only one of those things in mind. Shopping for a lipstick or eyeshadow color without taking into account the other items in your makeup wardrobe is a mistake. Instead, decide what kind of makeup wardrobe you want to create and then go about choosing compatible colors, products, and the application techniques to fit that concept. Think of the makeup staples you will need, such as black mascara, a healthy blush color, taupe or tan eyeshadow, and a suitable red lipstick. These items are akin to wardrobe staples such as a crisp white shirt, blue jeans, or the standard black dress—always fashionable and classic.

The way you see yourself, the way you want to be seen, what you do for a living, what you do in your leisure time, what colors are in your wardrobe, what style of clothing you are comfortable in, and how much time you are willing to spend creating a particular look all affect the way you choose and wear makeup. Those elements should set your course for choosing the right colors and products. It's imperative to think a bit about the image you want to create before you head out and shop for makeup. Questions to ponder include: How do you want to be seen? What do you do for a living? What occupies most of your time during the day? The external image you want to project in your business life and personal life is what wearing makeup is all about.

BEFORE YOU START

Because makeup goes on poorly over skin that isn't perfectly clean and smooth, the first step in applying beautiful makeup is to start with a gently cleaned face. Following the skin-care recommendations described in the first part of this book will help you get your skin to where it needs to be in order for makeup to look beautiful.

Either your daytime moisturizer or your foundation must be rated SPF 15 and contain the UVA-protecting ingredients of avobenzone (butyl methoxydibenz-oylmethane), titanium dioxide, zinc oxide, ecamsule (Mexoryl SX), or Tinosorb. Makeup without sun protection is only going to set your skin up for an unattractive future.

LESS IS BEST!

Never use more than you have to—either in the intensity of the colors you choose or the number of products you wear. Many steps in applying makeup can be consolidated or eliminated without affecting your overall makeup look in any way.

Frequently a salesperson at the cosmetics counter insists that you need an absurd number of products to be properly and attractively made up. Yet a more complicated routine doesn't mean you will look any better. If anything, a more complicated makeup routine can mean more chances for mistakes, which can cause you to look overdone—along with wasting your valuable time and money.

Speaking of doing too much, so-called foundation primers, eyeshadow bases, blemish cover-ups, eyeliner sealants, and color correctors—to name just a few—can be completely unnecessary. More often than not a foundation, concealer, and pressed powder are all you need. All the other extras tend to complicate the process of applying makeup, and also make it more time consuming. When you test specialty makeup products, be sure they are providing the benefit claimed on the label and that the extra step makes a difference for you.

PRIMERS

Foundation primers are seen in many makeup artistry lines, such as Laura Mercier, Vincent Longo, and NARS. Basically, these "primers" are nothing more than lightweight, silicone-based moisturizers. The silicone allows the product to spread easily over the skin, and to some extent can help smooth the skin's texture and remedy mild dry patches that could spell trouble when you apply most types of foundation. These primers also tend to have a soft matte finish on the skin once they dry down, and that can make your foundation a bit easier to control and blend because the skin will be much less slippery than if you had applied an emollient moisturizer.

Still, primers are truly optional and their benefits do not outweigh the extra step and expense. The only reason to consider one is if you have normal to oily skin and need the extra smoothness these can provide in order to make your foundation look its best. It is best to test these out via sampling before investing in a full-size tube so you can be sure you're making the purchase because you like what it does for your skin—not because you get suckered into the marketing pitch that makes it sound so important for skin. One more point: Lots of brilliantly formulated serums offer the same benefits as a foundation primer, but with the added bonus of giving your skin some truly helpful ingredients. In contrast, most foundation primer formulas lack these bells and whistles—and you definitely don't need a serum and a foundation primer!

Eyeshadow primers are sold to the consumer to help eyeshadows stay in place longer. The eye area is indeed a tricky place to get color to last, but there are ways to make it stay without specialty products. Besides, most eyeshadow bases are very similar to cream-to-powder concealers or foundations. Placing a matte or semi-matte foundation or concealer on your eyelid and applying loose powder over it works just as well. Also, if your eyeshadows tend to smear or slip into the eyelid crease, you can greatly reduce the problem by not placing a moisturizer or greasy foundation on your eyelid.

THE CLASSIC FACE

Classic makeup encompasses all of the following elements: concealer, foundation, powder, contour (optional), blush, eyeshadow, eyeliner, eyebrow color (if needed), lip liner (optional), and lipstick. For each of these steps, you want to find a corresponding product that is best for your skin type and the coverage or look you want. Each step also requires an application and blending tool so you can achieve a smooth, flawless appearance. Along the way, you can eliminate steps that seem excessive or too complicated, and decide how much makeup you want to wear and what colors are suitable to your needs.

The first two steps in applying a complete makeup are to reduce the darkness under the eyes and to apply a foundation to even out the skin. Once that's done, the eyeshadows and blushes can blend on smoothly over an even palette instead of over varying skin textures and colors. Whether you start your application with the concealer or the foundation depends more on personal preference than anything else, although the color of the concealer is another factor. For the sake of organization, I'll start with the concealer.

CONCEALER

The primary purpose of concealers is to offset the natural shadows that occur under the eyes, and, in more elaborate makeup applications, to highlight certain areas of the face such as the center of the nose, forehead, top of the cheekbones, or center of the chin. Principally, the under-eye area needs concealer most because the eye is set back in its socket, which lies in a shadow created by the surrounding bone structure. In addition, the skin around the eye tends to be thinner than the skin on the rest of the face, so pigment discolorations and surface veins show through easily, making the under-eye area look dark and dull. The first thing you need, then, is a lightweight, flesh-tone concealer that is a shade or two lighter than your foundation.

However, if you don't have dark circles under the eye area, you don't need a concealer. The same is true if your foundation is opaque enough to even out the skin tone under the eyes: you don't need an extra product for that area.

The logic behind using a lighter flesh-tone color is the same basic rule you learned in Art 101: When you need to make paint a lighter color, you add a lighter color than you started with. Any other color, or the same color, or a darker color would defeat the purpose. Blue, yellow, or shades that are the same as your foundation color will not make the under-eye area lighter. Standard shades can cover discolorations, which is fine, but applying a lighter shade is the only way to correct the darkness caused by shadows. Also, a slightly lighter under-eye area can make the face look brighter and more awake. Foundation may be all you need to even out minimal discolorations under the eye, cheeks, and nose, or to hide minor facial discolorations.

When you shop for an effective concealer, it is critical that the concealer be the same basic, natural skin tone as your foundation, only one or two shades lighter. That way you can be assured that the foundation and concealer will blend together under the eye. If you choose a concealer that is a very different color than your foundation, you will simply end up with a third color where they overlap and intersect.

The only time you wouldn't use a lighter concealer is when the area under the eye is naturally lighter or the same color as the rest of the face. In that case, it's fine to apply your foundation with no concealer. In fact, it may sometimes be necessary to apply a concealer that is slightly darker than your foundation to reduce having a whitish goggle effect around the eye.

I prefer to apply concealer first and then the foundation. You can apply your concealer in a small arc around the inside corner of the eye or, for a more involved makeup application, you can apply it in a sweep under the entire eye and out on the upper cheekbone. Blend this out evenly, taking care not to spread it onto areas where you don't want it. Be sure you are using a pat-and-blend method of application, as this will ensure that the concealer covers where it is supposed to and is not inadvertently wiped away. The foundation is then applied lightly over this area and blended out over the face. You may also want to try applying your foundation first and then sparingly applying concealer to the under-eye area if it is still dark. The trick is to make sure the foundation and concealer edges merge imperceptibly on the skin.

The most typical problem with a concealer is applying it smoothly over the under-eye area without making it look too white. It is important to always blend the edge of the concealer away from the eye until it disappears. Also, try to concentrate the concealer along the inside corner of the eye and down, as opposed to out. The less concealer you put at the back or outside corner of the eye (unless that area is dark), the lower your chances of looking like a raccoon with a white mask over the eyes.

At times when you wish to wear as little makeup as possible, try using only a minimal amount of concealer that is closer to your true skin tone than the concealer you normally use. Or try a lighter shade of foundation than you normally wear and apply it only in the under-eye area. This can make a world of difference in making you look rested and polished, but not made up. Again, the trick is to blend extremely well so that there is no discernible edge between the concealer area and the part of the face where there is no makeup.

Many cosmetics lines have excellent concealers, whether your preference is for a liquid, cream, or cream-to-powder texture. When shopping for a concealer, the primary things to look for are (1) a neutral skin tone that is one or two shades lighter than your foundation, but not so light that it looks obvious when blended on in the under-eye area, (2) a smooth texture to ensure easy blending, (3) coverage that suits your needs, and (4) staying power, so it doesn't crease into the lines around the eyes.

TYPES OF CONCEALERS

Concealers come in six different forms: stick concealers, creamy liquid concealers, cream concealers, matte-finish liquid, matte-finish cream-to-powder, and finally the ultra-matte liquid concealers, which blend on smoothly and creamily and dry quickly into an unmovable layer.

Stick concealers: Stick concealers come in swivel-up tubes similar to lipstick.

Examples: L'Oreal Infallible 16-Hour Concealer, Cle de Peau Beaute Concealer

Application: Stick concealers are applied to the under-eye area much the way a lipstick is applied to the mouth. They can be applied over or under your foundation, depending on how much coverage you want—under the foundation provides less coverage and over the foundation provides more. Dab the stick over the area in dots and then blend with clean fingers or a concealer brush. Avoid wiping it on from the stick in an opaque streak of color. That tends to build up too much makeup and it also pulls the eye area, causing sagging. If the skin under the eye area is dry or wrinkled, it does help to first apply a lightweight moisturizer and then apply the concealer. Be careful the moisturizer isn't too greasy and that you don't put it on too heavily to ensure that the concealer doesn't slip into facial lines. If you have applied too much moisturizer, use a tissue to dab off any excess before you apply the concealer.

Pros: Depending on their consistency, stick concealers can provide more complete coverage and control for very dark circles under the eye. They tend to go on thickly and don't spread easily, which means you can better control the application.

Cons: The texture of many stick concealers is rather dry and thick, which makes them difficult to blend without pulling the skin under the eye. They also go on too heavily, which can create an obviously made-up look. Other stick concealers are quite greasy; they can look less obvious because they blend so easily, but the texture often causes slippage into the lines around the eyes. For these reasons, this is the least common type of concealer you will encounter.

Creamy liquid concealers: Creamy liquid concealers generally come in small, squeeze-tube containers or long, thin tubes with wand applicators.

Examples: Prescriptives Camouflage Cream, Maybelline New York Instant Age Rewind Double Face Perfector

Application: Use your finger or the wand applicator to transfer the liquid concealer in small dots or to place a light coat of color under the eye area. Blend gently along the under-eye with either your finger or the sponge applicator, concentrating the largest amount of concealer over the darkest areas. If the skin under the eye area is dry or wrinkled, it helps to first apply a lightweight moisturizer and then apply the concealer. Be careful the moisturizer isn't too greasy and that you don't put it on too heavily or it will ensure that the concealer slips into facial lines.

Pros: Depending on their consistency, creamy liquid concealers provide very light, even coverage and have the least tendency to settle into creases in the eye area. They can also be easily layered if more coverage is needed, and they tend to not cake up on the skin.

Cons: Depending on their consistency, creamy liquid concealers can have too much movement and be hard to control. When applying an under-eye concealer, it is important to keep the color and coverage just where you want it. If the concealer is too greasy or slippery, it can spread too easily, highlighting parts of the face you don't want highlighted. Some liquid concealers go on too thinly, offering very little coverage.

Cream concealers: Cream concealers usually come in small pots and typically have a smooth and creamy texture. Occasionally these may have a dry, thick texture.

Examples: M.A.C. Studio Sculpt Concealer, Revlon Age-Defying Concealer SPF 20

Application: Depending on their consistency, cream concealers can go on easily with your fingertips, a concealer brush, or a sponge, placing the color in dots under the eye area. Blend the concealer out under the eye area, concentrating the application over the darkest areas. If the cream concealer has a dry, thick texture, it can be very difficult to blend and can look heavy and obvious on the skin. If the skin under the eye area is dry or wrinkled, it does help to first apply a lightweight moisturizer and then the concealer. If the cream concealer is very emollient, use minimal moisturizer under the eye area and dab off the excess. Most moisturizers can make cream-type concealers slip even more easily into facial lines. The emollient cream concealers should be set with loose powder immediately after blending to help promote crease-free wear.

Pros: Cream concealers can have a pleasing, creamy-moist consistency, but they can also be rather thick and heavy. Depending on the consistency, they can go on well and provide even, often opaque, coverage. They are especially good for someone with very dry skin who wants more coverage. In a pinch, cream concealers can also be used as foundations.

Cons: If the cream concealer is too thick or greasy it will crease into the lines on your face. If it is dry and thick it can be difficult to blend, and can also easily crease into facial lines. This is never the type of concealer to use over breakouts.

Matte-finish liquid concealers: Matte-finish liquid concealers typically come in a squeeze tube or a tube with a wand applicator.

Examples: Elizabeth Arden Flawless Finish Concealer, Benefit Lyin' Eyes

Application: Use your finger or the wand applicator to transfer the liquid concealer in small dots to the under-eye area, then quickly blend using a soft patting motion. If the skin under the eye area is dry or wrinkled, it helps to first apply a minimal amount of lightweight moisturizer and then apply the concealer. Although these are not as tricky to apply as ultra-matte concealers, they still demand adept blending for the best results.

Pros: Depending on their consistency, matte concealers can provide light to full coverage. They typically do not crease or migrate, and they tend to outlast cream and cream-to-powder concealers. They also work well as a base for eyeshadow if you have trouble with your eyeshadows fading or creasing. Matte-finish concealers work well over blemishes.

Cons: If you have prominent lines around and under the eyes, matte-finish concealers can make them look more pronounced. Some matte concealers go on quite thick and dry, and are difficult to blend easily or dry too quickly.

Matte-finish cream-to-powder: Matte-finish cream-to-powder concealers usually come in compact form and often look like small versions of cream-to-powder foundation.

Example: Lancome Photogenic Concealer SPF 15

Application: Use your finger, a concealer brush, or a sponge to dab the concealer onto the under-eye area or over other discolorations.

Pros: This type of concealer is very easy to apply. It provides the glide and blendability of a cream concealer with the long wear of a matte concealer. Concealers like this work well anywhere on the face, especially if more extensive coverage is needed.

Cons: Despite the initial matte finish, the ingredients that create the creamy texture tend to cause it to eventually crease—and to keep on creasing. The powder finish can make wrinkles look more pronounced, and this type of concealer is not the best to use over blemishes or dry, flaky skin.

TECHNIQUES FOR BLENDING CONCEALER

Regardless of the type of concealer you use, the application remains basically the same. Dab the color on with your fingertips, the wand applicator, or the tube concealer itself in a half-inch crescent from the inside corner of the eye out to approximately one-third of the way under the eye. Apply the concealer only where the eye area is dark. If it's dark all the way out under the eye, then that's where the concealer should go. You can apply concealer to the eyelid too if that area is also dark and could use some lightening. Unless you are using a matte finish concealer, set the concealer with a light dusting of loose or pressed powder. This will ensure a smooth finish and longer wear—but be careful not to overdo powdering under the eye area because this, too, can make lines look more pronounced.

If you want a more elaborate makeup application, you can apply the concealer along the flat bridge of the nose, along the laugh lines, out along the entire under-eye area, on the top of the cheekbone, and in the center of the forehead and chin for accent and enhancement. These options tend to be complicated and time-consuming, even for women adept at applying their makeup, and you can get almost the same results by applying the rest of your makeup correctly. If you do choose to highlight these areas, place your highlighter in dots over or under your foundation in these areas and blend well, controlling the color so it does not spread all over your face. Keeping the color contained is the goal if you wish to try this extra step.

CONCEALER MISTAKES TO AVOID

1. If you have noticeable lines around the eyes, do not wear a concealer that goes on too thickly or is too dry; it can cake under the eye and exaggerate wrinkles.

2. Consider my recommendations on www.Beautypedia.com for specific concealers that don't crease into the lines around eyes and have impressive wearability.
3. If the concealer is obvious, you've chosen the wrong shade, applied it too heavily, or didn't overlap as you blended it with your foundation.
4. Do not wear a peach, orange, green, rose, or ash shade of concealer.
5. Do not forget to blend the foundation and concealer together so there are no edges where one stops and the other starts. This is best done with a makeup sponge.

FOUNDATION

I totally understand when women complain about feeling "made up" when they wear a foundation. So why do I recommend using foundation at all? Because of the flawless, even base a foundation can provide. If the skin has a uniform color, texture, and appearance, the blush and eyeshadow colors you apply will look smooth instead of choppy. However—and here's the tricky part—to the extent possible, the face should never look like it has a layer of foundation on it.

If you are already blessed with a totally even, perfect complexion, you will nevertheless want to consider wearing a foundation because of the way it helps eyeshadows and blushes go on more evenly. If you try to blend blushes and eyeshadows without foundation, they will most likely go on choppily or wear unevenly during the day. Foundation keeps those powdered colors in place. Skin itself has no real adhesive properties (think about what would adhere to it if it did!). Foundation, therefore, gives the rest of the makeup something to hold on to evenly. By themselves, blushes and eyeshadows have some ability to cling, but not all that much. Besides, today's foundations offer some incredible options for creating the illusion of even, flawless skin without looking like makeup, and many of the best ones contain effective sunscreen.

FINDING THE PERFECT FOUNDATION COLOR

I cannot stress this point enough: Your skin and foundation should match exactly. If you are pale, that's OK—accept the fact that you are pale and buy a light foundation that matches exactly. Whether you have red hair and fair skin or black hair and dark ebony skin, the foundation must match your underlying skin color exactly. Do not buy a foundation that will make your face look even a shade or two darker or lighter or change its underlying color in any manner. Even with a difference that slight, you run the risk of a more obvious makeup application than you really want, particularly for daytime wear. Find a foundation that matches your skin perfectly and goes on softly and smoothly.

When I tell you to match the foundation with your underlying skin color, you may be asking yourself, "Exactly what is meant by skin color?"

Traditionally, skin color has been defined by the basic underlying tone. These tones are described as olive when the skin appears ashen or green in color, sallow when the skin has a yellow or golden shade, and ruddy when the skin has overtones of pink or red. These categories hold true for all women, including women of color; your underlying skin color will always relate to one of those skin tones. You may have been told that you are a particular "season" and your wardrobe and foundation color should be a specific undertone, either cool (blue tones) or warm (yellow tones). Unfortunately, all that information surrounding skin tone can be misleading when it comes to choosing a foundation color.

If you are told your face has cool undertones, meaning blue undertones, should you wear a blue-toned foundation? Of course not. If your skin color is ashen, choosing an ashen foundation will just make you look greener. If your face is strongly pink or red, applying a pink foundation all over will make you look like you're wearing a pink mask. If you have a sallow skin tone, applying a strong yellow-looking foundation will make you look more sallow. None of those would look natural and flawless the way foundation should look, and none of them would come close to matching your skin's underlying, basic color.

So what to do? When you're purchasing a foundation, it is important to identify your overall, exact skin color and find a foundation that matches it, regardless of the underlying tone. For the most part, regardless of your race, nationality, or age, your foundation should be some shade of neutral ivory, neutral beige, tan, dark brown, bronze brown, or ebony, with a slight, and I mean very slight, undertone of yellow but without any orange, pink, green, or blue tones. There are no orange, pink, green, or blue people, and buying foundations in those colors is absurd.

Why a slightly yellow undertone? Because skin color, more often than not, always has a yellow undertone—that's just what the natural color of melanin (the pigment in the skin) tends to be. There are a few exceptions to this rule. Native North American or South American women, a tiny percentage of African-American women, and some Polynesian women do indeed have a red cast to their skin, and in those instances this information about neutral foundations should be ignored. Because their skin has a slightly reddish cast, they need to look for foundations that have a slightly reddish cast to them—but that's only a hint of brownish red, and not copper, orange, or peach.

A few makeup lines are aimed at African-American women. Many lines also claim to meet the needs of darker skin colors, but often these lines actually have poor color selections or poor foundation types. It is best to find a foundation color and type that works for your skin type rather than limiting yourself to a special line claiming to serve a specific skin color.

EXCEPTION TO THE RULE OF MATCHING SKIN COLOR

Although you are attempting to exactly match the skin color of your face when you choose a foundation, in some cases it is more important to match the foundation to the color of your neck. If your face is darker than your neck and your foundation matches the face, it will look like a mask because of the difference in color. The opposite is also true. If your face is lighter than your neck and you put on a foundation that matches the face, it will still look like a mask because of the difference in color. In situations like this, match the foundation more to the neck color or to a color in between the color of the neck and the face.

For some women who have serious facial discolorations or scars it can be hard to ignore the need for a heavy foundation application that provides opaque, full, concealing coverage. Unfortunately, a heavy or thick foundation is the only way to achieve this effect. Foundations that make claims about providing superior coverage that also looks natural are not telling the truth. You can't cover your face with foundation and camouflage the imperfections without seeing what is providing the coverage. But that doesn't mean you shouldn't consider a heavier foundation—just be aware that you are essentially exchanging one problem for another. The advantage is you do get to choose between two options, and even if that's a dilemma, you are still the best judge of what works and feels best for you.

THE FINAL DECISION

Once you have selected a foundation color, there is only one way to be absolutely sure it is right for you: Apply the color all over your face and check it outside in the daylight. Check it from all angles and decide if it matches your skin exactly. If you applied it carefully but there are lines of demarcation at the jaw area; or if it looks too thick or too greasy, or gives the face an orange, pink, rose, or ashen tint; or if it looks heavy and opaque instead of sheer and light, wash it off and go back to the testers. In fact, you may need to test several types before you find the right foundation.

One practical guideline to narrow down your choices is to test many different colors at once. Begin with several that look like good possibilities and place stripes of each one in a row over the cheek area. The best choice is the one that blends almost perfectly with your skin color. The wrong choices will stand out, with obvious edges that don't disappear into your skin. This technique is a reliable way to eliminate some choices, but I've also seen it go wrong more times than I can count because it doesn't go far enough. Use it only as an elimination process; it does not replace the need to check out the color on your face in the daylight, nor the need to blend the foundation shade over a larger area of your face.

Keep trying on foundations until you find the best one. Once you've made a selection you feel good about, apply it all over your face, wait at least two hours, and check it again in the daylight. How a foundation wears during the day—does it change color or become too greasy or dry as the day passes?—can be evaluated only after you've worn it for awhile. Once you've assessed all these details, in the daylight, you can safely make a final determination as to whether this is the right color or type of foundation for you. Please take the time to follow this procedure. This advice will guide you in the right direction, and, ultimately, **it is the only way to guarantee that you'll find the right foundation**. If you rely only on the salesperson and the lighting at the cosmetics counters, it will be pure luck if you end up with the right color. And if you get the foundation wrong, regardless of how perfectly you choose and apply everything else in your makeup wardrobe, those will all look wrong, too.

WHERE TO SHOP

Although there are many wonderful foundation options available at the drugstore, the almost universal lack of testers is incredibly frustrating. For budget-conscious consumers looking for a reasonably priced foundation this can be quite a challenge, as you're often left standing in the aisle (under horrendous lighting and with no mirrors in sight) to guess which shade is best for you. For this reason, I encourage you to begin your foundation search at a department store or cosmetics boutique (like Sephora) where testers are the rule, not the exception. You will end up spending more for foundation, but the convenience of testers, mirrors, take-away samples, and (at times) professional guidance is worth it. Once you become more skilled at knowing which shades work for you and which do not, you can venture back to the drugstore to try again. It can be helpful to bring along the foundation you are currently using—assuming the color is a great match—to compare with the drugstore options. Last, since you will still not be able to see the color on your skin until you purchase it and test it at home, be sure you buy only from drugstores or mass merchandise stores that allow you to return opened cosmetics. Safe bets in this regard are Rite Aid and Walgreens.

TYPES OF FOUNDATION

Cosmetics counters carry a mind-boggling assortment of foundations these days, including oil-free and matte foundations, water-based foundations, pressed-powder foundations, cream-to-powder foundations, liquid-to-powder foundations, stick foundations, so-called self-adjusting foundations, and foundations that have shine. Given this range of options, narrowing down your choices can be tricky.

Note: Many of the following foundation types have effective sunscreen protection with an SPF 15 or greater and the UVA-protecting ingredients of avobenzone, titanium dioxide, or zinc oxide (as of this writing, I am not aware of any foundations that contain Mexoryl SX or Tinosorb as active ingredients). That means you can rely on these for sun protection if they are applied liberally and evenly all over the face. If you prefer to wear a sheer, thin layer of foundation or don't want to wear foundation all over your face, then a moisturizer with sunscreen must be worn underneath. To ensure your foundation with sunscreen is protecting you all day, consider setting your makeup or touching up your makeup during the day with a pressed powder that contains sunscreen.

Oil-free and matte liquid foundations: Most of these contain oils (even though the names don't sound as though they do) or ingredients that act or feel like oils, such as silicones. These oils and oil-like ingredients are not necessarily bad for any skin type, but their presence demonstrates that the term "oil-free" is another cosmetics industry contrivance that won't necessarily help you find the best product for your skin type. Keep in mind that what most of these foundations have in common when they are well formulated is that they set to a matte finish, with no shine or dewy appearance whatsoever. On the skin, "oil-free" matte foundations look like a traditional liquid foundation, although they are often thicker in appearance and have no shine.

Examples: Clinique Stay-True Makeup Oil-Free Formula, Almay Nearly Naked Liquid Makeup SPF 15

Application: See the section "Blending Foundation" that follows.

Pros: These foundations are the best choice for women who want balanced coverage with no shine at all, and who like a smooth, matte look. They last much longer on oily skin or oily areas than most other foundations, which for some women is a very desirable, if not essential, effect.

Cons: There aren't many disadvantages to using this kind of foundation. Some of them can make the skin look or feel dry and flaky, but this is usually true only for those that contain a high amount of talc or other absorbent ingredients.

Water-based and standard liquid foundations: Water-based does not mean oil-free, even if the label says so; what it does generally mean is that the first ingredient is water and the second or third ingredient is some kind of oil or emollient slip agent. These foundations look like a somewhat thick liquid that pours slowly but easily out of the bottle. They are perfect for women with normal to dry skin, and the number of foundations fitting this description and performance is extensive.

Examples: Laura Mercier Moisturizing Foundation, M.A.C. Select SPF 15 Moistureblend

Application: See the section "Blending Foundation" that follows.

Pros: Most water-based foundations are best for those with normal to dry skin. They are perfect for these skin types to wear without a moisturizer, or they can be worn with a moisturizer or a moisturizer that contains an SPF. The oil or emollient part of these foundations gives them good movement, which makes blending a pleasure and allows blushes and eyeshadows to blend on effortlessly and evenly over the face. Mistakes are easily buffed away with the sponge.

Cons: If you have oily or combination skin, this is not the foundation type for you. Even the little bit of oil or emollient in a water-based foundation will show as shine almost immediately if you have oily skin. Those who do not have oily skin but have a paranoia about any shine on the face will not like the effects of a water-based foundation either; and for those with breakout-prone skin, the small amount of oil or emollients in this cosmetic may make you nervous. For the most part, I personally don't believe there are any disadvantages to using water-based foundations and I recommend them wholeheartedly. Water-based foundation is also a great option for women of color. The slight amount of emollient these contain helps create a nice glow on the skin, preventing darker skin tones from appearing dull or ashen. That same glow is also most attractive for women with dry skin.

If you are concerned about the small amount of shine that water-based foundations leave behind on the skin, try adding a light dusting of loose powder. After you've blended the foundation in place, you can apply the powder all over the face to reduce the shine.

Pressed-powder foundations: These foundations come in a compact and appear and perform much like any pressed powder, which is what they really are, only with a bit more coverage and ability to stay put. Almost all of them have a superior creamy, silky feel, but when applied to the skin they blend on as easily and lightly as any pressed powder.

Examples: Laura Mercier Foundation Powder, Clinique Almost Powder Makeup SPF 15

Application: You can apply these foundations, either with a sponge or a brush, all over the face, including the eyelids. This is the easiest way to get a smooth, light, and fast application. You might have to worry about a smooth application if you have dry skin, but these powder-based foundations go on evenly for other skin types, providing extremely sheer to medium coverage. For more specifics about blending techniques, see the section "Blending Foundation" that follows.

Pros: Powder foundations are great for women with normal to oily or combination skin. They blend on easily and quickly, last all day, generally don't change color, and feel exceptionally light on the skin. They are best for those who want a minimal feel and appearance from their foundation. They also work very well over sunscreens, and can help reduce the shine some sunscreen ingredients (even those in a matte base) leave on the skin. Pressed-powder foundations also work well as a late-day touch-up over liquid foundation.

Cons: Women who have dry skin should not wear powder foundation. This is also not a good option if you have flaky skin, regardless of your skin type. The powder content makes this type of foundation too drying for someone with dry skin, and the way it goes on can make the skin look more dry and flaky. Also, women with very oily skin might want to be cautious, because powder-based foundations can get a thickened, pooled appearance as oil resurfaces on the face during the day.

Cream-to-powder foundations: These foundations are an interesting cross between a pressed powder and a creamy liquid foundation. They come in a compact and have a very creamy, sometimes greasy appearance. When you blend them on, the creamy part disappears and you are left with a slightly matte, powdery finish. Cream-to-powder foundations provide much better coverage than pressed-powder–based foundations.

Examples: Clarins Perfectly Real Compact Makeup, Estee Lauder Resilience Lift Extreme Ultra Firming Creme Compact Makeup SPF 15

Application: Cream-to-powder foundations are best applied with a sponge. Some women have success using a brush, but I think this is a difficult, messy technique. See the section "Blending Foundation" that follows.

Pros: Cream-to-powder foundations blend on quickly and easily and provide a semi-matte, soft, medium coverage. They work great for someone with normal to slightly dry or slightly combination skin. The consistency doesn't require powdering after you apply it. If you wish to use powder, make sure you apply it as lightly as possible to avoid a caked, heavy look.

Cons: Cream-to-powder foundations can blend on slightly thick, providing a made-up look rather than a sheer, natural appearance. They don't work well for someone with oily skin because the cream components can be too creamy, making skin look more oily, and they don't work well for dry skin because the powder part can be too powdery looking and cause more dryness.

Liquid-to-powder foundations: These liquidy powders with a gel-like wet feel apply easily and dry to a satiny-smooth, sheer, slightly matte finish. They typically contain water as the first ingredient, along with a slip agent such as glycerin. In contrast to cream-to-powder foundations, liquid-to-powder foundations feel significantly lighter on the skin. They also tend to last longer over combination or oily skins because the creamy, waxy ingredients are either decreased or altogether absent.

Examples: Vincent Longo Water Canvas Foundation, Cover Girl Aqua Smooth Makeup SPF 15

Application: Liquid-to-powder foundations are best applied with a sponge. Some women have success using a brush, but I think this is a difficult, messy technique. See the section "Blending Foundation" that follows.

Pros: Liquid-to-powder foundations blend on quickly and relatively easily and provide a semi-matte to matte finish with sheer to medium coverage. They work great for someone with normal to oily or slightly combination skin. The consistency means that it doesn't require powdering after you apply it. If you wish to use powder, make sure you apply it as lightly as possible to avoid a caked, heavy look.

Cons: Liquid-to-powder foundations dry quickly and can, therefore, blend on choppy, making application tricky. This type of foundation does not work very well over dry skin because the water portion tends to cling to dry areas, leaving a powder finish that is not easily moved. If you have dry skin and want to try this type of foundation, use an emollient moisturizer or sunscreen beforehand. The product itself must be kept tightly closed between uses because the water component will evaporate if left exposed to air for long periods. Some of the compact liquid-to-powder makeups can chip or break apart if you are not careful while swiping your sponge over the makeup.

Stick foundations: These foundations are essentially cream-to-powder foundations in stick form, and the application, pros, and cons mentioned in that section are the same. The main difference between stick and cream-to-powder foundations is the variety of coverage available from sticks. Whereas cream-to-powder makeups typically provide medium coverage, stick foundations come in formulas that range from full to sheer coverage with either matte to creamy texture. Some stick foundations also feature effective sunscreens, making them a great all-in-one option. In addition, they can do double duty as a concealer.

Examples: Stila Perfecting Foundation, Shiseido Stick Foundation SPF 15

Application: These can be swiped onto the skin right from the stick and then blended with a sponge, fingers, or a foundation brush.

Pros and Cons: Refer to the section for cream-to-powder foundations.

Self-adjusting foundations: These foundations supposedly can absorb oil, stop oil production, and also prevent moisture loss. I've yet to see one perform as promised, though it would be great if someone came up with one that could! Do not rely on these foundations to perform as claimed, but they're often a good choice for combination skin due to their lighter texture and soft matte finish.

Custom-blended foundations: If a foundation is blended for you and you only, will that get you the best shade? This style of selling makeup is very enticing. The customer-service interaction is impressive. Your foundation is supposedly mixed and matched for your exact skin color and needs. The premise is that there are only so many ready-made shades and you might be better off having one custom-blended. Unfortunately, the idea sounds better than the reality. The major problem with custom-blended cosmetics is that the success of the match depends on the expertise of the salesperson—and there are huge variations in skill.

As tempting as custom-blended foundations sound, the formulations are not necessarily superior to (or sometimes even as good as) standard products. The foundation may be too greasy or too dry and it might turn to rose or peach as you wear it. With so many off-the-shelf foundation products available, in many excellent colors, custom blending turns out to be more an expensive gimmick than anything else.

When should you try a custom-blended product, particularly foundation? When you have tested many standard foundations and are still frustrated with the color of your foundation.

BLENDING FOUNDATION

When it comes to blending foundation over your face, keep one mantra in your head: Blend, blend, and blend again, and then, just to be sure, blend one more time. All the other details are, well, just details, and not anywhere near as important as buffing off the excess foundation and smoothing out the edges to be sure you have the smoothest possible layer of foundation over the skin.

Exception to the rule: If you are using a foundation that contains an effective sunscreen, a thin or sheer application will not provide adequate protection from the sun. To ensure you will be getting the stated SPF, it is essential to apply the foundation liberally and in an even layer all over the face. If you prefer a sheer or spot application, then you will need to wear a separate sunscreen underneath your foundation or consider a tinted moisturizer with sunscreen or a pressed powder that contains sunscreen.

Keep in mind that the goal of wearing foundation is to create the illusion of smoother-looking skin, not a noticeable mask of color. Of course, the best place to check your blending technique is in broad daylight. Unfortunately, most of us apply foundation in bathroom light, with only minimal exposure to sunlight. Once you get into daylight, even on a cloudy day, the areas you missed, particularly next to the ears, mouth, jawline, sides of the nose, and temples, often look streaked, show a line of demarcation (even when the color matches perfectly), or appear blotchy or smudged. This is not the effect you are trying to achieve! Smoother-looking skin takes diligence and daylight, or the very best lighting you can create in your home where you apply your makeup. Always check your foundation in daylight before showing your made-up face to the world!

I recommend blending foundation with a sponge rather than using your fingers. The flat, smooth surface of a sponge is the best way to get a smooth application. The best tool is a flat, square, or round one-quarter-inch-thick sponge that doesn't have holes and is not made of synthetic foam rubber. Together, the shape and density of this kind of sponge provide the smoothest application possible. I know that some makeup artists advocate finger application of foundation. The rationale is that the warmth of your fingers will help the foundation mesh with the skin and provide a more natural look. If you feel more comfortable finger-painting than using a sponge, go for it. But humor me and make sure you always smooth out the edges of your finger-applied foundation with a sponge. I think you will find the results will be well worth the effort!

The sponges frequently found for sale or in use at most cosmetics counters are the thick, wedge-shaped, foam-rubber ones. These sponges are compact, but they drag over the skin, and that makes blending difficult. Also, because they're so thick, most of the foundation is absorbed into the sponge, where you can't get to it, which can waste a lot of product. Wedge sponges are used for traditional theatrical makeup. They are great for applying grease stick or pancake foundations, which require more "pull" across the face to apply them evenly, but that is the last thing you need when you're wearing a lightweight foundation. Shiseido,

Sephora, Sonia Kashuk, and Paula's Choice make some excellent makeup sponges—and these can be washed repeatedly without falling apart.

To achieve an even application with your sponge, shake some of the foundation from the bottle onto the sponge, then transfer the foundation to the face and over the eyes by dabbing the sponge over the skin. You can also use your fingers to transfer the foundation in dots from the bottle to the face and then use the sponge to blend the dots. Start by placing the foundation generously over the central area of the face, including the eyes but avoiding the sides of the face near the hairline, jaw, and chin. The foundation can go on in large patches or small dots all over the nose, eyelids, cheeks, and forehead, but only in this central area. Avoid placing the foundation all over the face unless you want a full makeup application or are using a foundation that contains sunscreen as your only source of sun protection. By concentrating the foundation over the central part of the face, as you blend down and out from the center there will be less foundation at the jaw and hairline. When applying a foundation with sunscreen, apply an even layer all over the face, and then use the clean side of your sponge to softly feather the edges of the makeup at the jaw and hairline. The objective is to soften, but not wipe off, the foundation.

Once the foundation is on your face, begin using your sponge to blend the foundation evenly. Holding the sponge between your fingers and thumb, spread the foundation down and out over the entire face with a stroking, buffing motion, going in the direction of the hair growth. (Going against the direction of the hair growth on your face coats the hair with too much foundation.) The idea is to blend the foundation color out from the center of the face, where you initially placed it, to the perimeter of the face, leaving no line of demarcation at the jaw or hairline. Use the edge of the sponge *without* foundation (or turn the sponge over to the clean side) to dab or buff away any of the excess that tends to collect under the eye or around the nose. You can also use the sponge to wipe away any of the excess that gathers at the jaw or hairline. When blending the foundation, do not try to force it into the skin. There is a fine line between blending something on and wiping something off. Instead, blend a thin layer over the face, smoothing it with your sponge as you go. Using this technique, you can build coverage as desired. At this point your sponge should not be full of foundation; if it is, you've used too much.

If you did not apply a concealer before the foundation, you can apply it now and blend that into place. Apply the concealer over the under-eye area and other areas you want to highlight, then dab it into place with your finger or a sponge.

Watch out for the jaw and neck. This is very important. Never, ever put makeup of any kind on the neck; you do not want your makeup to end up on your collar. Always double-check your blending. Places on the face that you are likely to miss with foundation include the corners of the nose, the tip of the nose, the corners of the eyes (especially over the concealer), and the edge along the lower eyelashes. Also, some places are likely to end up wearing foundation that shouldn't, including the ears, the jawline, and the hairline— especially blonde hairlines. Be careful to remove this foundation if you've gone past your mark. Both situations can cause your makeup to appear sloppy.

Your sponge is an exceptional blending tool that you should keep near you at all times. When the edges of your blush or eyeshadow need softening, you can blend out the hard edges with the side of the sponge that was used to spread the foundation over the face. Using the side of the sponge that has foundation on it as opposed to the dry edge allows the sponge to glide over the blush or eyeshadow without streaking or rubbing it off.

BLENDING OVER THOSE FINE LITTLE WRINKLES

If you've started to notice that foundation or concealer is sinking into some of those little wrinkles on your face, especially the laugh lines, lines under the eyes, or near the crow's feet, you have to be even more meticulous about how you blend your foundation into place. In this regard, less is best. Blend, blend, and blend again, being sure to remove the excess in those areas with the clean side of the sponge.

Minimize your use of moisturizers over the areas where you have lines, and use a foundation or concealer that's neither greasy nor too emollient. Anything with lingering movement and slip gives the foundation a free ride into the lines.

As for those concealers and foundations that claim to deflect, reflect, or somehow improve the appearance of wrinkles—they don't. And those foundation primers sold by various cosmetics lines, which are usually just moisturizers with extra film-forming agents (hairstyling-type ingredients), don't work all that well either, plus they just add another layer of product to the face, which increases the likelihood of clogging pores, exacerbating breakouts, or creating dull-looking skin.

The truth is that a face without foundation always looks less wrinkled. I'm not sure why this has to be so, but it is. You can test this for yourself. Go to the cosmetics counter, find the most expensive foundation with the most elaborate claims about making the skin look less wrinkled, apply a sample to one side of your face, and leave the other side naked with just a dab of moisturizer over dry areas. Then check out your face in the daylight. You will be amazed how much more noticeable the lines on the foundation side of the face are. Of course, the foundation side will look smoother and will have a more even tone, the redness and blotchiness will be gone, and the pores will have virtually disappeared. But the wrinkles will be more noticeable than on the side without foundation. That's the agony and ecstasy of foundation!

FOUNDATION MISTAKES TO AVOID

1. Do not buy a foundation before trying it on and checking it in the daylight.
2. Do not wear foundation unless it matches your skin color.
3. Do not wear pink, peach, rose, orange, or ash-colored foundation.
4. Cream-to-powder foundations work best for normal skin. The cream part can be too greasy for oily skin and the powder can be too dry for dry skin.
5. Do not apply a thick layer of foundation; thin and sheer are the operative words when it comes to applying foundation unless you are wearing a foundation with sunscreen, in which case liberal, even application is essential.

6. Do not use your fingers to blend your foundation over the face unless you're willing to go over your handiwork with a sponge.

BRUSHES

Before we go on to powders, eyeshadows, and blushes, it is crucial to discuss the most important blending tools you can use (besides the sponge for blending on foundation)—brushes. Brushes are simply the best way to apply almost all types of makeup, and you'd be hard put to find a makeup artist anywhere who disagrees. Moreover, nowadays we have a profusion of brushes to choose among. Whether they're from M.A.C., Prescriptives, Bobbi Brown, Trish McEvoy, Stila, Maybelline New York, Aveda, Lorac, BeneFit, Paula's Choice, or other lines, good brushes are available in an impressive array of sizes, shapes, and sensual textures that facilitate makeup application in ways that feel artistic and effortless. As with anything related to cosmetics, though, a high price does not always mean superior performance. And having more brushes does not mean you will be able to apply your makeup better.

The personal set of brushes you choose is determined strictly by how you prefer to apply your makeup. If your makeup application is elaborate and nuanced, involving several eyeshadows, contour, and highlighting, you need a variety of brushes. If your makeup application is uncomplicated and basic, you need fewer brushes. It's that simple. (The reason makeup artists carry an arsenal of brushes is because they see a vast assortment of eye and face sizes.) All you need is a group of brushes that match the areas of your face and the kinds and colors of makeup you apply.

As a general guideline, it is best to not purchase a prepackaged set of brushes unless you know you will use all of them and the particular shapes and sizes will meet your needs.

The general rule to follow when considering what size brush to purchase is: Does the size of the brush match the size of the area you are working on? Too small and it will take longer to apply your makeup and it can end up looking striped. Too large and you can end up with a messy application. If you are lining the eye, a tiny thin brush with just a few hairs and that doesn't scratch or feel stiff is best. If you are filling in the brow, a small angle brush with a slight amount of stiffness to control the color is best. (It should be small and stiff enough to fit through the spaces in the hair and follow the edge of the brow with pencil-like control.) For the eyelid, choose a brush size that fits the curve of your lid, and the same reasoning applies for the crease area. Both should be determined by the size of your eye, and there are countless eyeshadow brush sizes to choose from. To highlight along the brow, a soft, small wedge brush (less stiff than the brow brush), fitting just that area, is best. Try not to use the same brush for both lighter and darker shades of eyeshadow.

How many and which brushes do you need? A full makeup application can require three basic eyeshadow brushes: An eyeliner brush (for liner and brows), a blush brush, contour brush, large powder brush, a lash brush (an old clean mascara wand will do), a brow brush (here a toothbrush will do nicely), and a lip brush.

If you don't use a pencil for eyelining, a tiny, thin eyeliner brush is best for building either a thick or thin line along the upper and lower lashes. While some makeup artists use thicker brushes that are more square or wedge-shaped for this purpose, I think they are harder to control (they can make a thick line, but it's hard to get them to create a thin line, while a tiny thin brush can do either). If you're unsure, experiment with both styles and see which you prefer. A wedge-shaped brow brush can be used just for the brow to apply eyeshadow powder or to smooth out the line of an eyebrow pencil. Personally, I use a tiny eyeliner brush to fill in the brows to keep the shading soft by creating hair-thin strokes. An old toothbrush is still the best tool for combing through the brows. For combing through the lashes, I strongly recommend a good, densely packed used mascara wand that you wash clean, like the ones in L'Oreal Voluminous, Maybelline XXL (any of the versions), and Lancome Definicils mascara. Most lash brushes that are sold separately have bristles that are too far apart to be helpful for easy unclumping and separating. Avoid metal eyelash combs—these can be incredibly painful and damaging if you accidentally poke yourself in the eye. Plastic eyelash combs are a much better, safer option.

Both the blush brush and powder brush should have a soft, firm texture and not splay out when placed on the skin or into the color (no brush should be so loose as to splay when used either on the face or in the product). They should also feel soft and silky, yet hold their shape. If a brush is too wobbly, it will be hard to control the color. I often recommend getting two good blush brushes in the same size and using one for powder and one for blush (you don't want to dust color over the face). Many powder brushes, though they may feel incredibly soft and luxurious, are too large, cumbersome, and hard to control. It's nearly impossible to maneuver some of these behemoth brushes under the eye, along the corner of the nose, or along the cheek without hitting other areas of the face that may not need powder, and using too much powder is extremely likely.

If you are looking for a contour brush to shade along the temple, jaw, or cheekbone, a smaller blush brush is a great choice. Brushes specially designed for this area come in a variety of sizes, but the flat edge of these specially designed brushes, though impressive in appearance, can create just that, a hard edge, which takes more blending to soften than necessary. Simply use a small, half-inch-wide version of your blush brush; the idea is that this contour/blush brush should fit the hollow of the cheekbone.

I'm not among those who diligently apply lipstick with a lipstick brush. I just don't have the time. Generally, I save this precision for special occasions or when I want to use up every last drop in the tube. But if you like this option, look for a brush with bristles that are strong and slightly stiff. Tug hard on the brush and make sure the hairs don't move in the least. Look for a brush the size of your lips. Too small and it can take forever; too big and you'll be applying lipstick to your face. You know those retractable metal brushes you see almost everywhere and in every price range? They are all the same, and they are excellent! Retracting the bristles neatly back into place beats trying to keep the little plastic protective sheath on a wood-handled brush. (They never stay on and lipstick ends up getting all over your purse and makeup bag!)

I am not an advocate of foundation brushes, despite the fact that many lines now offer these as part of their brush collections. Quite simply, using foundation brushes takes longer than using a sponge (or fingers if you're so inclined), and they require more maintenance between uses. Depending on the type of foundation being used, these brushes can create a striped or streaked appearance. If you are tempted to try them, experiment with them before making a purchase so you can be sure you like the final result with whatever foundation you use.

BRUSH QUALITY AND CARE

As you check out the different lines of brushes, the first thing you will hear about is the so-called quality of the bristles, and the salespeople will use this to justify the cost. Depending on the line, you will hear pretentious claims about squirrel, sable, pony, goat, and several other animals that did not give up their coats voluntarily. Synthetic brush hair is an option for those who are 100% vegetarian. However, synthetic brush hair is not preferred for most makeup application other than foundations and concealers. The most reliable synthetic brushes are from Origins, The Body Shop, and Shu Uemura.

Although natural bristles are definitely softer (and often more expensive) than synthetic, it does not take sable to make the perfect brush, and mixed-hair bristles can make for a stronger, more pliable brush that doesn't lose its shape. Natural hairs tend to get softer over time, which means a firm, well-controlled brush can eventually become floppy and too soft. Salespeople who encourage you to buy the expensive brushes will claim that synthetic hairs get coarser and stiffer, or fall out after a year or two of usage, but that is not true. Synthetic hair brushes hold up as well if not better than natural hair brushes.

Ignore the claims about hair quality and trust your own **touch and feel tests**. Brush the bristles along the nape of your neck and ask yourself, "Is it smooth? Do the bristles hold their shape? Does it feel too loose, too stiff, or too soft? Does the brush feel densely packed, meaning lots of hairs, or flimsy?" Once you decide which feel you prefer, you can determine which brushes you want to work with.

Use the touch test to ascertain how the brush will hold up. Simply tug at the bristles, pulling away from the handle end, to see if there is any give. Do any hairs fall out? If you feel any release whatsoever, this is not a well-constructed brush. Some brushes are not well anchored and bound into the base of the brush. For example, Maybelline's incredibly inexpensive brushes beautifully pass the feel test (they are wonderfully soft and firm), but fail the touch test (the bristles tend to pull out). In the short term they are a superior bargain, but they won't hold up over the long haul.

When it comes to the shape of the brush, generally it is best to avoid blunt brushes and brushes with the bristles lined up flat with a severe edge. For most brushes—eyeliner, lip, eyeshadow, blush, and powder—look for ends that are more dome-shaped. Not only do these have a softer feel, but they also allow for a softer, less hard-edged application, which is almost always the goal. The only exception is the wedge brush for the brows or under the eyebrow.

When I'm doing my own makeup for media appearances or doing someone else's makeup, I personally favor brushes with long, elegantly tapered wood handles. But when I try to squeeze these long-stemmed beauties into the small makeup bag I travel with or keep in my briefcase, I realize how cumbersome they can be. For women who want to invest in only one set of brushes, short handles are not only more convenient, they are essential.

When it comes to caring for your brushes, some people claim you must wash them frequently. If you are a makeup artist working on lots of people, you should be washing your brushes every day. But for those of us who are working on ourselves only and not changing colors on a daily basis, once a month is just fine. Especially for natural-hair brushes, frequent washing breaks down the hair shaft and that breaks down the brush hairs. Also, washing too often can loosen the glue in the handle that holds the bristles together and keeps them in place. When you clean the brushes, concentrate your effort on the bristles, not the handle.

It is best to use a regular shampoo instead of a special brush-cleaning solution (which is just shampoo anyway). The shampoo shouldn't contain any conditioning agents, which can build up on the brush just like they do on the hair. Neutrogena Anti-Residue Shampoo and Paula's Choice All Over Hair and Body Shampoo are great inexpensive options. A conditioner is not necessary when caring for your brushes. Brush hair is extremely healthy. It isn't damaged from dyeing, perming, styling, brushing, and the other things people do to their own hair that make the use of conditioners required. When washing your brushes, carefully follow these steps:

- Gently but thoroughly wash the brush in tepid water.
- Meticulously rinse the brush, making sure the excess water is not running toward the base of the brush (where the hairs are secured).
- Carefully press out the excess water and dab the brush dry.
- Arrange the bristles back into their original shape.
- Let the brush air dry flat on a towel without the help of a blow dryer, which can damage bristles.

BRUSH TECHNIQUES

Brushes can be foolproof tools for applying makeup, yet it is definitely possible to use brushes incorrectly. I've seen enough women use their brushes in a rubbing or wiping motion on the face to know how often it can happen. Many women beat at their faces with a wild brushing motion as they attempt to apply their blush and eyeshadows. There truly is an easier and more effective method. When you wipe, beat, or heavily rub the brush against the face, it may be removing what you just put on, not to mention wiping off the foundation underneath, which can result in a streaky, uneven appearance. The best technique is to brush in short, light, purposeful motions that glide over the skin.

If there is a distinct line where the brushstroke was placed or if you feel an urge to use your finger to blend what you've just applied, most likely you are not using the brush properly or your brush is too stiff for a soft application. You should avoid blending anything with your fingers—use your brush or the flat, square, thin sponge you use to apply your foundation. Use your sponge for applying foundation and softening edges of your blush, contour, and eyeshadows.

Something else that is critical to using brushes effectively—even though it may seem insignificant at first—is the way you pick up the powder on your brush before you apply it. Never smash or rub your brush into the powder. Rather, gently place your brush into the powder without moving the bristles. You don't want to see the brush hair bend or splay. Always stroke through the powder evenly and always knock the excess powder off the brush before you apply it to the face. This prevents applying too much color to the first place your brush touches. When it comes to makeup, it is always easier to add than subtract!

BRUSH TIPS TO REMEMBER

1. Do not use brushes with hard or stiff bristles.
2. Do not use a brush that is too big or too small for the area of the face you are working on.
3. Do not use brushes that are too soft or ones with bristles that are too sparse; they won't hold up over time.
4. Do not forget to knock the excess powder off the brush before you apply the color to your face.
5. Do not wipe or rub the brush across the face; instead, gently brush on the color with short, even strokes.
6. Do not forget to use your sponge to blend out hard edges and soften your color application.
7. Do not forget to gently wash your brushes every month or so, unless you are using them on a variety of people, in which case you should be washing or disinfecting them every day.

POWDER

A classic makeup application requires powdering after you've applied your foundation, but powdering doesn't work for all types of foundation. Powdering works best after applying a water-based, creamy, or matte foundation that isn't all that matte. It can be either unnecessary or even problematic to apply powder over most oil-free or matte foundations, or over any of the pressed-powder, cream-to-powder, or liquid-to-powder foundations. Some stick foundations that dry to a powder finish do not need extra powder, but those that remain creamy do.

As a general guideline, the less powder you build up on your face, the less made-up you will appear. Overpowdering can also make the face look dull and dry, especially if you have dry skin or a darker skin tone. Some amount of natural, dewy shine to the face is very attractive. After a foundation is applied, the slight shine that is left behind (except with oil-free, matte, and pressed-powder foundations) gives the face a radiant glow. Powder is great for touch-ups as the day goes by to tone down excessive shine. The trick is to apply it in sheer layers so you don't look overdone.

TYPES OF POWDER

Loose powder and pressed powder: Loose powder is exactly what the name suggests. It tends to provide a sheerer, light application and can be best for someone with normal to oily skin. Pressed powder is merely loose powder with added waxes, binding agents, or emollients to keep the powder in a solid form. While pressed powder is heavier than loose powder, it is more convenient and a lot less messy. Both loose and pressed powders are perfectly fine options and it is a matter of personal preference which you use. What is essential, though, is to choose a powder that is the same color as your foundation. If your powder is lighter than your foundation, you can end up looking pasty and pale; if your powder is darker, you will look like you're wearing a mask.

Pressed powder with sunscreen: A few cosmetics lines, including Paula's Choice, Jane Iredale, Neutrogena, Stila, and Chanel, offer pressed powders that contain effective sunscreens. These powders are nearly identical to regular pressed powders except that they have a slightly thicker texture and provide more substantial coverage, along with an SPF 15 or greater, and include UVA-protecting ingredients, the most typically used being titanium dioxide and/or zinc oxide. Because sunscreens must be applied liberally to ensure sun protection, I generally do not recommend relying on pressed powders with sunscreen as your sole source of UV protection. Most women simply would not use enough of the powder to get the designated SPF number, and overpowdering is not an attractive option. Therefore, pressed powders with effective sunscreens are an excellent way to add to the UV protection you get from your sunscreen or foundation with sunscreen, particularly for those with oily skin. For longer days in the sun or times when it is not feasible to redo your makeup to maintain sun protection, pressed powders with sunscreen can be very convenient and extremely practical.

Talc is the basic element in almost all loose and pressed powders, but some companies opt to use mica (which lends a shiny finish), cornstarch, or rice starch (both starches have a light but very dry feel). Keep in mind that using powders made from corn or rice is not the best option if you're prone to breakouts. The bacteria that cause acne thrive on food ingredients like this, so why would you give something you don't want (blemish-causing bacteria) what it needs to survive?

Application: Apply the powder with a large (but not too large), full, round brush. Avoid using a sponge or powder puff, which can put too much powder onto the face. Pick up some of the powder on the full end of the brush, knock off the excess, and brush it on using the same motion and direction as you did for the foundation. Apply everything in the same direction to help retain a smooth appearance.

If you are touching up your makeup later in the day, before powdering, use your sponge, a facial tissue, or oil-blotting paper to dab away excess oil from the face. Then apply the powder.

Some makeup artists use a powder puff to press the powder into the skin for a very flat, matte finish. As professional a touch as this may be, it is best only for photographs. A powder puff places too much powder on the skin and the result can look thick and heavy in real life. Powdering with a makeup sponge has the same effect as using a powder puff, although the pores of the sponge do allow for a slightly less matte look. However, this can still lay too much powder on the skin.

Pros: If you want to reduce shine or moisture on the face, powdering is the fastest, easiest way to get the job done. Sans foundation, powder can lend a polished, sophisticated look to the skin.

Cons: There are really no drawbacks to wearing powder, but cautions exist: Don't overdo it, use the wrong color, or build up too much powder on the skin via frequent touch-ups.

Powder with shine: If you want to use something to make the skin look luminescent and shiny, one of the best ways to do this is with powder that has shine. Apply this after your foundation and regular powder, and only dust it over the areas you want to glow, such as the cheeks, chin, center of the forehead, shoulders, neck, and décolletage. Most makeup lines offer at least one shiny powder, and some lines offer several. If you want to try a shiny powder, be sure to check the finish in daylight so you can really see how shiny it is and decide if this is the look you had in mind. The best look is a soft, low-glow shimmer rather than obvious sparkles or, even more obvious, flecks of glitter.

TALC IN FACE POWDERS: FRIEND OR FOE?

Talc is often maligned as an awful cosmetic ingredient that should be avoided, but I do not agree in the least with that assessment when it comes to makeup products. The concern about talc is not about how it is used in makeup, but, rather, when it is used in pure, large concentrations in the form of talcum powder. Part of the story here dates back to several studies published in the '90s that found a significant increase in the risk of ovarian cancer from vaginal (perineal) application of talcum powder. (Sources: *International Journal of Cancer*, May 1999, pages 351–356; *Seminars in Oncology*, June 1998, pages 255–264; *Cancer*, June 1997, pages 2396–2401; and *American Journal of Epidemiology*, March 1997, pages 459–465.)

However, subsequent and concurring studies have cast doubt on the way these studies were conducted and the conclusions they reached. (Sources: *American Journal of Obstetrics and Gynecology*, March 2000, pages 720–724; *Journal of the National Cancer Institute*, February 2000, pages 249–252; and *Obstetrics and Gynecology*, March 1999, pages 372–376.)

None of the research about the use of talc is related to the way women use makeup. There is no indication anywhere that there is any risk for the face when using products that contain talc. That means you need not avoid using eyeshadows, blushes, or face powders that contain talc. But it absolutely means you should consider never using talcum powder on your children or on yourself in the vaginal area. If you still wish to avoid talc in makeup, it is easy enough to do so simply by checking the ingredient list.

MINERAL MAKEUP

Mineral makeup is such a sizzling, overly hyped, hot topic that it deserves its own section. Everyone wants to know if it is really the miracle answer for skin. Infomercials glorify its attributes, demonstrating magic results with a swift, brushed-on applications, and there are online chat rooms dedicated to the topic. With all this buzz it's no wonder that cosmetics companies of all sizes are creating their own versions as they jump on the mineral makeup bandwagon.

When all is said and done, mineral makeup is truly nothing all that revolutionary or even fail-safe. The claims are so inane it's plain that they are nothing more than fabrication and lies. It is nothing less than bizarre that they have garnered so much attention from the consumer. Because, by any name, "mineral makeup" is simply a type of powder foundation. If you wear a light layer it is a finishing powder; if you put a little more on it works more like a layer of foundation, providing light to medium coverage. In essence, mineral makeup is merely loose or pressed powder created from a blend of "powdery" substances.

While the minerals in many mineral makeup products are not the standard run of the mill, it is important to know that most pressed powders, whether they are called mineral makeup or not, are made of minerals. Talc is the primary ingredient in most standard powders, and talc, most assuredly, is as natural a mineral as you can get. However, the clamor over "mineral makeup" argues that the minerals being used in those special products are unique, natural, and far better for skin, and that is absolutely not the case!

The claims for mineral makeup, more than for any other makeup product, revolve around what it does not contain, rather than what it does. The companies that sell mineral makeup often warn consumers about how other companies' loose or pressed powders are tainted by the presence of talc (even though it's a natural earth mineral), fragrance, fillers, and "harsh chemical dyes," and that is also not true. According to most of the catalogs and Web sites selling mineral makeup I've seen, they all want you to believe that theirs is the ideal product, and that it contains only the good and none of the "bad," while simultaneously being the perfect choice for every skin type and skin-care problem or concern.

Here is what you need to know: Of the more popular mineral makeup lines—such as Bare Escentuals, Jane Iredale, Monave, Larenim, Baresense, Sheer Cover, Glominerals, Pur Minerals, Emani, Colorflo, Skin Alison Raffaele, Aromaleigh, Colorscience, Neutrogena, L'Oreal, and Everyday Minerals, and whether their powder is pressed or loose powder—almost all of them tend to contain the same basic ingredients: bismuth oxychloride, mica, titanium dioxide, and zinc oxide.

The standard primary ingredient in most mineral makeups is bismuth oxychloride, which is not found in nature and is not any better for skin than talc. In fact, talc is natural, and in many ways a far more unadulterated and pure ingredient than bismuth oxychloride. Bismuth oxychloride is manufactured by combining bismuth (which rarely occurs in its elemental form in nature), obtained as a by-product of lead and copper metal refining (dregs of the smelting process if you will), with chloride (a compound of chlorine) and water. And the *International Cosmetic Ingredient Dictionary and Handbook* (11th Edition, 2006) lists bismuth oxychloride as a synthetic ingredient. It's used in cosmetics because it has a distinct shimmery, pearlescent appearance and a fine, white powder texture that adheres well to skin. On the downside, bismuth oxychloride is heavier than talc and can look cakey on skin. And for some people, the bismuth and chloride combination can be irritating.

Bismuth itself is a metallic element chemically similar to poisonous arsenic. That is more shocking than it is significant, but it's also the kind of fact that mineral makeup companies use to scare you about the ingredients in other powders not deemed "mineral makeup." Just like cosmetic-grade mineral oil is not related to the crude petroleum from which it originates, neither is bismuth oxychloride identical to bismuth, and therefore, its association to arsenic is irrelevant. So the bismuth oxychloride used in cosmetics is indeed non-toxic. This is just a good example of how skewed a company's definition of "natural" can be, and how companies twist factual information to make other cosmetics companies' ingredients sound harmful.

It is interesting to note that bismuth oxychloride can cause skin irritation (Source: www.sciencelab.com/xMSDS-Bismuth_oxychloride-9923103). Although talc has the same potential for slight irritation, bismuth oxychloride is more likely to cause an allergic contact dermatitis because of its pearlescent nature (Source: www.emedicine.com/derm/topic502.htm). This is more of a concern when bismuth oxychloride is the main ingredient in a cosmetic, as it is for many mineral makeups.

Companies that sell mineral makeup (that is, mineral makeup that does not contain talc) often claim that the talc other companies use in their pressed and loose powders is harmful and carcinogenic. Let me assure you that there is absolutely no research to support that hysteria—far from it. A comprehensive review of several studies in *Regulatory Toxicology and Pharmacology* (August 2002, pages 40–50) notes that "Talc is not genotoxic, is not carcinogenic when injected into ovaries of rats. There is no credible evidence of a cancer risk from inhalation of cosmetic talc by humans."

Dismissing talc as a cheap, inelegant, less desirable, or filler material is inaccurate because talc is in fact the essential backbone for a number of the most luxurious-feeling powders from dozens of lines ranging from L'Oreal to Chanel. The best among those powders have a softness and virtually seamless finish on the skin that most mineral makeup lines should envy. The higher grades of talc are not "filler" materials, they are essential to creating a powder's gossamer texture and skin-like finish.

Some mineral makeup powders contain a 25% concentration of titanium dioxide and/or zinc oxide for sunscreen protection, and that's great because these are excellent non-irritating sunscreen ingredients. (Sources: *Cutis*, September 2004, pages 13–16 and 32–34; and *Cosmetics & Toiletries*, October 2003, pages 73–78.)

Most, but definitely not all, mineral makeups provide opaque coverage (which can be blended to achieve light to medium coverage), yet the claim is that they do so while looking extremely natural, like a second skin or better than your own skin. This does appear to be the case in pictures and on TV infomercials (just like every other makeup application created for advertising), but in real life that is not what you will actually see. These powders (most of which are tricky to blend because they tend to "grab" onto skin and don't glide very well once they are in place) can be applied sheer, but the very nature of their ingredients results in a textured application that can look powdery and "made-up" on the skin. This is especially true if you have patches of dry skin because these mineral powders exacerbate dryness and flaking, despite the fact that many claim to be moisturizing, which is just ludicrous given the properties of all powder materials, which are absorbent, not moisturizing.

For those with oily skin, mineral makeup can pool in pores and look thick and layered just like any powder. Generally speaking, mineral makeup is best for normal to slightly oily skin (meaning no signs of dryness and little to no problem oily areas).

Most of the skin-care attributes ascribed to mineral makeup are due to some tangential research about zinc oxide. There is no question that zinc oxide has healing properties for skin (it is FDA-approved as a skin protectant, and is a common active ingredient in oint-ments to treat diaper rash), but those healing properties have to do with skin whose barrier has been compromised, such as with wounds, ulcers, or rashes. In those cases, zinc oxide facilitates healing (Source: *Wound Repair and Regeneration*, January/February 2007, pages 2–16). But those studies don't use other minerals, such as mica or bismuth oxychloride, or have anything to do with healthy, intact skin. Zinc oxide is definitely a great sunscreen ingredient and protects skin from both UVA and UVB sun damage, with minimal to no risk of irritation, and that has immense value. But that can be said of any product that contains enough zinc oxide to earn a decent SPF rating.

Mineral makeup is often recommended for those with rosacea, but the irritation potential from bismuth oxychloride is something to pay attention to. Many women may have success using powder as a foundation, and mineral makeup is included in this category. Mineral makeup, especially those rated SPF 15 or greater, can be a three-in-one product (founda-tion/powder/sunscreen) that can be somewhat easy to apply once you get the knack of it, but it is not a slam-dunk or panacea for all skin types.

One word of warning: As is true for any product with an SPF rating, to get the right amount to ensure thorough protection, liberal application is essential. And that means a sheer, light layer of mineral makeup, no matter its SPF rating, won't provide your skin with enough protection from the sun.

POWDER MISTAKES TO AVOID

1. Never buy powder without testing it over your foundation first. Even if the powder is translucent, it always has some amount of color to it, and that color and its extra texture over the skin can greatly affect the appearance of your foundation. Powder should match the color of your skin (and foundation) and not change the color of either.
2. Never powder with a white, orange, pink, or coral shade of powder; it will make you look either pale or overly made-up.
3. To help prevent a caked appearance don't forget to dab any excess oil from the face before you apply your powder during the day to touch up your makeup.
4. Do not apply more than the sheerest layer necessary to take away excess shine; the face can handle only so much powder before it starts looking thick and heavy.
5. Do not powder more than necessary during the day. Powder only once or twice a day to prevent buildup, even if you are using a pressed powder with sunscreen.

EYESHADOW

I've been watching and evaluating other makeup artists and their eyeshadow techniques for years. Though there are myriad alternatives, eyeshadow design is usually built on an application sequence that allows you to create a flow of colors in either one, two, three, or four steps. The four steps involve applying a succession of colors that can be anything you want them to be. But if your goal is a classic makeup application, the colors proceed gradually from light to darker. The basic technique is to apply the lightest shade either just on the eyelid or all over the entire eye area (including the crease and up under the eyebrow) and then to place each progressively darker shade in a more specific section of the eye area, such as the crease and/or the back corner of the eye.

TYPES OF EYESHADOW

Aside from powder eyeshadows, which are by far the most common type, other types available include liquids, pencils, cream-to-powder, and creams. Though these can be fun and easy to use, they are often hard to blend and control. Makeup artists rarely, if ever, use the liquids or pencils, though some opt for creams as a change of pace from powder eyeshadows. Overall, I don't recommend them over powder eyeshadows. I admit they're fun, but I just wish they worked better to create a more sophisticated blend of colors. Almost without exception, cream eyeshadows crease and fade. They're also not the type to choose if you have trouble making mascara or eyeliner last, because their emollient consistency can cause smearing and smudging of these other products. If you're curious to try some non-powder eyeshadows, I review the best ones on my Web site, www.Beautypedia.com.

USING BRUSHES TO APPLY EYESHADOW

Eyeshadow should be applied exclusively with brushes, and it's best to use brushes that are designed specifically for eyeshadow. Never use sponge-tip applicators—they drag across the eye and tend to blend colors in streaks. Once you get used to good brushes, you will never go back to the sponge-tip applicators again.

When applying eyeshadow, use the flat side of the brush against the eye. Gently wipe the brush across the eyeshadow, tap the excess off the brush, and apply it with long, stroking motions across the eyelid, crease, or under the eyebrow area. This motion of laying strips of color that overlap and blend together over the eye as opposed to beating the brush back and forth across the eye is the way to achieve an even, well-blended design.

Remember that the size of the brush should match the size of the eye area you are working on. If you have a large eyelid area, use a brush that is wide and full. If your eyelid is small, use a smaller brush that's the same width as the lid. The same rule is true for the crease area (if a specific color is being placed just there) and the under-eyebrow area. Using brushes that match the job is essential to applying makeup effectively and efficiently. Do not purchase or use brushes that have hard, coarse bristles or you will end up with hard edges where the eyeshadow can't be blended, not to mention irritated skin.

DESIGNING THE EYE MAKEUP

Keep this fact in mind: The most beautiful makeup applications, the ones you see and admire the most on models and actresses, are neutral, not colorful. Look at any fashion magazine. You're not going to see pastel or vivid eyeshadows on many faces, unless it's a purposely eccentric or bizarre montage. Too many competing pastel or vividly colored shadows make the eye design distracting. Pastel and primary colors (green, blue, red) are hard to blend together, so they stand out. Besides, the general purpose of eyeshadows is to shape and shade the eye, not color it. The only way to shape the eye is by shading it with neutral shades such as taupe, brown, gray, ash, beige, tan, mahogany, redwood, caramel, sable, charcoal, and black. Eyeshadows are called *shadows* for a reason—they build shape, movement, and interest via shading, not with color.

The list of appropriately neutral colors and tones available is actually quite extensive. Yet color on the eyelid is best kept as subtle as possible, or you will end up creating an eye makeup design that is more noticeable than your eye. As a general rule, for a classically applied makeup, the lips and cheeks provide color on the face. More color standing out around the eyes can be overkill.

Be cautious about thinking you need to choose a design based on the need to correct a perceived facial problem, such as your eyes being too close together, too far apart, too round, or not round enough. There are no standard facial dimensions that define how attractive you or your eyes are. You can end up with a contrived look that allows the makeup to be more noticeable than your eyes.

The best way to choose which design to wear is to decide what image you want to project. The more shading you use, the more dramatic and formal the eye makeup design; the less shading, the more subtle and casual the design. Other considerations when choosing one eye-makeup design over another involve your skill at applying makeup, your personal preference, and the amount of time you want (or have) to spend. For example, if you are new or unaccustomed to wearing makeup, keep your entire makeup look simple until you become adept at the different application techniques. The same thing goes if you have only a few minutes in the morning to put your makeup on—it is best to keep your routine simple. Trying to apply full makeup very quickly can result in mistakes or a sloppy application.

APPLYING AN EYE-MAKEUP DESIGN

Options for building an eye design are almost too numerous to list. The basic concept is to shade the eye to accent its shape, or to change its shape by using a progression of light to dark colors across the eye, blending one over the other so that you can't see where one stops and another starts. Here I will explain, step by step, how you can use one eyeshadow or several different eyeshadows to create a well-blended, classic eye-makeup design. Even for the most formal eye-makeup design, four different colors should be plenty. Whether you use one, two, three, or four different eyeshadows, they become a full design when worn with eyeliner, temple contour (see the "Contouring" section later in this chapter), and mascara.

One-color eye-makeup design: This design blends one soft, subtle color all over the eye area, from the lashes to just under the eyebrow, with no patches of skin showing through. You should not wear only a splash of color over the eyelid and ignore the rest of the eye area.

Application: When applying a single color, first place it from the lashes to the crease, making sure that you do not extend the color into the inside corner of the eye (off the lid area) or out beyond the lid onto the temple. Also be certain there are no patches of skin showing through on the lid next to the eyelashes. The entire lid at this point is one solid color.

Next, place the color from the crease up to the brow, following the entire length of the eyebrow from the nose out to the temple area. Avoid leaving a hard edge at the back (outside) corner of the eye where the eyeshadow stops. If desired, fade the eyeshadow as you blend up and out from the crease. This will create subtlety and a soft highlight under the eyebrow. Because the eyeshadow for the one-color eye-makeup design is so soft and subtle, blending and application is quite easy. The best colors for this design include light tan, neutral taupe, beige, pale mauve brown, pale gray, light golden brown, camel, and light auburn. Whatever the color, it should definitely not be obvious.

Two-color eye-makeup design: This is one of the most common, practical eye designs for many women. You can approach this design by applying the lighter color to the eyelid and the deeper color from the crease up to the brow, or you can apply the deeper color to the lid and the lighter color from the crease to the brow. Generally speaking, the under-eyebrow color should be a shade or two darker than the lid color. You do not want it to be a distinctly different color, just a different shade. The lid can be taupe, beige, tan, camel, gray, light auburn, golden brown, or any light neutral shade, and the under-eyebrow color would be a deeper shade of the same color. Women with darker skin tones can wear muted rose, mauve, or peach as long as it doesn't make their eyes look irritated or isn't too obvious. Bright, shiny, or whitish shadows can look dated and make the brow bone look more prominent and heavy.

Which color and what shades go where? The general rule is that the larger or more prominent the eyelid area is compared with the under-brow area, the darker or deeper the eyelid color can be; the smaller the eyelid area is compared with the under-brow area, the brighter or lighter the eyelid color can be. The notion is that if the eyelid area is already prominent or large, it isn't necessary to make it appear any bigger by applying a light color to it. If the eyelid area is small, it is appropriate to make it more prominent by wearing a lighter color.

Application: Whichever way you choose to apply this design, the lid and under-brow shades should meet—but not overlap—at the crease. As an option for the two-color eye-makeup design, you can apply the light shade to the lid and the darker shade from the crease up to the brow. Then, using a small wedge brush, you can use the light color again as a highlight just along the lower edge of the eyebrow. This can bring dramatic, but subtle, attention to the shape of the brow and the eye without the need for another eyeshadow color. You can also apply the lighter color from the lid to the under-brow area and use the darker color in and slightly above the crease. Then take the brush and use the darker color to softly shade the back corner of the eye, being sure this shading is an extension of the crease color. For more dramatic variations on this theme, see the descriptions below.

Three-color eye-makeup design: Start by applying either of the two-color eye-makeup designs mentioned above. Once you have done that, the third shade, an even deeper color than the two previous colors, is added to the back (outside) corner of the lid or in the crease, or over both the crease and the back corner of the lid.

In this design, the lid and under-brow colors are softer and less intense than the color at the back corner of the lid or in the crease. Regardless of where you place this third, darker color, it can be a beautiful deep shade of brown, charcoal, cedar, mahogany, sable, red-brown, slate, chocolate brown, camel, deep taupe, or even black.

Application: If you apply the third eyeshadow in the crease, the trick is to not get the crease color on the lid, but rather to blend it slightly up into the under-eyebrow area and out onto the temple. When sweeping the crease color across the eye, be sure to not follow the down-curving movement of the shape of the eye. The best look is achieved if you blend the crease color out and up into the full back (outer) corner of the eye, and up onto the back of the brow bone.

When you apply the crease color, be sure to watch the angle of your brush as you blend the color from the crease out and up toward the under-brow area. If you place your color with the brush straight up at a 90-degree angle, you will look like you drew on wings. The softer the angle and the fuller the sweep, the softer the appearance, so be certain you blend *out* and slightly *up* from the lid area toward the under-brow area.

If you apply the third color at the back corner of the eye, the color hugs a small section of the lid, blending out and up into the crease and temple area. I explain this step in more detail for the four-color eye-makeup design.

Four-color eye-makeup design: In this design, you again start with the two-color eye-makeup design, then add a darker color to the crease and an even darker color such as black or deepest gray to the back corner of the eye. Shading the back corner of the eyelid involves the arts of placement and blending. Because this area almost always requires a dark color, blending is essential to make it look soft, with no hard edges.

Why bother with a crease color and more shading at the back corner of the eye? The best part of this full eye-makeup design is that it shades, defines, and creates movement by adding a shadow in a curved, flowing motion that follows the natural shape of the eye. The difficult part of this design is blending the crease color across the entire length of the eye without making it look obvious, choppy, or smeared. The goal is to tuck the color just in the crease at the fold nearest the nose and have it hug the crease until you get to the back corner of the eye, where you start the movement of the eyeshadow up and out onto the brow bone. Again, this sweep of color should not look like a stripe across the eye.

Application: Be sure to tap the excess eyeshadow off your brush, and apply the color with very small strokes over the back corner of the lid only. The problem here is keeping the color on the back of the lid only. If you don't know how to handle the brush, the back wedge can take up more than half of the eyelid (looking more like a mistake rather than carefully blended shading) or look like a stripe across the temple.

As mentioned above, when you apply the crease color, be sure to watch the angle of your brush as you blend the color from the crease out and up toward the under-brow area. If you place your color with the brush straight up at a 90-degree angle, you will look like you drew on wings. The softer the angle and the fuller the sweep, the softer the appearance, so be certain you blend out and slightly up from the lid area toward the under-eyebrow area.

Remember, the center or fold of the crease area is always the darkest, so start your brush there and blend out in each direction. Concentrate your efforts on how much of the crease area you want to shade. You can start all the way at the front part of the eye area under the front third of the brow, then follow the crease through the center, blending slightly up toward the brow. As you approach the back corner of the eye, begin your movement up and out toward the temple, aiming toward the eyebrow.

EYESHADOW TIPS

1. Matte powder eyeshadows in an array of neutral tones from light to dark are your best bets for a classic, sophisticated eye design that accents the shape and color of your eyes.
2. Unless you're using just one eyeshadow color, use at least two eyeshadow brushes for application.
3. Prime the eyelid and under-brow area with a matte-finish concealer, foundation, and/or powder before you apply eyeshadow. This helps to ensure a smooth, even application and (if you have fair to medium skin) will also neutralize the red and blue coloration of the eyelid.
4. Tap off any excess eyeshadow from your brush before applying—this will prevent overapplication as well as flaking eyeshadow.
5. If you really want to make the color of your eyes pop, choose a contrasting color in a soft tone and apply this to the lids. Blue eyes come alive with pale peach or cantaloupe hues, green eyes seem richer with light bronze or caramel tones, hazel eyes become more alluring with chestnut and golden brown shades, and brown eyes are nicely accented by almost all neutral tones.

EYE-DESIGN MISTAKES TO AVOID

1. Do not overcolor the eyes; too many bright colors can be distracting, not attractive.
2. Do not create hard edges; you should not be able to see where one color stops and another starts. Practice your application and blend well!
3. Do not wear bright pink or iridescent pink eyeshadows; they make eyes look irritated and tired. Muted or pale pink is an option, but be very, very careful. If it makes the eye look irritated or "red," it isn't the color for you.
4. Do not wear shiny eyeshadows of any kind if you are concerned about making the skin look more wrinkled because they exaggerate the appearance of lines. If you have smooth, unlined eyelids and prefer a touch of shine, apply it sparingly and look for a low-wattage glow instead of distracting glitter.
5. Do not apply lipstick or blush over the eye area; it might sound like a time-saver, but if you have a lighter skin tone, it can make you look like you've been up all night crying. However, most bronzing powders can work as eyeshadows.
6. Do not match your eyeshadow to your clothing or your eye color. If you have blue eyes, blue eyeshadow would make the blue of your eyes look duller. And complementing your clothing is at best dated; besides, what do you do if you're wearing red or black?

7. Unless your goal is short-lived, messy eye makeup, avoid eye glosses and other greasy colors at all costs. These may look intriguing in photographs, but are more annoying than alluring in real life because they smear and smudge all over the place in a very short period of time.

EYELINER

Eyeliner is a basic part of an eye-makeup design because it shapes and defines the eyes and makes the eyelashes look thicker. If you are wearing only mascara and not eyeshadow, or if you want an extremely soft look, eyeliner is not necessary. If you do decide to wear eyeliner when you are wearing mascara and no eyeshadow, be sure to line the eyes with only a very soft, well-blended eyeshadow color.

As with most aspects of makeup, eyeliner presents a host of options. There are eye pencils (both traditional and chunky), liquid liners, gel eyeliners, cake eyeliners, and powder eyeliners. When it comes to colors, what used to be a simple choice of black or brown has morphed into a range of hues that can be overwhelming. Depending on the look you're after and your personal taste, the color of your eyeliner can be anything from crimson to silver to gold, bronze, or even olive green. Although I strongly suggest staying with tried-and-true colors like black, brown, and gray, the final decision is yours.

TYPES OF EYELINER

What kind of eyeliner should you use? Eye pencils are a quick, convenient option, but they do have problems; many tend to smear or fade, and unless you are using a twist-up pencil they are tricky to keep sharpened.

For years my favorite option for applying a line was to use a tiny eyeliner brush with an appropriate color of traditional eyeshadow powder. Nowadays, I am very fond of the long-wearing gel eyeliners offered by many cosmetics lines, including mine. If you opt to use powder, I recommend using a dark-toned, matte eyeshadow color (almost any medium to deep eyeshadow color can work) and a tiny brush. I often apply the eyeshadow by wetting the brush and using it as "liquid" liner. The application is more controlled, but once it dries you have the soft look and the staying power of a powder without the hard edge that liquid eyeliners can create. A tiny, thin eyeliner brush allows absolute control over the thickness of the line around the eye.

Pencil eyeliners can often work well if you follow these basic rules:
- Self-sharpening pencils are by far the product of choice. Sharpening regular eye pencils is difficult, and keeping the point sharp without chewing up the pencil can be tricky.
- Remember that not all automatic pencils have a wind-down feature. That means if you wind the tip of the pencil up too high, it cannot be retracted and will likely break off.
- It is easier to apply pencil along the lower lashes than along the upper lid because the eyeshadows on the lid are harder for the pencil to stick to. You may want to

consider using a greasy pencil for the lid and a firmer, less greasy pencil for the lower lashes. (If a pencil flattens when you press it, it will blend on more easily—but also will tend to smear more easily.)

- Warm the pencil between your fingers to apply a softer line of color; just remember this is not a surefire way to get a smooth application.
- To get a more precise line, if you have the time, leave the pencil in the freezer for a minute or two.
- Apply matching or similar powder eyeshadow over pencil to get the best of both worlds.

Liquid eyeliner, in general, is the most dramatic option, and when applied correctly (meaning a well-controlled, even line with no patches of skin showing through) it can definitely have an impact! However, getting the application right is more than half the battle with liquid liners. Even those who have well-tapered and firm but flexible brushes can find it difficult to control and apply evenly to both eyes. Yet if you're intent on trying a liquid liner, the easiest (and I use this term loosely) way to apply it is after your eyeshadow design is done and before mascara. Do not blink excessively or touch your eye until you're sure the liner has dried. For best results, liquid liner should be used only on the upper lash-line. Powder eyeliner is a softer choice for the lower lash-line, and you will lose none of the oomph that comes with well-applied liquid liner. Make sure the liners meet at the outer corner of the eye.

Powder eyeliner can be applied with almost any eyeshadow you have, but by far the best products for this are those from Bobbi Brown, L'Oreal, M.A.C., Trish McEvoy, and Shu Uemura. Choose a dark shade of eyeshadow. Always line the eyes last—after all the other eyeshadows have been applied. Use a tiny, thin, slightly stiff brush. Whether you use your powder wet or dry (both are fine, dry is softer, wet is more dramatic), stroke the brush through the color, keeping the bristles together. Do not dab or rub the brush into the color. Move the brush across the eyeshadow in the direction of the bristles, making sure the form of the brush is not destroyed. Tap the excess color from the brush, then apply the color to the eyelid next to the lashes and under the eye near the lower lashes.

Gel eyeliner is similar to liquid liners in almost every respect, except that it is easier to apply and control—and the best ones offer the longest, most foolproof wear of any type of eyeliner. I was resistant to trying this type of eyeliner, but once I did it quickly became a favorite. Gel eyeliners are the only way to go if you have oily eyelids or have had difficulty getting various eye pencils or powders to last and remain neatly applied. Several major lines offer gel eyeliners, including L'Oreal, Bobbi Brown, Stila, M.A.C., and Paula's Choice.

Cake eyeliner has been around for years and most of us have either seen or tried it at some point. Compared to a well-pigmented powder eyeshadow or even a standard liquid liner, cake eyeliner is more of an antiquated choice that has no distinct advantages over other types of eyeliners. If you're a devoted user of cake liner and like the results, stick with it. Otherwise, I encourage you to try other types of liner before considering this one to achieve a softer look with more options for neutral color choices.

APPLYING EYELINER

Assuming you have a steady hand (if not, try this sitting down so you can steady your arm by placing your elbow on a table), position the brush, pencil, or applicator so it is as close to the lash-line along the eyelid as possible. Then draw a line from the inner to outer corner using one fluid stroke, following the curvature of the eyelid. Do not extend the line past the outer corner of the eye or hug the tear duct area of the eye. To start, keep the line as thin as possible, and if a thicker line is desired, repeat the process either across the entire lash-line or simply on the outer third of the lid along the lashes. Making the line along the eyelid a solid, even one, starting thin at the front third of the lid and becoming slightly thicker at the back third of the lid can be an attractive, classic look.

You can line all the way across the eyelid if you like, from the inside corner to the outer edge, or you can stop the line where the lashes stop and start. Along the lower lashes, line only the outer two-thirds of the eye. Be sure the lower liner is a less-intense color than the upper liner. Also make sure that the two lines meet at the back corner of the eye. As a general rule, avoid lining all the way across the lower eyelashes. Leaving some space on the inside corner of the eye where the lashes end near the tear ducts gives a softer, less severe look. Plus, wrapping a complete circle of eyeliner around the eye tends to create an eyeglasses look and can make the eyeliner a stronger statement than the eye itself.

Makeup artists sometimes recommend that women over 40 not line the inner corner of the eye either on top or on the bottom. I think that's a fine suggestion. Instead, highlighting this area with a light shade of matte eyeshadow can be a very attractive alternative.

How thickly should you line the eye? As a general rule, for a classic look, the thickness and intensity of the eyeliner is determined by the size of the lid—the larger the eyelid area, the thicker and softer the eyeliner should be. The smaller the eyelid area, the thinner and more intense the liner should be. If your lid doesn't show at all, forget lining altogether.

You may have seen or heard a dozen other ideas as to how to apply eyeliner. Halfway across the lid, or one-third, or one-fourth, and three-fourths of the way under the lower eyelashes, or one-third, or one-fourth, and on and on. You are more than welcome to experiment with all these placements, but I encourage you to try the classic way first and see how you like it. Because the major reason to wear eyeliner is to shape the eye and make the eyelashes look thicker and deeper, I believe it is important to line where the lashes are and not just arbitrary sections of the lid.

What about applying eyeliner in the rim of the eye? There are many reasons why this is not a good idea. The first is that this kind of application smears in a very short period of time and creates goopy dark specks in the eye. Applying any makeup that is destined to smear in less than an hour or two is not a good idea. Pencil applied along the rim of the eye usually causes the area to become irritated; after all you are putting a foreign substance next to the mucous membrane of your eye. I am equally concerned about the health of the eye area when this technique is used. While there are no studies indicating there are any risks associated with pencil being applied to the rim of the eye, it seems problematic to put cosmetic ingredients (which include coloring agents and preservatives) that close to the eye.

Which eyeliner color should you use? For a classic eyeliner application, choose shades of dark brown, gray, or black for the upper lid and a softer shade of those—tan, taupe, chestnut, soft brown, soft gray, or soft black—along the lower lashes. Eyeliner is meant to give depth to the lashes and make them appear thicker. If the liner is a bright color or a true pastel, attention will be focused past the lashes to the colored line, as opposed to the more subtle flow of color from dark lashes to dark liner. Test it on yourself. Line one eye with a vibrant color, the other eye with brown or black, and see which one looks like it has thicker lashes. Then, if all my attempts to convince you have failed, and you still prefer to use bright or pastel liners, go for it.

CHECKING FOR MISTAKES

After using powder eyeshadow as eyeliner, check for drippies under the eye and on the cheek. Drippies are those little powder flakes that fly off the brush and land on the cheek. Knocking off the excess from the brush every time helps prevent drippies, but there will always be flakes that end up where they don't belong. The best way to go after drippies is to use your sponge or a cotton swab and simply wipe them away. If you do this, your next step is to touch up your foundation if it has become smeared.

Some makeup artists recommend applying a thicker layer of loose powder under the eyes and onto the upper cheekbone to catch the inevitable drippies, allowing them to be whisked off with a powder brush. If you have relatively smooth, unlined skin in this area you may want to try this. Otherwise, it can make the under-eye area look dry and enhance lines and wrinkles.

Always double-check the intensity of your eyeliner application and blend away any thickness or color that is more dramatic than you intended. It is not possible to blend or correct mistakes with liquid liners, which is one of the reasons I generally don't recommend them. The gel eyeliners have a similar tendency, but you can fix some mistakes if you catch them before the liner sets.

If you do choose to wear pencil eyeliner, check for smears under the eye as the day goes by. This is annoying, but letting it go without blending away the smears can make any well-applied eye-makeup design look like a mess.

EYELINER MISTAKES TO AVOID

1. Do not use greasy or slick pencils to line the lower lashes; they smear and smudge.
2. Do not use brightly colored pencils or eyeshadows to line the eye; they are distracting and automatically look like too much makeup. All you'll see is the color and not your eye.
3. Do not extend the eyeliner beyond the corner of the eye (no wings).
4. Do not make the eyeliner the most obvious part of the eye-makeup design.
5. Do not line the inside rim of the lids, between the lash and the eye itself; it is messy and can be unhealthy for the cornea.
6. If you do use pencil to line the eye, apply a small amount of eyeshadow over your pencil eyeliner to help set it and keep it from smearing.

7. Do not apply a thick line to small or close-set eyes.
8. Do not use eyeshadow as eyeliner unless you use the proper brush.
9. Do not line the eye with a circle of dark or bright color. Both are too obvious and create an eyeglass-style circle around the eye.
10. Do not overblend, spilling your eyeliner onto the skin under the lower lashes; it makes dark circles look worse.

MASCARA

Mascara is an amazing invention and is considered basic to any kind of makeup application. Many makeup artists, including myself, say that if you're not wearing any other makeup but still want to wear something, wear mascara. On the other hand, many of us—and I'm guilty of this, too—get carried away and wear way too much mascara.

Women overdo mascara in part because the cosmetics industry tells us loudly and clearly that long, thick lashes are to be coveted, but even unadvised we can covet someone else's long, beautiful lashes. When we apply mascara, visions of longer, thicker lashes sometimes come into view and then we get carried away and decide to apply more and more. Unfortunately, applying too much mascara increases the chances that the mascara will flake, chip, or smear, and that the lashes will appear hard and spiked. Also, the eyelashes can take only so much weight, and excess weight can break them. Lashes gunked-up with tons of mascara do not resemble long, thick lashes—they resemble gunked-up lashes!

The desire for longer, more noticeable lashes brings up the image of that ever-popular device that curls the lashes by squeezing them into a bent-upward shape. The problem with curling lashes is that it can bend the lashes into a severe angle that can look unnatural; and, although it can make them more noticeable (sometimes in an odd sort of way), it can also end up breaking them and pulling them out. Doesn't that defeat the purpose of making your lashes look longer? If you're still gung-ho on doing this, curl lashes only before you apply mascara, never after, or you will end up with broken, strangely bent lashes. The best lash-curlers are the ones with a sponge-tip section where the eyelashes are squeezed for protection. Squeeze gently with even pressure. Hold for a few seconds as you "walk" the curler along the length of the eyelashes, and release slowly. Some fashion magazines recommend heating the rubber pad of the eyelash curler by running your blow dryer over it for a few seconds. This may be worth trying, but be extremely cautious that the pad does not get too hot (touch it with your finger to be sure) because you don't want to fry fragile lashes or burn the eyelid skin.

TYPES OF MASCARA

Mascara comes in two basic types: waterproof and water-soluble. Mascaras should not smudge, flake, or clump, and it is not your fault if they do. As is true for every aspect of the cosmetics industry, price does not tell you anything about how well a mascara performs. Drugstore mascaras can be as good as the more-expensive department-store brands, and sometimes even better. Regardless of where you buy your mascara, you might find that it already seems dried up the first time you open it. This is a recurring problem in the cosmetics world. Take it back immediately and get a refund or another tube.

Because there are two types of mascara available, the one you choose should be based on your needs, both in terms of personal preference and where you'll wear it.

Water-soluble mascaras: This type of mascara is the most common. A great water-soluble mascara should go on beautifully and wash away easily. The problem with some water-soluble mascaras is that they don't come off all that easily with water, even though they should.

Waterproof mascaras: This type of mascara is, as the name states, waterproof. Waterproof mascaras cause problems because to remove them you usually need to pull and wipe at the eyes, which can pull out lashes. I understand the desire to go swimming while wearing your makeup, or to cry at weddings and not have mascara streaming down your cheeks, especially if you're the bride! Waterproof mascara is fine for occasional use, but wearing it every day can cause more headaches in the long run. Another drawback is that although most waterproof mascaras hold up well under water, they can still break down and smear when they meet the oil from your skin or emollients from your moisturizer or foundation. Do not make the mistake of thinking that waterproof means smearproof.

For those times when you do need waterproof mascara, the most effective way to remove it is with a silicone-based makeup remover that won't leave a greasy film on the skin. To be as gentle as possible, soak a cotton pad with the remover and lightly press and hold this against your lashes (make sure the eye is closed) for a few seconds. This helps loosen the mascara from lashes. Using very light pressure, move the pad down over the lashes and then back and forth, paying close attention not to pull or tug the skin. You can perform this step before or after cleansing.

APPLYING MASCARA

The traditional upper-lash application, made by rotating the mascara wand as you round-brush from the base of the lashes up to cover all the lashes around the entire eye is the most efficient, expedient method. Keep an old, cleaned-up mascara wand in your makeup bag to use for removing occasional mascara clumps (it can happen with the best mascaras) and separating lashes.

Apply mascara to the lower lashes by holding the wand perpendicular to the eye and parallel to the lashes (using the tip of the wand). This prevents you from getting mascara on the cheek. It also makes it easier to reach the lashes at both ends of the eye. If you want a softer application on the lower lashes, wipe the wand down with a tissue and then apply lightly.

Have you ever had mascara end up on the eyelid or under the eye while you're applying it? Wait until it dries completely and then chip it away with a cotton swab or your sponge. Most of it will just flake off, with very little repair work needed. Always check for mascara smudges; they can look very sloppy and distracting.

FALSE EYELASHES

Although I am not a fan of false eyelashes (primarily because you can almost always tell that they're fake), I realize that many makeup artists love to use them, and because they do, women wonder if they should try them, either to be doing the "proper thing" or for fun. Basically, false lashes are available in full sets or as individual lashes. Application always involves the use of an adhesive gel (such as Duo) and must be precise if you want the effect to look convincing. Removing false eyelashes can also be tricky, not to mention hazardous to your real lashes. Remember, there are lots of mascaras available that can come pretty close to giving a false-eyelash effect—you may want to experiment with these before ever considering falsies.

MASCARA MISTAKES TO AVOID

1. Do not wear colored mascara such as blue, purple, or green if you're going for a classic daytime look.
2. Do not wear mascara that smears or flakes; don't put up with those that do, because there are lots that don't.
3. Do not use waterproof mascaras on a daily basis; they can be difficult to remove and hard on fragile eyelashes.
4. Do not overapply mascara; your lashes will look clumpy or like thick-barred windows.

EYE MAKEUP—IS IT SAFE?

Mascara, eyeshadow, and eyeliner are intended to make women more attractive. One thing they shouldn't do is harm the eyes! Yet each year, many women suffer eye infections from cosmetics. At the time of purchase, most eye cosmetics are free from bacteria that could cause eye infections. Problems happen when they aren't adequately preserved against microorganisms or if they are misused by the consumer after being opened. Poor preservation or misuse of an eye cosmetic can allow dangerous bacteria to enter and grow in the product. Then, when the cosmetic is applied to the area around the eye, it can cause an infection.

The Food and Drug Administration has taken numerous steps to make sure that eye cosmetics are free from contamination when they reach you and that they contain preservatives to inhibit the growth of bacteria. The cosmetics industry generally makes products that will not harm you. Nevertheless, the FDA urges you to follow these 11 tips on the use of eye cosmetics.

1. Discontinue immediately the use of any eye product that causes irritation. If irritation persists, see a doctor.
2. Recognize that bacteria on your hands could, if placed in the eye, cause infections. Wash your hands before applying cosmetics to your eyes.
3. Make sure that any instrument you place in the eye area is clean.
4. Do not allow cosmetics to become covered with dust or contaminated with dirt or soil. Wipe off the container with a damp cloth if dust or dirt is visible.

5. Do not use old containers of eye cosmetics. If you haven't used the product for several months, it's better to discard it and purchase a new one.

6. Do not spit into eye cosmetics. The bacteria in your mouth may grow in the cosmetic, and subsequent application to the eye could cause infection.

7. Do not share your cosmetics. Another person's bacteria in your cosmetics can be hazardous to you.

8. Do not store cosmetics at temperatures above 85 degrees Fahrenheit. Cosmetics held for long periods in hot cars, for example, are more susceptible to deterioration of the preservative.

9. Avoid using eye cosmetics if you have an eye infection or if the skin around the eye is inflamed. Wait until the area is healed.

10. Take particular care in using eye cosmetics if you have any allergies.

11. When applying or removing eye cosmetics, be careful not to scratch the eyeball or other sensitive areas.

EYEBROW SHAPING AND SHADING

No aspect of makeup seems to go through such dramatic fashion changes as eyebrow styles. Eyebrows are as representative of each fashion decade as clothes are. We've gone from overtweezed, pencil-thin, tortured brows to overdrawn, thickly penciled brows, to a full, bushy natural look, and now we've settled on very soft, natural, but definitely shaped brows. The best idea is for the eyebrows to be natural in appearance but not bushy or thick, with an expertly defined, but not pointed, arch.

SHAPING THE EYEBROWS

Discovering the best shape for your eyebrows without sacrificing a natural appearance is what you want to accomplish. The eye is framed by the arch, length, and thickness of the eyebrow. Just as the shape of a mustache can change the appearance of a man's face, the shape of the eyebrows can affect the appearance of the eyes. For example, if you tweeze too much off the front part of the eyebrows (near the nose), the eyes will appear smaller. If you tweeze too much from under the eyebrows, increasing the distance between the eye and the eyebrow, you can look permanently surprised.

Which hairs you leave and which ones you remove makes all the difference between attractively shaped brows and misshapen ones. And go slowly—because for some reason, over time, eyebrow hair does not always grow back after it is tweezed (there is no known physiological reason for this, but that is what many women experience). You can use an eyebrow pencil and a diagram to help you line up the following parameters for shaping your eyebrow.

The beginning of the brow should align with the center of the nostril, the arch should fall at the back third of the eye, and, although the eyebrow should be as long as possible, it still shouldn't extend into the temple area. **The basic rule is that the front part of the brow should never drop below the back part of the brow.** Allowing this to happen, either with the way you tweeze your eyebrows or the way you draw them on, makes you look like you're frowning and overemphasizes the downward movement of the back part of the eye.

What are the best tools? The best tweezers are the ones from Revlon or Tweezerman with tips that are slightly rounded to a soft point. Tweezers that are too pointy can stab the skin; if they're too flat across the top they can grab skin along with the hair. There are lots of other tweezers around in all kinds of shapes or with handles that snap together, but these all pose problems when it comes to reliability and ease of use.

STEPS TO SHAPING A PERFECT BROW

1. Before you start tweezing, use a lip or brow pencil to heavily draw on the shape you want; you can adjust it as you decide on the look you want.
2. Once the shape is drawn on, tweeze any hairs that fall outside the line of the brow.
3. Next, brush the brows straight up with an old toothbrush. Any hairs that are too long and floppy should be trimmed with small scissors. Tweezing long brow hairs rather than trimming them can result in gaps in the eyebrow or a patchy look.

TYPES OF EYEBROW PRODUCTS AND APPLICATION

Powder eyebrow colors or eyeshadows used to fill in the brow should be applied using a soft-textured powder (either an eyeshadow or a powder designed for the brow; both work great) that matches the brow color exactly, and a soft wedge brush or a tiny eyeliner brush (I prefer the control of a small eyeliner brush). Follow the basic shape of the brow, using the same guidelines as for tweezing. Fill in only at the front or underneath the brow, or through the brow itself. Avoid drawing on color above the brow. For a softer look, brush through the eyebrows using a clean, old toothbrush.

Eyebrow pencils: These are a perennial option but be careful when deciding which one to use. Eyebrow pencils can produce a greasy, hard look and mat the eyebrow hair, and too often you end up looking like you live in another decade. If you are presently penciling your eyebrows, seriously consider changing to powder. If penciling doesn't look absolutely natural, don't do it. Better to go without any eyebrow makeup at all than to be adorned with a line of pencil above your eye.

Many makeup artists use both pencil and powder to create natural-looking brows for women with little or no eyebrow hair, and this can be a great alternative. This way you can get the control and delineation of a pencil, and then soften and shade the effect with a powder. If you decide to try this, look for brow pencils that have a firm but smooth texture and a slightly powdery finish. Avoid using any brow pencil that is painful or that applies color too dramatically or thickly.

Application: To apply the powdered brow color or brow pencil, brush the brow up with an old toothbrush and then apply the color with an angled wedge brush, filling in the shape of the brow between the hairs where needed. If your eyebrows are set high, away from the eye area, and you want to reshape them, place the color directly under the eyebrow. The closer the brow is to the eye area (meaning the height from the brow to the lid or eyelashes is small), the more you should fill in the color in the existing brow itself rather than shading just below the brow. As much as possible, work only with the hair that is there. The idea is to shade rather than draw on eyebrows. Do not place your brow color, whether it is pencil or powder, more than one-quarter inch away from where the natural hair growth stops. It simply looks fake and accentuates the fact that there is no brow there in the first place! What you want is the suggestion, the shadow of a brow—not a line and not an obvious application of color.

Colored eyebrow gels: These are a good option for making the most of sparse, light-colored eyebrows or for giving a thicker look to most other eyebrows. These products look like mascara but they have a much lighter consistency. Examples are Paula's Choice Brow/Hair Tint and Bobbi Brown Natural Brow Shaper.

Application: Brush the wand through your brows, being careful not to get the product on the forehead or other areas of the skin and not to leave the brows standing straight up. It will probably take you a few times to get the hang of it. You also might have trouble at first controlling the amount of gel from the tube to the brow. But if you want your brows to look fuller, give this one a try—it really works. The products mentioned above have dual-bristled brushes, which can be used for a soft, full look or for more definition. Be wary of brow gels and tints with single- or small-bristled brushes because these can make application trickier (they often produce a lined or spotted effect).

WHAT EYEBROW COLOR SHOULD YOU USE?

Generally, you should match the exact color of the brows rather than your hair color or a color you think would look better than what already exists. You don't want to see a difference between the eyebrow hairs and the shadow or gel used to fill them in. However, if you have pale eyebrows and want to darken the brow color, use a soft shade of tan or brown that is as close to your brows' natural color as possible. If you have red hair and brown eyebrows, using a red pencil or red-brown powder will look unnatural; just stick with brown. If you have blonde eyebrows, you could use a slightly darker blonde or taupe color on your brows to make them visible. For those with well-shaped, naturally full brows, a clear brow gel (Cover Girl and Jane have good ones) is a great option for lightly grooming the brows without adding any color. You can also spritz some hairspray on an old toothbrush and comb through your brows, or add a dab of non-sticky styling gel to keep unruly brow hairs in place.

What if you don't have any hair at all where the eyebrows are supposed to be? This is the only circumstance that requires applying a brow color that matches the hair on your head. It will look the most natural. Use the wedge brush and powder to follow the bone above the eye, applying to whatever hair is there. Usually there's enough shape to create a natural, shaded impression of a brow. Use a light touch, with short, quick motions, and avoid the temptation to exaggerate the shape by arching it severely or extending it into the temple area. Downplay the fact that there is no hair; it's better not to overexaggerate the area with a strong, eye-catching line. Also, don't place a highlighter or light-colored eyeshadow under the brow to further emphasize the brow. Putting something dark next to something light makes it look even more prominent. Once the brows are softly accented (or left alone), play up your lips or cheeks instead so that these will become the focus rather than your absent or too-sparse eyebrows.

EYEBROW MISTAKES TO AVOID

1. Do not over-tweeze, and never tweeze above the brow, only underneath. Tweezing above the brow can ruin its natural shape.
2. Do not overstate the shape of the brow; minimal brow alteration is best.
3. Do not pluck brows into a thin line thinking it will make your eyes look larger. It will only look strange, contrived, or even sinister. It can also give the face a surprised look, and none of this is attractive or natural—or easy to correct once the damage is done.
4. Do not use eyebrow pencil or eyeliner pencil to fill in your eyebrows unless you are adept at making it look very soft and shaded.
5. Do not apply eyebrow powders that are a different color than your own eyebrows; it is best to always match your existing brow color.
6. Do not apply brow color that is obvious or has a drawn-on look.
7. Be careful of brow colors that look red on the skin, which can make the eyebrow look fake and the skin look irritated. If you're in doubt when choosing between brow shades, go with the more muted option.

CONTOURING

Contouring is the art of creating or increasing shadows in certain areas so the face appears to have more structure and definition. It involves using brown tones of blush or pressed powder to contour along the sides of the nose, at the sides of the forehead, under the cheekbones, and in the center of the chin to add color, definition, and shape to the face. Although contouring is an optional step for most daytime makeup applications, it is still rather intriguing and is worthwhile for some women.

Today the popularity of using contouring to reshape the face has subsided to some extent. The likely reason for its decline is that believable-looking contouring is difficult to master (it's even more difficult than believable-looking blush). Contouring takes skill and patience, and very few women have the time to deal with it every morning. Women who do decide to take the time often end up with a brown stripe under their blush, and that is not the way contouring is supposed to look! Think twice before incorporating this step into your daily makeup routine, at least until you've practiced and developed the skill to apply this look softly. Without careful application and conscientious blending, what looks sculptural from the front may look odd from other angles.

Contouring is always done as a separate step, using a completely different brush and shade of powder than for the blush application. Shades of pink, red, and orange are used as blushes; only shades of brown are used in contouring. The safest contour shade to use if you have fair to medium-dark skin tones is one that looks like your skin color when it is tanned. A soft or rich golden shade of brown is generally the perfect color to use when trying to produce realistic shadows on the face. Shades of gray-brown can look dirty, and shades of red-brown and mauve-brown can look like bruising on women with fair to medium-dark skin tones. For women of color, particularly African-American women, either an extremely dark shade of golden brown or a deep chocolate brown color can work exceptionally well.

Types of Contour

Contour is essentially blush in a golden brown or reddish-brown color. For the varying types of contour, take a look at the "Types of Blush" section below. The easiest type of contour to work with is applied with powder-based color. Cream and cream-to-powder contour colors can be extremely difficult to control and blend, which can interfere with proper placement—a major no-no when it comes to natural-looking contour color.

Applying Contour

Use a full-size brush designed for blush or those indicating they are for contouring that have a softly angled (rather than flat or square-cut) brush head. Surprisingly, traditional contouring brushes are a poor choice for applying contour because they are usually too stiff, have a flat edge, and can leave visible edges when you apply your color; you want the full end of the blush brush when contouring. Or you can explore some of the softly-shaped contour brushes, which won't leave hard edges. Tapping off the excess powder before applying, and brushing on the color in short, quick motions going back to the ear will net the best results. Here are some rules of placement to help you most effectively contour your face.

Contouring under or along the jawline: Avoid contouring or shading along any portion of the jawline for daytime. Though this technique can make you look like you've lost a few pounds, you can end up with a line of demarcation around the jaw, negating the trouble you went through to find a foundation that leaves no such line. That means it will not look like natural shading. Nevertheless, shading the jawline or just under the chin can be passable for pictures or possibly for evening, but it must be applied very carefully. Shading under the jawline can also result in shading your collar at the same time. Be careful! Be sure to blend well and soften any noticeable edges or concentrations of color.

Contouring under the cheekbone: Place the center of your brush about one-quarter to one-half inch behind the laugh line, and stroke the color straight back, aiming toward the middle of the ear. The area of application should be approximately a half inch in width, with no definite edges visible. Use your sponge to soften hard edges. The starting point for under-cheekbone contouring is almost always the same regardless of the face shape, because the cheekbone corresponds nicely to the laugh line and middle ear area for most women. You can adjust the angle depending on your preferences. The steeper the angle going toward the top of the ear, the longer the face will appear. If you have a square or round face, you might want to try contouring at a steeper angle. The longer the face (as an oblong or triangular face might be), the more horizontal (straight back toward the middle of the ear) the line can be. This, in effect, deemphasizes the length of the face. All this takes experimentation, so be patient until you achieve the look you want. Be sure to blend well and soften any noticeable edges or concentrations of color.

Caution: When applying the under-cheekbone contour, be sure never to blend or place the contour color below the mouth area, below the middle of the ear, or onto the cheekbone itself. There is also no need to suck in your mouth to help find your cheekbones—that will only help you find the sides of the mouth, not the cheekbone.

Contouring the sides of the nose: Although most women think that contouring the nose is strictly to make it look smaller or narrower or longer, there is actually a more artistic reason for using this shading technique. If you're applying a full makeup, particularly for evening, and you ignore the nose, you will have color everywhere on your face except for a blank spot in the center of the face. Contouring the nose helps to achieve color balance for the whole face when you choose to wear a formal, full-makeup application. It isn't essential, but it's a great trick—and one that can be seen on models gracing the covers of almost every fashion magazine out there.

The goal is to make the contour color look absolutely as soft as possible. The challenge is to restrict the color to the sides of the nose. You never want to accidentally blend the color of the nose contour onto the area under your eyes or onto your cheeks. Take extra care to blend only a small amount of contour color on such an obvious focal point.

The best technique for applying the nose contour is to place the brush itself between your fingers and thumb, so the brush tip becomes somewhat flattened. This way the brush tip can more easily follow along the sides of your nose. (You can use the same brush you use for contouring or a very large, flat eyeshadow brush.) Now, take the index finger of your other hand, place it flat down the center of the nose, and apply the contour color along the side of your finger. Where the brush falls against your finger is the area to be contoured. Once you've done this, remove your finger and softly apply the contour fully around the tip of the nose and on the flare of the nostrils. Continue the contour in a narrow, soft line up under the eyebrow, avoiding the corner of the eye and the area between the eyebrows. Be sure to blend well and soften any noticeable edges or concentrations of color. Blend using very soft, short strokes and pay careful attention so that you do not spread the contour color onto the cheeks.

Contouring the temple area: Temple contour is a traditional step that is as basic as applying blush. The difference is that most women don't know about it. Take a look at the cover of any fashion magazine or ad for designer clothes, and you will notice this contouring on most of the models. When temple contour is neatly applied, the eyeshadows at the back of the eye can be blended into it so they don't end abruptly with a harsh edge of color. Without temple contour, the forehead becomes a great bare wall against the colored background of the cheeks and eyes.

The temple contour is placed next to the back third of the eye near the brow bone, directly out and up onto the forehead like a pie wedge, but without the edges. Temple contour can be applied either before or after the eye-makeup design is in place. If you apply the contour after the eye-makeup design, it is important to place the brush directly over the eyeshadows at the back third of the eye and then brush the contour all the way back to the hairline. If you do the contour first, apply it in the exact same place and in the same way, but when you apply the eyeshadows, blend them directly over and onto the temple contour. Either way, the contour softens the back edge of the eyeshadows.

When temple contour looks wrong or unnatural, it's usually for one of three reasons:

1. Forgetting that this step begins at the back third of the under-eyebrow area, right on top of and over the back third of the entire eye area. It does not float on the forehead unconnected to the back corner of the eye.
2. Not brushing the contour directly over the eyebrow itself, which can make the application look choppy instead of smooth and even (you should apply the eyebrow color after the temple contour).
3. Applying the color in a straight, one-inch strip next to the eye instead of in a softly blended, two-inch pie wedge that is partially blended onto the forehead. Temple contour is a shaded area, like the blush area, and it should never look like a stripe. Be sure to blend well and soften any noticeable edges or concentrations of color.

CONTOUR MISTAKES TO AVOID

1. Do not use a blush color to contour any part of your face. Contour only with golden brown, chocolate brown, or dark brown shades.
2. Do not use contour under the jaw or at the chin area during the day; it can look too obvious and possibly get on clothing.
3. Do not apply contour as part of your regular makeup routine until you get used to blending it on softly; it should never look like stripes or brown lines on the face.
4. Do not forget to blend hard edges; contour should always look soft and as natural as possible on the face.

BLUSH

Knowing how to choose a great blush color and applying it correctly are essential to successful makeup application. Blush adds life and a hint of healthy color to the face and its importance should not be overlooked when you're deciding how to go about doing your makeup.

Blush is one of the more prominent parts of any makeup routine, so if you do make a mistake—such as applying it too close to the lines around the eye, applying it like a stripe of color across the cheek, applying the wrong color, or applying it underneath the cheekbones as if it were contour—it is very noticeable. I urge you to take time to learn how to apply blush properly.

There's no universal consensus about where you are supposed to place blush. There are many opinions on where it should start, where it should end, and how high or low to place it along the cheekbone. My strong preference—one that is shared by many, as is evident in fashion magazines—is to keep the blush on the cheekbones and away from the eye area, blending the color just on the cheekbones and starting it about one-half inch behind the laugh lines. Some women start the blush no farther into the center of the face than the center of the eye. That can make the blush look very strange. The idea is to blush the entire cheekbone, and that means full across the cheek.

TYPES OF BLUSH

Powder blushes: Powder blushes are an excellent choice for all skin types. They go on easily, blend beautifully, and are available in great colors. A brush is essential for applying these smoothly, softly, and evenly.

Application: To find the area to be blushed, place the full end of your brush about one-quarter to one-half inch behind the laugh line. Starting here, brush downward and back toward the center of your ear, being careful not to place any color below the level of the mouth. Applying your blush by brushing down as opposed to back and forth eliminates a stripe effect. The blush area should be about two inches across, with no hard edges. Always use your sponge to soften edges.

Pros: There are only pros to this type; it works for just about everyone! The only possible negative for powder blushes is due to powder's naturally drier texture, making it sometimes appear to sit on top of the surface of the skin, although this effect is usually short-lived. It can be eliminated altogether by choosing a silky-smooth, perfectly soft powder blush.

Liquid, gel, cream, and cream-to-powder or stick blushes: These are not my favorites and I recommend considering these carefully. The only real advantage they have over powder blushes is that they tend to mesh better with the skin, which on some women can look more natural—as if it were a glow from within. Yet in spite of this minor positive point, liquid, gel, and cream-type blushes don't perform reliably for most skin types. They can be very awkward to blend evenly, and many tend to streak whether you use your fingers or a sponge. Liquid and gel blushes can also stain the pores, making the face look dotted with color, and they don't work well over foundation—the foundation gets wiped off as you apply the blush. Still, if you have near-flawless, smooth skin (no dryness and not oily), no visible pores, and have a deft touch at blending, you are a candidate for liquid, gel, or cream blush. It does help that many of today's cream blushes are silicone-based, which allows a clean, smooth application and a soft powder finish. Just don't buy anything until you check it out in the daylight and see how it wears during the day.

Application: There isn't one best way to apply these types of blushes. A sponge is my first choice, but some women do fine using their fingers, or even a synthetic brush. Use whatever works best for you and always double-check to make sure there are no hard edges to soften. Gel blushes can be the hardest to blend evenly, so you may want to start with cream or cream-to-powder formulas.

APPLYING BLUSH AND CONTOURING

If you are applying both blush and under-cheekbone contour, apply the contour color first and then blend the blush on top of and gradually down into the contour color. Then, using your sponge, blend until you meld the colors together into an attractive design. The hallmark of an attractive design is not being able to see where one color stops and the other starts. When done properly, blush and contour add color, depth, and dimension to a face—and that's always attractive.

CHOOSING A BLUSH COLOR

In the long run the color that looks best and most natural to your skin tone is the best place to start. Think of the color your cheeks turn when you've exercised and consider that as a starting point (but not necessarily the definitive color your blush should be).

An option to consider when choosing blush color is to go neutral; a soft golden brown or tannish-looking color is a great foolproof choice for many skin tones. I personally use this look for the summer. For darker skin colors, a deeper golden brown works perfectly. Whatever option you choose, be sure your lipstick colors match the underlying tone of your blush. In other words, if you are wearing a blush with a blue undertone, the lipstick should be in that same color family; rose blush means rose lipstick; coral blush coordinates with coral or coral/tan lipstick, though a soft-tan looking blush works with almost any color of lipstick. You absolutely do not want to wear pink blush and coral lipstick or mauve blush with orange lipstick. The point is for lipstick and blush colors to work together and not look like opposite, clashing ends of a rainbow.

Your blush color does not need to match your clothing, shoes, or any other accessories, although if you wear vivid clothing colors (fuchsia, turquoise, royal blue) your blush should ideally be in the same tonal family as your clothing to prevent an overly contrasting look.

BLUSH MISTAKES TO AVOID

1. Blush and lipstick colors should never clash; they should either complement each other or be in the same color family.
2. Never put blush close to or on the lines around the eye; it makes them look more evident, and if you are using a pink, peach, or coral shade of blush, the eye area can also look red and irritated.
3. Do not apply blush below the mouth or the laugh lines; blush is for the cheekbones only.
4. Do not blush your nose, forehead, hairline, or chin; it can make the face look overly pink or red, or made-up. It may look great in professional photographs, but can look blotchy and uneven in daylight.
5. Do not forget to use your sponge to blend out hard edges or smudges of blush. Blush should always be well blended, with no visible edges where the blush starts and stops.

LIPSTICK AND LIP PENCIL

I'd hardly lose the bet if I said most of you already know about lipstick, but I've talked to enough women to know that my next sentence needs to be said. Luckily, it's not complicated: If you're wearing makeup, your lips need lipstick—not lip gloss, but lipstick. Lip gloss doesn't last, but lipstick does. Lip gloss provides a sheer, temporary look that can be great, but it doesn't go with a full or classic makeup look. Lipstick (cream, matte, or semi-matte lipstick) provides a polished and put-together look that can last at least until your second cup of coffee. If your lips are naked while your eyes and cheeks are made up, you will look like you forgot you had a mouth when applying your makeup. For the sake of balance, remember lipstick.

TYPES OF LIPSTICK

There are vast differences among lipsticks. As you probably already know from experience, lipstick colors and textures can vary even within the same cosmetics line. Some are creamy; others are dry, greasy, shiny, or flat. Some melt easily; others go on stickily, evenly, thickly, thinly, and all combinations thereof. I recommend lipsticks that go on creamily, in an even layer that doesn't smear or look thick or greasy. Whether or not to go with a matte or creamy finish is your own personal preference. True matte-finish lipsticks do last noticeably longer than creamy (and especially sheer) lipsticks. The only way to find out which ones you prefer is to be patient and try on various formulas in the colors you like and see how they feel and look. But whatever you do, avoid wearing overly shiny or glittery lipsticks, particularly if you are an adult with a serious career. Glaring iridescence is best reserved for evening, not for daytime. A lipstick with a soft shimmer is perfect for daytime wear.

Note: If your lipstick has a tendency to cake or to dry out as the day goes by, avoid reapplying more lipstick over semi-worn-off lipstick. Wipe off all your lipstick first and then reapply. You may also want to apply a bit of lip balm under your lipstick if the problem of caking persists.

What about lipsticks with sunscreen? When it comes to sun protection, ignoring the lips is problematic. Not only is the skin on the lips very thin, it does not contain any melanin—which essentially provides the rest of the skin's built-in defense against UV radiation. Although conventional, opaque lipsticks do provide a barrier (which is one of the reasons skin cancer on the lips is markedly higher in men than in women), for true sun protection a lip balm with sunscreen applied underneath lipstick, or better yet a lipstick with built-in sunscreen is a must. A few cosmetics companies offer wonderful lipsticks with effective UVA/UVB sunscreens. My favorites are Chanel Aqualumiere Sheer Color Lipshine SPF 15, Clinique High Impact Lipstick SPF 15, Neutrogena Moisture Shine Lipstick with SPF 20, and Paula's Choice Sheer Cream Lipstick SPF 15. You can read reviews of these lipsticks and others I rate highly on my Web site, www.Beautypedia.com.

Note: When checking an SPF-labeled lipstick, make sure the UVA-protecting elements of avobenzone, titanium dioxide, or zinc oxide are listed as one of the active ingredients. If they don't appear, or if they are listed anyplace other than in the active ingredient list, you can't count on getting reliable sun protection.

CHOOSING LIP COLORS

When choosing lipstick colors, there are three basic rules. (1) Thinner or smaller lips look best with brighter, more vivid colors. Brighter colors may take a bit of getting used to, but they truly make a smaller mouth more noticeable. Occasionally I read about or hear makeup advisors suggesting that women should wear a neutral color on small lips and instead play up the eyes (as if the notion is ever to play down the eyes or ignore the mouth!). Test this technique for yourself before you give in to this nonsense. (2) Avoid darker colors on thin lips; they make the mouth look severe and harsh. (3) Larger lips can wear just about any color, but softer shades look better because darker or vivid colors can make large lips look too prominent.

APPLYING LIP COLOR

A lip brush or lip pencil is an optional accessory. You can use a lip pencil to draw a definitive edge around the mouth to follow when applying lipstick, and a lip brush to control your application. A tube of lipstick makes too wide a mark for some lips and too narrow a mark for others. If your lips are small, it is best to use a lip brush; if your lips are large, the only reason to use a lip brush is to improve your accuracy.

If you do choose to work with a lip pencil, always place the color on the actual outline of your mouth. Do not use corrective techniques that make the mouth look larger or longer, especially for daytime makeup. If you try to change the outline of your mouth with a lip pencil by drawing outside the lips, some time later, when your lipstick wears off, the lip liner, which almost always lasts longer than the lipstick, will still be in place and it will look like you missed your lips. Always line the lips following their actual shape, then fill in the lipstick color, using either the tube or a lip brush.

What about the center outline of the mouth? Do you round the point of the lips or make the point more obvious? As a general rule, a softer appearance is better than a hard one. Leave the points neither rounded nor pyramid-like—someplace in between with a soft arch is best.

To prevent lipstick from gunking up in the corners of the mouth, don't place lip liner or pencil in that area. Stop before you get to the very corners of the mouth. If you feel doing this makes you look as if you have missed a spot, carefully fill in this area with color using a lip brush, applying only the smallest amount.

Lip pencils should never create a contrasting dark, brown, or clearly visible line. Your lip pencil should not appear to be an obvious line that shows up as a colored border around the lipstick. The goal is to have the lipstick and lip pencil meld so that you can't see where one starts and the other stops.

If you wear lip liner and you want to help your lipstick last longer, apply the lip pencil all over the lip area, including the outline of the lips, and then apply your lipstick over it. This extra step puts a more permanent color on the lips so the lipstick won't wear off as quickly as it normally does. Beyond that, and with the exception of the various lip paints available (such as Max Factor Lipfinity or Cover Girl Outlast), all-day lipstick doesn't exist. Even these formidable lip paints can present some reapplication issues if you eat oily foods, and there is still the issue of touching up with the moisturizing top coat that accompanies each of these paints. For years the cosmetics industry has been proclaiming new "all-day" or "long-wearing" lipsticks, yet women continually need to reapply their lipstick. To date it remains impossible for 99.9% of all lipsticks to make it past lunch, or even past midmorning, still looking the same as when you first put them on.

How can you stop lipstick from traveling into the lines around your mouth? The first step is to stop wearing greasy lipsticks and lip glosses. The greasier the lipstick or lip pencil, the faster the color will slip into the lines around your mouth. The drier-feeling lipsticks are best for conquering this problem. Powdering the mouth with loose powder before applying the lipstick also helps, but can be a bit messy. Lip pencil will not stop greasy lipsticks from traveling, but it can slow them down.

Several years ago, some cosmetics companies came out with new products that were supposed to prevent lipstick from bleeding. I tried a lot of them and many never worked, but I finally found three that changed the way I wear lipstick. Regrettably, all of the options I used to love are no longer made. Refusing to be dismayed by this, I simply found out which company produced the formula (there are only a handful worldwide that make almost all cosmetic pencils) and added the formula I loved to my own line. If you have trouble with lipstick migrating into lines around your mouth, I strongly recommended my Long-Lasting Anti-Feather Lipliner in Clear.

LIPSTICK AND LIP PENCIL MISTAKES TO AVOID

1. Do not use a lip pencil that contrasts with your lipstick; it has been unfashionable since the '80s. Not only does it almost always looks severe, but it also gives a contrived appearance to the mouth area.
2. Do not wear lipstick that is a different color tone from the rest of your makeup. For example, if you are wearing a rose-toned blush, wear a rose-toned lipstick.
3. Do not use lip gloss in place of lipstick during the day; it can bleed and won't last as long as lipstick.
4. Do not exaggerate or change the shape of your mouth with your lip pencil or lipstick; it will look like you missed your mouth.
5. If you want your lipstick to last, wear more of it and don't blot it; blotting takes off several layers before you've even left the house.

TOUCHING UP

As the day goes by, even the best-applied makeup can slip, fade, and get phone- or finger-printed. Long days call for a few quick touch-ups to revive beautifully applied makeup. Following the steps below, in order, will revive the look you started with.

- If you have oily skin, blot away the excess oil by laying either a tissue or oil-blotting paper on it. Perm endpapers also work well. Do this before reapplying any makeup.
- Remove all of your lipstick so you can start over after you have touched up your face makeup. Apply a light layer of lip balm if your lips feel dry.
- Once the excess oil on your skin has been absorbed, take a fresh sponge and smooth out the foundation, blush, and contour (women with dry and normal skin should also follow this step). Use a gentle, buffing motion, making sure to smooth things as you go.

- Apply a little extra concealer under the eyes if that area looks a bit dark or if the concealer has faded.
- If you need a little more foundation over blemishes or discolorations, blend it on now, avoiding the blush and contour area.
- Dust a light layer of pressed powder over the face. A pressed powder with sunscreen that includes the UVA-protecting ingredients of avobenzone, titanium dioxide, or zinc oxide is an excellent option to ensure all-day sun protection.
- Apply more blush or contour if needed, but only if needed, and be careful; color "grabs" more over makeup that has been on the face awhile.
- If you want to touch up your eyeliner, particularly under the eyes where it might have smeared, use a powder shadow instead of a pencil. Use the corner or side of your makeup sponge to remove any smeared eyeliner.
- If your eyeshadows have creased, blot the area gently with a tissue or blotting paper and then use a brush to smooth out the color. Apply a powder over the area to even out the shadows and add whatever color is needed to make the eye makeup look balanced.
- Finally, reapply your lipstick and lip liner.

TURNING DAYTIME MAKEUP INTO NIGHT

All right, you've touched up your makeup, but suppose you now want to change it from your office or daytime look to a knockout evening visage? Here are some ideas to consider:
- Add a dark or black shade of eyeshadow to the back corner of the lid or in the crease.
- Use the same shade of dark or black eyeshadow to create a more dramatic line around the eye.
- Use a wedge or angle brush to add extra definition to the arch of your eyebrows, or add a bit more brow powder to the ends of your brows (but don't overdo it).
- Use a powder or liquid that has shine to add some shimmering highlights to the cheekbones, center of the forehead, chin, neck, shoulders, or décolletage.
- A vivid red lipstick always makes a dramatic evening look, especially if you are wearing black.
- Avoid overdoing your blush. Making the cheeks look overly colorful doesn't improve an evening look.
- Avoid applying more mascara, unless you're adept at doing so without creating a clumpy, spiky mess.

BALANCE, PROPORTION, AND DETAIL

Have you ever wondered exactly what it is you admire when you see a well-made-up woman? You may not be able to pinpoint what it is you find appealing, but you probably envy her skill and wish you could figure out how she did it. At the airport several years ago, I noticed such a woman and watched other women (and a few men) turn their heads and take notice. It wasn't just that she was attractive and her clothes were stylish; but that her makeup in particular was impeccable. Her face looked smooth and was accented with rich, though subtle, blush and contour tones. All the colors, from her lipstick to her eyeshadows, softly mingled into a harmonious sweep of light to dark, with just the right amount of shading—not too much and not too little.

That's when it occurred to me that any woman can revitalize her makeup by going over a list of everyday makeup guidelines and just omitting the mistakes that detract from, rather than enhance, her appearance. Recognizing the nuances of a well-done makeup application versus one that is not so good can make all the difference in helping a woman look great all day long. Considering all the time most women spend buying makeup and wearing it, putting it on wrong just doesn't make sense.

Besides the essential rules regarding application and blending techniques, there are only three basic concepts you need to keep in mind to achieve a flattering look: balance, proportion, and detail. **Balance** is about making sure the different elements of your makeup go together and that no one aspect is more prominent than any other. In other words, if you are wearing a dark, rich, brownish red lipstick, you must choose blush in a harmonious color (shiny pink blush is not going to work with a lipstick in that color range). Meanwhile, make sure your eyeshadows accent the eyes so they don't get lost because too much attention is directed toward the lips. When colors and tones are in balance and no one aspect of the makeup shouts over another, you don't notice the makeup as much as you notice the woman.

Proportion is about the total package of selecting what to wear. It's about paying attention to symmetry, to how your makeup colors, wardrobe, and hairstyle work together. If you are wearing a classic, tailored business suit and the eyeshadows you have on range from tan to black, with a wine-colored lipstick and blush, that may indeed be a stunning combination, but a bit too dramatic and overpowering with what you're wearing. The same is true for someone with very light hair and fair skin: the color combination may be dramatic and beautiful, but it will look out of place in sunlight or office light. Proportion is making sure that everything works together, with nothing looking out of synch, so your makeup doesn't upstage you.

Detail is the most essential and perhaps the most difficult area because it takes so much effort and concentration. Pay attention to every nuance of your makeup. If necessary, apply your makeup using a magnifying mirror so you don't leave the house with eyeshadow sprinkles on your cheek or mascara smudges at the back corner of your eyelid. Do not be satisfied with doing a ten-minute makeup application in only five minutes when you're in a hurry. If you don't have enough time to do your normal makeup routine, be ready to change your look; do only what you have time to apply well.

I can't tell you how often women have asked me what they can do differently with their makeup, and my responses were that they needed to blend their foundation better because it looked patchy and uneven, or the eyeshadow area looked uncertain or too obvious. Often these women reply, "Things were just frantic this morning, and this was the best I could do." I then say, "I notice you have your blouse buttoned and your skirt zipped up." Typically their answer is, "Of course!" I in turn comment, "Well, even though you didn't have much time, you didn't leave the house undressed. You should apply the same rule to your face." It doesn't mean being late because of your makeup; it means doing less so it goes faster. But whatever you do, take the time to do it right. Because when makeup is sloppy, it just looks wrong.

As I mentioned above, I use several levels of makeup application, depending on the time I have and what the makeup is for. For me, and I've done this a lot, full makeup for a television appearance takes 20 to 25 minutes. Makeup for a business meeting or a formal event takes 15 minutes. Makeup for casual daily business or informal get-togethers takes 5 to 10 minutes. Makeup for running to the gym to work out takes a minute and a half (lipstick and mascara only).

CHOOSING COLOR

Finally, we come to the most difficult subject of all to discuss, at least on paper. I would love to have the time to sit down and create a makeup look that works for everyone. That isn't humanly possible, but I do have some rules that can help you create the makeup look you want.

- Foundation must match the skin exactly so there are no lines of demarcation. (I know this is getting repetitive, but I can't emphasize this point enough.)
- Concealer is only a shade or two lighter than the foundation.
- Powder should match the foundation exactly or go on transparent so it does not affect the color of foundation in the least.
- Eyeshadow colors should be neutral shades ranging from pale beige to tan, brown, dark brown, and black (and the thousands of shades in between).
- Eyebrow color should match the exact shade of the existing brow hair, unless your brows are naturally blonde, in which case the brow color should be slightly darker.
- Eyeliner on the upper lid should be a darker color (all the way to black, depending on the look you want) than the line along the lower lashes, which should be a softer shade of brown or gray.
- Blush can be almost any color as long as it coordinates in some logical fashion with the lipstick color, but it must be blended on softly, without any noticeable edges whatsoever.
- Lipstick can be bold to neutral—there is a fantastic range of great colors. When you're choosing, remember that smaller lips should wear brighter shades than larger lips.
- To create a tanned appearance, use golden brown and chestnut shades for your blush, eyeshadows, contour, and lipstick. Never apply a foundation or bronzer all over the face if that means you'll end up with a line of demarcation at the jaw or hairline.

COLOR MISTAKES TO AVOID

- Don't wear white or very pale lipstick with a white cast to it. This can look ghostly and ghastly.
- Don't wear blue, green, or overly pastel anything, including eyeliner, eyeshadow, and mascara.

- Avoid navy blue eyeshadow. (Stick with black—it looks smoky, while navy just tends to look sooty.)
- Don't wear overly shiny eyeshadows (they exaggerate any wrinkles around the eye); they may be fun occasionally, but only if you have smooth, unlined eyelids.
- Don't wear rainbow-style eyeshadow designs (think Cyndi Lauper in the mid 1980s).
- Don't wear blush and lipstick colors that clash; they should be in the same color family, not glaring opposites.
- Use shine sparingly rather than making every part of your makeup routine include it.

CORRECTING SOME POPULAR MAKEUP MYTHS

- Some makeup artists declare that you shouldn't be afraid to touch your makeup. The truth is you should be very careful about touching it. After you've taken the time to apply your foundation smoothly with a sponge and your eyeshadows evenly with brushes, there's no reason to use your fingers unless it's absolutely necessary, and only lightly at that.
- Don't spray water or toner on makeup to set it or freshen things up. It doesn't work. A mist of water can streak foundation, powder, and mascara. How this makeup myth got circulated is anyone's guess!
- Don't change every part of your makeup with every season. If you want to go softer during the spring and summer, that's fine, but it isn't an absolute must. Makeup should reflect how you want to be seen by the world and what makes you feel good—and that's not dictated by the seasons.
- Don't use makeup to correct the shape of anything on your face, especially the lips. Close up and in person you can absolutely tell when lipstick has been applied beyond or inside the natural lip line.
- Don't use foundation or color correctors to change the color of your skin. Foundation must match the underlying skin tone exactly. That will soften any skin discoloration or redness. If you have yellow or olive skin there's nothing you can or should do to change it. It's best to accept it and work with it for your own look. Even if you succeeded in changing the color of your face, it would look strange next to your neck and along the hairline.
- To keep pencil eyeliner in place, many makeup artists recommend going over it with a matching powder eyeshadow. That works, but why do two steps when only one is needed? Forget the pencil and just use dark eyeshadow to begin with.
- Glowing skin does look nice, but mostly just in pictures. In real life, the same skin looks like it is covered with glitter. That isn't bad, but it isn't as appealing as the pictures make it seem, and any wrinkles will be illuminated, too. It is an option for an evening out, but that's about it.
- No single set of colors is absolutely right for any skin color. The days of being typed into one color grouping are long gone. Just because you have red hair doesn't mean

you have to wear corals and avoid blue-red lipstick. It's all up for experimentation and finding what looks best. Quite honestly, most women can wear just about any color they want to, as long as they pay attention to color intensity and application and adjust the details accordingly.

THE BEAUTY INDUSTRY'S EFFECT ON GIRLS

In our society, for young girls on the perilous journey from preadolescence and adolescence to young adult status, one of the emotional pitfalls is the social pressure and self-awareness that precipitates wearing makeup. Putting on blush, lipstick, mascara, and eyeshadow has become one of the primary rites of passage that marks the moment when changing hormones begin to influence both mind and body. As this new style of expression is developing, teenage anxiety begins to take on a whole new depth (witness a teen's explosive desperation at a single perceived insult or problem). What do you do when the little girl in your life (who is looking less and less like a little girl) wants to start wearing makeup? Particularly when her sensitivities are overflowing but her sophistication is lagging? And it isn't just that she *wants* to wear makeup—she *has* to. To make things even more confusing, teenagers continually demonstrate an inexplicable duality of fierce individualism, while at the same time buying only what everyone else is wearing. How many times have you heard the teen in your life proclaim loudly that she doesn't care what anyone else thinks, while at the same time she refuses to wear anything else but the same style of makeup, shoes, skirts, blouses, sweaters, and dresses her friends or her latest rock-star idol are wearing? Too many to count!

Feeling attractive is an overwhelmingly important aspect of life for many teenage girls. It is often complicated by well-meaning adults who don't quite know what to do or say. "You look beautiful, you don't need to wear makeup" is just as irksome as "A little pink blush, rose lipstick, and brown mascara will make you look beautiful." The first statement, "You look beautiful just the way you are," comes off as a thunderous lie. It discounts what the teenager sees all around her on television and in magazines—that women can look more exciting and glamorous with makeup on (or why else would Mom and the rest of the world be wearing it?). The other comment about adding just a little color here and there suggests that the girl is unattractive and would be better off hiding her face behind a layer of cosmetics (albeit a small one). Then there's the ever-popular, "You can start wearing makeup when you're 16 and that's that." At best, an arbitrary date like this ignores the specific needs and development of each teen.

What to do? I wouldn't recommend any of the above approaches, that's for sure. Instead, I suggest incorporating all three positions into a compassionate compromise. The goal is to acknowledge the teenager's needs, letting her know they are valid and important. Tell her something along the lines of "I know wearing makeup is important to you and it could look lovely on you. But at the same time I want you to know that I think you are beautiful just the way you are." Then the two of you can decide together what is appropriate, giving in a little as you go. Remember, what you think is important may not be what the teen thinks is important. Gloss yes, lipstick no; blush yes, but only a little; mascara yes, but only brown; concealer yes, but foundation no; and so on. Mostly this process is about being gentle and respectful of the teen's feelings as they arise (and not about trying to control or contradict).

Another option is going together to a professional makeup artist or makeup demonstration. This can be a positive experience as long as you are careful to ward off any attempt on the part of the salesperson to foster insecurity and vulnerability via sales techniques. Let the salesperson know ahead of time, in no uncertain terms, that you don't want her to use any language that suggests something is unattractive or wrong with any aspect of your teen's appearance. If the salesperson wants to introduce something different she can easily say, "I think a softer blush can be an attractive look," instead of "The blush you have on is all wrong for you." Don't let the counterperson get away with "You have small lids and a bright color will make them look larger," when a simple statement such as "A pale brown eyeshadow on the lid is a good color choice for you." Instead of encouraging an addiction to makeup brought on by insecurity, that phrasing can go a long way to build self-esteem.

If the age of your teen is of great importance to you in making your decision about when to allow makeup, you can put off the inevitable by intervening with an emphasis on skin care (which is a good starting point in general). Encouraging the everyday use of UVA-protective sunscreen, regular cleansing with a water-soluble cleanser, exfoliating gently with an AHA or BHA product, and using 2.5% benzoyl peroxide over blemishes is a great way to start paying attention to beauty issues without getting into makeup, except maybe for mascara or lip gloss. At the same time, it is essential that you take the time to share information about how the cosmetics industry can take advantage of women and stress why it is a waste of money to buy expensive products. That combination is an excellent and beautiful introduction to the world of cosmetics.

You and your teen can even read one of my books or visit my Web site together, marking areas to discuss. If you reach a crossroads and cannot agree, seek out an impartial third party to mediate (preferably not male unless you're looking for a "Who cares?" response!).

Most of us grown-ups started off on the wrong foot with makeup and skin care, somehow learning incorrectly from the outset that it would make us perfect and correct all our flaws (of which there were always too many—eyes too close together or too far apart, nose too broad or too narrow, face too square or too round, skin too yellow or too pink, and on and on). We are now in a good position to hand the next generation a new measure of self-worth and to tell them the truth about cosmetics and what they can and cannot do. That's something the cosmetics industry probably isn't expecting.

CHAPTER 30
ANIMAL RIGHTS

BEAUTY VERSUS ANIMAL RIGHTS

Politically, I'm a moderate. I haven't always been. I grew up in the 1960s, and my politics have ranged from idealistic liberal to confused bipartisan. Now, as I stand loosely planted in the new millennium, I can earnestly say I am convinced that few, if any, issues in life are black and white, or all or nothing. I find more and more often that there is truth on both sides of the issues and the middle ground is often the only reasonable position. At least the middle ground is the only position that acknowledges the whole picture and not just one side.

This middle position also reflects my perspective on animal testing as it pertains to cosmetic products and the health-care industry. While I unquestionably advocate the humane and ethical treatment of all life, especially unprotected and dependent life, I am not in favor of eliminating all forms of animal testing when it comes to health-care issues or human safety issues.

I feel terrible pain and anguish when I think of animals suffering in any way so that I can put on mascara or clean my face. Many animal tests that are used to ascertain whether a cosmetic will hurt people are cruel and gratuitous. No one is ever going to eat 50 pounds of mascara. Forcing animals to do so in order to demonstrate how much mascara people can eat before they die makes me want to resign from the human race. How can anyone put an animal through such torture?

On the other hand, my older sister who had breast cancer, my father who had prostate cancer, my friends whose parents have suffered through Alzheimer's, my friends who have multiple sclerosis, and my brother-in-law who has diabetes all take or have at some point taken medication or undergone medical procedures that improved their quality of life or facilitated recovery. All of these medications and procedures had been proven effective and safe as a result of animal testing. I absolutely do not want to see even one animal die by being force-fed foundation or eyeshadow to prove a favorable formulation. Yet, if sacrificing an animal's life can help find the cure for Alzheimer's, prevent more cancers, or reduce the risks of high blood pressure and a host of other illnesses, I would and do support that research.

Most of us are aware of the dramatic pictures distributed by animal-rights groups showing the terrible torment of animals in research laboratories. They have exposed conditions that are indeed grotesque and painful and that all of us should be sickened by and do our best to change. But this narrow, shocking display does not address the positive results of animal research (the creation of safe products and medical treatments), nor does it represent the labs that treat animals humanely by caring for them and anesthetizing them.

Children who survive leukemia owe their lives to animal testing. Arthritis patients who can walk again owe their agility to animal testing. Successful excisions of brain tumors are due to animal testing, and on and on. Human health-care advancement and the use of animals to test various protocols and risks are inextricably linked and cannot be separated. This is the dilemma of animal testing.

There are many arguments surrounding this issue from both points of view. On one side are the animal-rights activists who claim there is no need or reason to ever use animal testing (or eat meat, use leather goods, or use animals for any purpose other than as pets). When it comes to animal testing, they point to alternative methods of research assessment that can be used. Spokespeople for People for the Ethical Treatment of Animals (PETA) and the National Anti-Vivisection Society (NAVS) claim that a preponderance of research proves that all animal testing is inconclusive and has no relation to what takes place in humans. Animal activists insist that all animal testing is motivated by financial profit and stubborn, old-fashioned doctors or "good old boys" who refuse to change. Their reasoning is that animal testing is big business, and no one wants to alter what they are doing and potentially lose money.

On the other side are the vast majority of physicians, medical research groups from most major universities, national medical organizations representing everything from cancer to heart disease, and pharmaceutical companies, all of which believe the use of animal models for research is essential to evaluating new and old medical treatments and procedures. These physicians and organizations often agree that in vitro (test tube–oriented) tests and computer model studies can replace some animal testing, but definitely not all of it.

No one among these countless medical professionals would concede that all or even most animal testing is futile and immaterial. They can point to thousands of chemical substances and operations that were first determined to be safe and effective or dangerous and deleterious because of animal testing. Suggesting that these be stopped would halt most medical research, from AIDS to Alzheimer's, and the development of any new drug. Even physicians deeply involved in finding alternative research methods to replace animal testing would not agree that we should close the door to the ultimate goal or eradicating many diseases.

The truth probably lies somewhere in the middle. Medical, pharmaceutical, and cosmetics industry experts freely admit that, in the past, they were doing far more animal experiments than were needed to prove safety. Animal-rights activist campaigns inspired a vocal consumer base to force a major change in the number and type of animal tests being done. Many companies responded by reducing animal testing, changing to alternative methods whenever possible, and instituting humane treatment of their animals. Yet all or nothing is the goal of animal activists, and it may not be the goal of all consumers buying makeup, taking medicines, or considering medical procedures. Consumers should look at the whole issue, not just at shocking pictures.

For example, according to an article in the January 1997 issue of *Drug and Cosmetics Industry* magazine (Drug and Cosmetics Industry magazine's name has been changed to *Global Cosmetic Industry*), Gillette has been a boycott target of PETA since 1986. What PETA does not acknowledge is that, since its boycott, Gillette has reduced tests on animals by over 90%, has contributed millions of dollars to alternative research, and has donated over $100,000 to the Humane Society. You would think PETA would ease up on Gillette, but that isn't the case. It still lists Gillette among its companies to boycott. As long as a company does any animal testing, humane or otherwise, it is a target for PETA's condemnation. That is regrettable, because as a consumer you get only a limited perspective.

Most of us are against animal testing, but we also have the right to safe products and straight information about how that can best be accomplished. It would be wonderful if alternative, computer-based, and test-tube models were sufficient to establish a cosmetic, drug, or medical procedure's safety, but that doesn't seem to be true, at least not now or in the near future. If alternatives do become common practice, that will probably happen in the world of cosmetics first, mainly because cosmetics are not ingested and alternative research methods for irritation studies are in use.

I will continue to earnestly support the humane and ethical treatment of animals, but I do not at this time support a complete ban on animal testing. I personally do not use animal testing for any of my Paula's Choice skin-care products, either directly or indirectly (meaning I don't hire third-party testing facilities to do my testing for me). I use only proven, long-established formulations and ingredients, as do many other companies that make claims about no animal testing. But because all of the cosmetic ingredients currently in use have at some point been tested on animals, including everything from vitamin C to sunscreen ingredients, no one can claim that the ingredients in their products involved no animal testing. It's great that they don't test on animals, but at least some of the ingredients they use were tested at some point in the ingredient's history.

By creating products that are not tested on animals and by my supporting through financial contributions such organizations as animal welfare groups and legal groups that fight for animal causes, I feel I am doing my part to help create a world where fewer and fewer animals will be used for testing, and those that are will be treated humanely and ethically every step of the way.

I want my readers to know that I believe their decisions and consumer activism in this area have been and continue to be vital. Cosmetics companies only started changing and looking for alternative methods because you, the consumer, brought pressure to bear and forced them to change. It is important to keep up this pressure. However, I feel it would be foolish to follow organizations like PETA and NAVS blindly unless you truly agree completely with their goal of abolishing all animal testing and creating a completely vegetarian or vegan society.

Instead, I encourage you to support organizations fighting for the welfare and safety of all animals, for limited and humane animal testing, and for continued research to find alternatives to animal testing in hopes that someday no animals will have to be used in any research experiments. This is completely in your power, because you, the consumer, have everything to say about what you buy and whom you buy it from, and your actions speak loudly and clearly to all kinds of corporations and enterprises the world over.